COMPASS

To Direct First Years

The Complete First Year MBBS Practical Manual

COMPASS

To Direct First Years

The Complete First Year MBBS Practical Manual

Anto Jose MBBS (Pursuing)
MES Medical College
Perinthalmanna, Malappuram
Kerala, India

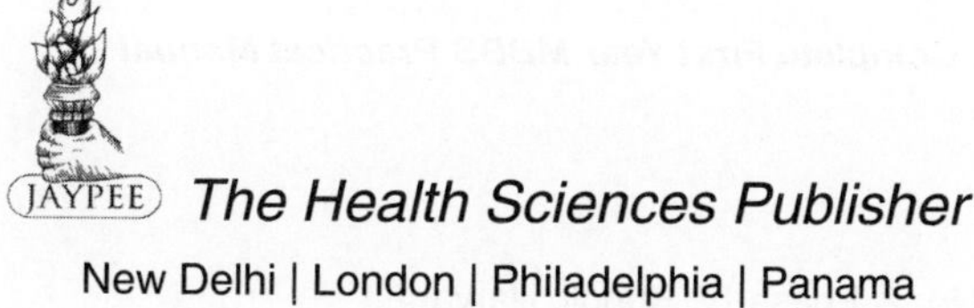

The Health Sciences Publisher
New Delhi | London | Philadelphia | Panama

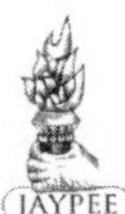

Jaypee Brothers Medical Publishers (P) Ltd.

Headquarters
Jaypee Brothers Medical Publishers (P) Ltd.
4838/24, Ansari Road, Daryaganj
New Delhi 110 002, India
Phone: +91-11-43574357
Fax: +91-11-43574314
E-mail: jaypee@jaypeebrothers.com

Overseas Offices

J.P. Medical Ltd.
83, Victoria Street, London
SW1H 0HW (UK)
Phone: +44-20 3170 8910
Fax: +44 (0)20 3008 6180
E-mail: info@jpmedpub.com

Jaypee-Highlights Medical Publishers Inc.
City of Knowledge, Bld. 237, Clayton
Panama City, Panama
Phone: +1 507-301-0496
Fax: +1 507-301-0499
E-mail: cservice@jphmedical.com

Jaypee Medical Inc.
The Bourse
111, South Independence Mall East
Suite 835, Philadelphia, PA 19106, USA
Phone: +1 267-519-9789
E-mail: jpmed.us@gmail.com

Jaypee Brothers Medical Publishers (P) Ltd.
17/1-B, Babar Road, Block-B, Shaymali
Mohammadpur, Dhaka-1207
Bangladesh
Mobile: +08801912003485
E-mail: jaypeedhaka@gmail.com

Jaypee Brothers Medical Publishers (P) Ltd.
Bhotahity, Kathmandu, Nepal
Phone: +977-9741283608
E-mail: kathmandu@jaypeebrothers.com

Website: www.jaypeebrothers.com
Website: www.jaypeedigital.com

Inquiries for bulk sales may be solicited at: jaypee@jaypeebrothers.com

COMPASS (To Direct First Years): The Complete First Year MBBS Practical Manual

First Edition: **2015**

ISBN: 978-93-5152-670-4

Printed at Rajkamal Electric Press, Plot No. 2, Phase-IV, Kundli, Haryana.

Dedicated to

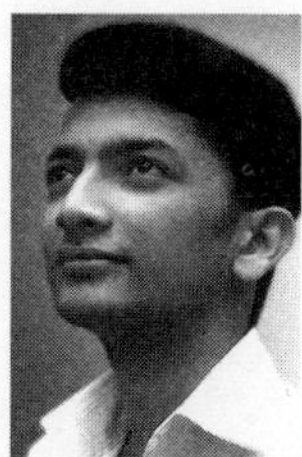

Lebin Najeeb

You may be far from our reach,
but you will be close to
our heart always...

Preface

As the name *COMPASS: The Complete First Year MBBS Practical Manual*, it aims at directing the first year MBBS students to overcome the mighty path of completing the first year. *COMPASS* is an exam-oriented material and cannot substitute any standard textbooks. It helps in easy grasping and understanding the basics of all the topics in the syllabus as directed by the Kerala University of Health Sciences (KUHS), Kerala, India.

COMPASS includes all the necessary topics which a MBBS student should know with its root basics. The book stands unique in its way of presentation.

The book emphasizes on all the practical aspects of Anatomy, Physiology and Biochemistry and includes:

- All practical aspects with explanations
- Chapterwise question bank
- Essential diagrams and tables
- Expected theory viva questions
- Standard exam-oriented questions and answers
- Normal values
- Model question papers.

The book is prepared as such that students can memorize important topics in a short time and avoid mugging up. *COMPASS* is preferred for last time revision and helps the students to present them in the most appropriate way and score good marks in the examination.

I am really thankful to God, my parents, teachers, seniors and my friends, without them the book would not have reached this present state.

Anto Jose

Acknowledgments

It is deep sense of gratitude and thanks to all persons, their thoughts, inspirations incepted the seed of the idea of the book *COMPASS: The Complete First Year MBBS Practical Manual.*

First and foremost, I bow my head before God Almighty, who is source of all inspirations and actions of the universe. I thank Him for His blessing conferred on me to accomplish this work.

No words are sufficient to express my acknowledgments to my parents, my brothers Seby Jose and Lijo Jose, for their endless support.

I express my thanks to seniors Jobin, Derin, Jithin, Soja Raj, Chinnu, Jyothis Merry, Annie, Ancy, for their endless care and support.

I also express my gratitude to all my batchmates, especially Mohammed Musthafa, Ahamed Thameem, Ameera Hussain, Anagha Peethambaran, Anumol Jai Joseph, Ashna Pulikkal Asgar, Balil Afsath, Hameedha, Cinda S Ukken, Farsana Kondeth, Jeslin Mohammed, Sejna, Musthakeemath, Shahina, for their support given to me during the preparation of the book, without which the book would have never been a reality.

My sincere thanks to Shri Jitendar P Vij (Group Chairman), Mr Ankit Vij (Group President), Mr Tarun Duneja (Director–Publishing), and Ms Samina Khan (PA to Director–Publishing) of M/s Jaypee Brothers Medical Publishers (P) Ltd, who readily accepted for publishing the book.

Contents

1. Anatomy 1

2. Physiology 167

3. Biochemistry 241

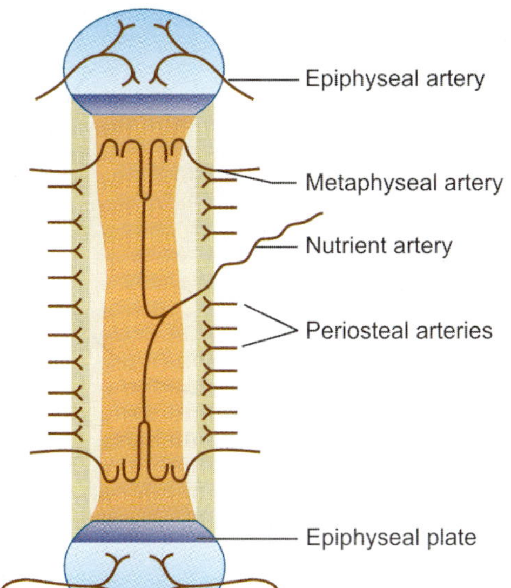

- *Nutrient artery:* It enters the shaft through a nutrient foramen. On reaching bone marrow cavity they divide into ascending and descending branches.
- *Epiphyseal artery:* Several in number and enter the bone near its ends.
- *Metaphyseal artery:* Enters along the line of attachment of capsular ligament.
- *Periosteal artery:* Numerous and enter the bone along its attachment.

Fig. 6 Blood supply to a growing long bone

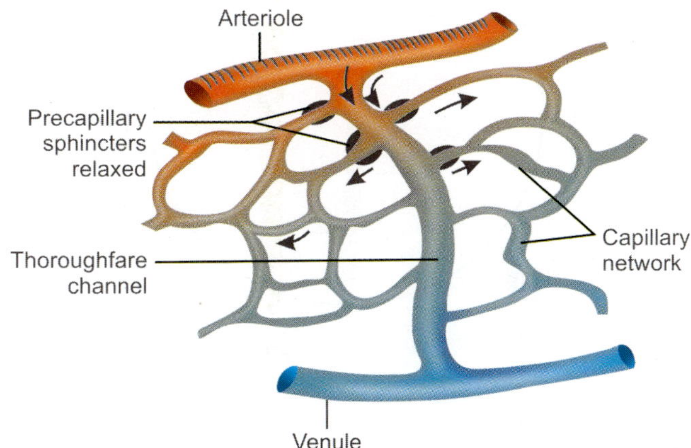

Fig. 21 Anastomosis

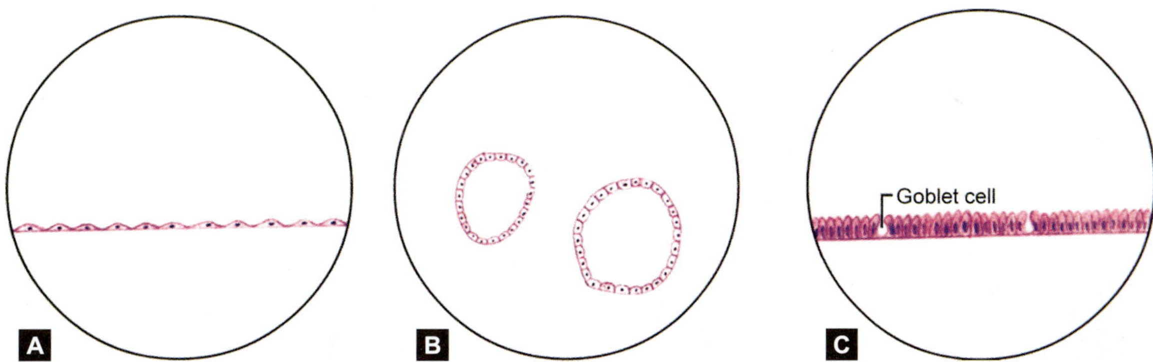

Figs 107A to C (A) Simple squamous epithelium; (B) Simple cuboidal epithelium; (C) Simple columnar epithelium

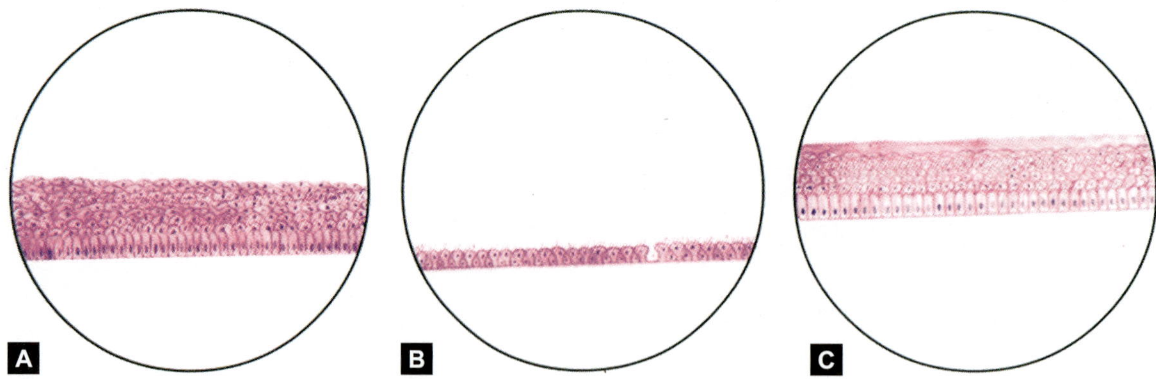

Figs 108A to C (A) Pseudostratified epithelium; (B) Stratified squamous non-keratinized epithelium; (C) Stratified squamous keratinized epithelium

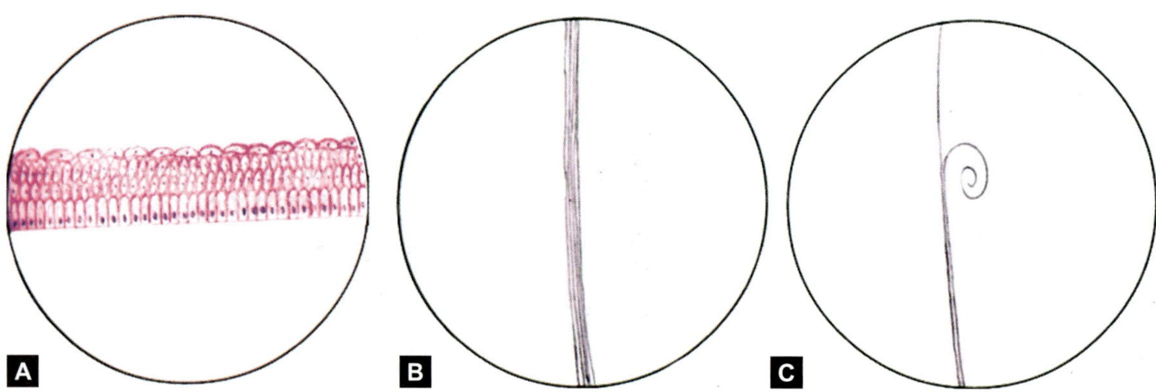

Figs 109A to C (A) Transitional epithelium; (B) Collagen fiber; (C) Elastin fiber

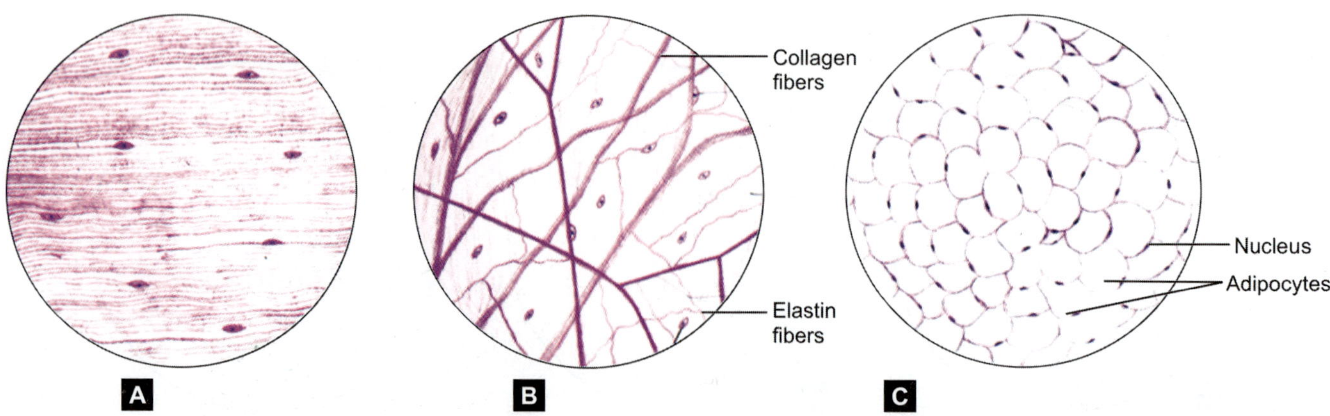

Figs 110A to C (A) Dense regular connective tissue; (B) Loose connective tissue; (C) Adipose tissue

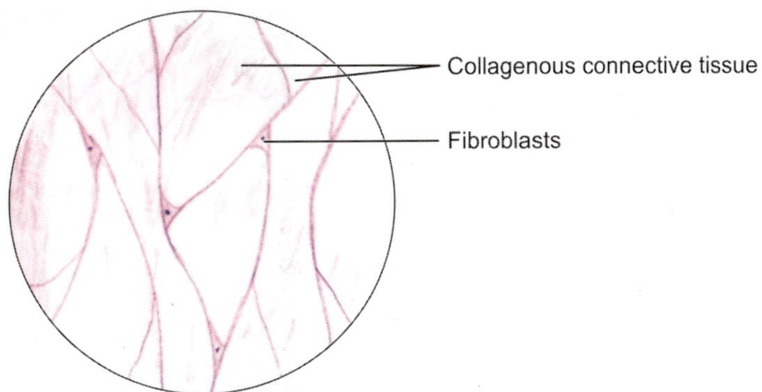

Fig. 111 Mucoid tissue

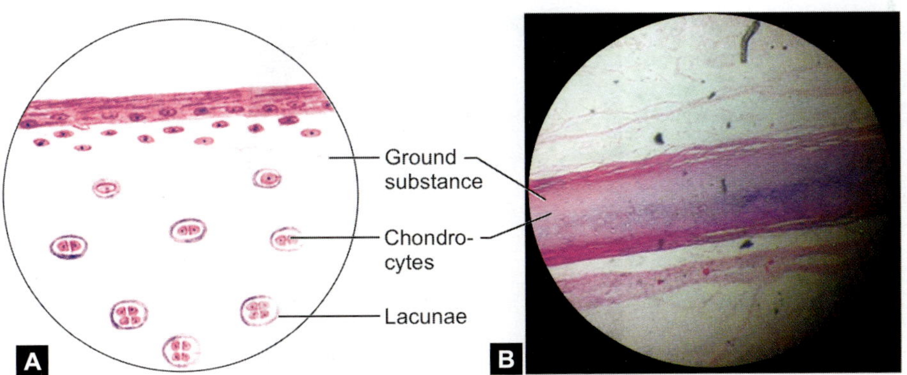

Figs 112A and B Hyaline cartilage

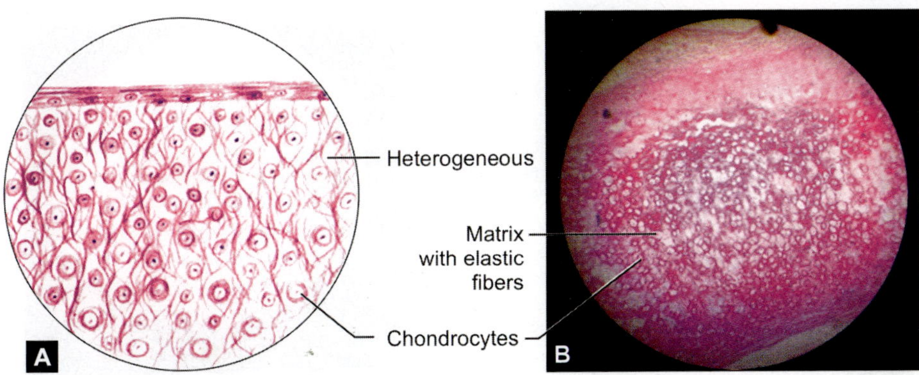

Figs 113A and B Elastic cartilage

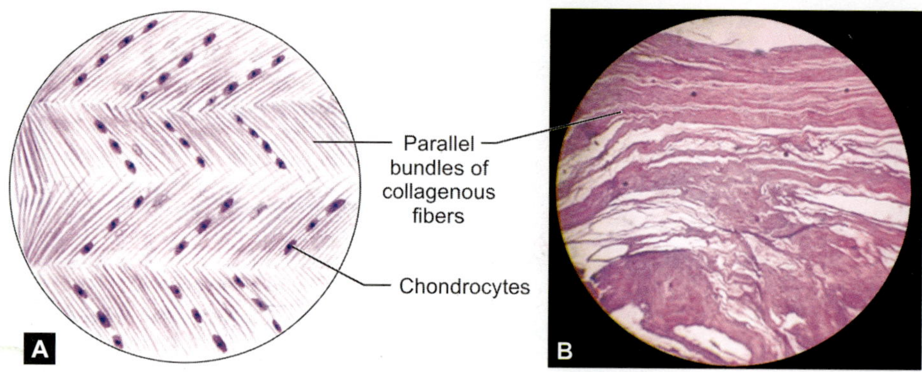

Figs 114A and B Fibrocartilage

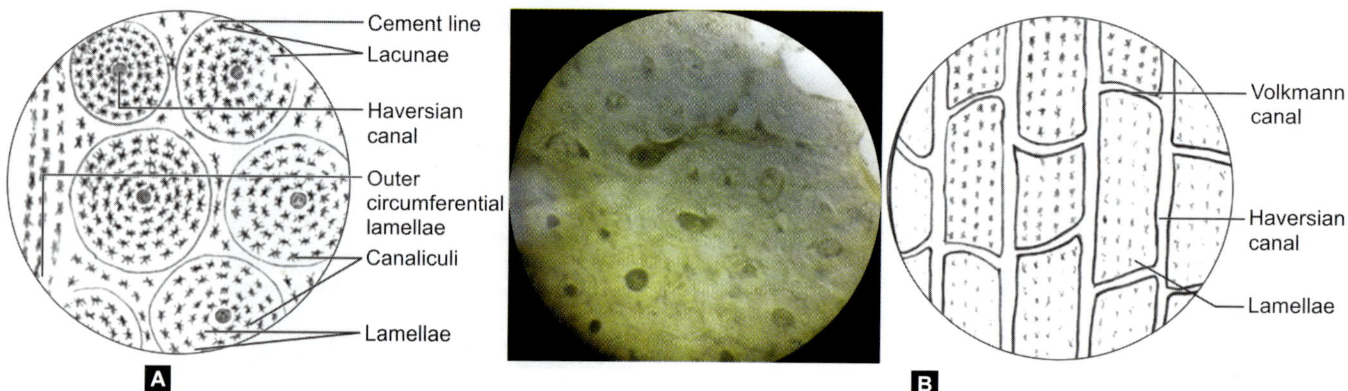

Figs 115A and B (A) Transverse section of bone; (B) Longitudinal section of bone

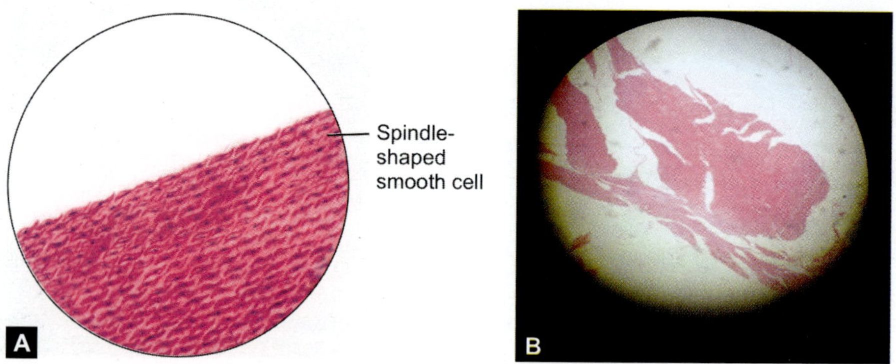

Figs 116A and B Smooth muscle

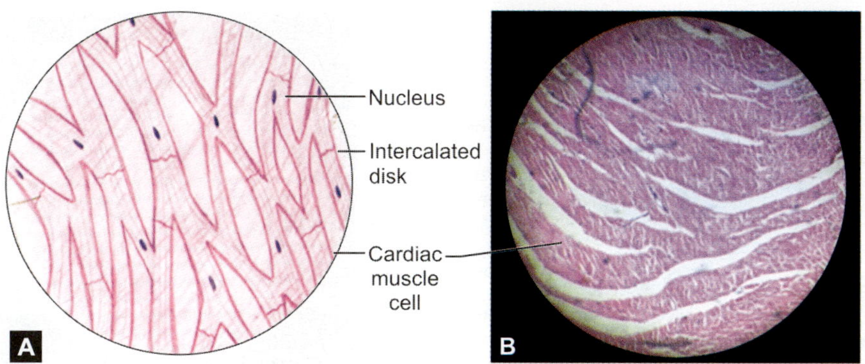

Figs 117A and B Cardiac muscle

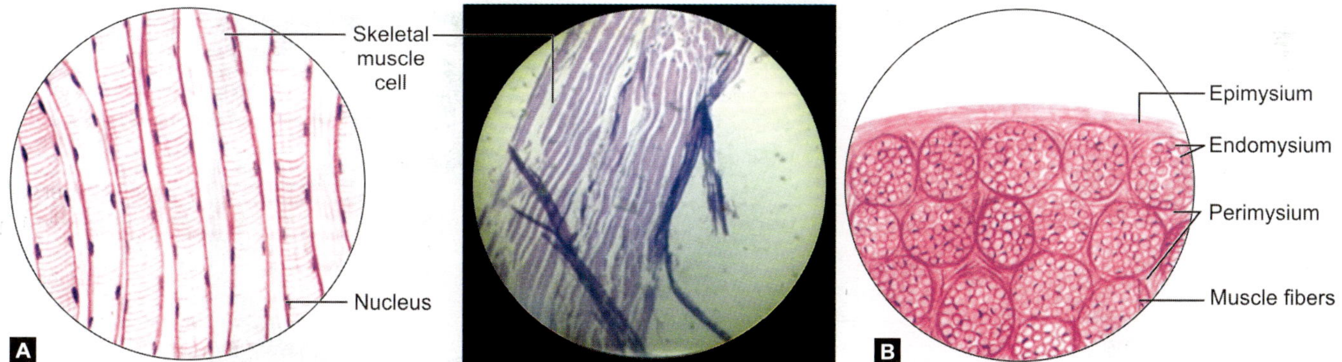

Figs 118A and B Longitudinal section of skeletal muscle; (B) Transverse section of skeletal muscle

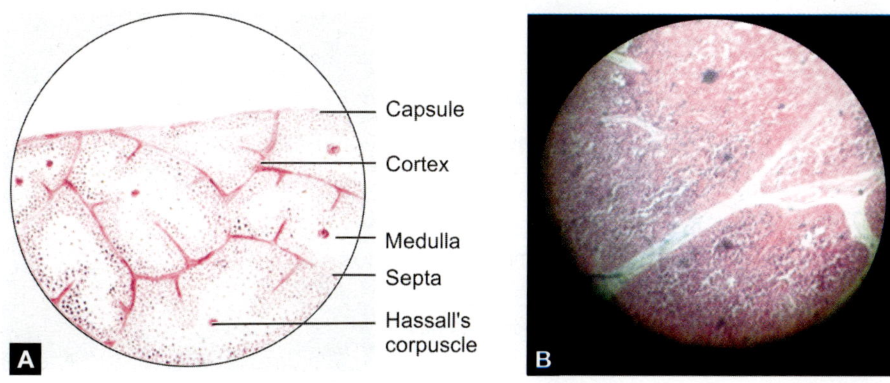

Figs 119A and B Thymus

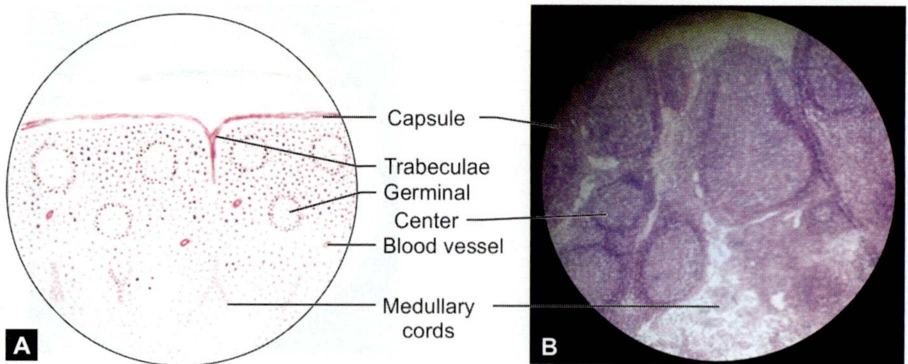

Figs 120A and B Lymph node

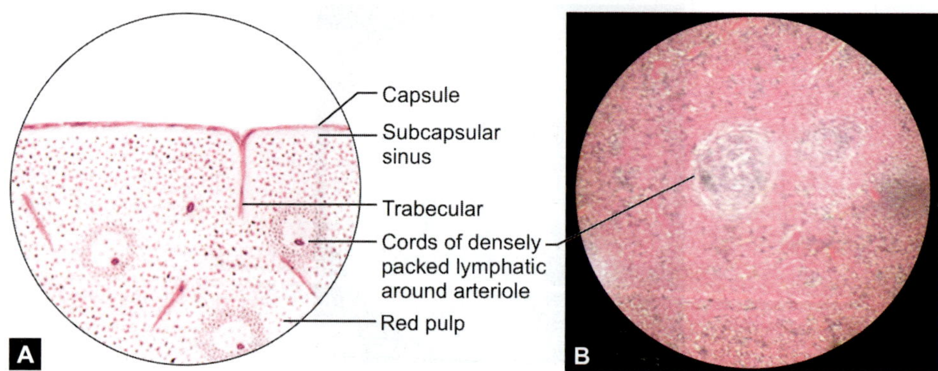

Figs 121A and B Spleen

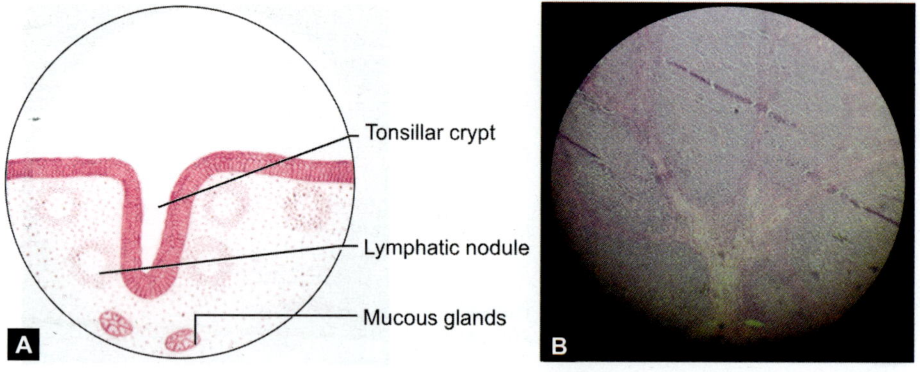

Figs 122A and B Tonsil

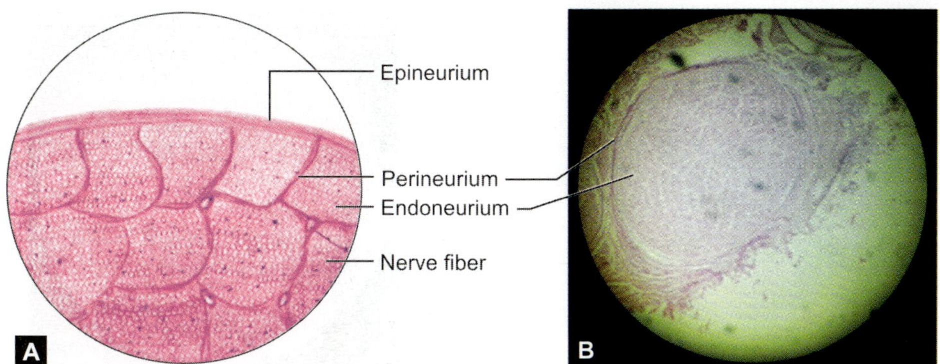

Figs 123A and B Peripheral nerve

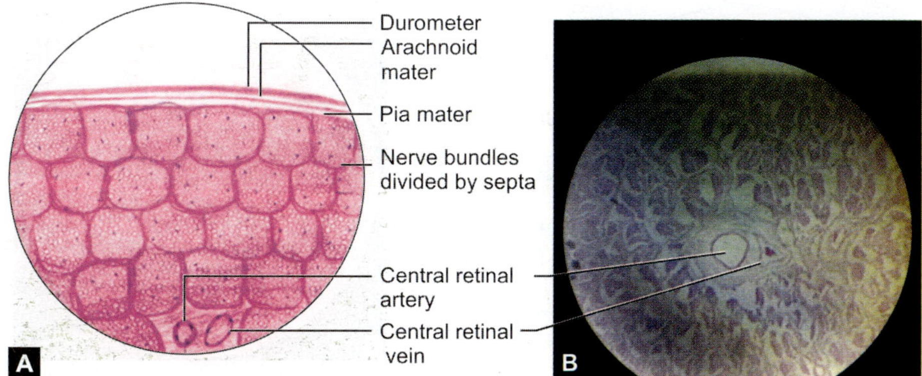

Figs 124A and B Optic nerve

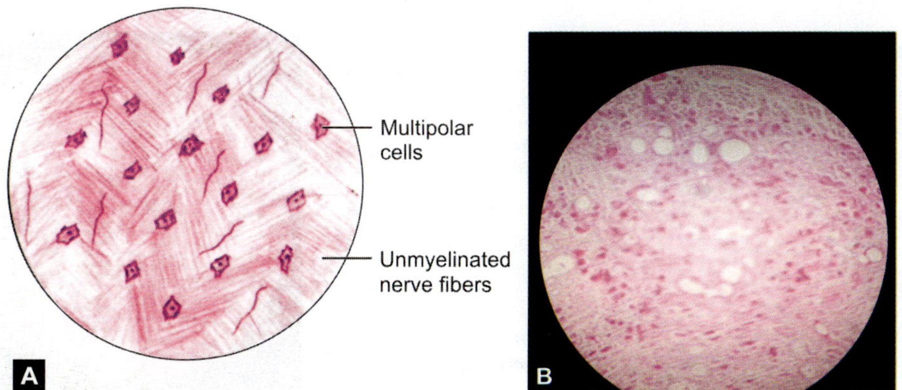

Figs 125A and B Sympathetic (Autonomic ganglion)

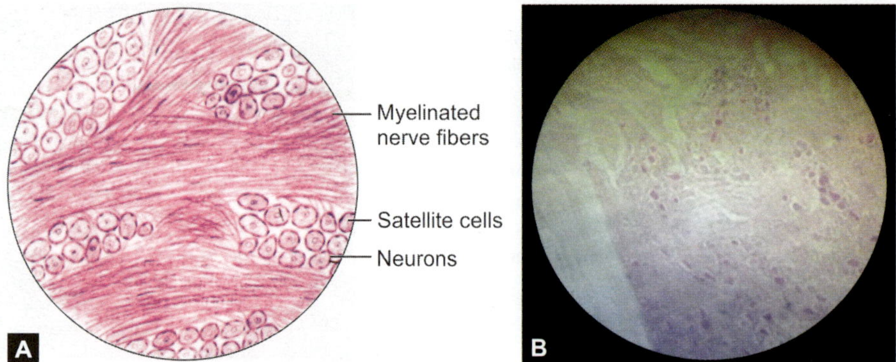

Figs 126A and B Dorsal root (Sensory) ganglion

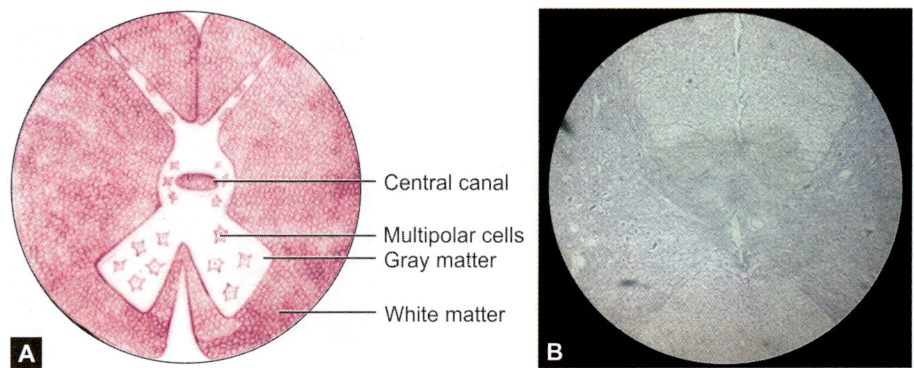

Figs 127A and B Spinal cord

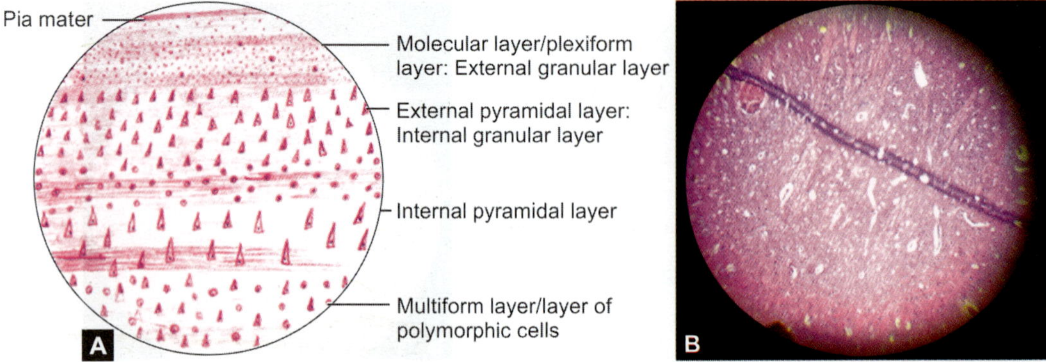

Figs 128A and B Cerebral cortex

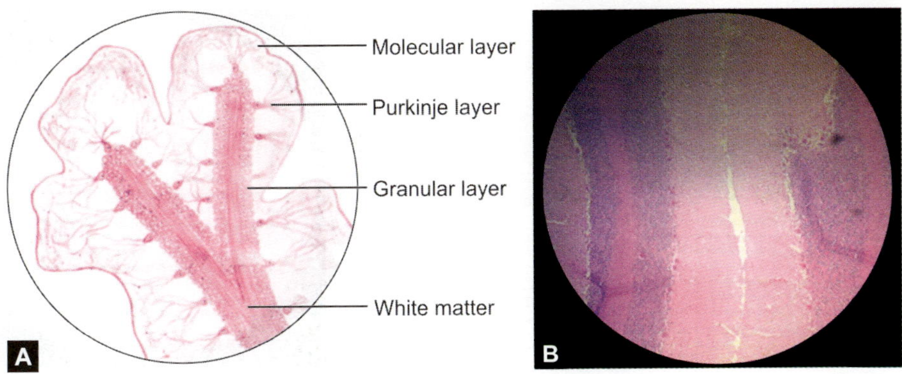

Figs 129A and B Cerebellum

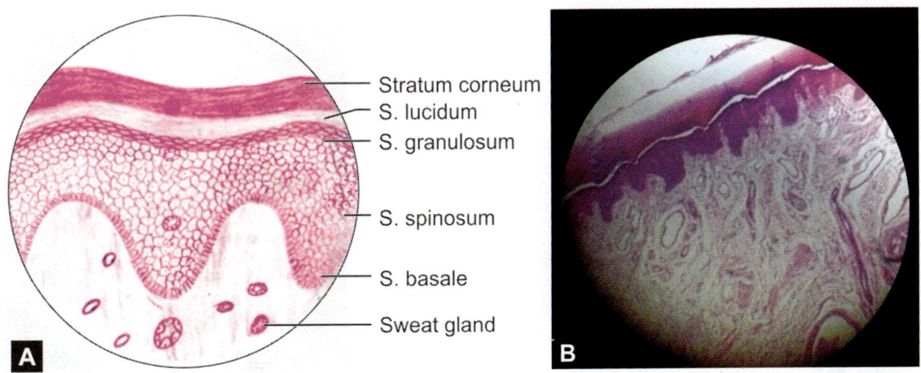

Figs 130A and B Thick skin

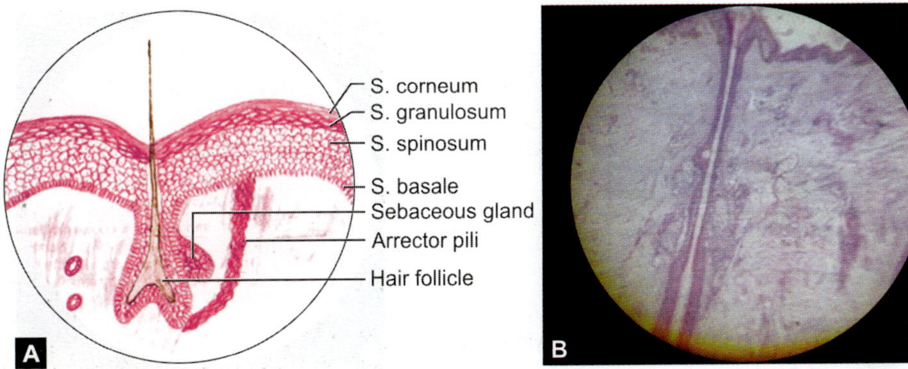

Figs 131A and B Thin skin

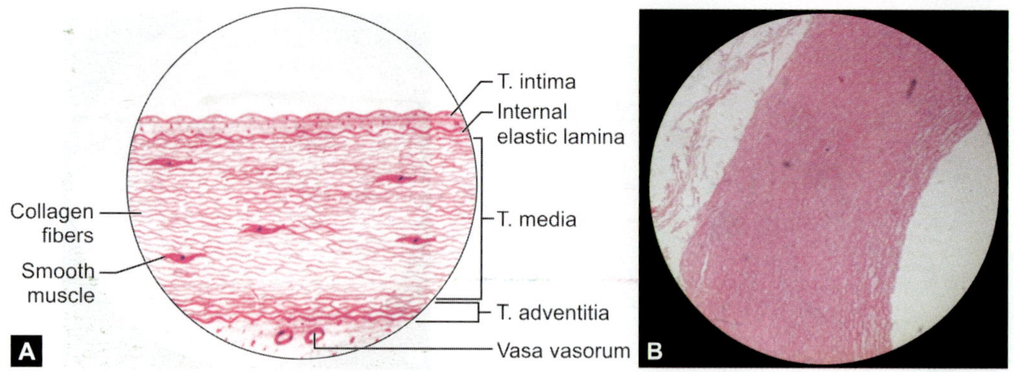

Figs 132A and B Large/elastic artery

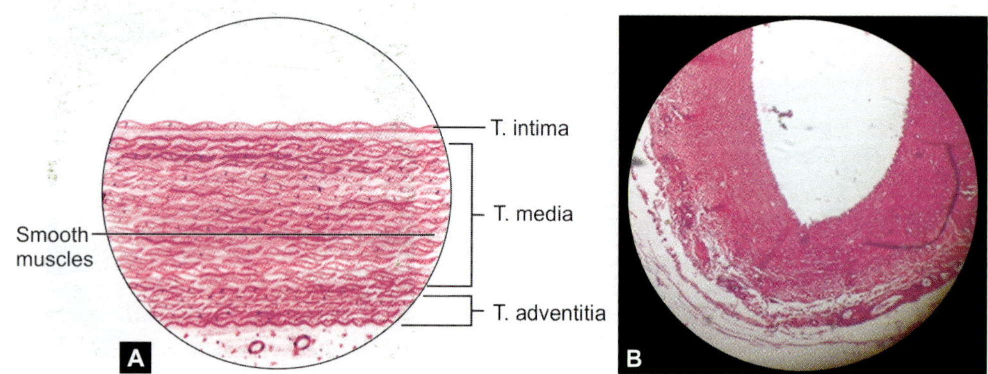

Figs 133A and B Medium sized/muscular artery

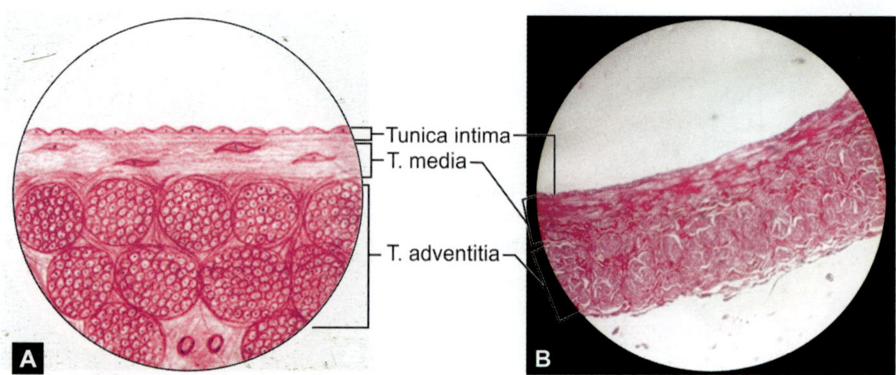

Figs 134A and B Large vein

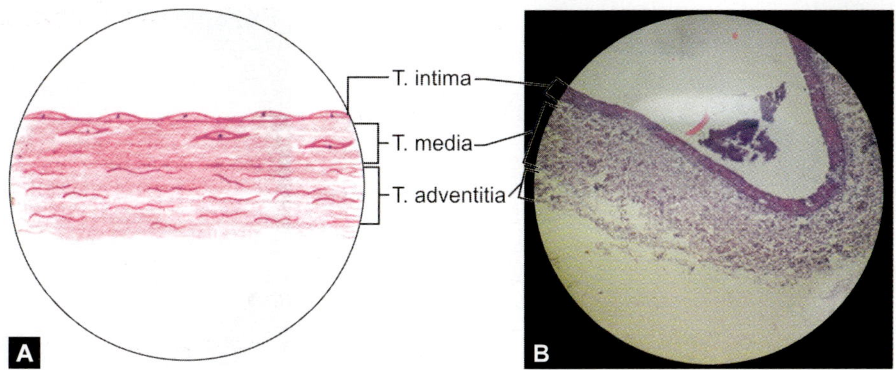

Figs 135A and B Medium-sized vein

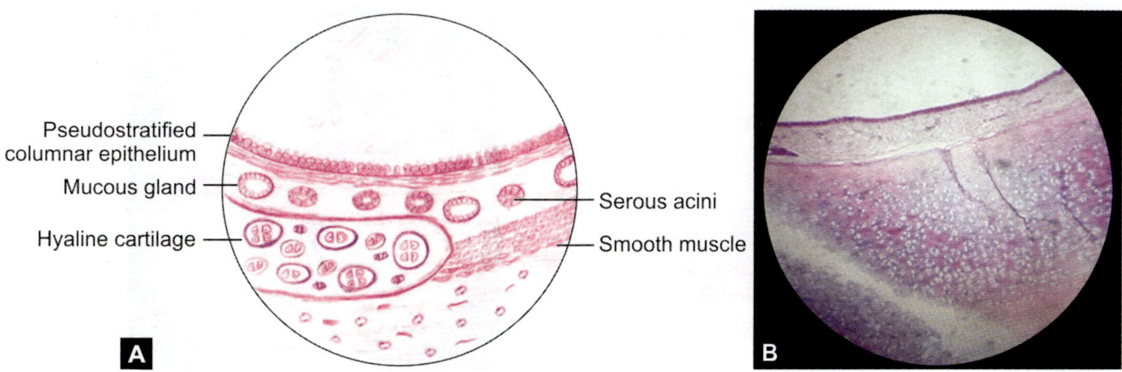

Figs 136A and B Trachea

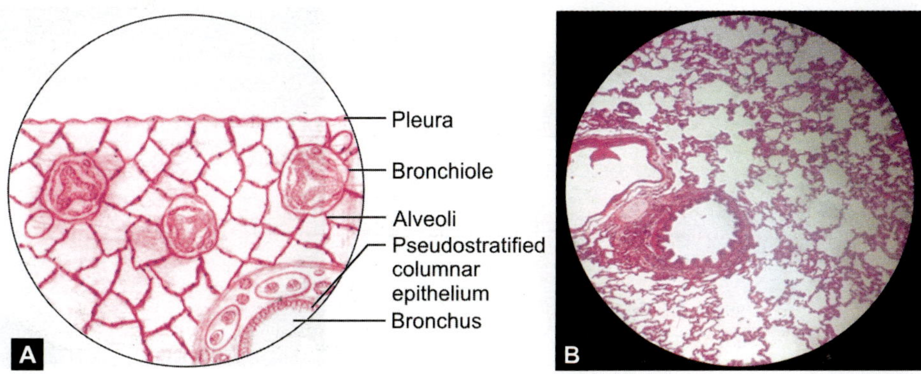

Figs 137A and B Lungs

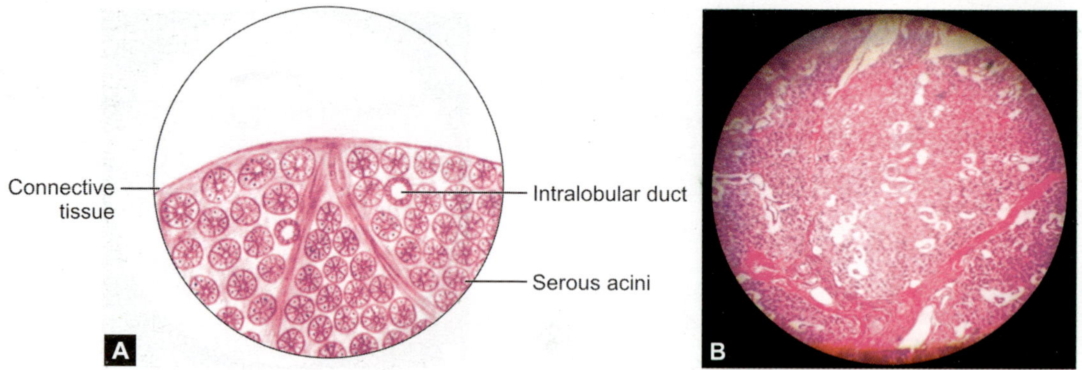

Figs 138A and B Serous salivary gland—parotid gland

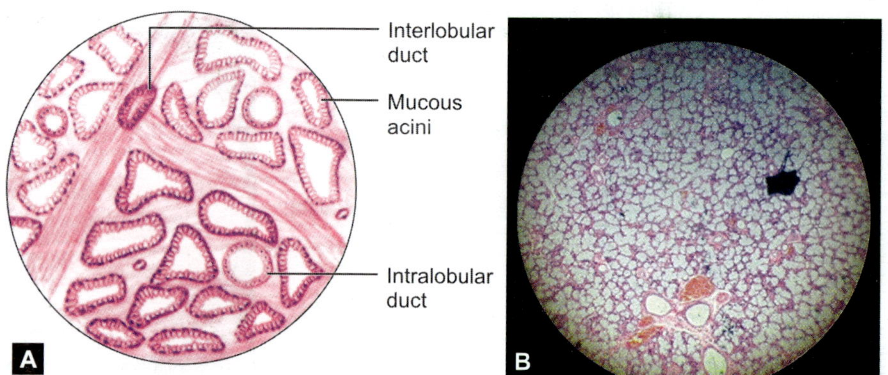

Figs 139A and B Mucous salivary gland—sublingual gland

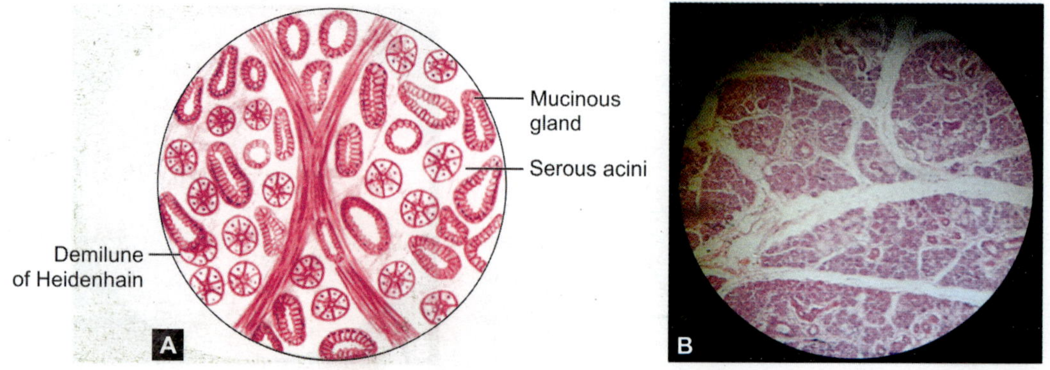

Figs 140A and B Mixed salivary gland—submandibular gland

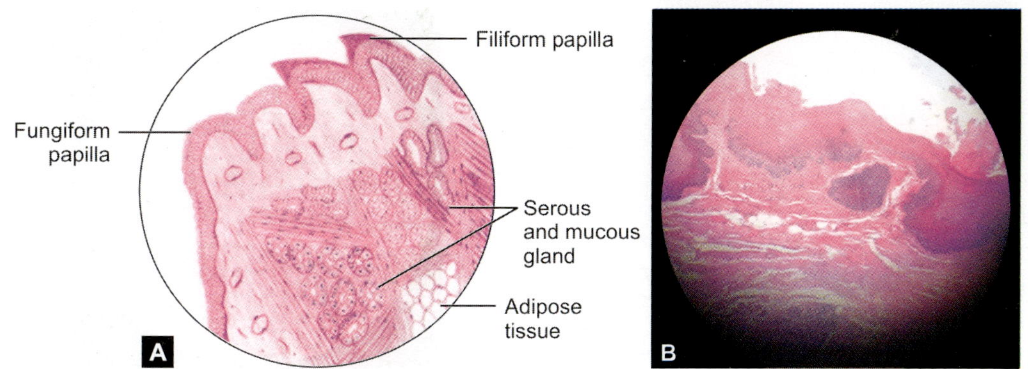

Figs 141A and B Filliform and fungiform papillae

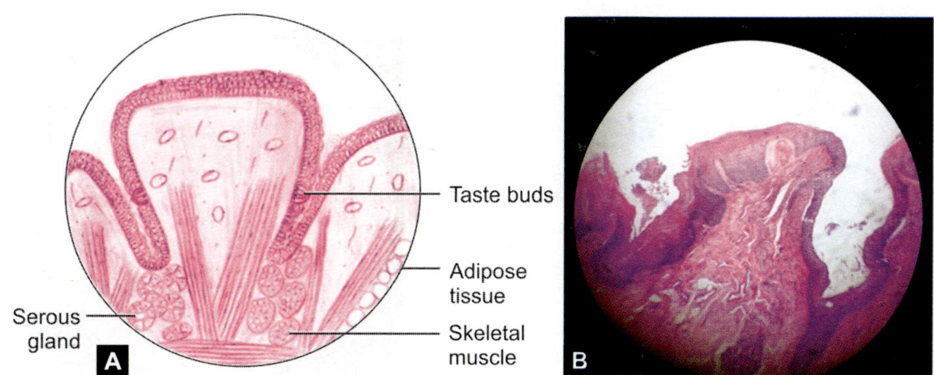

Figs 142A and B Circumvallate papillae

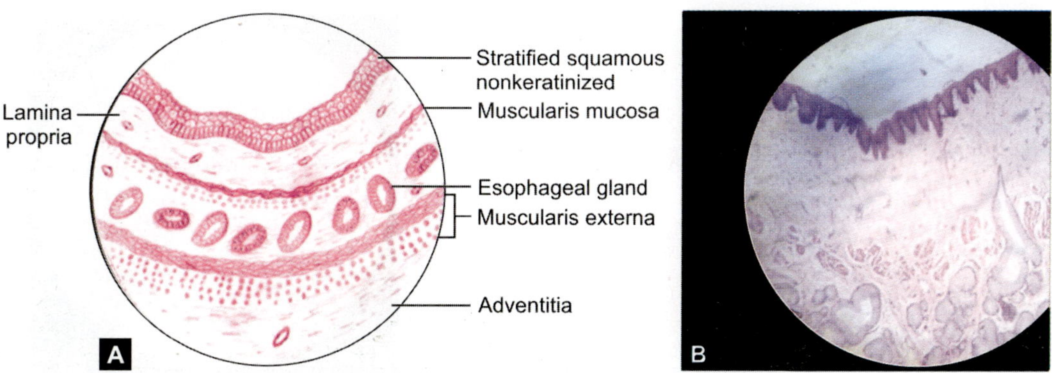

Figs 143A and B Esophagus

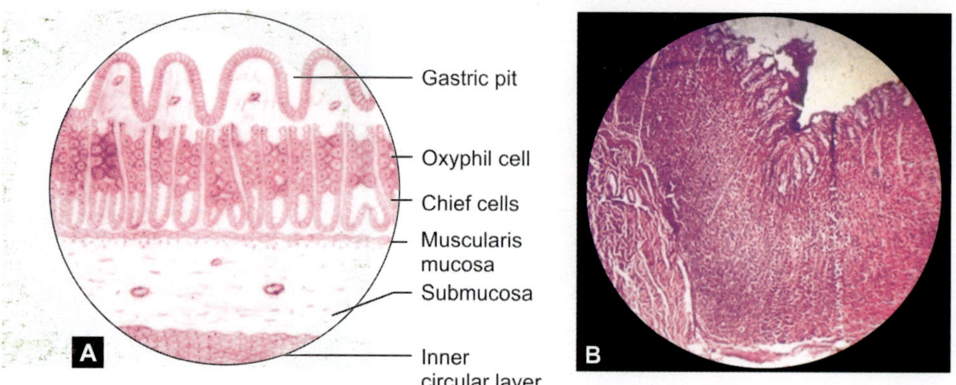

Figs 144A and B Stomach—fundus

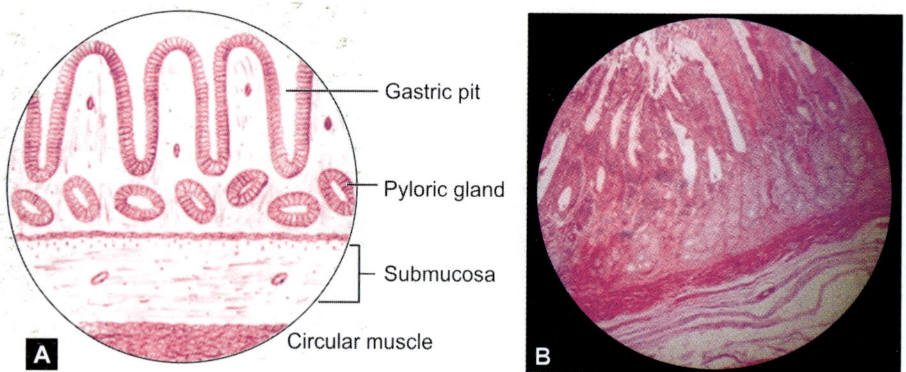

Figs 145A and B Stomach—pylorus

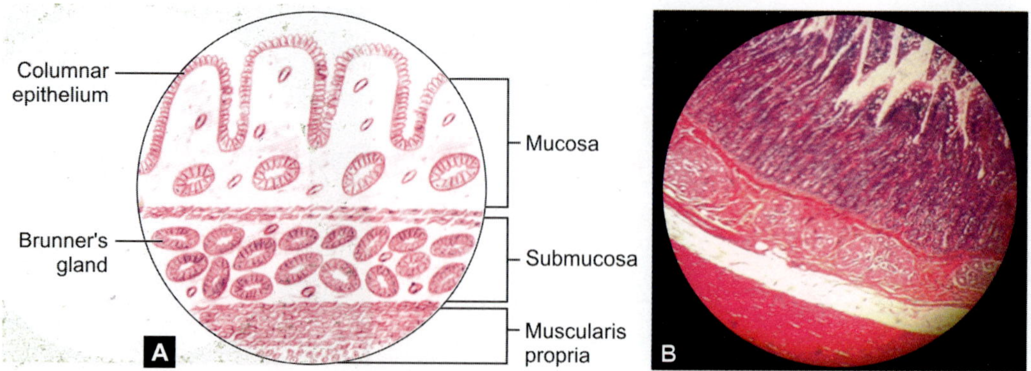

Figs 146A and B Duodenum

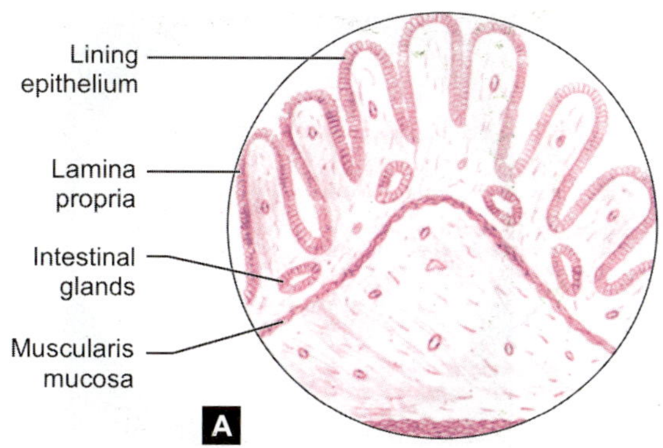

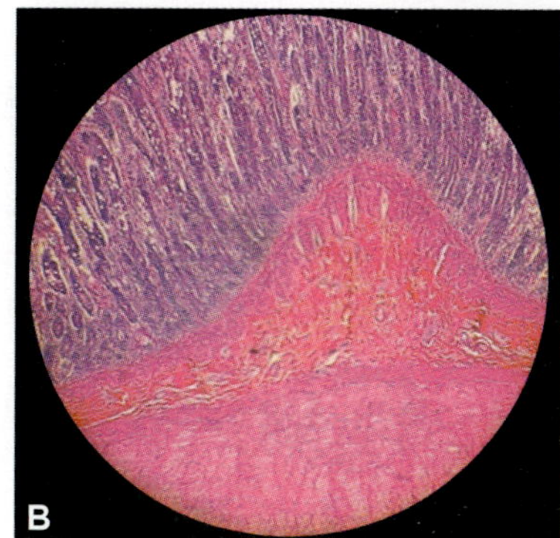

Figs 147A and B Jejunum

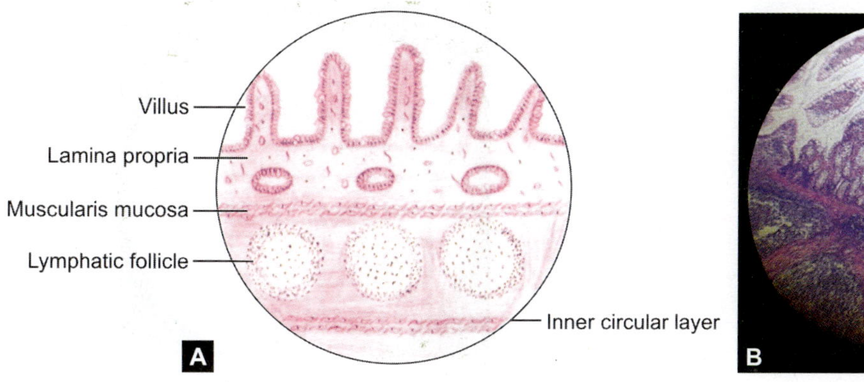

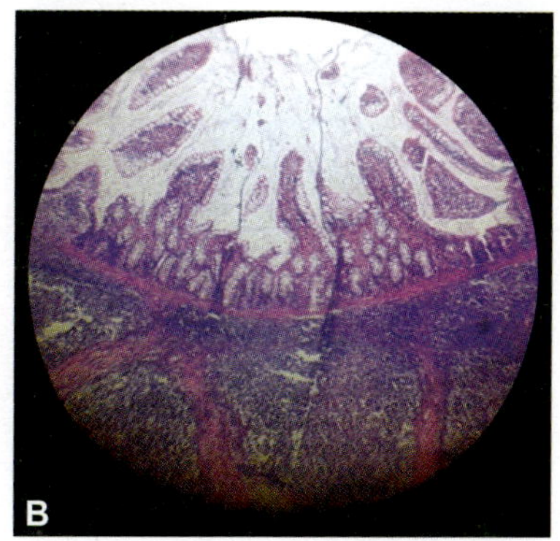

Figs 148A and B Ileum

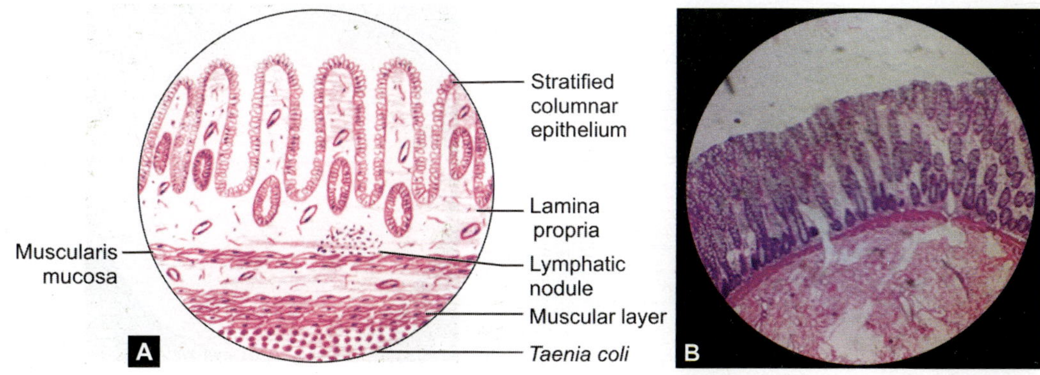

Figs 149A and B Large intestine

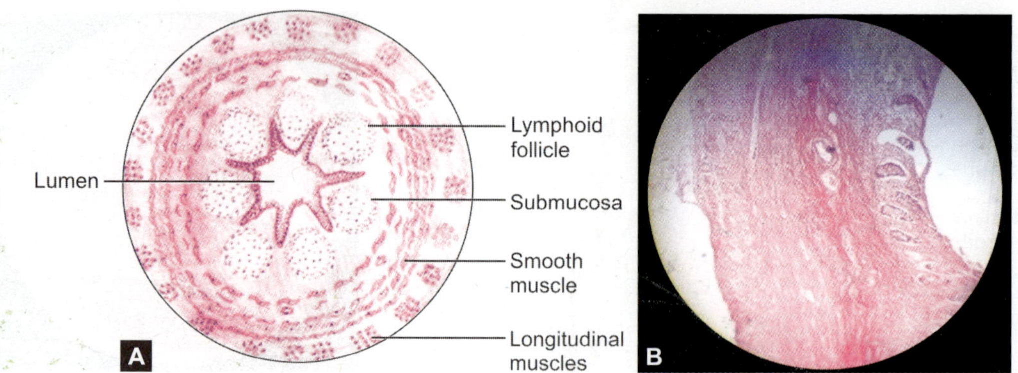

Figs 150A and B Vermiform appendix

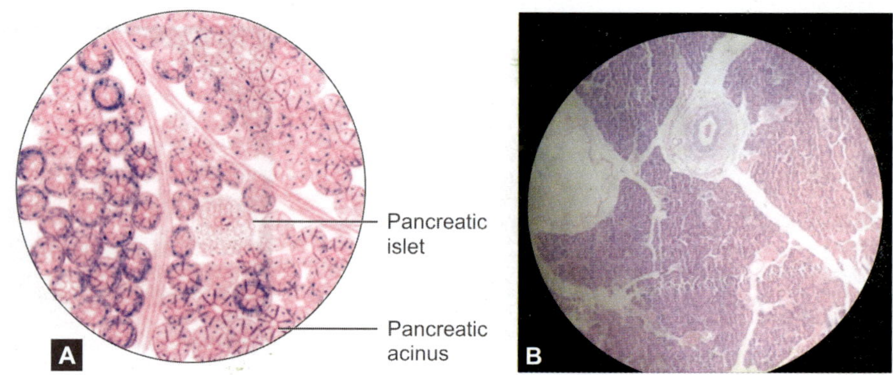

Figs 151A and B Pancreas

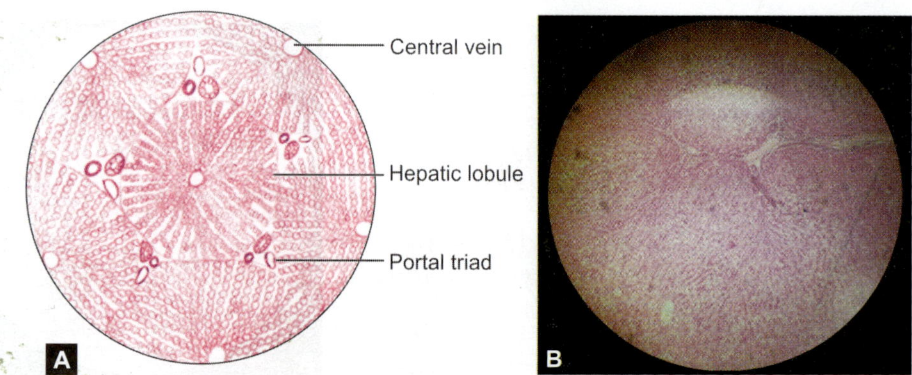

Figs 152A and B Liver

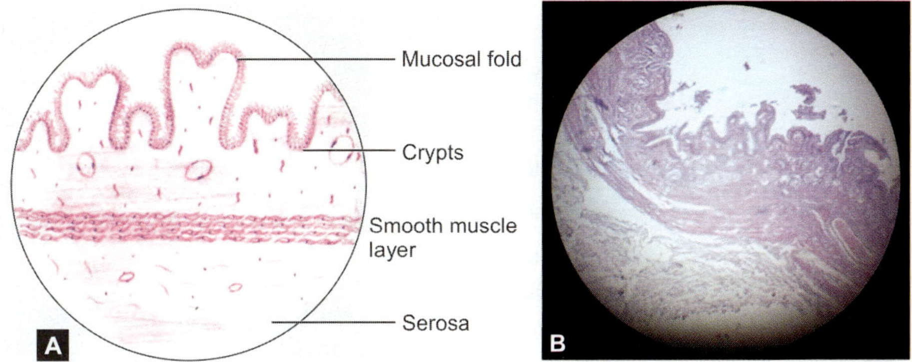

Figs 153A and B Gallbladder

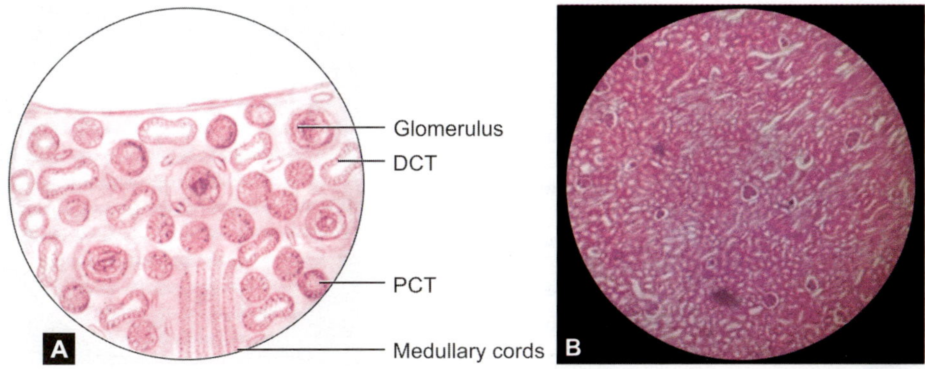

Figs 154A and B Kidney

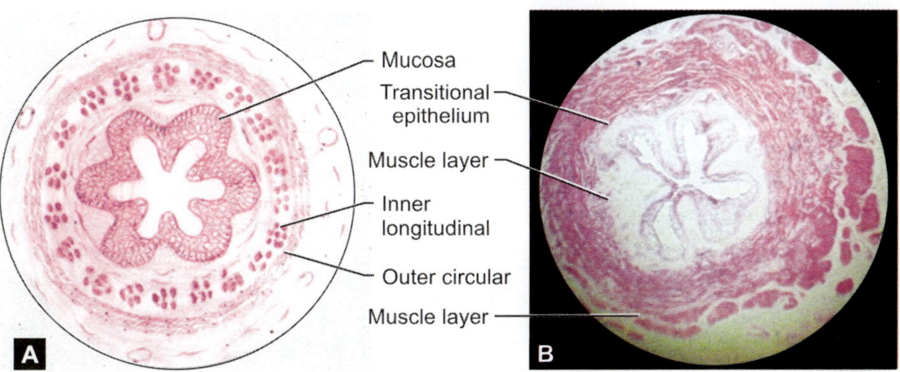

Figs 155A and B Ureter

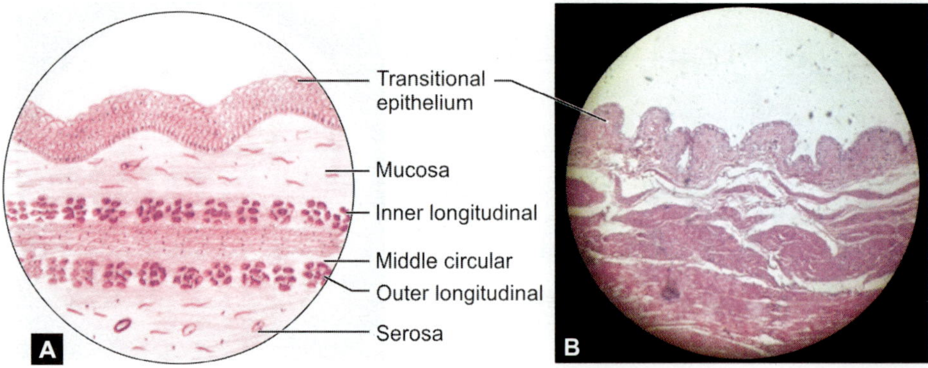

Figs 156A and B Urinary bladder

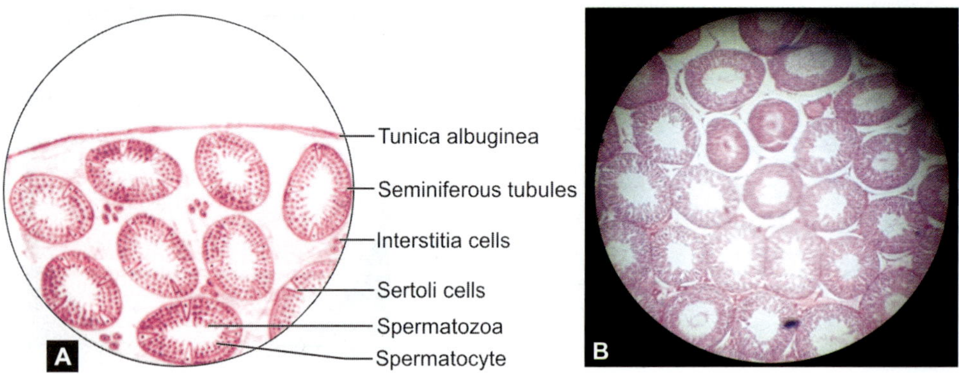

Figs 157A and B Testis

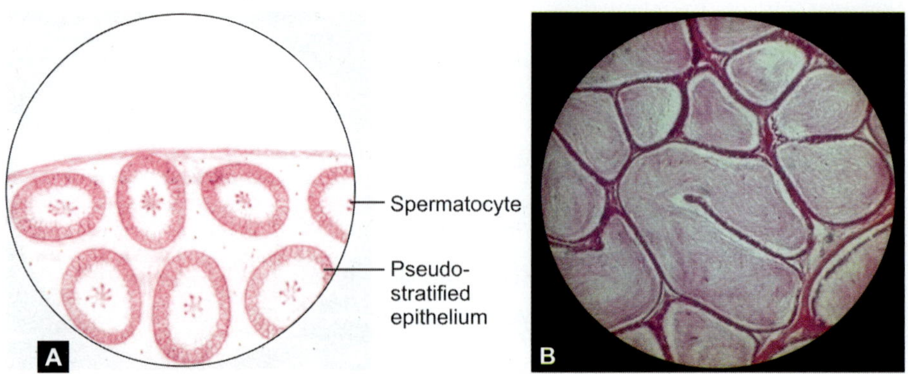

Figs 158A and B Epididymis

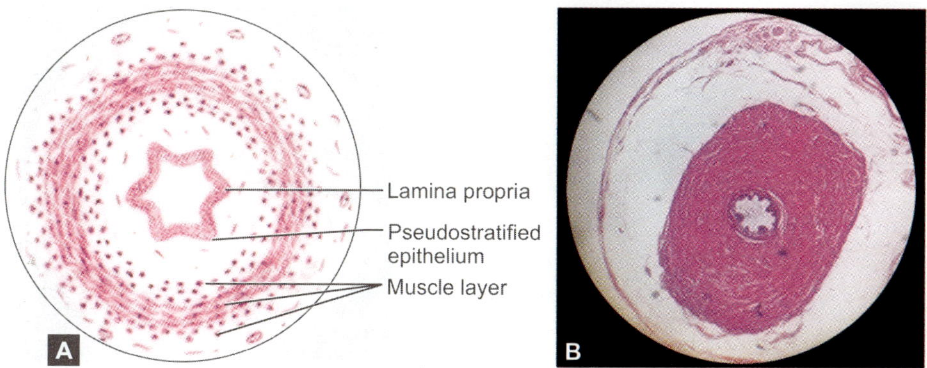

Figs 159A and B Ductus deferens

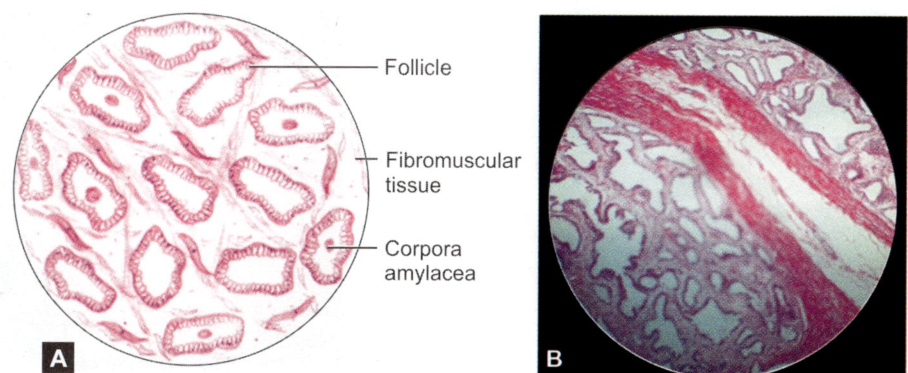

Figs 160A and B Prostate

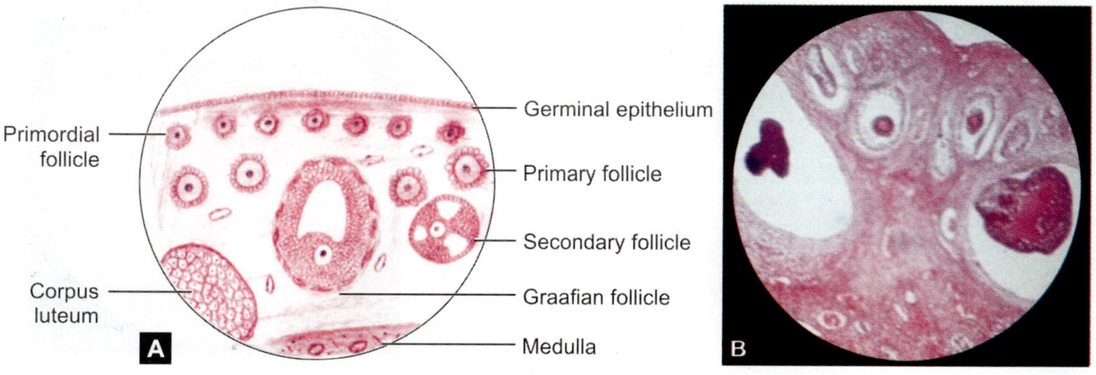

Figs 161A and B Ovary

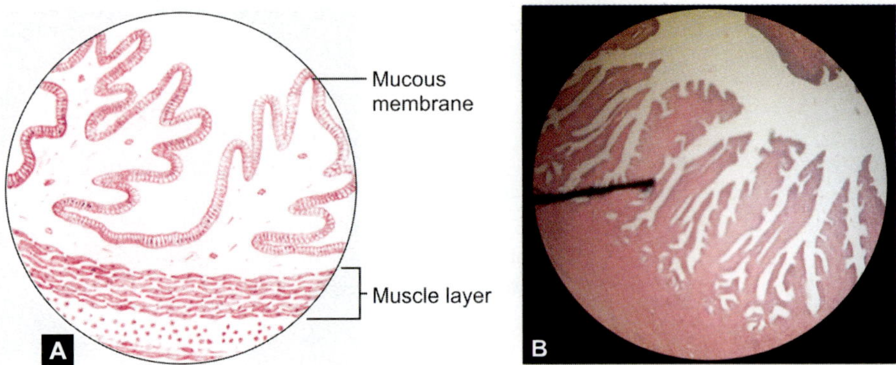

Figs 162A and B Fallopian tube

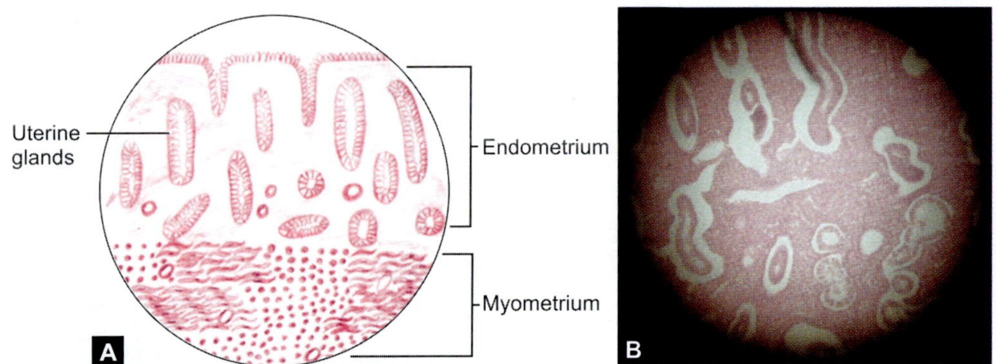

Figs 163A and B Uterus—proliferative

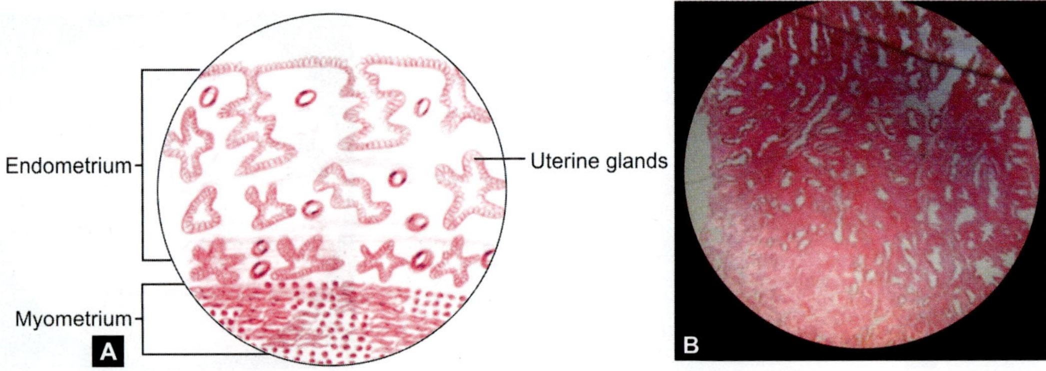

Figs 164A and B Uterus—secretory

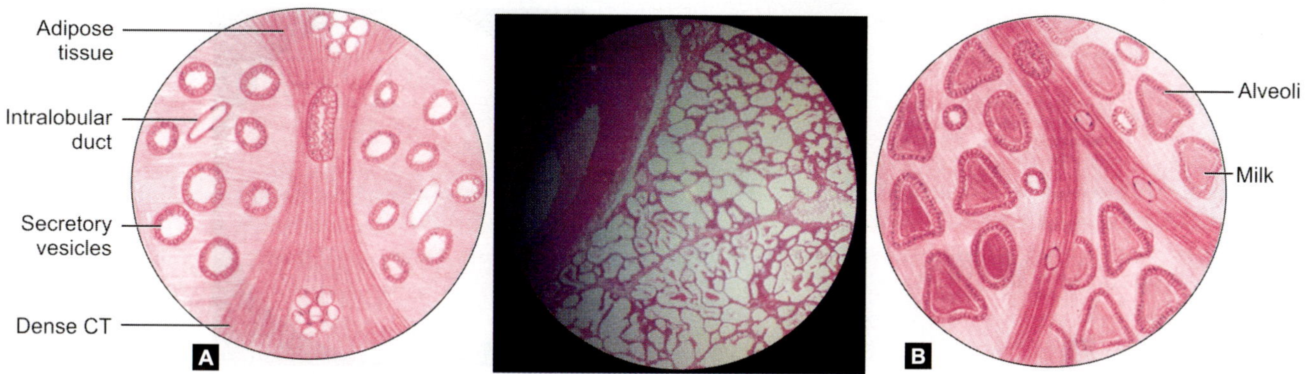

Figs 165A and B (A) Inactive mammary gland; (B) Active mammary gland

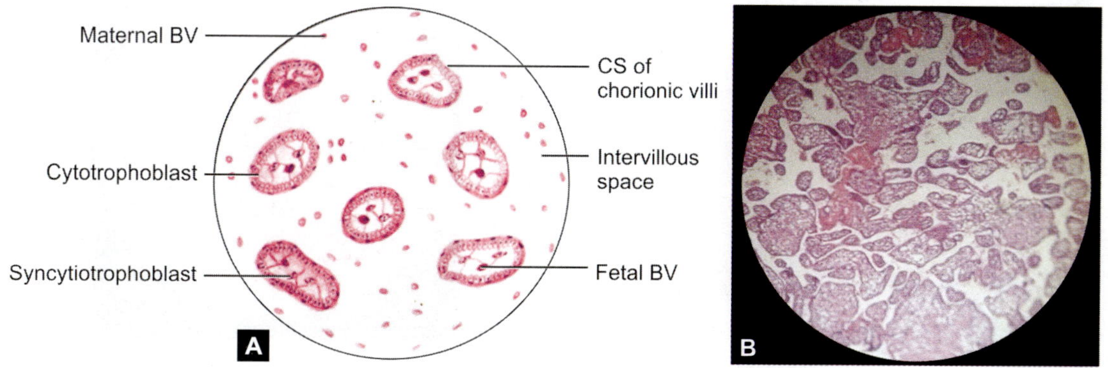

Figs 166A and B Placenta

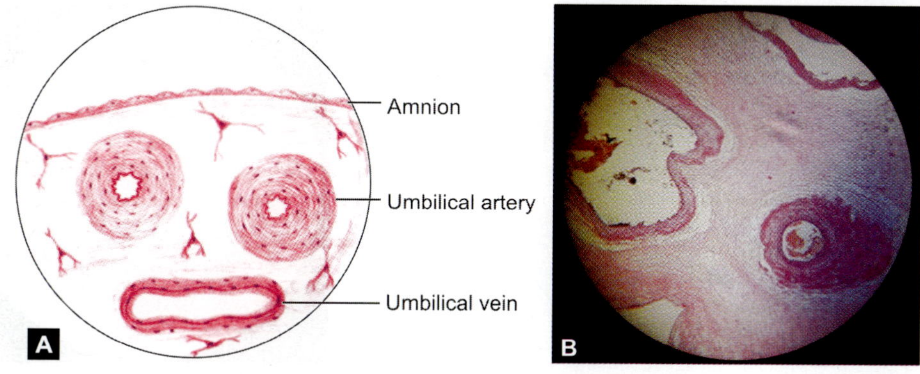

Figs 167A and B Umbilical cord

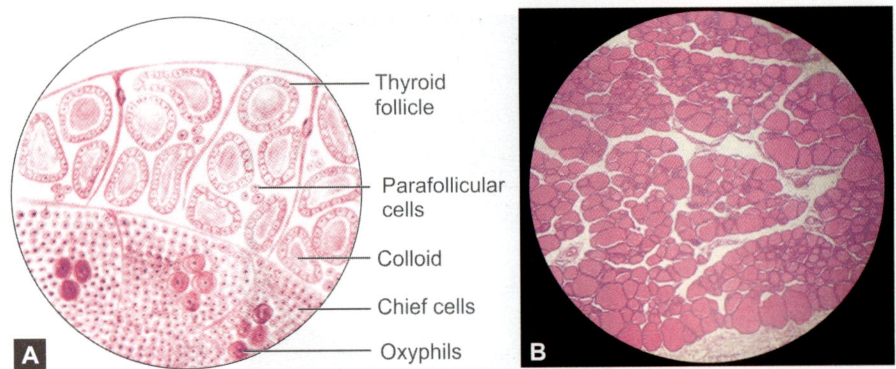

Figs 168A and B Thyroid and parathyroid glands

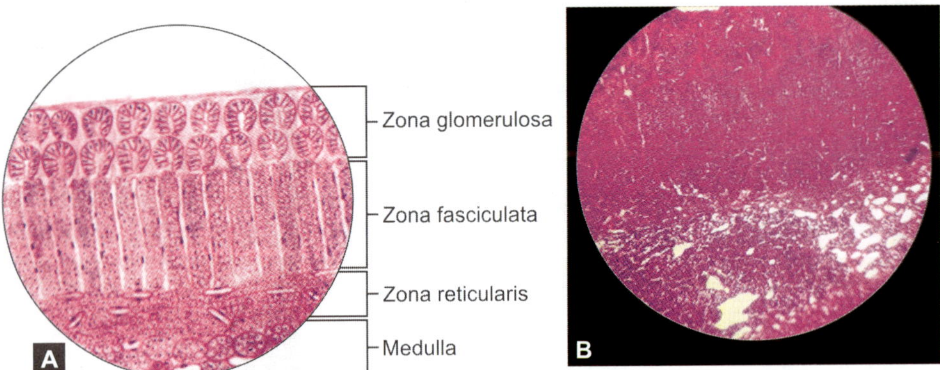

Figs 169A and B Suprarenal gland

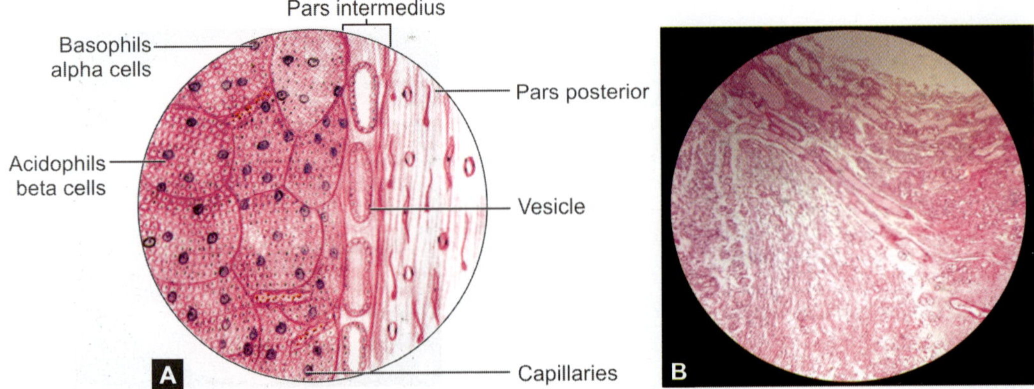

Figs 170A and B Pituitary gland

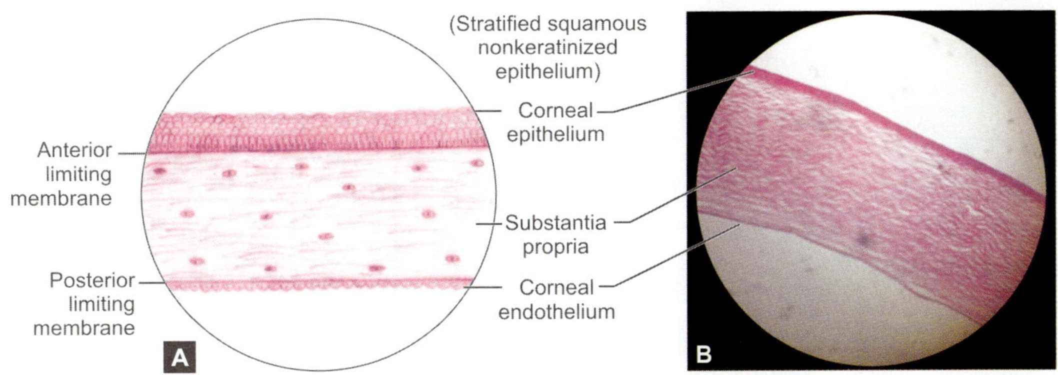

Figs 171A and B Cornea

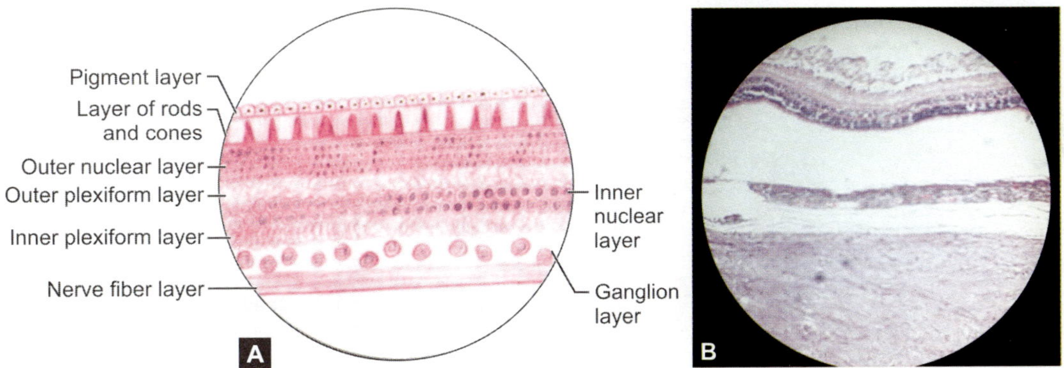

Figs 172A and B Retina

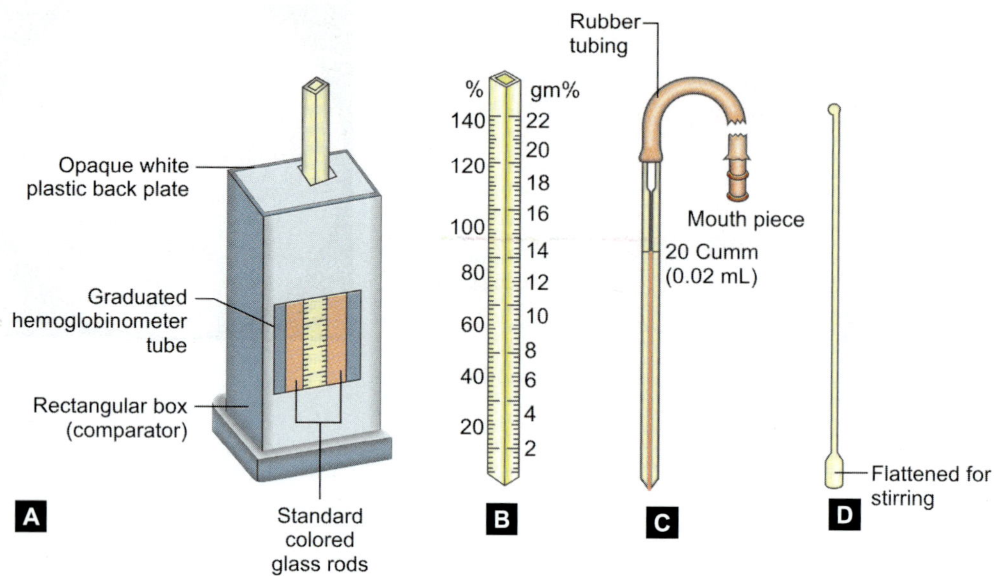

Figs 1A to D (A) Sahli's hemoglobinometer; (B) Graduated hemoglobinometer tube; (C) Hemoglobinometer pipette; (D) Glass rod (stirrer)

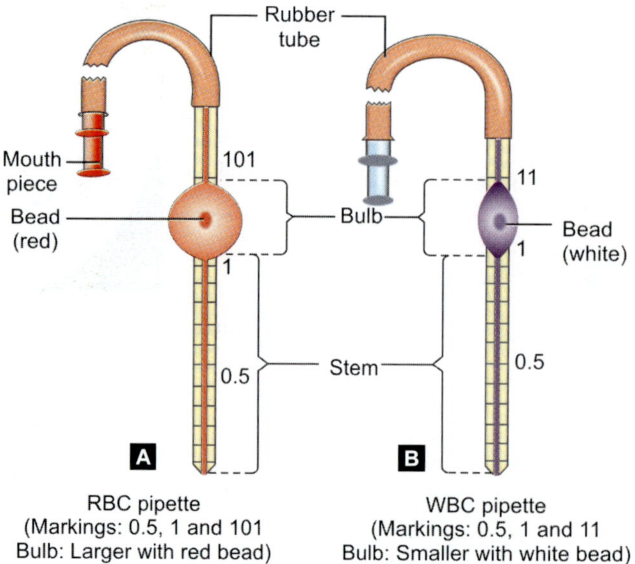

Figs 2A and B RBC and WBC pipettes

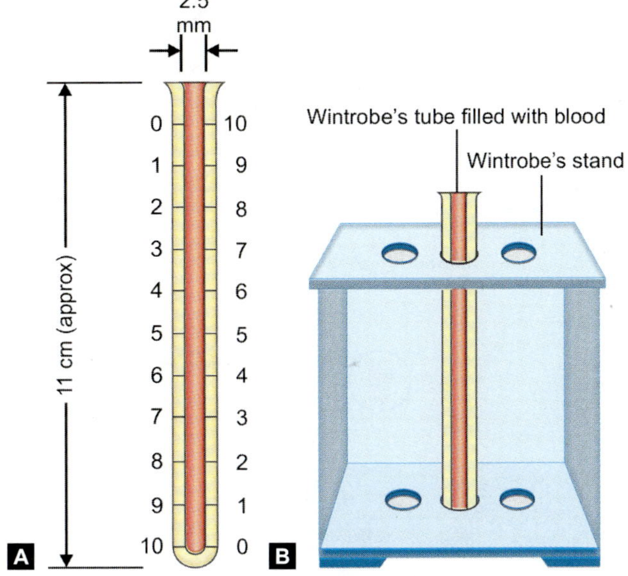

Figs 6A and B (A) Wintrobe's hematocrit tube with its stand (B)

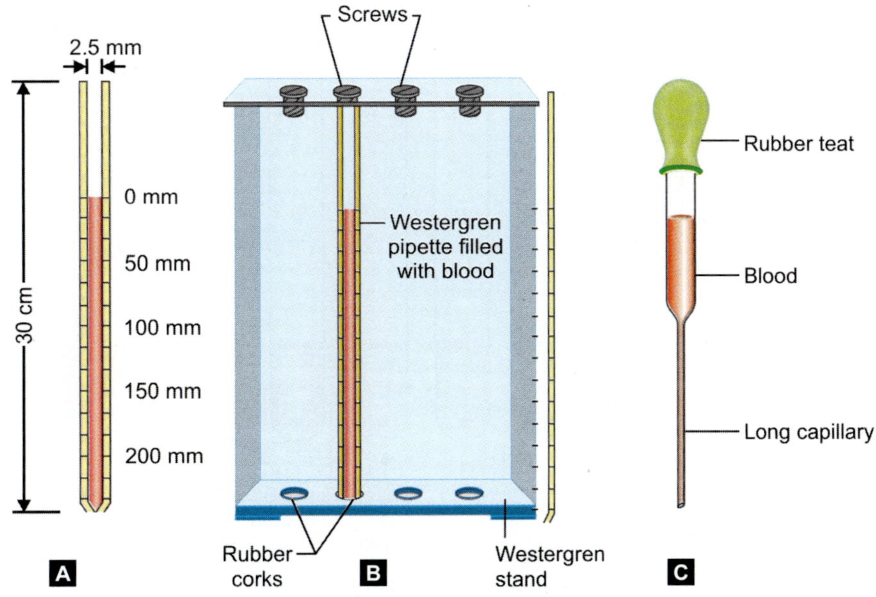

Figs 7A to C (A) Westergren's pipette; (B) with it stand; (C) Pasteur pipette

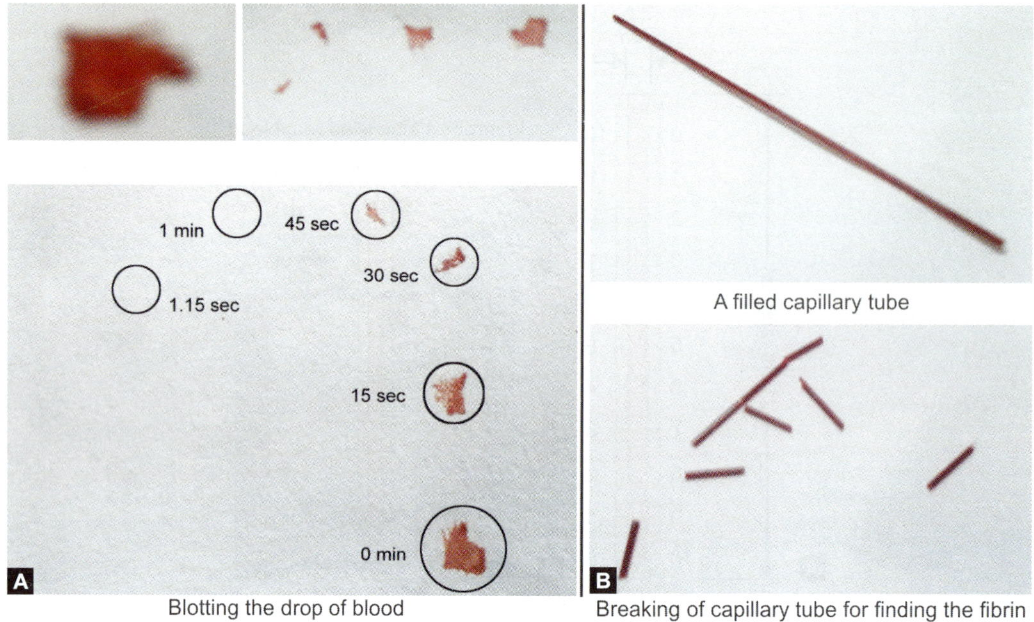

Figs 8A and B (A) Estimation of bleeding time by Duke's method; (B) Clotting time by capillary tube method

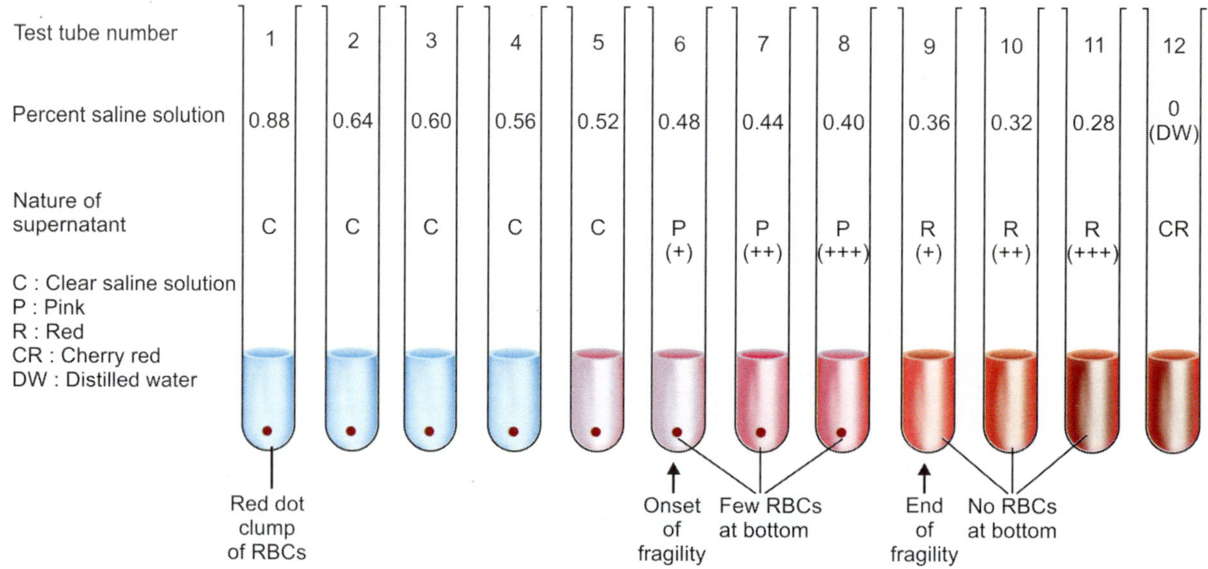

Fig. 9 Osmotic fragility of erythrocytes

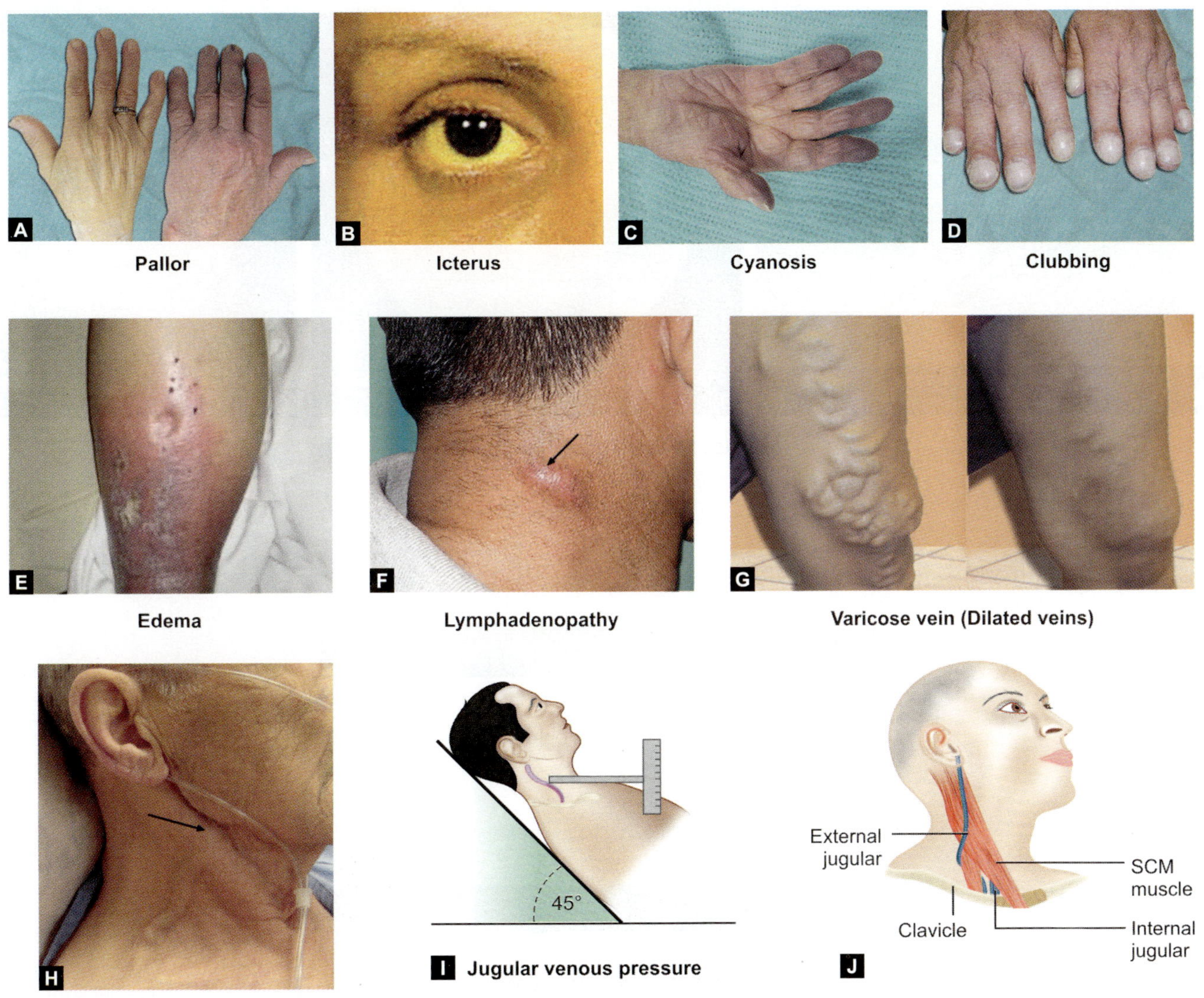

Figs 11A to J General examination

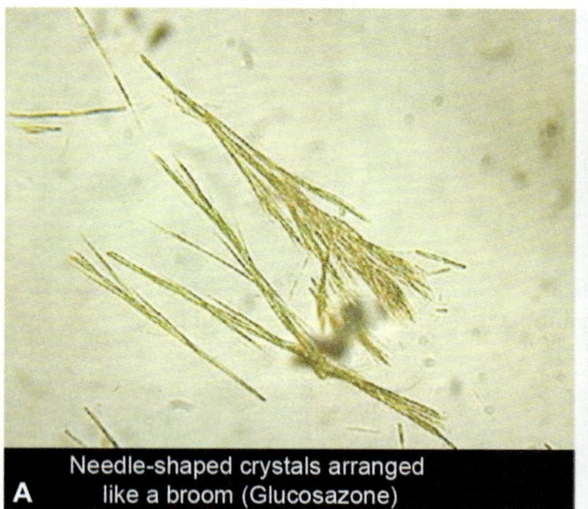
A Needle-shaped crystals arranged like a broom (Glucosazone)

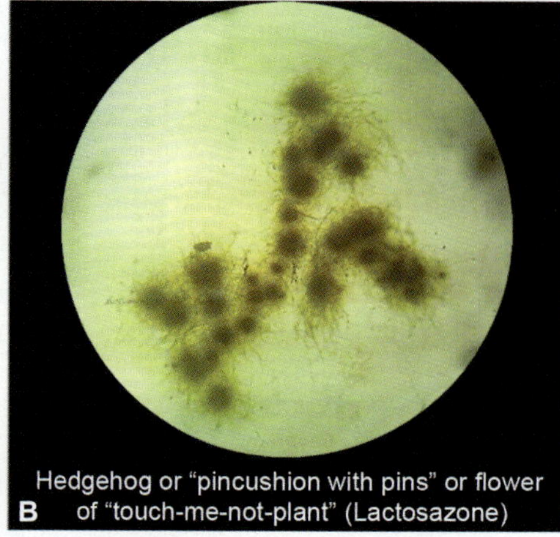
B Hedgehog or "pincushion with pins" or flower of "touch-me-not-plant" (Lactosazone)

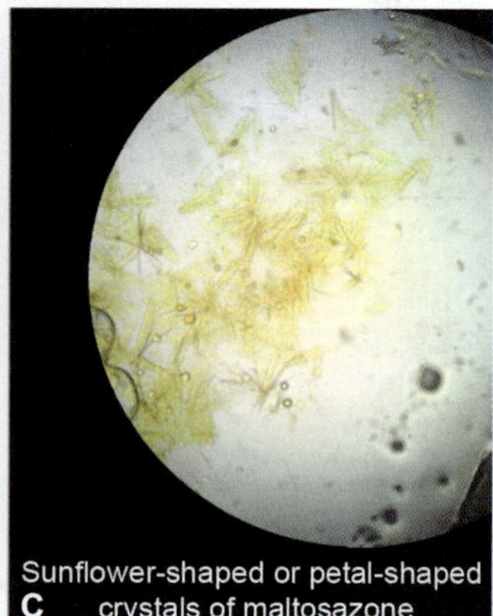
C Sunflower-shaped or petal-shaped crystals of maltosazone

Figs 1A to C Osazone crystals

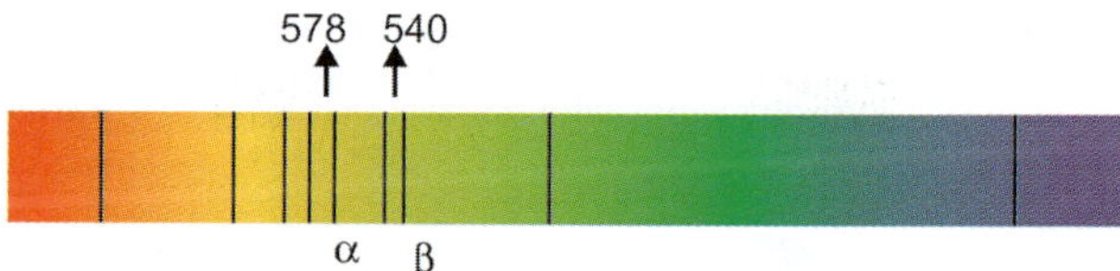

Fig. 7 Oxyhemoglobin

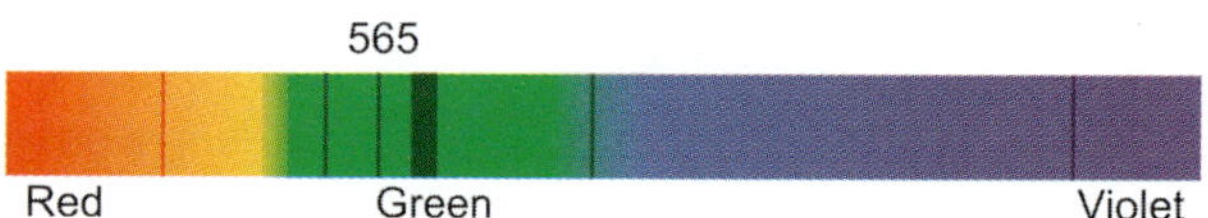

Fig. 8 Deoxyhemoglobin

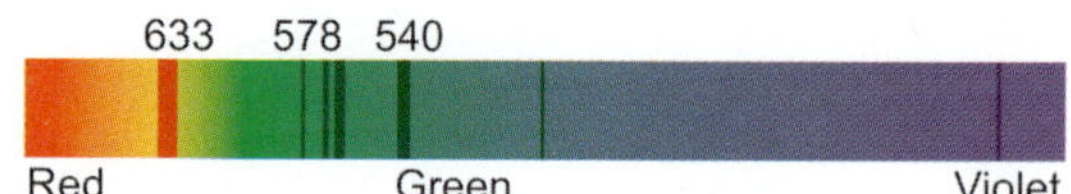

Fig. 9 Methemoglobin

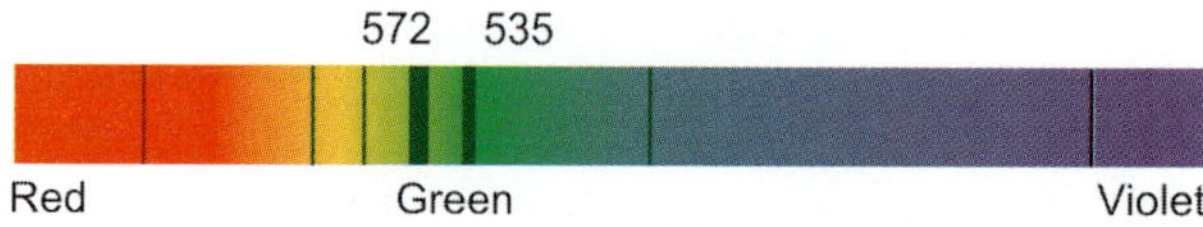

Fig. 10 Carboxyhemoglobin

1

Anatomy

KERALA UNIVERSITY OF HEALTH SCIENCES (KUHS) SYLLABUS

Theory Paper I	50
Theory Paper II	50
Theory: Internal Assessment	20
Practicals I	20
Practicals II	20
Practicals: Internal Assessment	20
Practical: Viva Voce	20
TOTAL	200

Theory	
Paper I	General Anatomy
	General Embryology
	Genetics
	Upper Limb
	Lower Limb
	Thorax
Paper II	Head and Neck
	Abdomen and Pelvis
	Neuroanatomy

Model Question Paper			
I	Long Essay	10 × 1	10
II	Short Essays (3 Nos)	5 × 3	15
III	Short Answer Questions (5 Nos)	3 × 5	15
IV	Short Answer Questions (3 Nos)	2 × 3	6
V	Labeled Diagram (One CS and One Gross)	2 × 2	4
	TOTAL		50

Practicals				
Practical I: Gross Anatomy				40
A	Spotting (20 Stations)		20 × ½ = 10	
B	Discussion with Specimen	Above Diaphragm	8	
		Below Diaphragm	7	
Practical II: Histology				
A	Spotting (14 Station -13 Slide + 1 Genetic Chart)		14 × ½ = 7	
B	Discussion with Slides	One from General Histology	4	
		One from Systemic Histology	4	

Viva Voce			
I	Embryology	5	20
II	Radiology	5	
III	Osteology	5	
IV	Surface Markings	5	

THEORY: IMPORTANT QUESTIONS

UPPER LIMB

NK—Neetha Kulkarni 2nd edition
CH—BD Chaurasia 6th edition
IBS—Inderbir Singh 8th edition
*—Important Questions

Essays

- Breast*(NK-87;CH-39)
- Brachial plexus*(NK-98;CH-54)
- Shoulder joint*(NK-115;CH-140)
- Ulnar nerve (NK-130,176;CH-171,160)
- Median nerve (NK-130,174;CH-109,159)
- Radial nerve (NK-131,179;CH-159,170)

Short Notes

- Clavipectoral fascia*(NK-86;CH-46)
- Rotator cuff*(NK-117;CH-140,80)
- Intermuscular spaces(NK-110,CH-82)
- Cubital fossa*(NK-133;CH-92)
- Palmar aponeurosis (NK-161;CH-112)
- Anatomical snuff box (NK-157;CH-102)
- Flexor retinaculum*(NK-156;CH-123)
- Extensor retinaculum*(NK-158;CH-125)
- Carrying angle*(NK-137;CH-145)
- Superior radioulnar joint (NK-151;CH-146)
- Interosseous membrane*(NK-152;CH-145)
- Supination and pronation (NK-153;CH-146)
- Wrist joint (NK-155;CH-147)
- First carpometacarpal joint*(NK-172;CH-149)

Vascular Systems

- Axillary artery*(NK-102;CH-55)
- Lymphatic drainage of breast*(NK-89;CH-42)
- Cephalic vein*(NK-122;CH-72)
- Median cubital vein (NK-123;CH-73)
- Anastomosis around scapula*(NK-104;CH-83)
- Anastomosis around elbow joint*(NK-134;CH-90)
- Brachial artery*(NK-127;CH-89,174)
- Profunda brachii artery (NK-131;CH-97)
- Anterior interosseous artery (NK-134;CH-175)
- Superficial palmar arch*(NK-164;CH-119,158)
- Deep palmar arch (NK-165;CH-120)
- Axillary lymph nodes (NK-96;CH-58)

Nerves

- Axillary nerve*(NK-111;CH-82,159,169)
- Deep branch of ulnar nerve (NK-170;CH-58)
- Erb's paralysis (NK-101;CH-58)
- Klumpke's paralysis*(NK-101;CH-59)
- Musculocutaneous nerve (NK-129;CH-88,169)
- Anterior interosseous nerve*(NK-143;CH-110)

PNEUMONICS

- Branches of lateral cord of brachial plexus
  Love Means Love
  Lateral pectoral nerve
  Musculocutaneous nerve
  Lateral root of median nerve
- Branches of medial cord of brachial plexus—**M4U**
  Medial pectoral nerve
  Medial cutaneous nerve of arm
  Medial cutaneous nerve of forearm
  Medial root of median nerve
  Ulnar nerve
- Branches of posterior cord of brachial plexus—**ULTRA**
  Upper subscapular nerve
  Lower subscapular nerve
  Thoracodorsal nerve
  Radial nerve
  Axillary nerve
- Structures piercing clavipectoral fascia—**TALC**
  Thoracoacromial vessels
  Apical lymphatics
  Lateral pectoral nerve
  Cephalic vein
- Contents of **AXILLA**
  A-axillary artery and its branches
  X-axillary vein and its tributaries
  I-infraclavicular part of brachial plexus
  L-long thoracic nerve
  L-lymph nodes (axillary)
  A-axillary pad of fat
- Rotator cuff formed by—**SITS**
  S-supraspinatus
  I-infraspinatus
  T-teres minor
  S-subscapularis
- Muscles supplied by musculocutaneous nerve—**BBC**
  Biceps
  Brachialis
  Coracobrachialis
- Cubital fossa—contents:
  MBBR—from medial to lateral
  M-median nerve
  B-brachial artery termination
  B-biceps tendon
  R-radial nerve
- Contents of anatomical snuff box—**CvRaN**
  C-cephalic vein
  R-radial artery
  N-nerve, superficial radial nerve

- Posterior interosseous nerve (NK-150;CH-128)
- Carpal tunnel syndrome (NK-158;CH-133,176)
- Cutaneous innervations of hand (NK-159;CH-67)

Muscles

- Pectoralis major (NK-85;CH-45)
- Serratus anterior (NK-95;CH-47)
- Deltoid*(NK-108;CH-77)
- Triceps (NK-130;CH-94)
- Supinator (NK-154;CH-129)
- Biceps brachii*(NK-154;CH-20,87)
- Coracobrachialis (NK-126;CH-87)
- Brachioradialis (NK-147;CH-16,20)
- Pronator teres (NK-153;CH-103)
- Lumbricals*(NK-168;CH-116)
- Interossei (NK-169;CH-116)

Diagram

- Lymphatic drainage of breast (NK-90;CH-42)
- Clavipectoral fascia (NK-87;CH-44)
- CS through arm (NK-126;CH-89)
- Brachial plexus (NK-99;CH-54)
- Anastomosis around scapula (NK-104;CH-83)
- Anastomosis around elbow (NK-127;CH-91)
- Superficial and deep palmar arch (NK-164;CH-115)
- Oblique section through hand (NK-162;CH-121)

LOWER LIMB

Essays

- Femoral artery (NK-850;CH-48)
- Popliteal fossa and contents*(NK-825,878;CH-76)
- Sciatic nerve (NK-863;CH-84)
- Saphenous vein (NK-836;CH-103)
- Hip joint*(NK-872;CH-136)
- Knee joint*(NK-883;CH-140)
- Arches of foot*(NK-922;CH-159)

Short Notes

- Adductor canal*(NK-848;CH-55)
- Femoral triangle*(NK-846;CH-45)
- Fascia lata (NK-843;CH-44)
- Iliotibial tract*(NK-845;CH-44)
- Femoral sheath (NK-845;CH-47)
- Femoral canal*(NK-845;CH-47)
- Extensor retinaculum (NK-904;CH-93)
- Plantar aponeurosis (NK-914;CH-114)
- Flexor retinaculum (NK-905;CH-104)
- Iliofemoral ligament*(NK-873;CH-137)
- Intra-articular ligaments of knee joint (NK-886;CH-141)
- Ligamentum patella (NK-884;CH-142)
- Cruciate ligaments (NK-886;CH-141)

- Anterior dislocation of lunate may cause *median nerve compression*
- Radial nerve palsy and chronic nerve palsy can lead to *wrist drop*
- Palmar interossei-adduct the finger—**PAD**
- Dorsal interossei-abduct the finger—**DAB**
- All muscles of hand; thenar, hypothenar, interossei and lumbricals are supplied by C8 and T1
- Attachments on medial side of tibia

  Girls between 2 super stars

  Gracilis between sartorius and semitendinosus
- Inversion and eversion muscles

  Eversion

  p**E**roneus longus

  p**E**roneus brevis

  p**E**roneus tertius

  Inversion

  t**I**bialis anterior

  t**I**bialis posterior
- Structures under extensor retinaculum

  Tom Has A Nice Dark Pen

  Tibialis anterior

  extensor **H**allucis longus

  deep peroneal **N**erve

  extensor **D**igitorum

  Peroneus tertius
- Deep inguinal ring lies ½ inch above mid inguinal point
- Superficial inguinal ring lies ½ inch below mid inguinal point
- Saphenous opening lies 4 cm below and lateral to the pubic tubercle
- Abductors of hip are:

  Short Tense Middle class Men

  Sartorius

  Tensor fascia lata

  Minimus gluteus

  Medius gluteus
- Structures in the tibial intercondylar area

  From anterior to posterior

  Medical College Lucknow, Lucknow Medical College

  Medial meniscus (anterior horn)

  Cruciate ligament (anterior)

  Lateral meniscus (anterior horn)

  Lateral meniscus (posterior horn)

  Medial meniscus (posterior horn)

  Cruciate ligament (posterior)

- Locking and unlocking of knee joint (NK-892;CH-146)
- Deltoid ligament (NK-908;CH-148)
- Spring ligament (NK-921;CH-149)
- Inversion and eversion (NK-921;CH-153)
- Longitudinal arches of foot (NK-922;CH-159)
- Tendocalcaneous (NK-899;CH-105)

Vascular Systems

- Great saphenous vein (NK-836;CH-143)
- Saphenous opening (NK-844;CH-42)
- Inguinal lymph nodes (NK-840;CH-43)
- Trochanteric and cruciate anastomosis*(NK-79;CH-73)
- Profunda femoris artery*(NK-870;CH-55)
- Anastomosis at back of thigh*(NK-871;CH-88)
- Popliteal artery (NK-879;CH-78)
- Anterior tibial artery (NK-896;CH-94)
- Dorsalis pedis artery (NK-912;CH-97)
- Peroneal artery (NK-901;CH-110)
- Plantar arch (NK-918;CH-160)

Nerves

- Femoral nerve (NK-845,849;CH-52)
- Obturator nerve*(NK-869;CH-61)
- Tibial nerve (NK-881,902;CH-79)
- Common peroneal nerve (NK-882;CH-80)
- Medial plantar nerve*(NK-919;CH-116)
- Lateral plantar nerve (NK-920;CH-117)
- Cutaneous sensation of leg and foot (NK-911;CH-103)
- Deep peroneal nerve*(NK-896;CH-95)

Muscles

- Sartorius (NK-852;CH-111,53)
- Quadriceps femoris (NK-853;CH-53)
- Adductor muscles of thigh*(NK-867,868;CH-59)
- Gluteus maximus and structures under it*(NK-856; CH-106)
- Piriformis (NK-858;CH-68)
- Peroneal muscles (NK-897;CH-68)
- Popliteus*(NK-902;CH-80)
- Tibialis posterior (NK-904;CH-94)

Diagrams

- Femoral triangle (NK-847;CH-45)
- Adductor canal (NK-848;CH-55)
- TS through thigh (NK-856;CH-85)
- TS through middle of leg (NK-895;CH-93)
- Knee joint (NK-886,891;CH-142)
- Popliteal fossa (NK-878;CH-77)
- Longitudinal arches of foot (NK-922;CH-160)
- CS through thigh (NK-844;CH-53)
- Cutaneous sensation of dorsum of foot (NK-910; CH-104)

- Calcaneonavicular/spring ligament is most important ligament for maintaining the median longitudinal arch but it has nothing to do with stability of ankle joint because it is not around ankle joint.
- Gastrocnemius and plantaris acts by plantiflexing ankle joint and flexing knee joint
- Structures passing deep to flexor retinaculum

  The Doctors Are Not Here

  Tibialis posterior tendon

  flexor **D**igitorum longus

  posterior tibial **A**rtery

  tibial **N**erve

  flexor **H**allucis longus
- Quadriceps femoris, i.e. (rectus femoris, vastus lateralis, vastus medialis, vastus intermedius) is strong extensor of knee
- Extension at knee produced by quadriceps femoris (main) and tensor fascia lata (accessory)
- Anterior cruciate ligament

  APLLe

  Origin—**A**nterior intercondylar area of tibia

  Direction of fiber—**P**osterior, **L**ateral

  Insertion—**L**ateral femoral condyle
- Posterior cruciate ligament

  PAMM

  Origin—**P**osterior intercondylar area of tibia

  Direction of fiber—**A**nterior, **M**edial

  Insertion—**M**edial femoral condyle
- Structures in costal groove

  VAN

  Vein

  Artery

  Nerve
- Structures at lung roots (above downwards)

  Left lung

  Are Brahmins Vegetarians?

  Artery, **B**ronchi, **V**ein

  Right lung

  Brahmins Are Born Vegetarians

  Bronchus

  Artery

  Bronchus

  Vein

THORAX

Essays

- Typical intercostal space (NK-202;CH-211)
- Pleura and pleural recesses*(NK-216;CH-223)
- Lungs*(NK-219;CH-222)
- Heart (right atrium)*(NK-255;CH-245)
- Blood supply of heart (RCA,LCA)**(NK-263;CH-252)

Short Notes

- Openings in diaphragm*(NK-231;CH-336)
- Suprapleural fascia/Sibson's fascia (NK-217;CH-225)
- Impressions on mediastinal surface of lung* (NK-222; CH-230)
- Root of lung*(NK-224;CH-231)
- Pulmonary ligament (NK-224;CH-225)
- Left atrium*(NK-254;CH-248)
- Left coronary artery*(NK-264;CH-252)
- Ligamentum arteriosum*(NK-247;CH-265)
- Bronchopulmonary segment*(NK-226;CH-233)
- Superior mediastinum*(NK-209;CH-237)
- Posterior mediastinum*(NK-210;CH-238)
- Sinuses of pericardium (NK-250;CH-242)
- Thoracic duct*(NK-282;CH-270)
- Esophagus (NK-286;CH-279)

Vascular Systems

- Internal thoracic artery*(NK-206;CH-217)
- Azygos, hemiazygos and accessory hemiazygos vein* (NK-218,278;CH-218)
- Blood supply and nerve supply of lung (NK-226;CH-232)
- Arch of aorta*(NK-274;CH-278)
- Superior vena cava*(NK-277;CH-278)

Nerves

- Typical intercostal nerve (NK-203;CH-287)
- Thoracic sympathetic trunk (NK-284;CH-219)

Muscles

- Intercostal muscles (NK-202;CH-211)

Diagrams

- Typical intercostal space (NK-202;CH-214)
- Lungs—mediastinal surface of left and right lung (NK-222;CH-230)
- Bronchopulmonary segments (NK-225;CH-230)
- Interior of right atrium (NK-255;CH-246)
- Blood supply of heart (NK-263;CH-253,254)
- CS at the level of T3 (NK-287;CH-263)
- CS at the level of T4 (NK-275;CH-262)
- CS at the level of intervertebral disk between T5 and T6

- Bronchopulmonary segment of left lung

  A PALM Seed Makes Another Little Palm

  A - Apical

  P - Posterior

  A - Anterior

  L - Lateral

  M - Medial

  S - Superior

  M - Medial basal

  A - Anterior basal

  L - Lateral basal

  P - Posterior basal
- Orbit-medial wall formed by:

  uSMLE

  S - Sphenoid (body)

  M - Maxilla (frontal process)

  L - Lacrimal bone

  E - Ethmoid (orbital plate)
- Orbit-lateral wall formed by—**ZyGS**

  Z - Zygomatic (frontal process)

  G,S - Greater wing of sphenoid
- Orbit-floor formed by:

  Pa Ma Zy

  Pa - Palatine (orbital process)

  Ma - Maxilla

  Zy - Zygomatic
- Structures pierced by parotid duct

  BBBB

  Buccinators

  Buccopharyngeal fascia

  Buccal pad of fat

  Buccal mucosa
- Layers of **SCALP**

  S - Skin

  C - Connective tissue

  A - Aponeurosis

  L - Loose connective tissue

  P - Periosteum
- Nerve supply of extrinsic muscles of eyeball

  $LR_6(SO_4)_3$

  Lateral rectus - 6th CN

  Superior oblique - 4th CN

  All others muscles - 3rd CN

HEAD AND NECK

Essays

- Scalp*(NK-320;CH-60)
- Face (NK-323;CH-64)
- Deep cervical fascia (NK-343;CH-81)
- Cavernous sinus*(NK-504;CH-193)
- Parotid gland*(NK-338;CH-106)
- Temperomandibular joint*(NK-393;CH-121)
- Submandibular gland (NK-360;CH-133)
- Mandiblar nerve (NK-388;CH-125)
- Thyroid gland*(NK-368;CH-140)
- Palatine tonsil*(NK-435;CH-229)
- Lateral wall of nose*(NK-424;CH-245)
- Tongue (NK-415;CH-266)
- Middle ear*(NK-448;CH-277)
- Pituitary gland (NK-508;CH-197)

Short Notes

- Dangerous area of face (NK-329;CH-72)
- Vertebral artery (NK-475;CH-165)
- Carotid sheath (NK-346;CH-99)
- Digastrics triangle*(NK-357;CH-96)
- Carotid triangle*(NK-354;CH-96)
- Suboccipital triangle (NK-474;CH-179)
- Filum terminale (NK-487;CH-339)
- Falx cerebri*(NK-501;CH-328)
- Tentorium cerebelli*(NK-501;CH-328)
- Sigmoid sinus (NK-504;CH-196)
- Styloid apparatus (NK-314;CH-159)
- Palate (NK-420;CH-222)
- Waldeyers lymphatic ring*(NK-437;CH-228)
- Constrictors of pharynx and Killian's dehiscence (NK-433;CH-232)
- Auditory tube (NK-452;CH-278)
- Nasal septum*(NK-425;CH-240)
- Little's area (NK-426;CH-242)
- Frontal air sinus*(NK-427;CH-245)
- Maxillary sinus*(NK-428;CH-245)
- Vocal cord*(NK-442;CH-259)
- Nerve supply of pinna (NK-446;CH-273)
- Tympanic membrane*(NK-449;CH-278)
- Medial wall of middle ear*(NK-451;CH-279)
- Eye ball*(NK-406;CH-288)
- Cavity of larynx*(NK-441;CH-256)

Vascular Systems

- Facial artery*(NK-327;CH-71)
- Superior sagittal sinus (NK-351;CH-195)
- Middle meningeal artery*(NK-507;CH-201,120)
- Maxillary artery*(NK-392;CH-119,313)
- Blood supply of thyroid (NK-370;CH-143)

- Branches of external carotid artery

  SLiPy FOAMS

  S - Superior thyroid artery

  L - Lingual artery

  P - Posterior auricular artery

  F - Facial artery

  O -Occipital artery

  A - Ascendimg pharyngeal artery

  M - Maxillary artery

  S - Superficial temporal artery

Abductors and abductors of eye

- **BOLR**

  a**B**ductors—superior and inferior **O**blique, **L**ateral **R**ectus
- **MIS RED**—**M**edial, **I**nferior, **S**uperior **RE**ctus are a**DD**uctors
- **BORD**—in a**B**ducted eye, **O**bliques are chief tortors; in a a**DD**ucted eye **R**ecti are chief tortors
- Anterior 2/3rd of tongue is supplied by chorda tympani (taste) and lingual (general)
- Posterior1/3rd of tongue is supplied by glossopharyngeal nerve (taste and general)
- Posterior most tongue is supplied by internal laryngeal branch of vagus nerve (taste and general)
- All muscles (genioglossus, hypoglossus, styloglossus) except palatoglossus are supplied by hypoglossal nerve
- Waldeyers ring—by palatine tonsil, lingual tonsil, pharyngeal tonsil, tubal tonsil
- a**DD**uctors of vocal cord—**TILaC**

  T - Thyroarytenoids

  I - Intertransverse arytenoids

  LaC - Lateral cricoarytenoid
- Muscles of mastication—**MTP** Act

  M - **M**asseter

  T - **T**emporalis

  P - **M**edial and lateral pterygoid
- Secretory motor pathway for parotid gland

  I Sailed 9 Typically Less Pet Of AuTm

  I sailed - **I**nferior **Sali**vary nucleus

  9 - **9th**/glossopharyngeal nerve

  Typically - Tympanic **branch** and **plexus**

  Less Pet - **Less**er **Pet**rosal nerve

  Of - Otic ganglion

  AuTm - **Au**riculo**tem**poral nerve

- Internal jugular vein (NK-380;CH-153)
- Vertebral artery (NK-475;CH-165)

Nerves

- Mandibular nerve*(NK-388;CH-125)
- Lingual nerve (NK-388;CH-126)
- Nerve supply of face*(NK-325;CH-69)
- Trigeminal ganglion (NK-602;CH-199)
- Otic ganglion*(NK-390;CH-311)
- Submandibular ganglion (NK-363;CH-309)
- Pterygopalatine ganglion (NK-391;CH-310)
- Ansa cervicalis*(NK-382;CH-103)
- Ciliary ganglion*(NK-404;CH-311)

Muscles

- Orbicularis oculi (NK-329;CH-225)
- Orbicularis oris (NK-331;CH-66)
- Buccinators (NK-331;CH-66)
- Extraocular muscles (NK-401;CH-206)
- Superior oblique muscles*(NK-402;CH-206)
- Sternocleidomastoid*(NK-346;CH-89)
- Digastric muscles*(NK-358;CH-132)
- Hyoglossus*(NK-359;CH-132,133)
- Muscles of mastication*(NK-396;CH-116)
- Mylohyoid (NK-359;CH-132)
- Scalene anterior (NK-385;CH-165)
- Muscles of larynx (NK-443;CH-258)
- Cricothyroid (NK-444;CH-258)
- Posterior cricoarytenoid (NK-444;CH-258)
- Tongue muscles (NK-416;CH-266)

Diagrams

- Cavernous sinus (NK-504;CH-101)
- Thyroid gland (NK-370;CH-173)
- BS and NS of lateral wall of nasal cavity (NK-426; CH-230)
- Distribution of cutaneous nerve to head and neck
- TS at the level of C6

NEUROANATOMY

Essays

- Sulci, gyri and functional areas of brain*(NK-548; IBS-178)
- Internal capsule*(NK-564;IBS-197)
- Cerebellum (NK-532;IBS-131)
- Corpus callosum*(NK-563;IBS-173)
- Ventricles of brain*(NK-568,336;IBS-202)
- Blood supply of brain (circle of Willis*) (NK-555;IBS-248)
- Superolateral surface of brain*(NK-549;IBS-172)

Short Notes

- Lateral ventricle (NK-568;IBS-202)
- Floor of 4th ventricle*(NK-537;IBS-206)
- Third ventricle (NK-545;IBS-204)

- **RISE—Inferior** thyroid artery (branch of thyrocervical trunk) is closely related to **Recurrent** laryngeal nerve. **Superior** thyroid artery (branch of external carotid artery) lies in close association with **External** laryngeal nerve.
- Cerebellar nuclei
  DEFG
  D - **D**entate nucleus
  E - **E**mboliform nucleus
  F - **F**astigal nucleus
  G - **G**lobose nucleus
- Auditory pathway—**SLIM**
  S - **S**uperior olivary nucleus
  L - **L**ateral lemniscus
  I - **I**nferior colliculus
  M - **M**edial geniculate body
- **M**edial geniculate body—**A**uditory path (**MA**)
- Lateral geniculate body—Optic tract
- Structures involved in pathway of hearing—**Totally SLIM**
  Totally - **T**rapezoid body
  S - **S**uperior olivary nucleus
  L - **L**ateral lemniscus
  I - **I**nferior colliculus
  M - **M**edial geniculate body
- The muscles of posterior abdominal wall are psoas major and minor, iliacus, quadratus lumborum.
- Deep inguinal ring is an opening in fascia transversalis. It is situated 1.25 cm above mid inguinal point and passes spermatic cord in males and round ligament in females.
- Phrenicocolic ligament and left colic flexure prevent downward displacement of enlarged spleen
- Sites of portocaval anastomoses
  PE BALU
  Posterior abdominal wall
  Esophagus
  Bare area of liver
  Anal canal
  Liver
  Umbilicus
- Structures related to hilum of kidney
  Anterior to posterior
  VAP
  Renal **V**ein
  Renal **A**rtery
  Renal **P**elvis

- Lateral geniculate body*(NK-593;IBS-218)
- Blood supply of superolateral area (NK-558;IBS-252)
- Cerebellar peduncle*(NK-534;IBS-134)
- Cerebellar nuclei (NK-534;IBS-140)
- Superior colliculus*(NK-531;IBS-75,106)
- Red nucleus (NK-529;IBS-106)
- Central sulcus (NK-549;IBS-171)
- Facial colliculus*(IBS-102)
- Blood supply of spinal cord (NK-496;IBS-57)
- Fornix (IBS-233)
- Thalamus*(NK-539;IBS-150)
- Basal ganglia (NK-570;IBS-190)

Diagrams

- Arterial supply of cerebral hemisphere (IBS-248)
- Circle of Willis (IBS-248)
- Transverse section of medulla at the level of pyramid (IBS-97)
- Transverse section of medulla at the level of sensory decussation (IBS-98)
- TS of medulla at the level of olive (IBS-99)
- TS of pons at lower part (IBS-102)
- TS of pons at upper part (IBS-103)
- TS of midbrain at the level of inferior colliculus (IBS-105)
- TS of midbrain at the level of superior colliculus (IBS-106)
- Floor of fourth ventricle (IBS-207)

ABDOMEN AND PELVIS

Essays

- Inguinal canal*(NK-649;CH-211)
- Rectus sheath (NK-643;CH-209)
- Stomach*(NK-666;CH-250)
- Duodenum (2nd part) *(NK-674;CH-259)
- Liver (NK-691;CH-304)
- Billiary apparatus*(NK-697;CH-287)
- Spleen (NK-700;CH-294)
- Pancreas (NK-687;CH-298)
- Portal vein*(NK-707;CH-289)
- Kidney*(NK-724;CH-312)
- Urinary bladder*(NK-748;CH-372)
- Uterus (development)*(NK-770;CH-387)
- Prostate*(NK-763;CH-401)
- Rectum and anal canal*(NK-745;CH-407,413)
- Portosystemic circulation*(NK-707;CH-283)
- Ishiorectal fossa*(NK-777;CH-352)

Short Notes

- Inguinal ligament*(NK-640;CH-205)
- Conjoint tendon (NK-643;CH-206)
- Lesser and greater omentum (NK-659,668;CH-234)
- Epiploic foramen*(NK-661;CH-240)

- 2nd part of duodenum (not 4th) is not anteriorly related to right kidney.
- **Right** suprarenal vein drain into **IVC**; and **left suprarenal vein** drain into **left renal vein.**
- The most common position of vermiform appendix is retro-cecal (12 o'clock = 65%) followed by pelvic or 4 o'clock position
- Cystic artery is a branch of right hepatic artery
- Structures passing through greater sciatic foramen—**PIN**

  P - Pudendal nerve

  I - Internal pudendal vessels

  N - Nerve to obturator internus
- Structures passing through lesser sciatic foramen

  PINTO

  P - **Pudendal** nerve

  I - **Internal** pudendal vessels

  NTO - **N**erve and **T**endon of **O**bturator internus
- Broad ligament contains suspensary ligament of ovary but not ovary.
- Broad ligament provides no support to uterus and round ligament provide week support to uterus.
- In females, anterior division of internal iliac artery has 7 (in spite of 6) branches. Inferior vesicle is replaced by vaginal artery; and uterine artery is 7th branch.
- Anterior division of internal iliac artery—**SI-V Obtained Middle Rank In-PG**

  SIV—**S**uperior and **I**nferior **V**esicle

  Obt - **Ob**turator

  Middle - **Mid**dle rectal artery

  In P - **Int**ernal **P**udendal artey

  In G - **In**ferior **G**luteal artery
- Posterior division of internal iliac artery—**ILS**

  I - **I**liolumbar artery

  L - **L**ateral sacral artery

  S - **S**uperior gluteal artery
- Anterior branches of abdominal aorta—**CIMS**

  C - **C**oeliac trunk

  I - **I**nferior mesenteric artery

  S - **S**uperior mesenteric artery
- Lateral branches of abdominal aorta—

  Inferior MS Ruin Gonads

  Inferior - **I**nferior phrenic artery

  MS - **M**iddle **S**uprarenal artery

  R - **R**enal artery

  Testicular or ovarian artery

- Rectouterine pouch (NK-662;CH-244)
- Porta hepatis (NK-693;CH-304)
- Ligaments of liver (NK-693;CH-305)
- Vermiform appendix*(NK-682;CH-269)
- Fascia transversalis (NK-645;CH-211)
- Inguinal hernia*(NK-651;CH-215)
- Testis*(NK-759;CH-223)
- Stomach bed*(NK-668;CH-252)
- BS of stomach (NK-669;CH-252)
- Transverse mesocolon (NK-659;CH-272)
- Ureter (NK-733;CH-318)
- Diaphragm (NK-230;CH-331)
- Suprarenal gland (NK-722;CH-326)
- Thoracolumbar fascia (NK-711;CH-343)
- Cystic duct (NK-698;CH-288)
- Renal angle and renal fascia (NK-727;CH-317)
- Cisterna chyli (NK-719;CH-341)
- Perineal body*(NK-785;CH-352)
- Perineal membrane*(NK-785;CH-357)
- Urogenital diaphragm*(NK-784;CH-354)
- Pudendal canal (NK-778;CH-362)
- Trigone of bladder (NK-751;CH-375)
- Superficial and deep peroneal pouch (NK-782;CH-355)
- Vas deferens*(NK-762;CH-399)
- Male urethra (NK-790;CH-376)
- Female urethra*(NK-788;CH-379)
- Uterine tubes*(NK-769;CH-385)
- Ovary (NK-766;CH-382)
- Supports of uterus*(NK-773;CH-390)
- Pelvic muscles and pelvic diaphragms (NK-738;CH-424)
- Levator ani*(NK-738;CH-425)

Vascular Systems

- Coeliac trunk*(NK-704;CH-275)
- Superior mesenteric artery (NK-705;CH-277)
- Inferior mesenteric artery (NK-706;CH-280)
- Vessels supplying stomach (NK-669;CH-252)
- Internal iliac artery (NK-741;CH-419)

Diagrams

- TS of anterior abdominal wall (NK-643)
- Visceral surface of spleen (NK-701;CH-296)
- Horizontal section of abdomen through pylorus and 4th lumbar (NK-622)
- Horizontal section of abdomen at the level of epiploic foramen (NK-661;CH-240)
- Structures forming stomach bed (NK-668;CH-252)
- Anterior and posterior surface of kidney (NK-728; CH-313,314).

GENERAL ANATOMY

TISSUES

Epithelial Tissue (Flow chart 1)

Epithelial tissue is detaily described in histology...

GLANDULAR EPITHELIUM*

Glandular epithelial cells are specialized epithelial cells that secrete bodily products, sometimes called simply glands. Glands include two types: endocrine and exocrine.

A comparison of endocrine and exocrine glands:

Endocrine glands	*Exocrine glands*
No duct system	Ducts to release products
Secretions directed into the extracellular fluid (basal side), move into vascular system	Secretions released to the apical cell surface, move out of ducts to outside environment

Exocrine glands are often the only glands associated with the term "glandular epithelium."

These glands are classified by the following morphological characteristics:

- Number of cells
- Type of secretion.

Serous	*Mucous*	*Mixed Serous-Mucous*
Thin, watery protein-rich secretion	Viscous secretion with lubricating or protective function	Serous demilunes (cells) secrete into space between mucous cells

- Mechanism of secretion

Merocrine	*Apocrine*	*Holocrine*
Only secretory product is lost	Secretory product and some membrane lost	Entire secretory product and membrane lost
For example, sweat glands	For example, milk secreting glands	For example, sebaceous glands

Flow chart 1 Types of epithelium

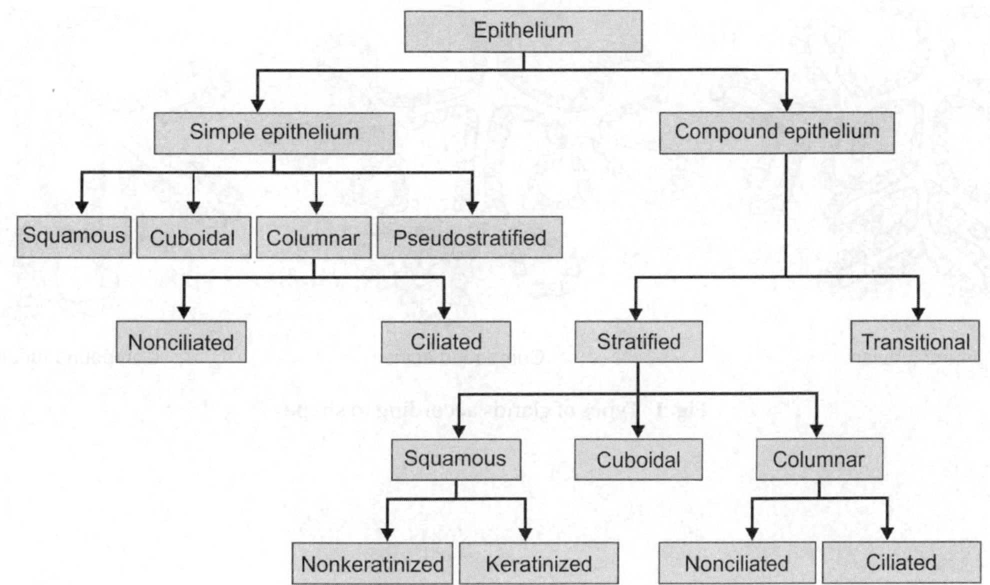

- Shape and arrangement (Fig. 1)

Shapes include tubular, coiled tubular, acinar or alveolar, or a combination of these. The arrangement could be simple, branched, or compound

Connective Tissue

- Connective tissue proper—**DAREL**
  - **D**ense regular connective tissue (tendons, ligaments)
  - **D**ense irregular connective tissue (deep fascia, periosteum)
  - **A**dipose connective tissue
  - **R**eticular connective tissue
  - **E**lastic connective tissue
  - **L**oose (areolar) connective tissue
- Specialized connective tissue
  - Bone
  - Cartilage
  - Blood

Composition of connective tissue (Flow chart 2)

- *Ground substance:* Colorless
  - Gel-like substance in which cells and fibers are embedded
- *Fibers* (Fig. 2A)*
  - *Collagen*—composed of protein, called collagen
    - Fibers are strong, inelastic but flexible in nature
    - Run in wavy nature
    - They do not branch
    - Each collagen fiber consists of small parallel fibrils
    - They are synthesized by fibroblast
  - *Elastic*—composed of protein called elastin
    - Fibers occur singly and not in bundles
    - Synthesized by fibroblast and smooth muscle cell
    - Branches and anastomoses forming a network
  - *Reticular*—are very thin immature collagen fibers
    - Structurally similar to collagen fibers
    - Composed of collagen type III
    - Form supportive framework of lymphoid organ and glands

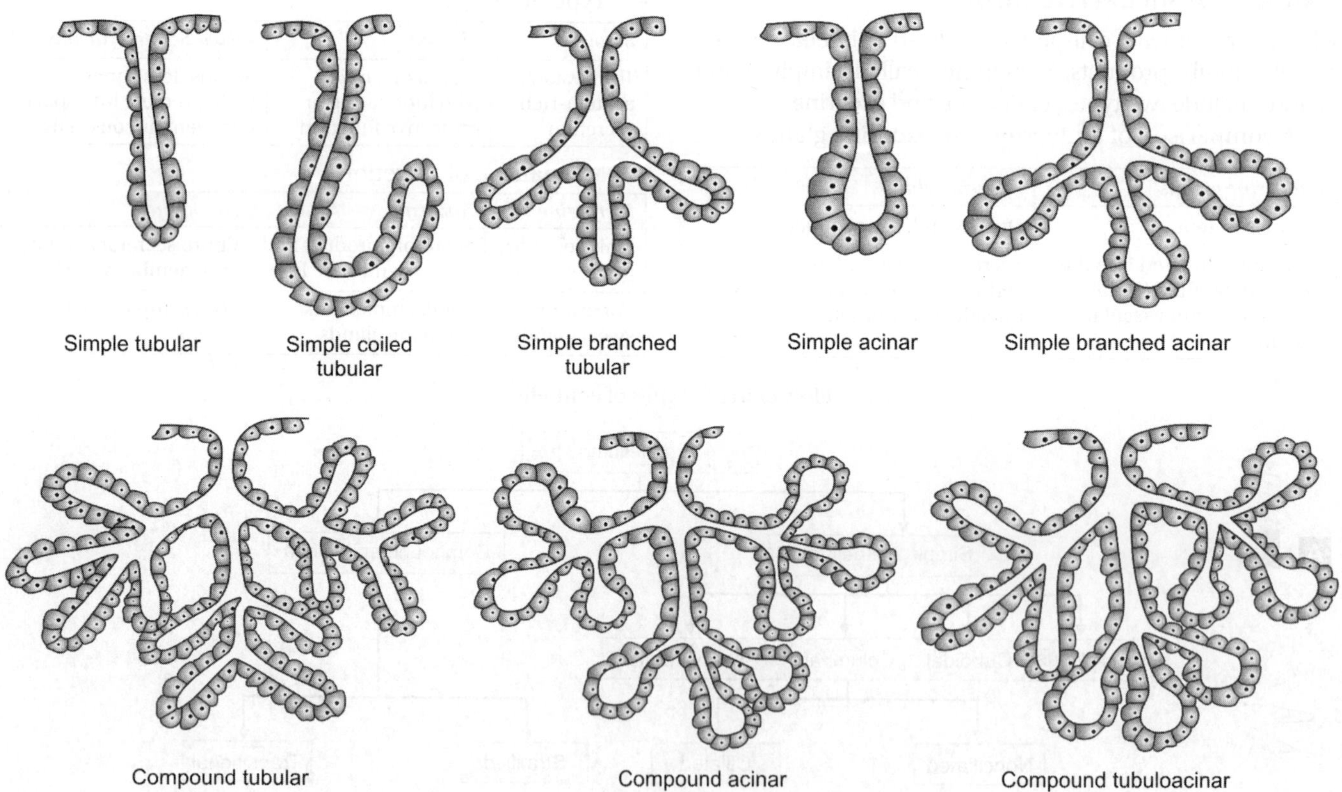

Fig. 1 Types of glands according to shape

Flow chart 2 Composition of connective tissue

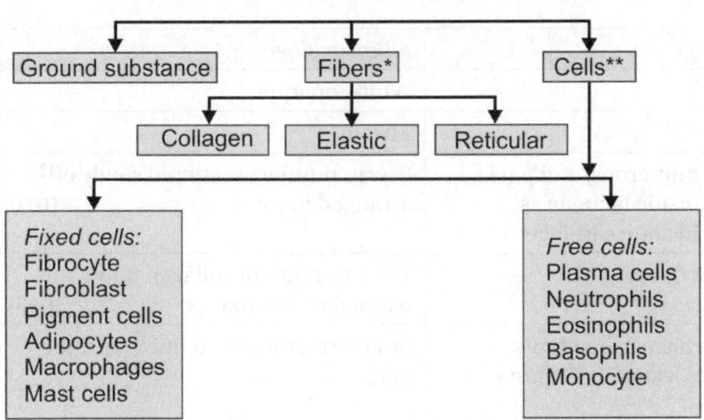

- *Cells** (Fig. 2B)*
  - *Fibroblast:*
    - Large, flat, spindle-shaped cells
    - They have many branching processes
    - Responsible for secretion of ground substance and all type of connective tissue fibers
    - Becomes very active during wound repair and synthesizes collagen fibers
  - *Fat cells/adipose cells:*
    - A fat cell is spherical in shape
    - Nucleus is flattened and displaced to the periphery
    - They synthesize and store large quantities of lipid
    - In H and E staining, fat is dissolved, hence cells appear empty
    - It stains orange with Sudan III stain
  - *Pigment cells:*
    - Cells are star-shaped with branching processes
    - Capable of synthesizing pigment—melanin
  - *Macrophages:*
    - Developed from monocytes of blood
    - Capable of eating bacteria by the process of phagocytosis
  - *Mast cells:*
    - They are small and oval in shape
    - Found mostly close to the blood vessels in connective tissue
    - The nucleus is centrally placed and cytoplasm contains many granules
    - They release histamine
  - *Plasma cells:*
    - They are ovoid in shape
    - Nucleus is round and eccentrically placed
    - They arise from B-lymphocyte
    - Synthesize antibodies against antigens
  - *WBC/leukocyte:*
    - Play important role in defence mechanism of body
    - Granulocytes (basophil, eosinophil, neutrophil) and agranulocyte (lymphocyte and monocyte).

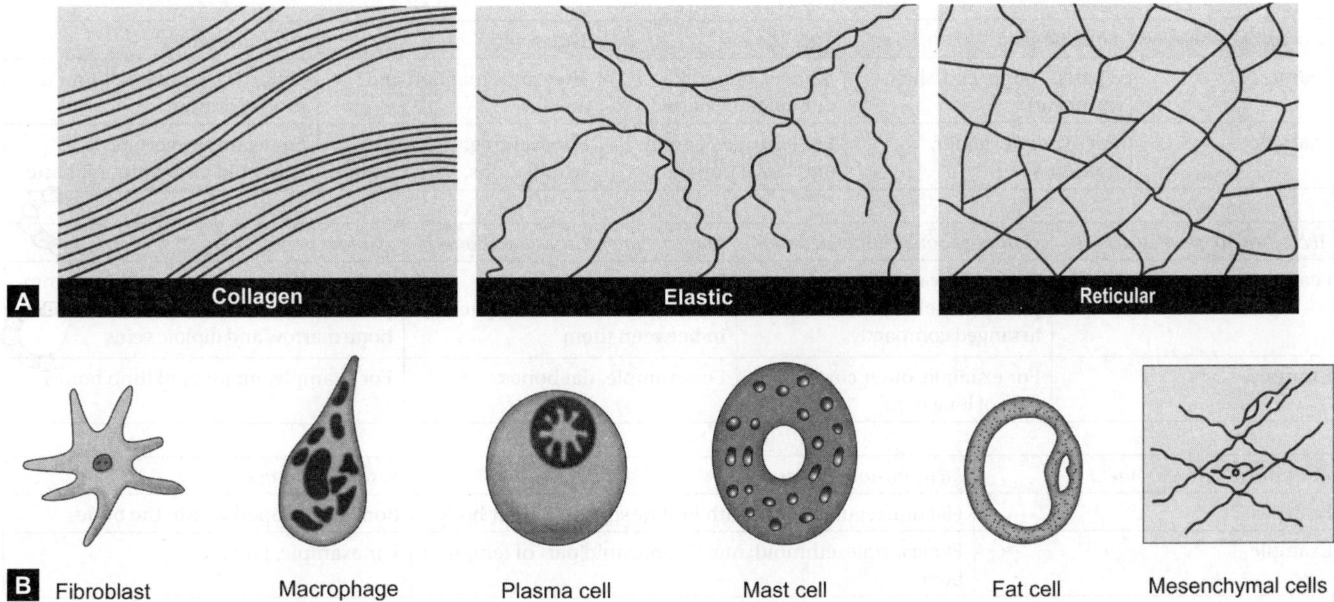

Figs 2A and B (A) Fibrous component of connective tissue—types*; (B) Cellular components of connective tissue—types**

CARTILAGE*

	*Hyaline cartilage**	*Elastic cartilage**	*Fibrocartilage*
Color	Glossy, bluish, transparent	Yellowish	White, opaque
Perichondrium	Present	Present	Absent
Chondrocytes	Present in large numbers, singly or in groups inside lacunae	Larger, more numerous, and packed more closely inside lacunae as compared to hyaline cartilage	Few in number, scattered singly or arranged in rows
Matrix	Homogeneous, basophilic, collagen fibers delicate and not visible	Rich in elastic fibers	Thick bundles of collagen fibers run parallel within matrix
Examples	Articular cartilage Thyroid cartilage, cricoids cartilage, tracheal rings, costal cartilages	Pinna of external ear, epiglottis, auditory tubes, external auditory meatus	Intervertebral disk, menisci of knee joint

BONE

- Human skeleton consists of 206 bones
- It is highly vascular living connective tissue in which the matrix is calcified by the deposition of calcium phosphate.

According to shape	*Long bones*	*Short bones*	*Flat bones*	*Irregular bone*
Features	3 parts—upper end, shaft, lower end	Smaller, generally cuboidal in shape	They are expanded and are flat	Shape is irregular without any proper outline
Example	For example, femur, humerus	For example, carpal and tarsal bones	For example, sternum, scapula, ribs, parietal bone	For example, vertebrae, sphenoid and temporal bone

According to gross structure	*Compact bone (lamellar bone)*	*Spongy bones (cancellous bones)*	*Diploic bones*
Features	Structurally made up of bony plates (lamellae) which are arranged compactly	Lamellae are arranged irregularly and leaving space in between them	Consists of inner and outer tables of compact bone and middle space occupied by bone marrow and diploic veins
Example	For example, outer cortical part of long bone	For example, flat bones	For example, majority of limb bones

According to development	*Membranous bones*	*Sesamoid bones*
Features	Flat or irregular bones with hollow spaces in their body	Bones developed within the bone
Example	For example, ethmoid, maxilla, mastoid part of temporal bone	For example, patella

Compact Bone*

- Compact bone is made up of compactly placed lamellae (collagen fibers embedded in ground substance)
- Most of the lamellae are arranged in the form of concentric rings that surround a Haversian canal, which is present at the center of each ring (Figs 3A to C).
- The lamellae are occupied by osteocytes
- The space between lamellae are called lacunae
- Adjacent lacunae are connected through canaliculi, which are occupied by cytoplasmic processes of osteocytes
- Haversian canals are placed parallel to medullary cavity and they are occupied by nerve fibers
- Adjacent Haversian canals are connected by Volkmann's canal
- Haversian canal and lamella around it constitutes Haversian system or osteon.

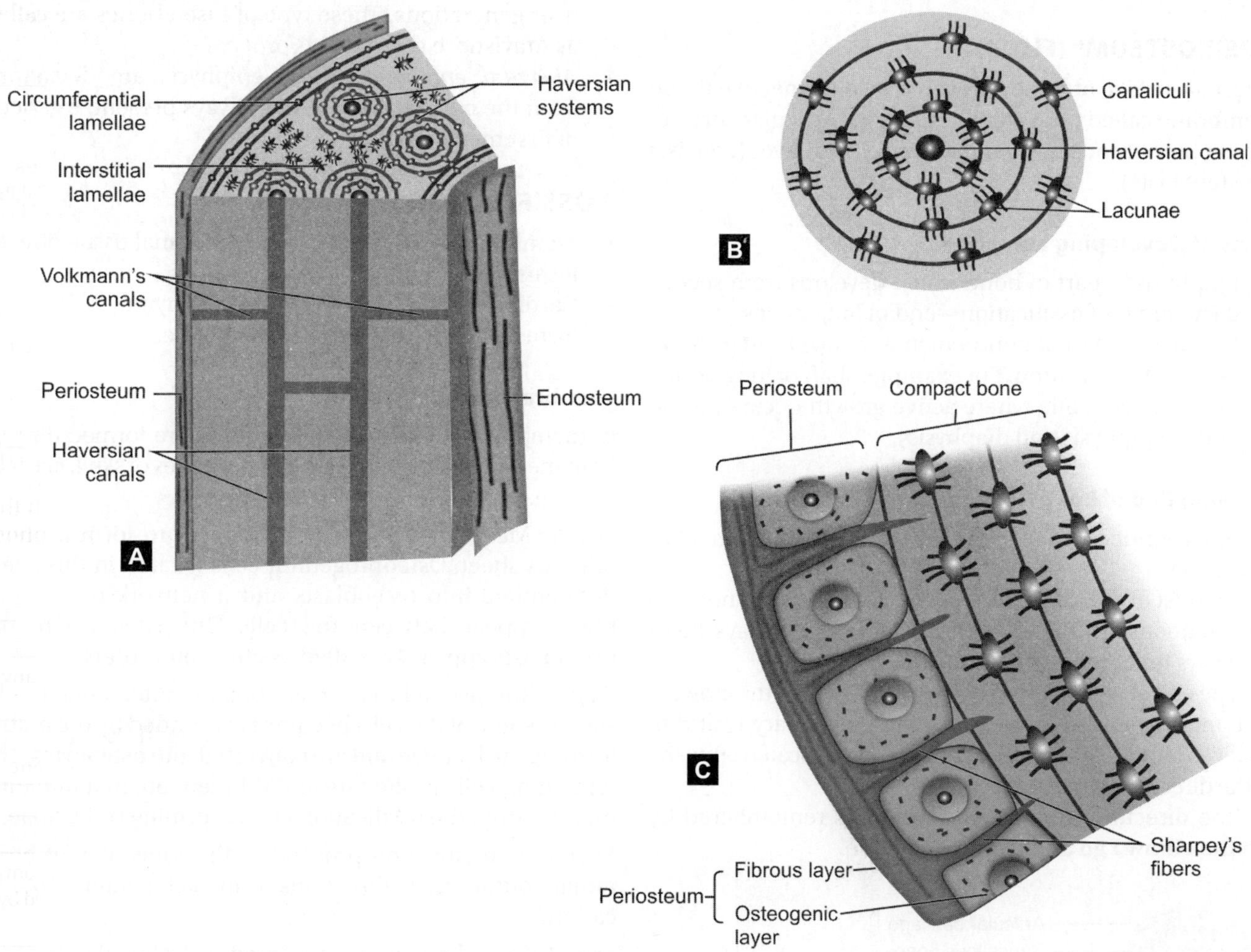

Figs 3A to C (A) Longitudinal section of bone; (B) Cross section of bone; (C) Cross section of bone (magnified)

Bone Cells

Osteoblast	*Osteocytes*	*Osteoclasts*
• These are bone-forming cell • Numerous in the periosteum • Responsible for calcification of matrix	• These are matrix bone cells • They maintain the integrity of lacunae and thus keep open the channels for diffusion of nutrients	• These are bone removing cells • Lysosome of their cytoplasm contains acid phosphates • They are stimulated by parathyroid hormone

PERIOSTEUM* (FIG. 4)

External surface of bone is covered by a connective tissue membrane called periosteum except the articular surface. It has outer fibrous layer and inner cellular layer (consists of osteoblasts).

Parts of Developing Long Bone

- Epiphysis*—part of bone which develops from secondary center of ossification—end of long bones
- Diaphysis—part of bone which develops from primary center of ossification. For example, shaft of long bones
- Metaphysis—zone where active growth occurs (at the end of epiphysis and diaphysis).

Growing End of Long Bone*

It is the rounded end of a long bone, at its joint with adjacent bone.

In most of the long bones the two epiphysis do not fuse simultaneously. The epiphysis at one end always fuses few years before that at the other end.

The end at which fusion occurs later is called the growing end and this is also the end at which secondary center of ossification appears first. The growing end is located opposite to the direction of nutrient foramen.

The direction of nutrient foramen is remembered by **'To the elbow I go and from knee I flee'.**

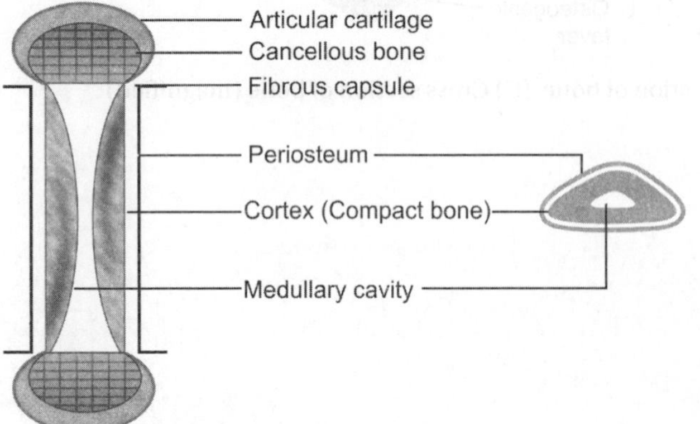

Fig. 4 Structure of long bone

*Epiphysis**

There are four types of epiphysis:

1. *Pressure epiphysis:* The region of the long bone that forms the joint is called pressure epiphysis, e.g. head of femur.
2. *Traction epiphyses:* The regions of the long bone which are nonarticular, that is, not involved in the joint formation is called as traction epiphysis, e.g. acromian, mastoid process.
3. *Atavistic epiphyses:* As evolution progresses, some of the bones together due to the change in functionality over generations. These type of fused bones are called as Atavistic, e.g. coracoids process.
4. *Aberrant epiphyses:* These epiphysis are deviations from the normal and are not always present, e.g. head of first metacarpal.

OSSIFICATION

- Membranous ossification—mesenchymal tissue directly forms bone
- Cartilaginous ossification—mesenchymal tissue first forms hyaline cartilage and then bone.

Membranous Ossification

In membranous ossification, the bones are formed directly from mesenchymal templates, e.g. flat bones of skull, clavicle, etc. (Fig. 5).

Step 1: Mesenchymal tissue condenses to form a membranous sheet. Osteoprogenitor cells located in this sheet differentiate into osteoblasts and a network of collagen fibers appear between the cells. The sites where the osteoblasts appear are called ossification centers.

Step 2: The osteoblasts secrete organic intercellular substance, some of the cells become surrounded by the matrix forming the lacunae and are converted into osteocytes. The remaining cells proliferate and differentiate in a radiating manner from the ossification center forming trabeculae.

Step 3: As ossification proceeds, thin trabeculae of bone radiate out in many directions from each center of ossification.

Step 4: Cancellous bone is formed as trabeculae join together to form interconnected network of trabeculae separated spaces.

Step 5: Cells within intertrabecular spaces specialize to form red bone marrow.

Step 6: At peripheral margins of membranous sheet, periosteum which contains osteoblasts, lay down bone matrix beneath periosteum to form an outer surface of the compact bone.

Step 7: The bones thus formed by intramembranous ossification consist of outer superficial plates of compact bone with cancellous bone within them.

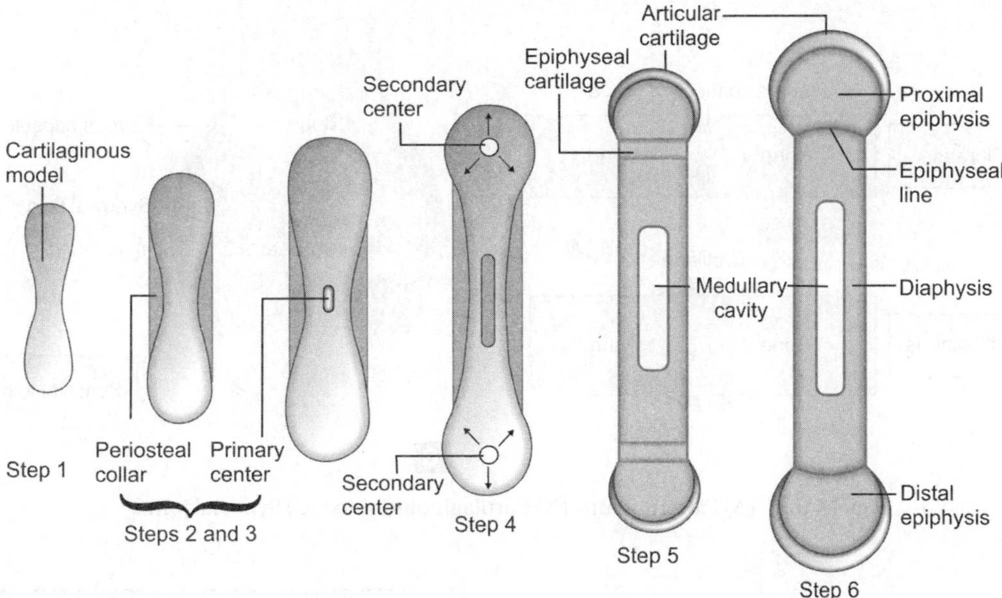

Fig. 5 Ossification of a long bone

Cartilaginous Ossification

All the long bones of the limb are ossified by this process.

Step 1: First the bone is laid down as a cartilaginous model which is approximately similar in shape to that of a adult bone. The cartilaginous model consists of hyaline cartilage, surrounded by perichondrium.

Step 2: A primary center of ossification then appears in the center of the shaft and this spread towards the ends to form diaphysis.

Step 3: At the same time, periosteum lays down a collar of bone (periosteal collar) around the circumference of the shaft.

Step 4: Later, one or more secondary centers of ossification develop at each end of the cartilaginous model and form the epiphysis.

Step 5: The epiphyseal cartilage separating epiphysis from diaphysis and articular cartilage at each end of bone are still cartilaginous.

Step 6: The epiphyseal plate of cartilage continues to produce new cartilage and thus enable the bone to grow in length. For this reason, epiphyseal plate of cartilage is also called growth plate.

Center of Ossification

The first step in ossification of the cartilage is that the cartilage cells, at the point where ossification is commencing and which is termed an ossification center, enlarge and arrange themselves in rows. The matrix in which they are embedded increases in quantity.

There are two types of ossification centers—primary and secondary.

1. A primary ossification center is the first area of a bone to start ossifying. It usually appears during prenatal development in the central part of each developing bone, i.e. center situated in the diaphyses.
2. A secondary ossification center is the area of ossification that appears after the primary. Most of which appear during the postnatal and adolescent years. Most bones have more than one secondary ossification center. It is situated in the epiphyses.

Blood Supply of Long Bones (Fig. 6)*

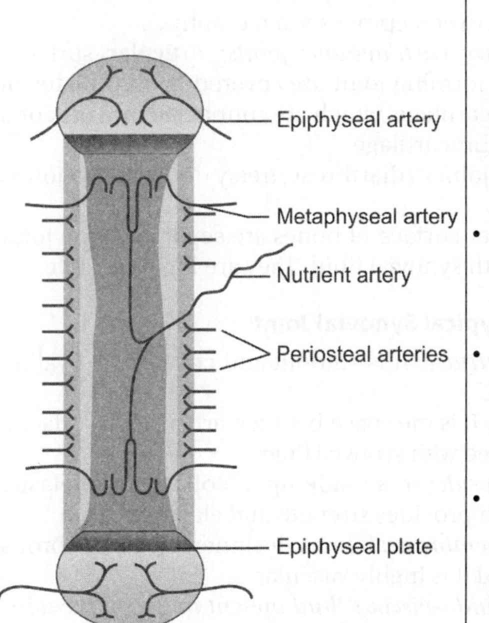

- *Nutrient artery:* It enters the shaft through a nutrient foramen. On reaching bone marrow cavity they divide into ascending and descending branches.
- *Epiphyseal artery:* Several in number and enter the bone near its ends.
- *Metaphyseal artery:* Enters along the line of attachment of capsular ligament.
- *Periosteal artery:* Numerous and enter the bone along its attachment.

Fig. 6 Blood supply to a growing long bone
(For color version, see Plate 1)

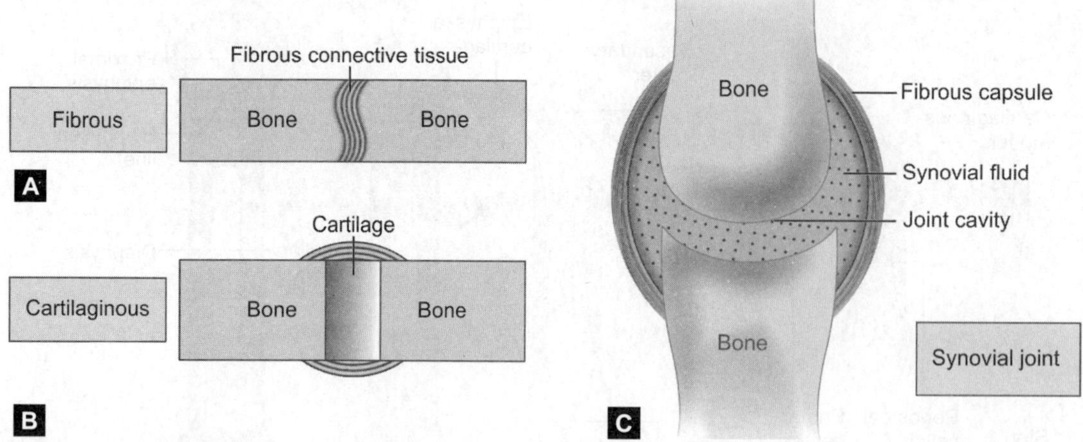

Figs 7A to C (A) Fibrous joints; (B) Cartilaginous joints; (C) Synovial joints

JOINTS*

- Fibrous joints/fixed/synarthroses joints (Fig. 7A)
  - Sutures—the articular surfaces are connected by sutural ligaments, e.g. many skull bones are held together by sutures
  - Syndesmosis—articulating parts are connected by interosseous ligaments, e.g. inferior tibiofibular joint
  - Gomphosis, e.g. tooth in bony socket
- Cartilaginous joints/amphiarthroses/slightly movable joints (Fig. 7B).

  Bones forming the joint are united by means of either hyaline cartilage/fibrocartilage:
  - *Primary cartilaginous joints:* Bones forming the joints are joined by a plate of hyaline cartilage, e.g. joints between epiphysis and diaphysis
  - *Secondary cartilaginous joints:* Articular surfaces of bone forming joint are covered by thin plates of hyaline cartilage, which are connected by a disk or a pad of fibrocartilage
- Synovial joints*/diarthrose/freely movable joints (Fig. 7C).

The articular surface of bones are separated by a joint cavity filled with synovial fluid. They are highly mobile.

Structure of Typical Synovial Joint

- *Articular surface:* It is smooth and covered by hyaline cartilage
- *Joint cavity:* It is the space between articulating surfaces, which is filled with synovial fluid
- *Fibrous capsule:* It is made up of collagen and elastic fibers and it provides strength and elasticity
- *Synovial membrane:* It lines the inner aspect of fibrous capsule and it is highly vascular
- *Synovial fluid—viscous fluid present in the joint cavity:* It provides nutrition and also lubricates the joint
- *Ligaments:* These will stabilize the joint and permits desirable movements and prevent undesirable ones.

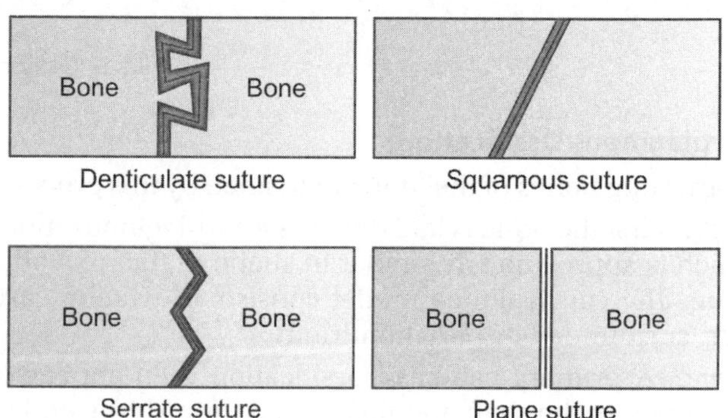

Fig. 8 Types of sutures in fibrous joints

Types of Synovial Joints* (Figs 8 to 11)

- *Plane joints:* Articular surfaces are flat and limiting only sliding movements. For example, acromioclavicular joint, joint between articular processes of vertebrae
- *Hinge joints:* Only flexion and extension movements are possible. For example, elbow, knee, interphalangeal joint, etc. (Fig. 9A)
- *Pivot joints:* In this joint, an axis surrounded by a bony or ligamentous ring (Fig. 9B).
  - Either the pivot or the ring rotates.
  - Only rotation is possible. For example, atlantoaxial joint, superior radioulnar joint
- *Condylar joints:* The round articular surface of one bone fits into socket type articular surface of another bone (Fig. 10A).
  - Permits movement in two directions. For example, right and left temporomandibular joint, knee joint, metacarpophalangeal joint
- *Ellipsoid joints:* There is an elliptical convex articular surface that fits into an elliptical concave articular surface (Fig. 10B). For example, wrist joint, atlanto-occipital joint, metacarpophalangeal joint

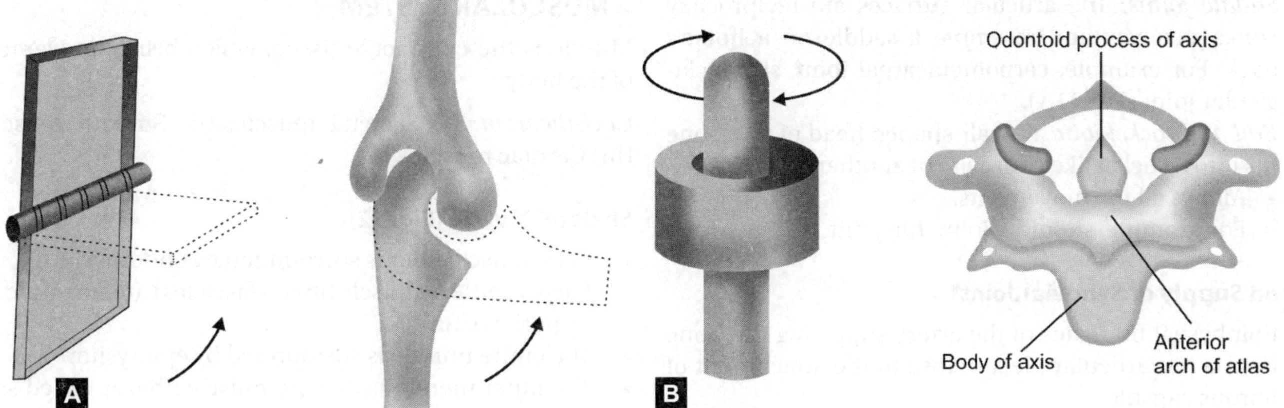

Figs 9A and B (A) Hinge joints; (B) Pivot joints

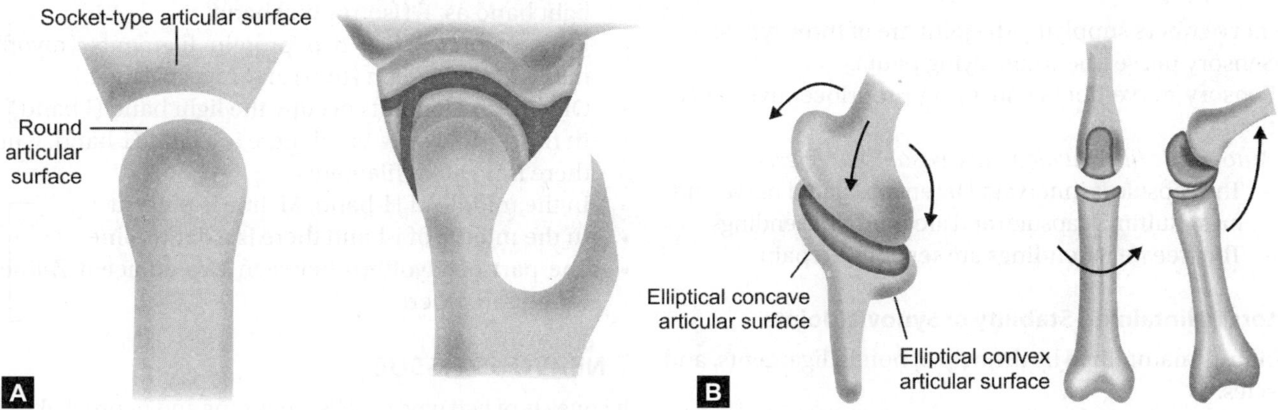

Figs 10A and B (A) Condylar joints; (B) Ellipsoid joints

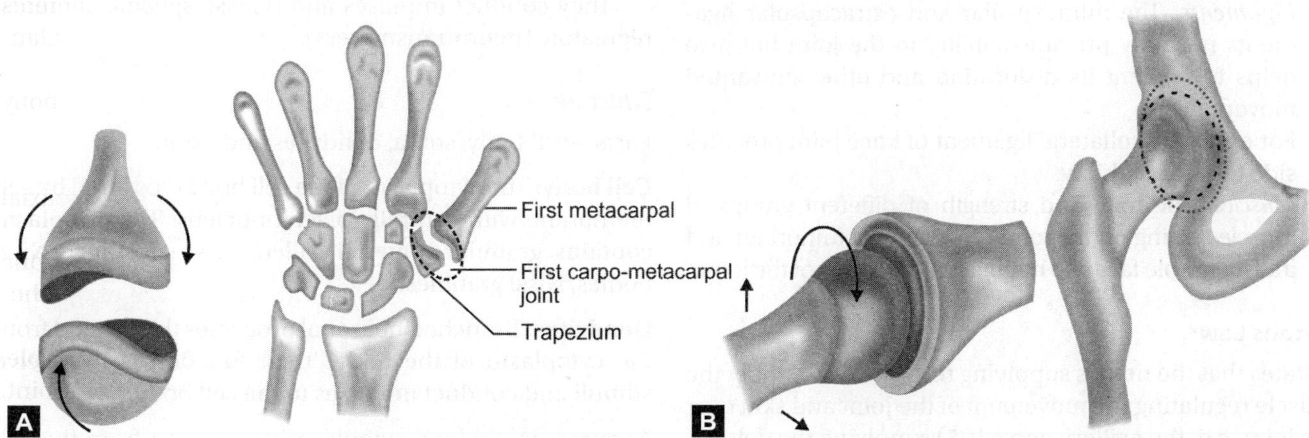

Figs 11A and B (A) Saddle joints; (B) Ball and socket joints

- *Saddle joints:* The articular surfaces are reciprocally concavoconvex and resemble a saddle on a horse's back. For example, carpometacarpal joint, sternoclavicular joint (Fig. 11A).
- *Ball and socket joints:* A ball-shaped head of one bone fits into a socket like concavity of another (Fig. 11B).
  - Allows all the movements.
  - For example, shoulder joint, hip joint.

Blood Supply of Synovial Joint*

- Epiphyseal branches of the artery supplying the bone from a periarticular plexus close to the attachment of fibrous capsule.
- Numerous minute vessels arising from it form a rich vascular plexus on the outer surface of synovial membrane.

Nerve Supply to Synovial Joint

The nerve fibers supplying the joint are of three types:

1. Sensory nerve fibers conveying pain
2. Sensory nerve fibers conveying proprioceptive sensations
3. *Autonomic fibers which have vasomotor effects:*
   - The capsule is innervated by encapsulated nerve endings (Ruffini's capsule) and are free nerve endings
   - The free nerve endings are sensitive to pain.

Factors Maintaining Stability of Synovial Joints

Stability is maintained by the help of bones, ligaments, and muscles.

- *Bones:* Important role in providing stability to certain joints.
  For example, in hip joint, the head of femur is perfectly fitted into the socket of hip bone, hence acquired dislocation of hip joint is rare.
- *Ligaments:* The intracapsular and extracapsular ligaments not only provide stability to the joint but also helps to prevent its dislocation and other unwanted movements.
  For example, collateral ligament of knee joint provides side too side stability.
- *Muscles:* The tone and strength of different groups of muscles acting on the joint provide most important and indispensable factor to maintain the stability of the joint.

Hiltons Law*

It states that the nerves supplying the joint also supply the muscle regulating the movement of the joint and skin over the joint, e.g. the axillary nerve (C5) supplying the deltoid, the shoulder joint and the skin over the joint.

MUSCULAR SYSTEM

Muscle is the contractile tissue, which brings movement of the body.

Classification: (i) Skeletal muscle; (ii) Smooth muscle; (iii) Cardiac muscle.

Skeletal Muscle (Fig. 12)

- Each muscle fiber is surrounded by endomysium
- Each bundle of muscle fibers (fascicles) are surrounded by perimysium
- The entire muscle is surrounded by epimysium
- The outer membrane of the muscle fiber is called sarcolemma and its cytoplasm is called sarcoplasm
- It shows many peripherally placed nuclei and large number of myofibrils
- Each myofibril shows alternate dark and light bands
- The dark band is known as 'A' (anisotrophic) band and light band as 'I' (isotrophic) band
- Each myofibril has two protein filaments (myofilaments), that is actin (thin) and myosin (thick)
- Only actin filaments occupy the light band (I band)
- In the middle of 'A' band there is a light H-band, where there is no actin filaments
- In the middle of H-band, M-line is present
- In the middle of I-band there is a dark Z-line
- The part of myofibril between two adjacent Z-line is called sarcomere.

NERVOUS TISSUE

It consists of two type of cells—neurons and neuroglial cells.

Neuron (Fig. 13)

These are basic structural and functional unit of nervous system.

They conduct impulses and release specific chemical regulators (neurotransmitters).

Structure

Parts—cell body/soma, dendrites and axon.

Cell body: The cytoplasm of the cell body is covered by cell membrane with centrally placed nucleus. The cytoplasm contains granular material called Nissl substance/Nissl bodies/Nissl granules.

Dendrites: Branched neuronal processes that extend from the cytoplasm of the body. Their function is to receive stimuli and conduct impulses to the cell body.

Axons: It is the long cytoplasmic extension from the cell body. It will conduct impulses away from the cell body.

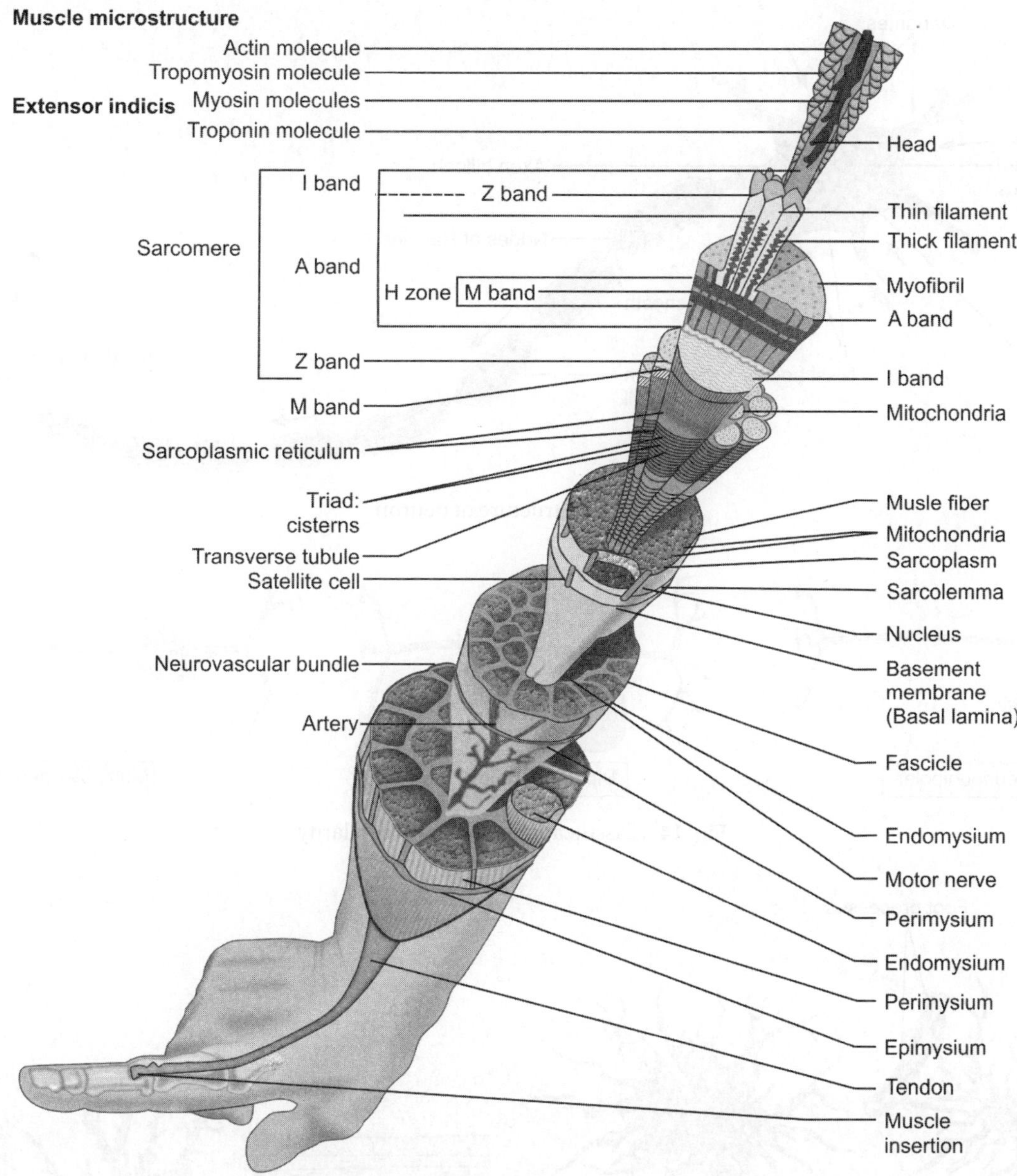

Fig. 12 Structure of skeletal muscle

Classification (Fig. 14)

According to polarity	*Pseudounipolar neurons*	*Bipolar neurons*	*Multipolar neuron*
Features	These neurons have a single process which divides like letter 'T'	They have an axon and dendrite	Several dendrites and only one axon
Examples	For example, dorsal root ganglia of spinal nerves	For example, retina of eye, olfactory epithelium	For example, motor neuron forming tracts of brain and spinal cord

According to length of axon	*Golgi type I*	*Golgi type II*
Features	With long axon	Without axon
Examples	For example, pyramidal cells of cerebral cortex	

Neuroglia (Glial Cells)* (Fig. 15)

These are nonexcitable supporting cells of nervous tissue. They produce CSF and phagocytose foreign substance. These are of two types, macroglia, and microglia.

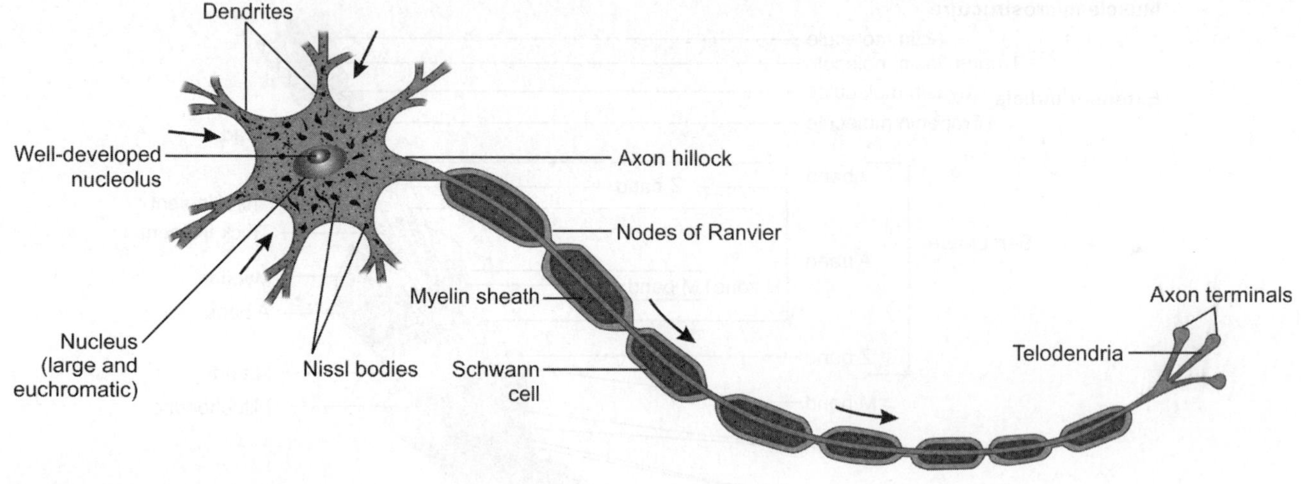

Fig. 13 Structure of neuron

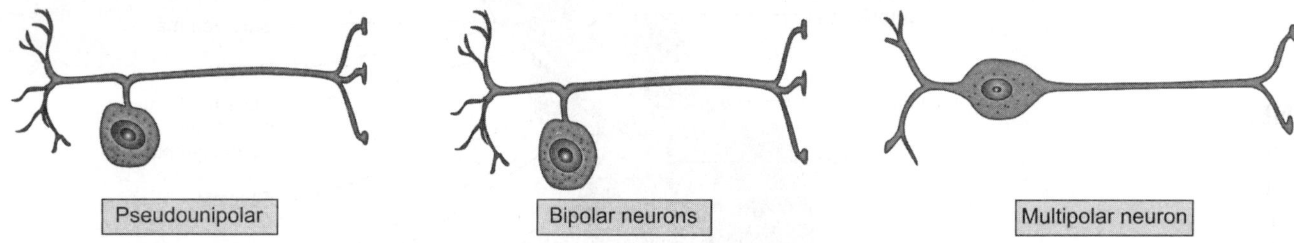

Fig. 14 Classification according to polarity

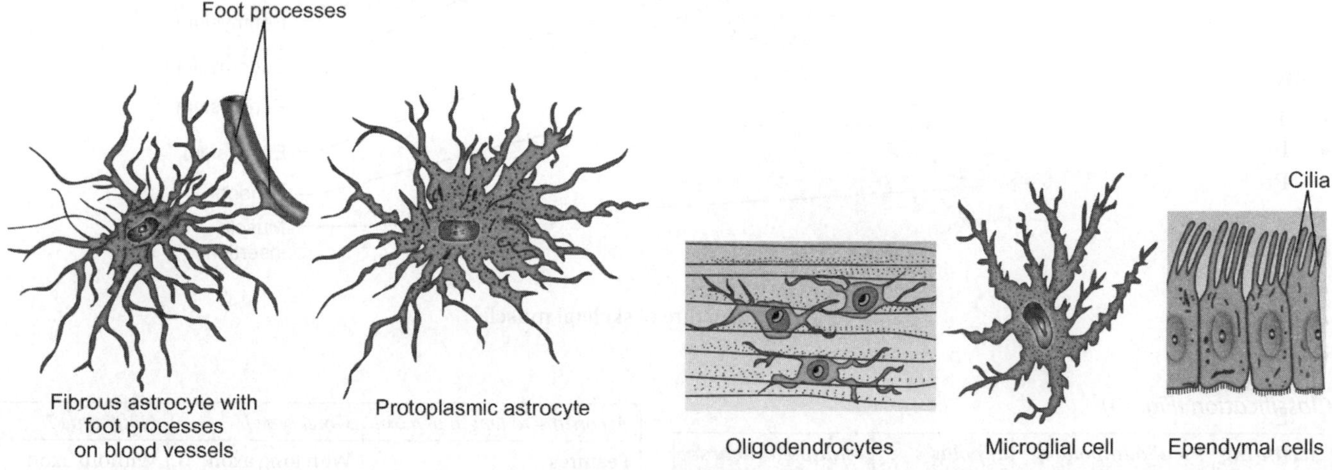

Fig. 15 Glial cells

Macroglia				*Microglia (Small glial cells)*
Astrocyte		*Oligodendrocytes*	*Ependymal*	
• They are star-shaped cells • Cells have a small body and many dendrites like processes		• Important for the formation of myelin sheath • Found among myelinated nerves	• Lines the ventricle of the brain and the central canal of spinal cord	Phagocytic cells
Protoplasmic	Fibrous			
Found in gray matter	Found in white matter			

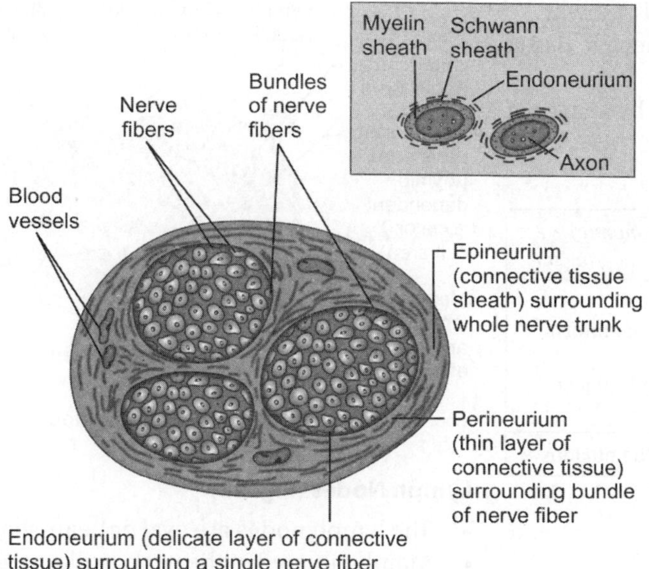

Fig. 16 Nerve fiber

Cranial nerve: There are 12 pairs of cranial nerves which arise from brain within the cranial cavity and come out through foramina.
Spinal nerve: Thirty-one pairs of spinal nerves which arise from the spinal cord within the vertebral canal and come out through intervertebral foramina.
C8 T12 L5 S5 C1

NERVE FIBER (FIG. 16)

- The nerve fibers are formed by axons.
- The axons are covered by myelin sheath and are called myelinated nerve fibers.
- Axons without myelin sheaths are unmyelinated.
- Myelin sheaths are interrupted at intervals and these are called nodes of Ranveir.
- The myelin sheaths are covered by Schwann cells.

Function of Myelin Sheath

- Thicker is the myelin sheath, faster is the conductivity.
- Prevents leak of impulses from one to another.
- Protects and nourishes the enclosed axon.

NERVES

- The term 'nerve' refers to peripheral nerve.
- Peripheral nerve consists of bundles of nerve fibers.
- Each nerve fiber is enclosed by a connective tissue sheath called endoneurium.
- Each group of nerve fibers (fasciculus) surrounded by perineurium.
- The entire nerve fiber is surrounded by epineurium.

Autonomic Nervous System

Autonomic nervous system (ANS) controls the involuntary activities of the body such as the activities of smooth muscle, cardiac muscle and glands.

It has two parts: Afferent (Body ⟶ CNS)
Efferent (CNS ⟶ Body)

Ganglia

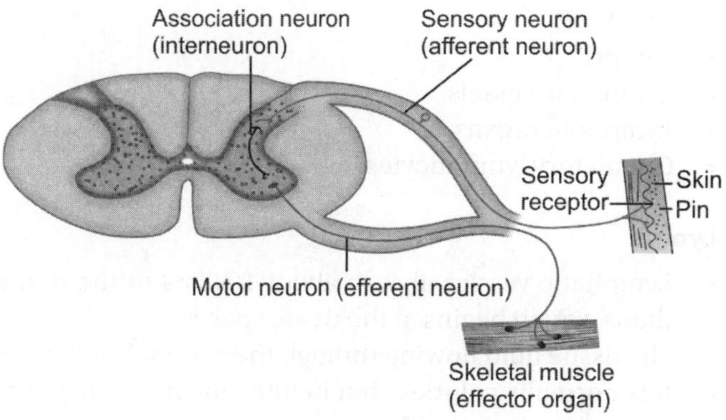

Fig. 17 Reflex arc

Ans: Sympathetic
Parasympathetic.

REFLEX ARC (FIG. 17)

- It is an automatic response to a stimulus without conscious thought.
- It is protective in nature.

For example, when a pin is pricked on the hand—sensory receptors stimulated—nerve impulse travels through sensory (afferent) neuron—reaches the spinal cord—association neuron (connector)—nerve impulse travels through motor (efferent) neuron—stimulates the effector organ—hand moves away from the pin.

GANGLIA

- These are oval bodies made of aggregation of cell bodies of neurons, outside the central nervous system.

- They serve as relay centers in the neuronal pathway.
- They are usually covered by a dense connective tissue capsule called epineurium.
- The cell bodies of neurons are enveloped by a layer of cuboidal cells called satellite.

According to morphology and function:

Sensory ganglion/(somatic) *For example, spinal ganglion*	*Motor ganglion/(autonomic)* *For example, sympathetic ganglion*
Pseudounipolar neurons • Large, rounded and with varying size • Nucleus is centrally placed • Found in groups	Multipolar neurons • Small angular and of uniform size • Nucleus eccentrically placed • Found scattered
Well-defined satellite nucleus	Poorly-defined satellite nucleus

LYMPHATIC SYSTEM

It is drainage system which is accessory to the venous system. It removes larger particles from the tissue fluid to the venous system.

It consists of:

- Lymph
- Lymphatic vessels
- Lymphoid organs
- Circulatory lymphocytes.

Lymph

- Lymphatic vessles absorb about 10–20% of the tissue fluids, which begins at the tissue spaces.
- The tissue fluid flowing through these vessels is lymph.
- It is normally colorless but in intestine it is milk-white due to absorption of fat.

Lymphatic Vessels

- The lymphatic capillaries begins blindly in the tissue spaces.
- Lymphatic vessels are connected to each other by forming a network.
- Lymphatic capillaries are absent in brain, spinal cord and BM.

Lymphoid Organs

- They are made up of lymphatic tissue and it contains reticular fibers, lymphocytes (mainly) and related plasma cells and macrophages.
  - Primary lymphoid organ—involved in the production of lymphocyte, e.g. thymus, BM
  - Secondary lymphoid organ—involved in activation of lymphocyte and initiation of immune response, e.g. lymph nodes, spleen.

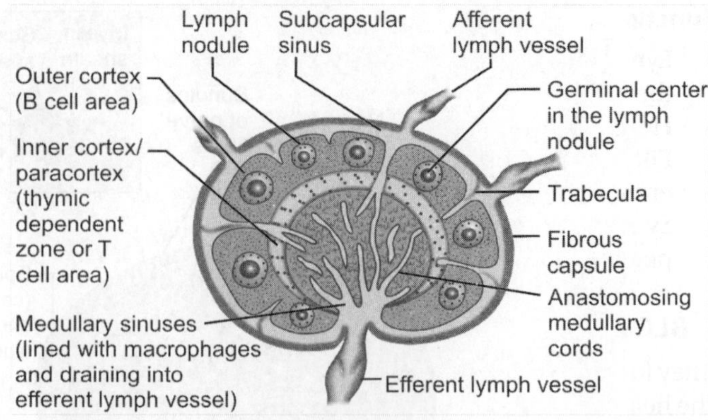

Fig. 18 Lymph node

Lymph Nodes (Fig. 18)

- The lymph nodes are oval or bean-shaped bodies.
- Mainly situated in the neck, axilla, mediastinum, abdomen, inguinal region, etc.
- They form important constituents of immunity of the body.

Structure

- *Capsule:*
  - Outer covering and it is made up of collagen and few elastic fibers.
  - The capsule send trabeculae into the substance of lymph node.
  - It provides a media for the passage of blood vessels.
  - Substance of lymph node is divided into outer cortex and inner medulla.
- *Cortex:*
  - It is absent in the hilum.
  - Lymphocytes are arranged in the form of follicles (or nodules) in the cortex.
  - Each lymphatic follicle consists of densily packed lymphocytes outside and large lymphocytes (lymphoblast) called germinal center in the middle.

Medulla

- It shows medullary cords where lymphocytes are arranged in irregular masses, with spaces in between them called medullary sinus.
- These medullary sinuses contain lymph fluid.
- Subscapular sinus—space between lymph nodule and capsule.
- The afferent lymphatic vessels entering the lymph node at multiple sites opens into the subscapular sinus.
- The subscapular sinuses are connecting with medullary sinuses through radiating cortical sinuses.
- The lymph collected in the medullary sinus is drained out from the lymph node by efferent lymphatic vessel.

Function

- Lymphatic vessels drain large protein molecules from the tissue plate.
- Helps in transportation of fat from the gut.
- Filter the lymph and prevent the foreign particles entering into the bloodstream.
- Synthesis of antibodies and maintaining immune competency of the person.

BLOOD VESSELS

They form closed system of tubes that carry blood away from the heart to the tissues of the body and then to the heart.
This includes:

- Arteries
- Capillaries
- Veins.

Arteries (Figs 19A and B)

Features: Thick-walled vessels which carry blood from heart. Their lumen is smaller than that of accompanying veins.
It has three layers:

1. *Tunica intima (innermost layer) three parts:*
   a. Endothelial layers—cells are polygonal and are arranged into folds.
   b. Subendothelial layer—formed by delicate elastic and collagen fibers.
   c. Internal elastic lamina—thick and flexible.
2. *Tunica media (intermediate layer):* Made up of circularly arranged smooth muscle fibers and elastic fibers. It is limited externally by external elastic lamina.
3. *Tunica adventitia (outer layer):* Thin but strongest of all coats. Made up of elastic and collagen fibers.

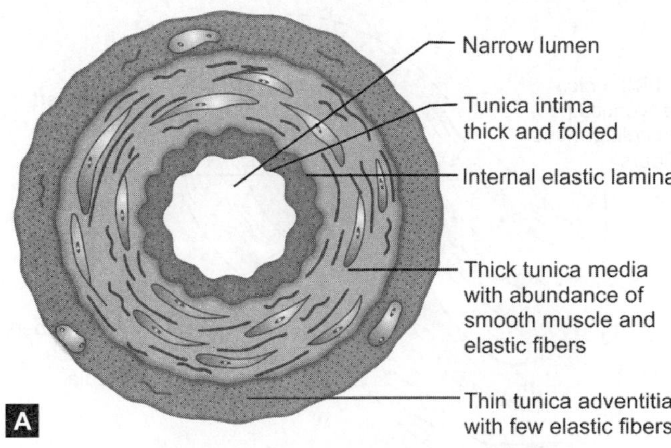

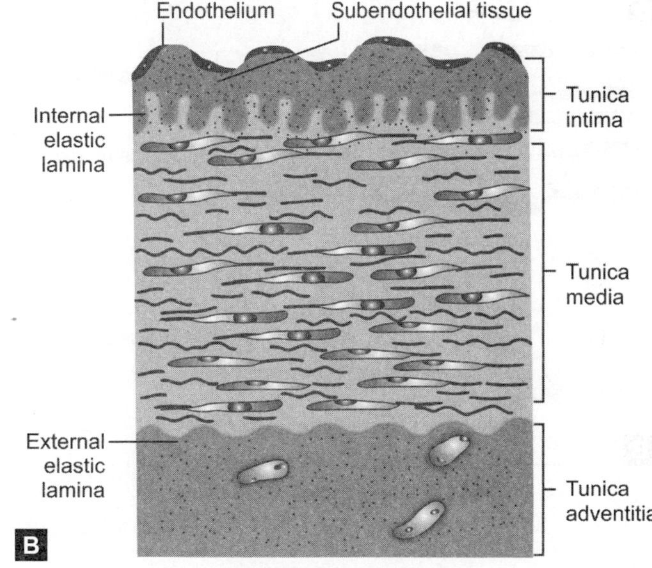

Figs 19A and B Artery

Capillaries

These are endothelium lined thin microscopic vessels, that connect arterioles and venules. Average diameter of capillary is 6–8 micrometer.

Sinusoids

These are large irregular vascular spaces which connects arteriole with venule or venule with venule.

- They replace capillaries in certain organs such as liver, spleen, bone marrow, suprarenal glands, parathyroid gland, etc.
- Their wall is thinner and incomplete with spaces between endothelial cells.

Veins (Figs 20A and B)

- These are thin-walled vessels that carry blood from capillaries to heart.
- Veins are formed by the union of many tributaries.
- Their lumen is larger.
- They have 'valves' which prevent the reflux of blood and thus maintain unidirectional flow of blood even against gravity.

Structure: It has three layers:

1. Tunica intima—made up of endothelium and subendothelial connective tissue
2. Tunica media—poorly developed
3. Tunica adventia—thickest and large amount of smooth muscle fibers along with collagen and elastic fibers.

BLOOD SUPPLY TO THE WALL OF BLOOD VESSEL

- Large arteries and veins are supplied by nutrient vessels called vaso-vasorum. They form a capillary network in tunica adventitia and outer part of tunica media
- Inner part of wall nourished directly by diffusion from luminal blood.

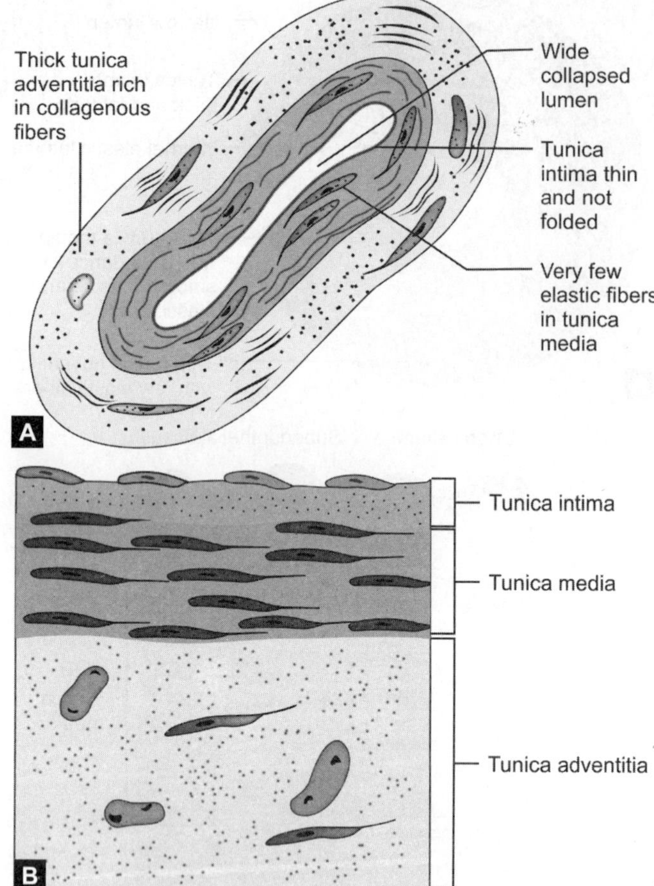

Figs 20A and B Vein

NERVE SUPPLY TO BLOOD VESSEL

Supplied by nonmyelinated sympathetic fibers which are vasoconstrictor in function.

Anastomosis

A precapillary or postcapillary communication between the neighboring vessels is called anastomosis (Fig. 21).

- *Arterial anastomosis:* Terminal branches of arteries or arterioles join with each other to form anastomosis, e.g. plantar arch, palmar arch
- *Venous anastomosis:* Communications between veins and tributaries of vein, e.g. dorsal venous arch of hand.
- *Arteriovenous anastomosis:* It is the direct communication between the arterioles and veins. It will help to regulate temperature, blood pressure and regional blood flow.

End Arteries*

Arteries which do not anastomose with their adjacent arteries are called end arteries. If these arteries are

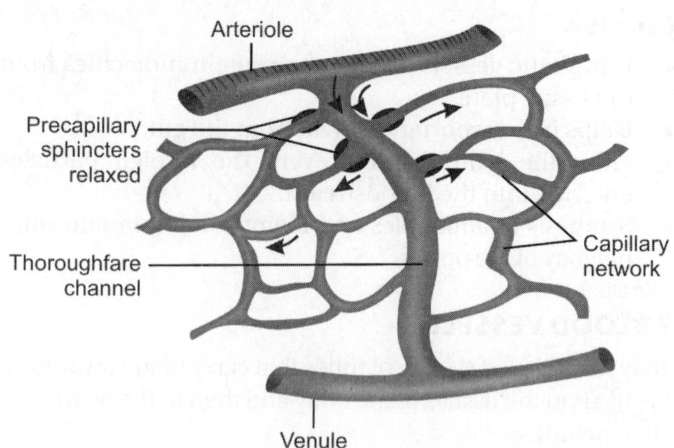

Fig. 21 Anastomosis (*For color version, see Plate 1*)

blocked, the area supplied will suffer from ischemia and that may lead to cell necrosis, e.g. central artery of retina; central branches of cerebral arteries.

SKIN

It is the outer covering of the body. It has two principal layers: (i) epidermis and (ii) dermis (Fig. 22).

Epidermis

It is a layer of stratified squamous keratinized epithelium, derived from ectoderm.

Layers—from superficial to deep:

- *Stratum corneum:* Most superficial layer. Consists of fully keratinized flattened scale-like dead cells. These anucleated cells are filled with protein called *keratin.*
- *Stratum lucidum:* It is a thin clear homogeneous glassy layer.
- *Stratum granulosum (granular layer):* It consists of 3 or 4 rows of flattened cells with pyknic nucleus showing signs of degranulation. The cytoplasm contains keratohyaline granulations.
- *Stratum spinosum (spiny layer):* It consists of several layers of polygonal cells. Centrally located large oval nucleus.
- *Stratum basale (stratum germinativum):* It consists of single layer of cuboidal or columnar cells. A thin basement membrane is situated between stratum basale and dermis.

Dermis*

It is the deep vascular layer of the skin derived from mesoderm. The smooth muscles of dermis are associated with hair follicles as 'erectores pili muscle'.

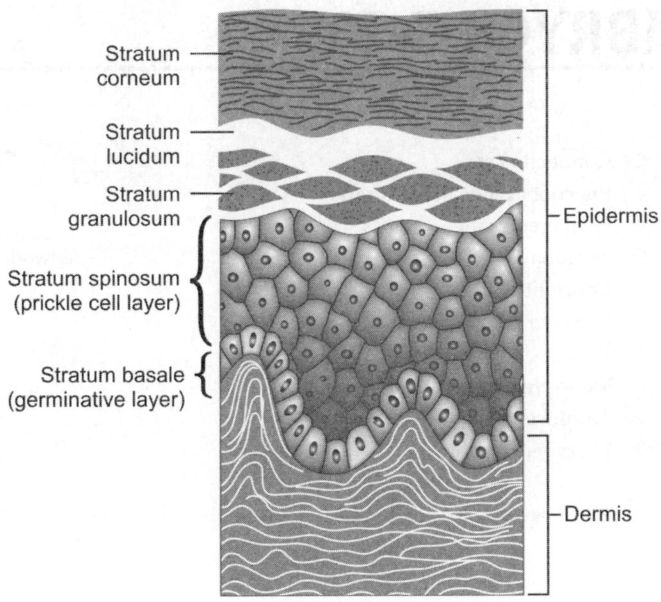

Fig. 22 Layers of skin

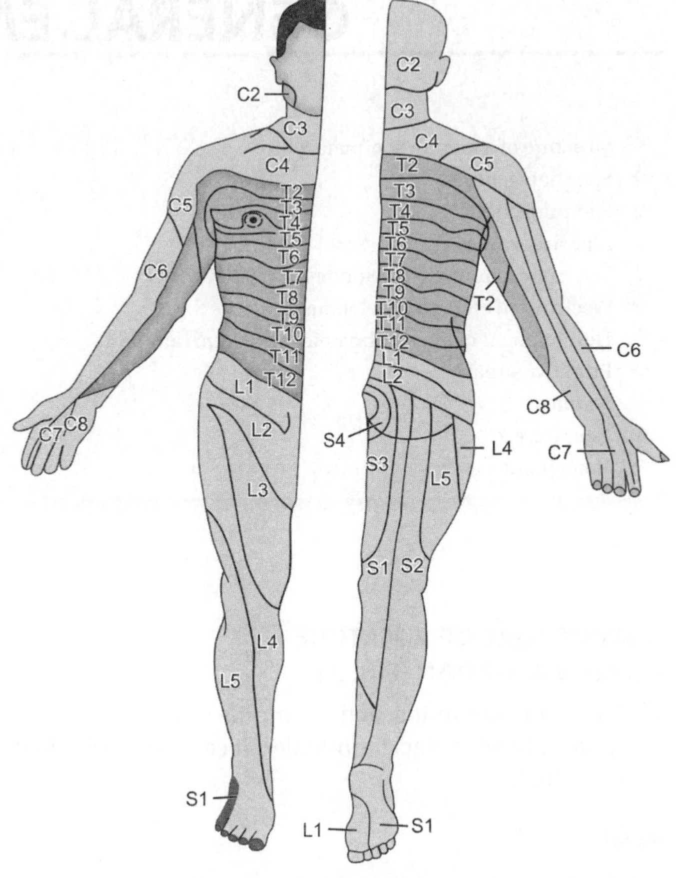

Fig. 23 Dermatome

Layers

Superficially	*Deep*
Papillary layer, account for about 1/5th of entire thickness of dermis	**Reticular layer**, composed of collagen fibers and arranged mostly in parallel bundles
It forms numerous conical blunt projections called dermal papillae	

Types

Thick skin	*Thin skin*
Present only in palms and soles	Present all over the body except in *palms and soles*
There is additional layer of stratum lucidum underneath the stratum corneum	No stratum lucidum
Hair follicles and sebaceous glands are totally absent but sweat glands are seen in abundance	Hair follicles, sebaceous and sweat glands are seen in abundance

Dermatome

A dermatome is an area of skin that is mainly supplied by a single spinal nerve. There are eight cervical nerves (C1 being an exception with no dermatome), twelve thoracic nerves, five lumbar nerves and five sacral nerves. Each of these nerves relays sensation (including pain) from a particular region of skin to the brain (Fig. 23).

Along the thorax and abdomen the dermatomes are like a stack of disks forming a human, each supplied by a different spinal nerve. Along the arms and the legs, the pattern is different: the dermatomes run longitudinally along the limbs. Although the general pattern is similar in all people, the precise areas of innervation are as unique to an individual as fingerprints.

GENERAL EMBRYOLOGY

- Structure of a mature spermatozoan
- Spermatogenesis*
- Spermiogenesis*
- Menstrual cycle
- Week one of human development
- Week two of embryo development
- Development of extraembryonic mesoderm (amnion)
- Primitive streak*
- Somites*
- Neural crest*
- Notochord*
- Connecting stalk
- Buccopharyngeal membrane
- Fetal membrane
- Decidua
- Chorionic villi*
- Placenta*
- Twins
- Monozygotic (identical) twins
- Amniocentesis
- Pharyngeal arches

STRUCTURE OF A MATURE SPERMATOZOAN (Fig. 24)

- It is a free swimming, actively motile cell
- It has a head, a neck, a middle piece, and a principal piece/tail.

Head

It is pyriform shaped and is derived from the nucleus:

- It is covered by a cap like structure called the acrosome/acrosomic cap
- The acrosome contains enzymes that help in penetration of spermatozoan into the ovum during fertilization.

Neck

It is narrow:

- It contains a funnel-shaped basal body and a spherical centriole.
- It helps to establish an intimate connection between the head and the remainder of the spermatozoan.

Axial Filament

It begins just behind the centriole.

- It passes through the middle piece and most of the tail.
- At the point where the middle piece joins the tail, the axial filament passes through a ring-like structure called the annulus.
- The part of the axial filament, which lies in the middle piece is surrounded by a spiral sheath made up of mitochondria.

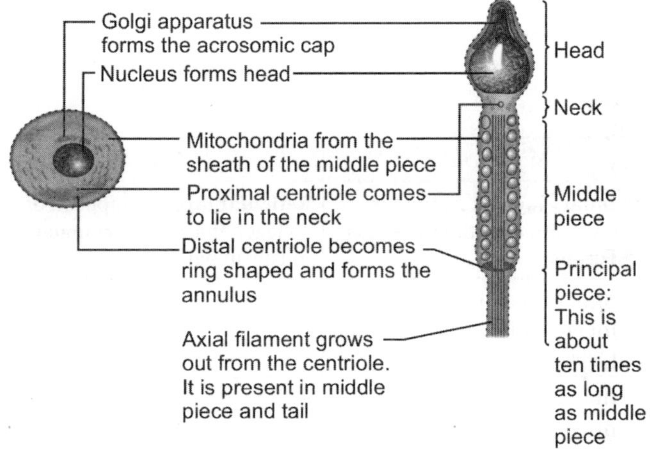

Fig. 24 Structure of a mature spermatozoan

SPERMATOGENESIS*

It is the process whereby the germ cell is converted into spermatids (Fig. 25).

Primordial germ cells (46, 2N) in the male are seen on the testicular cords and they remain there until puberty. At puberty, the testicular cords become canalized to form seminiferous tubules and the primordial germ cells differentiate into Type A spermatogonia (46, 2N). Type A spermatogonia undergo mitosis to provide a continuous supply of stem cells throughout the reproductive life of the male. Some Type A spermatogonia differentiate into Type B spermatogonia (46, 2N).

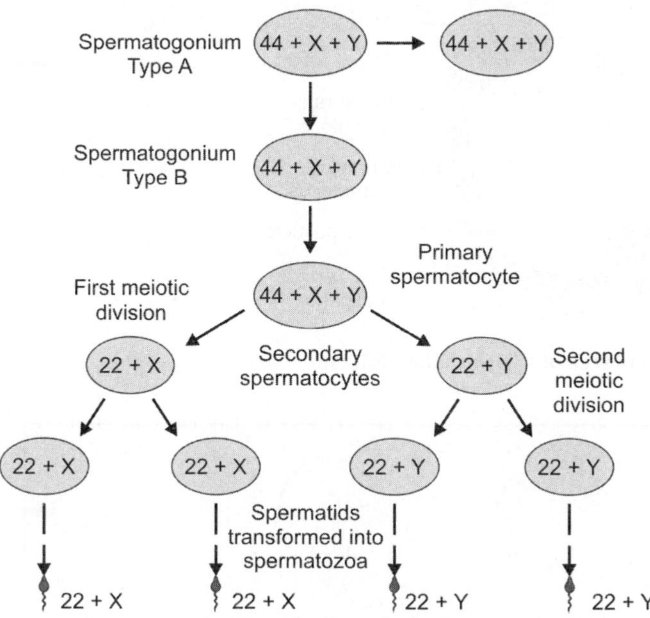

Fig. 25 Spermatogenesis

Type B spermatogonia enter meiosis I and undergo DNA replication to form primary spermatocytes (46, 2N). Primary spermatocytes complete meiosis I to form secondary spermatocytes (23, N). Secondary spermatocytes complete meiosis II to form four spermatids (23, N).

SPERMIOGENESIS* (Figs 26A TO E)

- Spermatids undergo a postmeiotic series of morphologic changes to form sperm (23, 1N).
- It involves: (i) formation of acrosome; (ii) formation of neck, middle piece and tail; (iii) condensation of the nucleus; (iv) shedding of most of the cytoplasm.
- The total time of sperm formation (from spermatogonia to spermatozoa) is about 64 days.
- Newly ejaculated sperm undergo capacitation, occurs in the female reproductive tract and after that they are capable of fertilization.

Graafian Follicle (Figs 27A and B)

- Ova develops from the oogonia (like the spermatogonia) present in the cortex of the ovary.
- The oogonia are surrounded by other cells that form the stroma.
- Some of the follicular cells surround the ova/oocyte to form primordial follicles.
- The zona pellucida appears between follicular cells and oocyte
- The follicular cells (now called granulosa cells) proliferates to form several layers to form membrane granulosa.
- A cavity (antrum) appears within the membrana granulosa.
- The oocyte then lies eccentrically in the follicle, surrounded by some granulosa cells and that are given the name cumulus oophoricus. The cells that attach it to the wall of the follicle are given the name discus proligerus.
- The stromal cells surrounding the membrana granulosa become condensed to form a covering called theca interna (*the cells of theca interna secretes estrogen*).

MENSTRUAL CYCLE

- The menstrual cycle is the physiological changes that can occur in fertile women for the purpose of sexual reproduction and fertilization (Fig. 28).

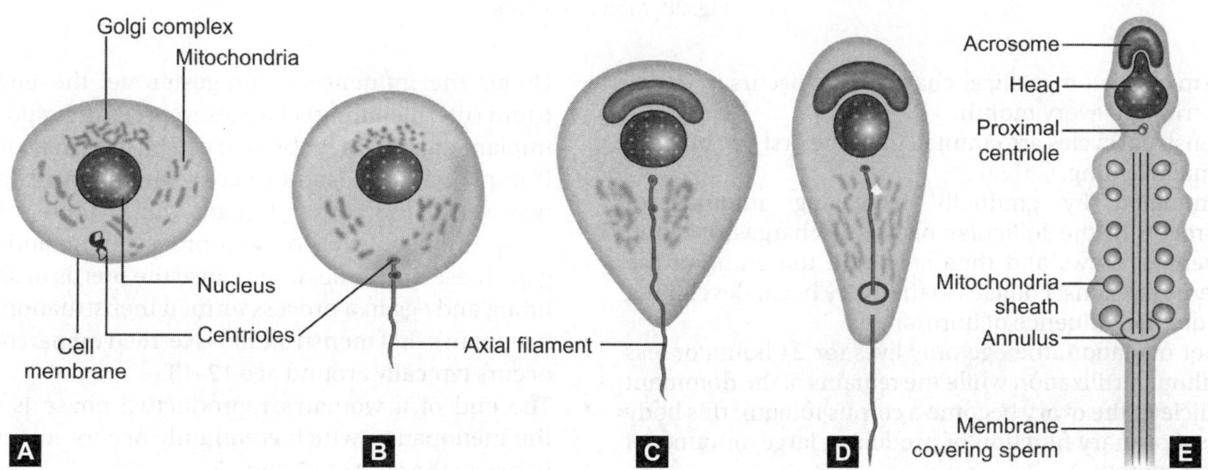

Figs 26A to E Stage in spermatogenesis

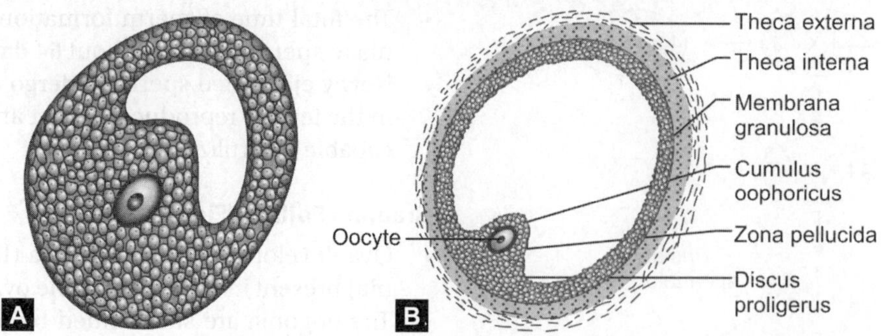

Figs 27A and B (A) Formation of follicular cavity; (B) Graafian follicle

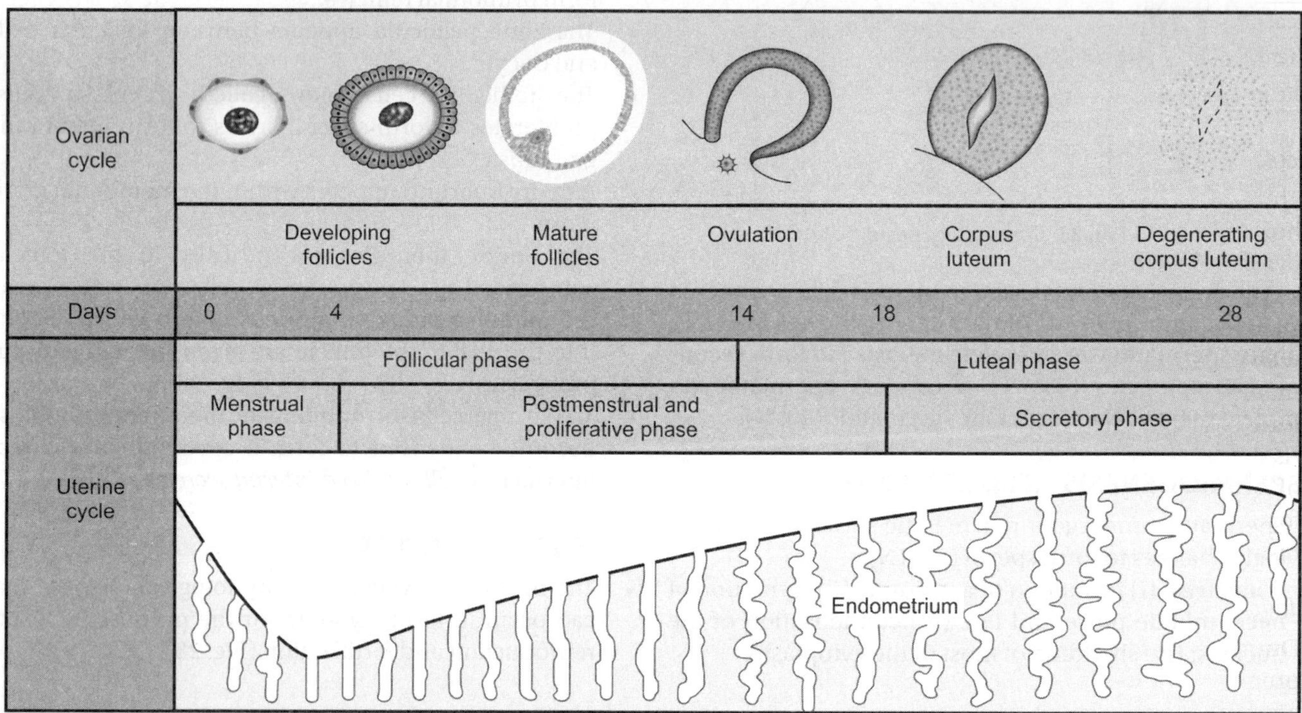

Fig. 28 Menstrual cycle

- Term applied to cyclical changes that occurs in endometrium in every month.
- Menstrual cycles are counted from the first day of menstrual bleeding.
- Stimulated by gradually increasing amounts of estrogen in the follicular phase, discharges of blood (menses) slows and then stop, and the lining of the uterus thickens. Follicles in the ovary begin developing under the influence of hormones.
- After ovulation, the egg only lives for 24 hours or less without fertilization while the remains of the dominant follicle in the ovary become a corpus luteum; this body has a primary function of producing large amounts of progesterone.
- Under the influence of progesterone, the endometrium (uterine lining) changes to prepare for potential implantation of an embryo to establish a pregnancy.
- If implantation does not occur within approximately two weeks, the corpus luteum will involute, causing sharp drops in levels of both progesterone and estrogen. These hormone drops cause the uterus to shed its lining and egg in a process termed menstruation.
- A woman's first menstruation is termed menarche, and occurs typically around age 12–13.
- The end of a woman's reproductive phase is called the menopause, which commonly occurs somewhere between the ages of 45 and 55.

Phases

The menstrual cycle can be divided into several different phases. The average length of each phase is shown below, *the first three are related to changes in the lining of the uterus whereas the final three are related to processes occurring in the ovary*:

Name of phase	*Average start day assuming a 28-day cycle*	*Average end day*
Menstrual phase (Menstruation)	1	4
Proliferative phase	5	13
Ovulatory phase (Ovulation)	13	16
Luteal phase or secretory phase	16	28
Ischemic phase	27	28
Follicular phase	1	13

Follicular Phase/Proliferative Phase

- Through the influence of a rise in follicle stimulating hormone (FSH) during the first days of the cycle, a few ovarian follicles are stimulated. Under the influence of several hormones, all except one of these follicles will stop growing, while one dominant follicle in the ovary will continue to maturity. The follicle that reaches maturity is called a tertiary, or Graafian follicle, and it forms the ovum.
- As they mature, the follicles secrete increasing amounts of estradiol, an estrogen. The estrogens initiate the formation of a new layer of endometrium in the uterus, histologically identified as the proliferative endometrium.

Ovulation

- During the follicular phase, estradiol suppresses production of luteinizing hormone (LH) from the anterior pituitary gland. When the egg has nearly matured, levels of estradiol reach a threshold above which they stimulate production of LH (Fig. 29).
- In an average cycle this LH surge starts around cycle day 12 and may last 48 hours.
- The release of LH matures the egg and weakens the wall of the follicle in the ovary, causing the fully developed follicle to release its secondary oocyte.
- The secondary oocyte promptly matures into an ootid and then becomes a mature ovum. The mature ovum has a diameter of about 0.2 mm.
- After being released from the ovary, the egg is swept into the fallopian tube by the fimbria. After about a day, an unfertilized egg will disintegrate or dissolve in the fallopian tube.
- Fertilization by a spermatozoan, when it occurs, usually takes place in the ampulla, the widest section of the fallopian tubes.

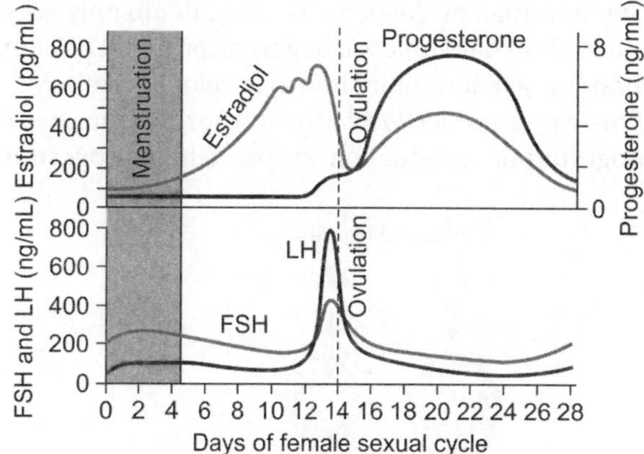

Fig. 29 Enzymatic changes in ovulatory cycle

- A fertilized egg immediately begins the process of embryogenesis, or development. The developing embryo takes about three days to reach the uterus and another three days to implant into the endometrium. It has usually reached the blastocyst stage at the time of implantation.

Luteal Phase/Secretory Phase

- An important role is played by the corpus luteum, the solid body formed in an ovary after the egg has been released from the ovary into the fallopian tube.
- This body continues to grow for some time after ovulation and produces significant amounts of hormones, particularly progesterone.
- Progesterone plays a vital role in making the endometrium receptive to implantation of the blastocyst and supportive of the early pregnancy.
- After ovulation, the pituitary hormones FSH and LH cause the remaining parts of the dominant follicle to transform into the corpus luteum, which produces progesterone.

*Corpus Luteum**

- The corpus luteum, which means yellow body in Latin, is what is left of the follicle after a woman ovulates.
- When a woman ovulates, the egg will burst from the follicle. Then what is left of the follicle will become the corpus luteum (Fig. 30).
- The luteal phase, named after the corpus luteum, is the second half of a woman's menstrual cycle.
- The corpus luteum produces progesterone. Progesterone makes the lining of the uterus thick for implantation and is necessary to sustain a healthy pregnancy.
- The progesterone production will prolong until the placenta begins to take over progesterone production around ten weeks gestation.

- After a woman ovulates, the corpus luteum only lasts for about 12–14 days unless it begins receiving hCG (human chorionic gonadotropin) from a developing embryo.
- *If the egg is not fertilized,* the corpus luteum dies and progesterone production stops. When progesterone levels drop, the uterus lining stops thickening and is consequently shed during menstruation.
- *If the egg is fertilized,* the corpus luteum will begin receiving hCG from the embryo. hCG tells the corpus luteum to keep producing progesterone. The corpus luteum lasts for about ten weeks after ovulation. After ten weeks the placenta takes over progesterone production through the end of pregnancy.

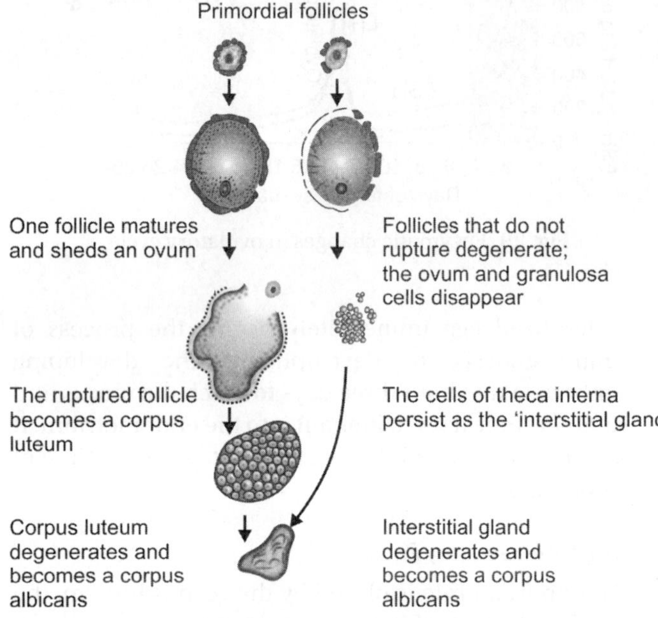

Fig. 30 Fate of ovarian follicles

WEEK ONE OF HUMAN DEVELOPMENT

Week one of human development is illustrated in Figure 31.

Fertilization

Fertilization occures in the ampulla of the uterine tube and includes three phases:

Phase 1: Sperm penetration of corona radiata is aided by the action of sperm and uterine tube mucosal enzymes.

Phase 2: Sperm binding and penetration of zona pellucida:

- Sperm binding occurs through interaction of sperm glycosyltransferases and ZP3 receptors located on the zona pellucida. Sperm binding triggers the acrosome reaction, which result in the release of acrosomal enzymes.
- Penetration of zona pellucida is aided by acrosomal enzymes, specifically acrosin.

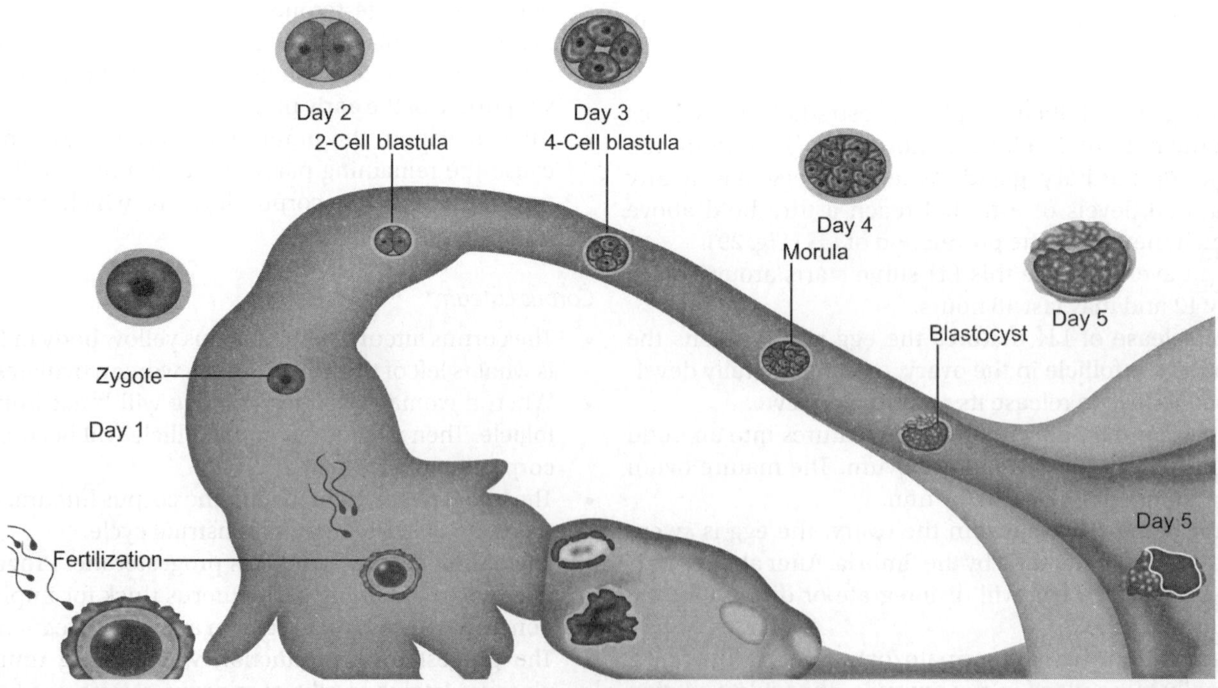

Fig. 31 Week one of human development

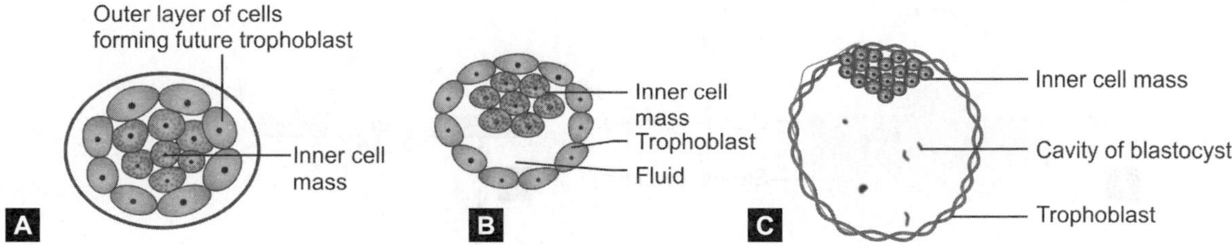

Figs 32A to C Formation of blastocyst

Phase 3: Fusion of sperm and oocyte cell membranes occurs with subsequent breakdown of both membranes at the fusion area.

- The entire sperm (except the cell membrane) enters the cytoplasm of the secondary oocyte arrested in metaphase of meiosis II.
- The sperm mitochondria and tail degenerate.
- The sperm nucleus is now called the male pronucleus. Since all sperm mitochondria degenerate, all mitochondria within the zygote are of maternal origin (i.e. *all mitochondrial DNA is of maternal origin*).
- The secondary oocyte completes meiosis II, forming a mature ovum and a second polar body. The nucleus of mature ovum is now called the female pronucleus.
- Male and female pronuclei fuse, thereby forming a zygote (a new cell whose genotype is an intermingling of maternal and paternal chromosomes, i.e. diploid).

Zona Pellucida*

- It is a glycoprotein membrane
- The strong membrane that forms around an ovum as it develops in the ovary.
- To fertilize the egg, a sperm must penetrate the zona pellucida.
- If fertilization takes place, the zona pellucida disappears, to permit implantation in the uterus.
- The membrane remains in place during the ovum's travel through the fallopian tube. It prevents the implantation at abnormal sites.

Cleavage and Blastocyst Formation Cleavage

- It is a series of mitotic divisions of the zygote within the zona pellucida.
- Zygote cytoplasm is successively partitioned (cleaved) to form a blastula consisting of increasingly smaller blastomeres (2-cell, 4-cell, 8-cell, and so on). Blastomeres are considered totipotent (capable of forming a complete embryo) up to the 4- to 8-cell stage.
- Blastomeres form a morula (16 celled stage) by undergoing compaction.
- Morula consists of an inner cell mass and outer layers of cells forming future trophoblast.

Blastocyst Formation (Figs 32A to C)*

- When fluid from uterine cavity passes into morula, it will partially separate the cells of inner cell mass from trophoblast, resulting in formation of blastocyst.
- The inner cell mass is now called the embryoblast (becomes the embryo).
- The outer cell mass is now called the trophoblast (becomes fetal portion of the placenta).

Implantation*

- The blastocyst usually implants within the posterior-superior wall of the uterus by day 7 after fertilization (Figs 33A to D).
- Implantation occurs in the functional layer of the endometrium during the secretory phase of the menstrual cycle.
- The trophoblast proliferates and differentiates into the cytotrophoblast and syncytiotrophoblast.

Abnormal Sites of Implantation

Implantation occurs in the *lower uterine segment* and this condition is called *placenta previa (Fig. 34A)*.

Various Degrees of Placenta Previa

- *First degree:* Attachment of placenta extends into the lower uterine segment, but not reaches the internal os.
- *Second degree:* Margin of placenta reaches the internal os, but does not cover it.
- *Third degree:* The edge of placenta covers the internal os but not when it is dilated.
- *Fourth degree:* The placenta completely covers the internal os, and occludes the os even after it has dilated.

Implantation outside the uterus (Fig. 34B)

When the ovum gets implanted at any site outside the uterus, this is called an *ectopic pregnancy*.

- Tubal pregnancy—the blastocyst gets implanted in the uterine tube.
- Interstitial tubal implantation—the blastocyst may get implanted in the part of the uterine tube passing through the uterine wall.

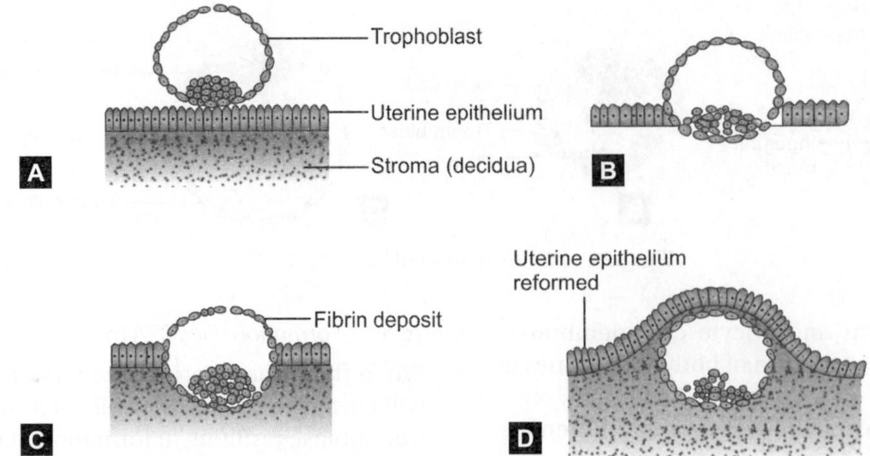

Figs 33A to D Stages in implantation of blastocyst

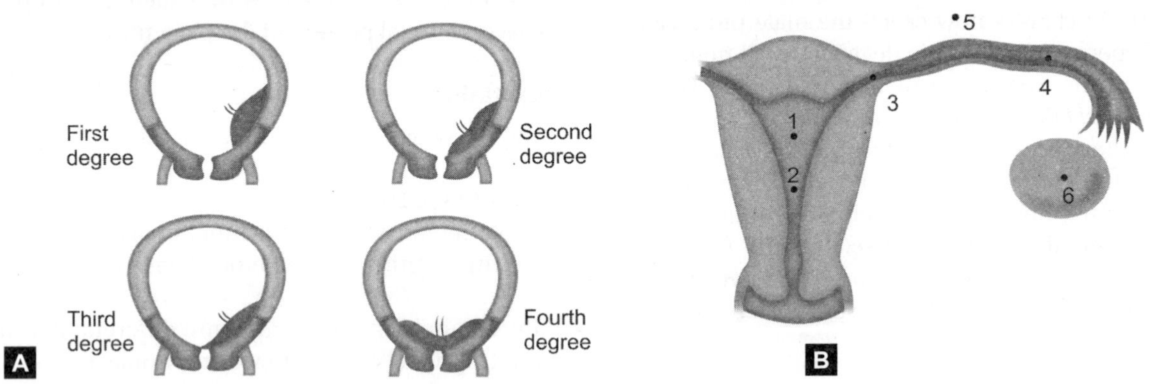

Figs 34A and B (A) Types of placenta previa; (B) Abnormal sites of implantation: (1) normal site, (2) placenta previa, (3) interstitial tubal implantation, (4) tubal implantation, (5) abdominal implantation, (6) ovarian implantation

- Implantation in the ovary—fertilization and implantation may occur while the ovum still in the ovary.

WEEK TWO OF EMBRYO DEVELOPMENT (FIG. 35)

Further Development of the Embryoblast (Inner Cell Mass)

- During week two, the embryoblast differentiates into two distinct cellular layers—the dorsal epiblast layer (columnar cells) and the ventral hypoblast layer (cuboidal cells).
- The epiblast and hypoblast together form a flat, ovoid-shaped disk known as the bilaminar embryonic disk. Within the epiblast, clefts begin to develop and eventually coalesce to form the amniotic cavity.
- Hypoblast cells begin to migrate and line the inner surface of the cytotrophoblast forming the exocoelomic membrane, which delimits a space called the yolk sac.
- At the future site of the mouth, hypoblast cells become columnar shaped and fuse with epiblast cells to form a circular, midline thickening called the prochordal plate.

Further Development of the Trophoblast* (Outer Cell Mass)

Syncytiotrophoblast

- The syncytiotrophoblast is the outer multinucleated zone of the trophoblast where no mitosis occurs (i.e. it arises from the cytotrophoblast).
- During this time period, the syncytiotrophoblast continues its invasion of the endometrium, thereby eroding endometrial blood vessels and endometrial glands.
- Lacunae form within the syncytiotrophoblast and become filled with maternal blood and glandular secretions. In addition, endometrial stromal cells (decidual cells) at the site of implantation become filled with glycogen and lipids and also supply nutrients to the embryoblast.

Cytotrophoblast

- The cytotrophoblast is mitotically active as new cytotrophoblastic cells migrate into the syncytiotrophoblast, thereby fueling its growth.

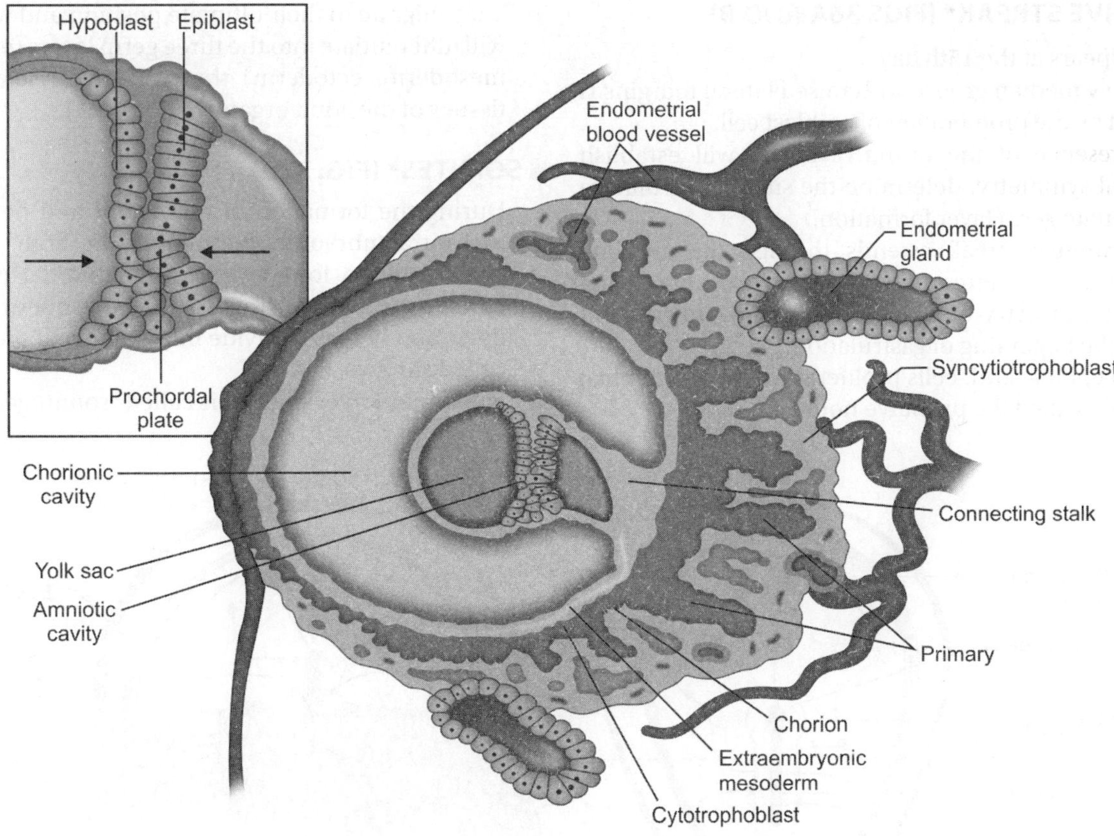

Fig. 35 Week 2 of embryo development

- In addition, cytotrophoblastic cells produce local mounds called primary chorionic villi that bulge into the surrounding syncytiotrophoblast.

DEVELOPMENT OF EXTRAEMBRYONIC MESODERM (AMNION)

- The extraembryonic mesoderm develops from the epiblast and consists of loosely arranged cells that fill the space between the exocoelomic membrane and the cytotrophoblast.
- Large spaces develop in the extraembryonic mesoderm and coalesce to form the extraembryonic coelom.
- Extraembryonic coelom divides the extraembryonic mesoderm into the extraembryonic somatic mesoderm and extraembryonic visceral mesoderm.
- The extraembryonic somatic mesoderm lines the trophoblast, forms the connecting stalk, and covers the amnion.
- The extraembryonic visceral mesoderm covers the yolk sac.
- As soon as the extraembryonic somatic mesoderm and extraembryonic visceral mesoderm form, one can delineate the chorion, which consists of the extraembryonic somatic mesoderm, cytotrophoblast, and syncytiotrophoblast.

Embryonic Period (Weeks 3–8)

Further Development of the Embryoblast

Gastrulation*: It is the process that establishes the three definitive germ layers of embryo (ectoderm), intraembryonic mesoderm, and endoderm), thereby forming a trilaminar disk by day 21 of development.

- These three germ layers give rise to all the tissues and organs of the adult.
- Gastrulation is first indicated by the formation of the primitive streak, caused by the proliferation of epiblast cell. The primitive streak consists of the primitive groove, primitive node and primitive pit.
- Located caudal to the primitive streak is the future site of the anus, known as the cloacal membrane, where epiblast and hypoblast cells are fused.
- The ectoderm, intraembryonic mesoderm and endoderm of the trilaminar embryonic disk all are derived from the epiblast.
- The term intraembryonic mesoderm describes the germ layer that forms during week 3 (gastrulation) in contrast to the extraembryonic mesoderm, which formed during week 2.
- Intraembryonic mesoderm forms various tissues and organ found in the adult, whereas extraembryonic mesoderm is involved in placenta formation.

PRIMITIVE STREAK* (FIGS 36A AND B)

- This appears at the 15th day.
- A narrow median groove with raised lateral margins is formed by the proliferation of epiblast cell.
- The presence of the primitive streak will establish bilateral symmetry, determine the site of gastrulation and initiate germ layer formation.
- The primitive streak extends through this midline and creates the anteroposterior body axis, becoming the first symmetry-breaking event in the embryo, and marks the beginning of gastrulation.
- At the cephalic end, cells proliferate to form knob like elevation called the primitive node.
- They migrate to their ultimate position and where they will differentiate into the three germ layers (endoderm, mesoderm, ectoderm) that will give rise to all the tissues of the adult organism (Fig. 37A).

SOMITES* (FIG. 37B)

- During the formation of notochord and neural tube, the intraembryonic mesoderm on both the sides proliferates to form a thick, longitudinal column of paraxial mesoderm. This paraxial mesoderm differentiates and begins to divide into paired cuboidal bodies called somites.
- The formation of somites is called "somitogenesis".

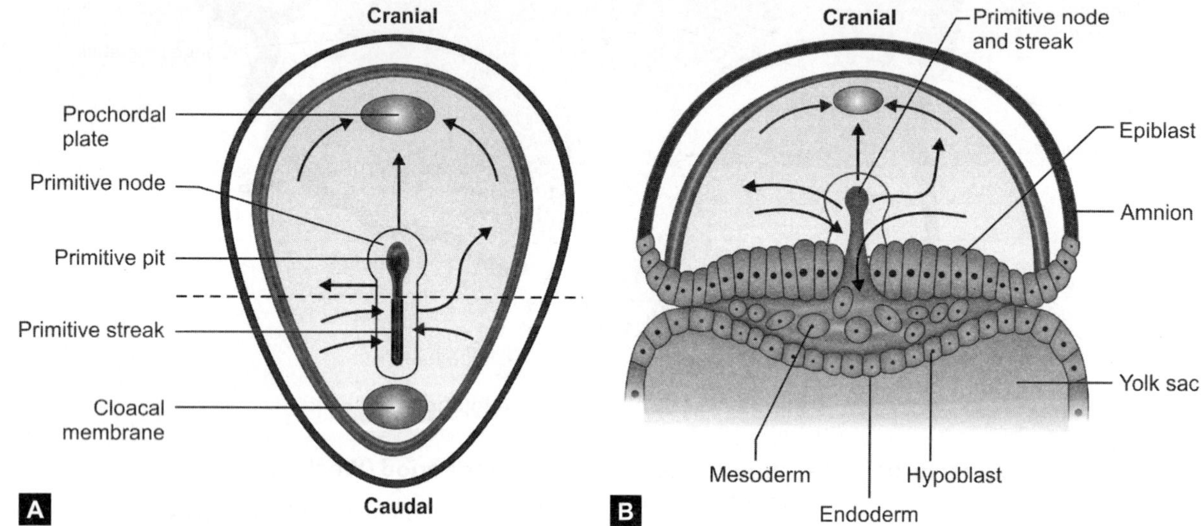

Figs 36A and B Formation of primitive streak

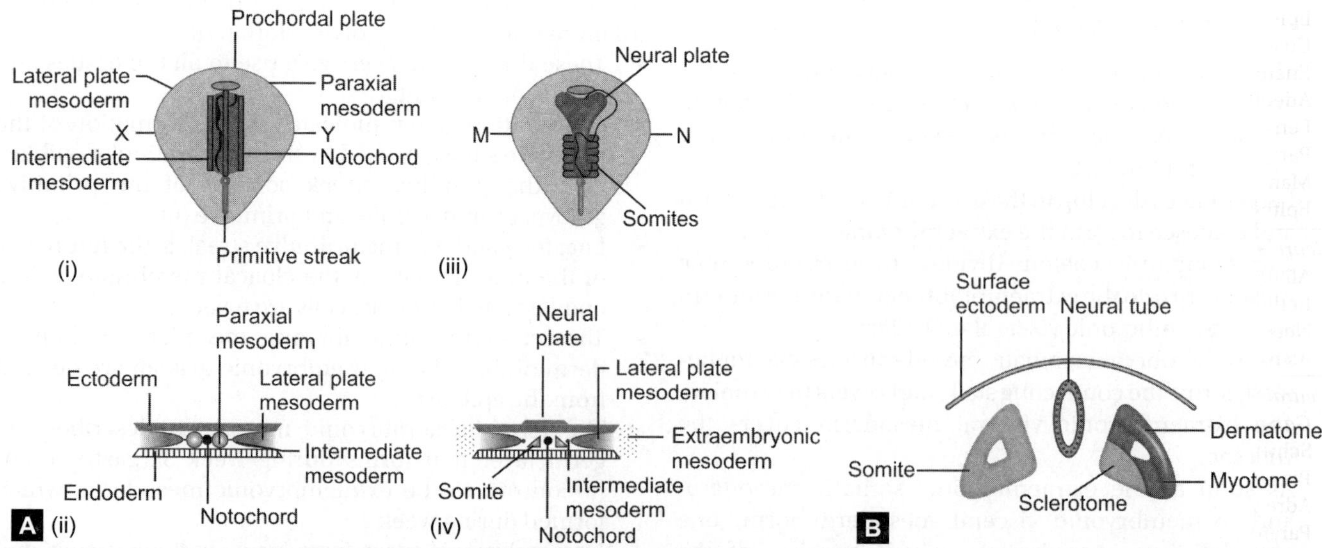

Figs 37A and B (A) Subdivisions of intraembryonic mesoderm. (ii) and (iv) are transverse, sections across axes XY [in (i)] and MN [in (iii)] respectively. Note that the notochord and mesoderm are deep to the ectoderm. Their position is shown diagrammatically; (B) CS of somites

- In around 20–30 days, 38 pairs of somites develop. By the end of 5th week, 42–44 pairs are formed
- Each somite is triangular in cross-section.
- Each somite is divisible into three parts:
  1. Ventromedial part is called sclerotome—forms vertebral column and ribs.
  2. Lateral part is called dermatome—forms dermis and subcutaneous area of skin.
  3. Intermediate part is called myotome—forms striated muscles.

NEURAL CREST*

- Neural crest cells are a transient, multipotent, migratory cell population unique to vertebrate that give rise to a diverse cell lineage.
- After gastrulation, neural crest cells are specified at the border of the neural plate and the non-neural ectoderm.
- During neurulation, the borders of the neural plate, also known as the neural folds, converge at the dorsal midline to form the neural tube.

Changes involving Intraembryonic Mesoderm*

- *Paraxial mesoderm:* It is a thick plate of mesoderm located on each side of the midline.
  - It becomes organized into segments known as somatomeres, which formed in a craniocaudal sequence.
  - Somitomeres 1–7 do not forms somites but contribute mesoderm to the pharyngeal arch.
  - The remaining somitomeres further condense in a craniocaudal sequence to form 42–44 pairs of somites.
  - Somites further differentiate into these components: sclerotome, myotome and dermatome.
- *Intermediate mesoderm* is a longitudinal dorsal ridge of mesoderm located between the paraxial mesoderm and lateral mesoderm.
  - This ridge forms the urogenital ridge, which is involved in the formation of the future kidneys and gonads.
- *Lateral mesoderm* is a thin plate of mesoderm located along the lateral sides of the embryo. Large spaces develop in the lateral mesoderm and coalesce to form the intraembryonic coelom.
  - The intraembryonic coelom divides the lateral mesoderm into two layers:
    1. Intraembryonic somatic mesoderm/somatopleuric).
    2. Intraembryonic visceral mesoderm/visceropleuric/splanchnopleuric.

NOTOCHORD*

- It is a solid cylinder of mesoderm extending in the midline of the trilaminar embryonic vertebral column.
- Embryonic disk from the primitive node to the prochordal plate. The notochord has a number of important functions, which include the following:
  - It induces the overlying ectoderm to differentiate into neuroectoderm to form the neural tube.

Ectoderm	*Mesoderm*	*Endoderm*
• Epidermis, hair, nails • Cochlear duct, semicircular ducts • Enamel of teech • Adenohypophysis • Lens of the eye • Parotid gland • Mammary glands • Epithelial lining of lower anal canal	• Musle (smooth, cardia, skeletal) • Extraocular musles (preotic somites) • Muscles of the tongue (occipital somites) • Connective tissue, dermis of skin • Bone, cartilage • Blood and lymph vessels • Heart • Adrenal cortex • Spleen • Kidney • Dura mater • Testes, ovaries	• *Epithelial lining of:* - Gastrointestinal tract - Trachea, bronchi, lungs • Biliary apparatus • Urinary bladder, urethra • Vagina • Auditory tube • Middle ear cavity • *Parenchyma of:* - Liver - Pancreas - Submandibular gland - Sublingual gland - Thyroid - Parathyroid
Neuroectoderm • All neurons within brain and spinal cord • Retina • Neurohypophysis • Astrocytes, oligodendrocytes		
Neural crest • *Ganglia:* Dorsal root, cranial, autonomic • Schwann cells • Pia and arachnoid • Adrenal medulla • Parafollicular cells (calcitonin) • Aorticopulmonary septum • Dilator and sphincter pupillae mm. • Ciliary musle		

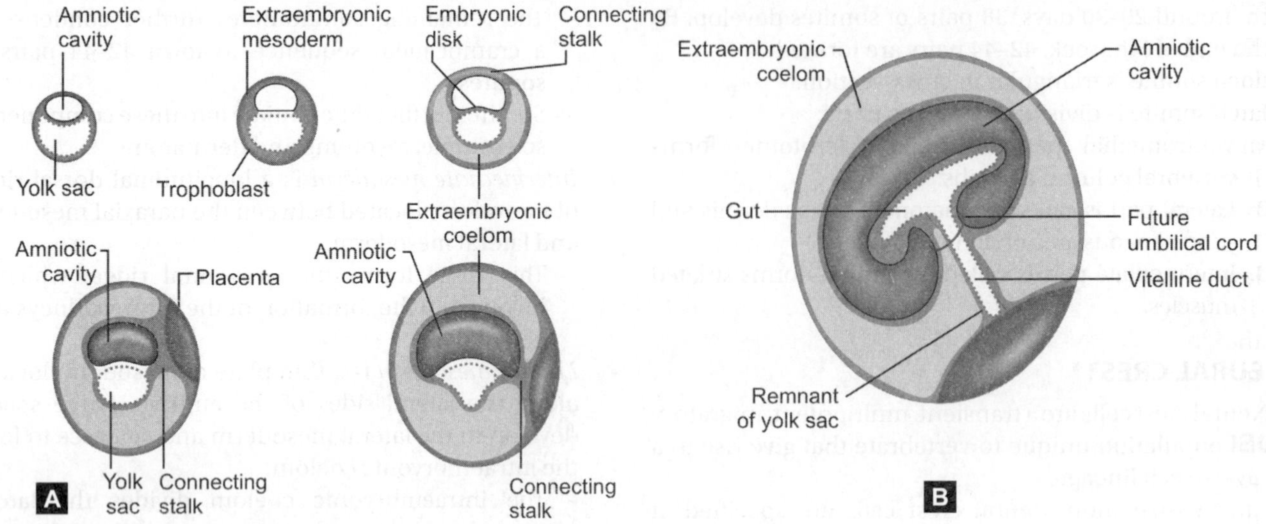

Figs 38A and B Stages in the establishment of the umbilical cord

- It includes the formation of each vertebral body.
- It forms the nucleus pulposus of each intervertebral disk.

CONNECTING STALK (FIGS 38A AND B)

- The connecting stalk is a yolk sac diverticulum.
- The amnion and yolk sac are attached by the connecting stalk to the trophoblast.
- It is derived from extraembryonic mesoderm.

BUCCOPHARYNGEAL MEMBRANE

- The region where the crescentic masses of the ectoderm and endoderm come into direct contact with each other constitutes a thin membrane, the buccopharyngeal membrane (or oropharyngeal membrane)
- It forms a septum between the primitive mouth and pharynx.
- In front of the buccopharyngeal area, where the lateral crescents of mesoderm fuse in the middle line, the pericardium is afterward developed, and this region is, therefore, designated the pericardial area.

FETAL MEMBRANE

Yolk Sac

- On the 9th day, the flattened mesothelial cells appear on the inner surface of the primary yolk sac and are called Heuser's membrane.
- This membrane is continuous with the primitive endoderm.
- With the formation of extraembryonic mesoderm, and later the extraembryonic coelom, the yolk sac becomes much smaller.
- It comes to be lined all round by cubical cells, and is then called the secondary yolk sac.

(The primary extraembryonic mesoderm increases in size and a number of cavities appear within it and coalesce to form the extraembryonic coelom. The coelomic cavity splits the extraembryonic mesoderm into somatopleuric layer, which lines the cytotrophoblast and amnion and a splanchnopleuric layer, which covers the yolk sac).

Allantois

- It arises as a tubular diverticulum of the posterior part of the yolk sac; when the hind-gut is developed the allantois is carried backward with it and then opens into the cloaca or terminal part of the hind-gut.
- This sac-like structure is primarily involved in nutrition and excretion, and is webbed with blood vessels.
- The function of the allantois is to collect liquid waste from the embryo, as well as to exchange gases used by the embryo.
- In mammals, it forms an axis for the development of the umbilical cord.

Amnion (Look Back...)

- It is the inner layer of the fetal membranes. Its internal surface is smooth and shiny and is in contact with liquor amnii.
- This membranous sac will surround and protect the embryo.
- It stems from parts of the mesoderm on the outer side and the ectoderm on the inner side.
- It will contribute to the formation of liquor amnii and facilitate dilation of cervix during labor.

Chorion

- The chorion consists of two layers: an outer layer formed by the primitive ectoderm or trophoblast, and an inner by the somatic mesoderm; with this latter the amnion is in contact.
- It is one of the membranes that exist during pregnancy between the developing fetus and mother.
- It is formed by extraembryonic mesoderm and the two layers of trophoblast.
- The chorionic villi emerge from the chorion, invade the endometrium, and allow transfer of nutrients from maternal blood to fetal blood.

DECIDUA (FIGS 39A AND B)

- Before the fertilized ovum reaches the uterus, the mucous membrane of the body of the uterus undergoes important changes and is then known as the decidua.
- The thickness and vascularity of the mucous membrane are greatly increased; its glands are elongated and open on its free surface by funnel-shaped orifices, while their deeper portions are tortuous and dilated into irregular spaces.
- These changes are well advanced by the second month of pregnancy.
- The mucous membrane consists of the following strata.
- Stratum compactum, next to the free surface; in this the uterine glands are only slightly expanded, and are lined by columnar cells.
- Stratum spongiosum, in which the gland tubes are greatly dilated and very tortuous.
- A thin unaltered or boundary layer, next to the uterine muscular fibers, containing the deepest parts of the uterine glands, which are not dilated, and are lined with columnar epithelium.
- The part which covers in the ovum is named the decidua capsularis.
- The portion which intervenes between the ovum and the uterine wall is named the decidua basalis or decidua placentalis.
- The part of the decidua which lines the remainder of the body of the uterus is known as the decidua vera or decidua parietalis.
- Coincidently with the growth of the embryo, the decidua capsularis is thinned and extended and the space between it and decidua vera is gradually obliterated.

CHORIONIC VILLI*

- It undergoes rapid proliferation and forms numerous processes, the chorionic villi, which invade and destroy the uterine decidua and at the same time it absorbs nutritive materials for the growth of the embryo.
- The chorionic villi small and nonvascular, and consist of trophoblast only, but they increase in size.
- Blood is carried to the villi by the branches of the umbilical arteries (deoxygenated blood), and after circulating through the capillaries of the villi, is returned to the embryo by the umbilical veins (oxygenated blood).
- Until about the end of the second month of pregnancy the villi cover the entire chorion, and are almost uniform in size but after this they develop unequally.
- Primary villi—consist of a central core of cytotrophoblast covered by a layer of syncytiotrophoblst. Adjoining villi are separated by a intervillous space (Figs 40A and 41B).
- Secondary villi—show three layers: (i) outer-syncytio-trophoblast, (ii) intermediate-cytotrophoblast, (iii) inner layer of extraembryonic mesoderm (Figs 40B and 41B).
- Tertiary villi—are like secondary villi except that there are blood capillaries in the mesoderm (Figs 41A and B).

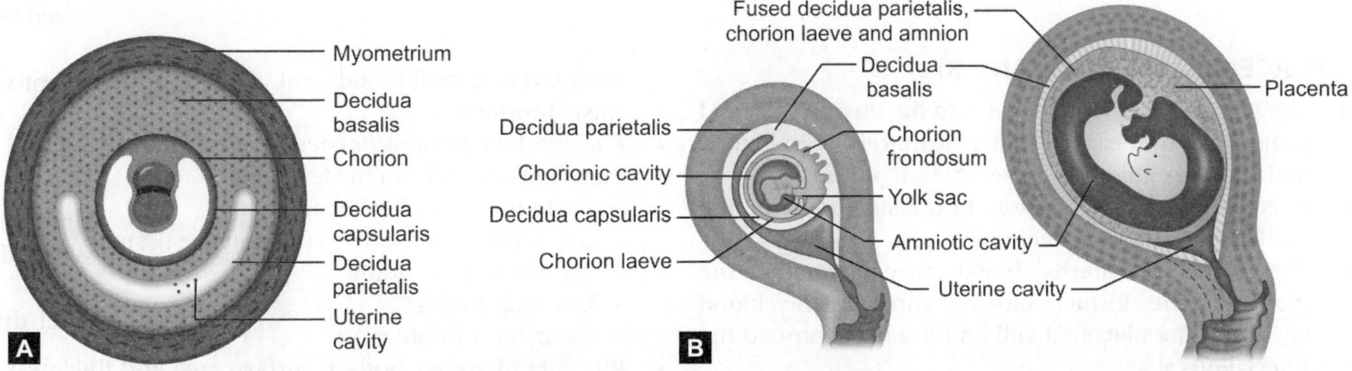

Figs 39A and B (A) Decidua; (B) Arrangement of fetal membranes with the uterine wall

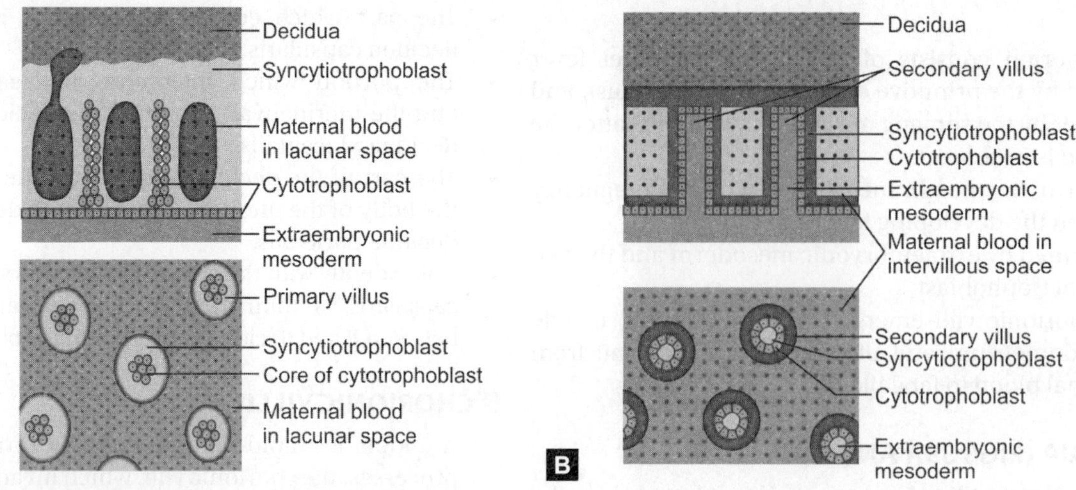

Figs 40A and B (A) Primary villi; (B) Secondary villi

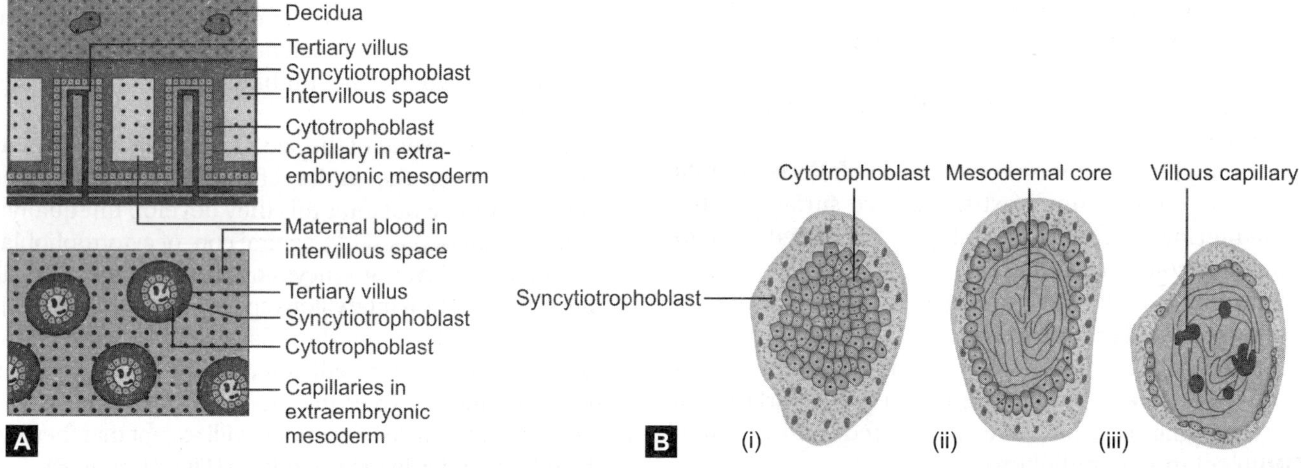

Figs 41A and B (A) Tertiary villi; (B) (i) Primary; (ii) Secondary; (iii) Tertiary

PLACENTA* (FIGS 42A AND B)

- The placenta connects the fetus to the uterine wall, and is the organ by means of which the nutritive, respiratory, and excretory functions of the fetus are carried on.
- It is composed of chorion frondosum (villi of the embryonic pole) and decidua basalis.
- The fetal and maternal blood currents traverse the placenta, the former passing through the blood vessels of the placental villi and the later through the intervillous space.
- The two currents do not intermingle, being separated from each other by the delicate walls of the villi. Nevertheless, the fetal blood is able to absorb, through the walls of the villi, oxygen and nutritive materials from the maternal blood, and give up to the latter its waste products.
- *Placental membrane/barrier*—this seperates fetal and maternal blood (from the fetal side)
  - Endothelium of fetal capillaries
  - Surrounding mesoderm (connective tissue)
  - Basement membrane
  - Cytotrophoblast
  - Syncytiotrophoblast
- Placenta increases both in surface area and thickness and this involves branching out laterally of the villi. By the 4th month, the placenta has two surfaces.
  - Maternal surface—formed by deciduas basalis, which then forms a decidual plate. A number of

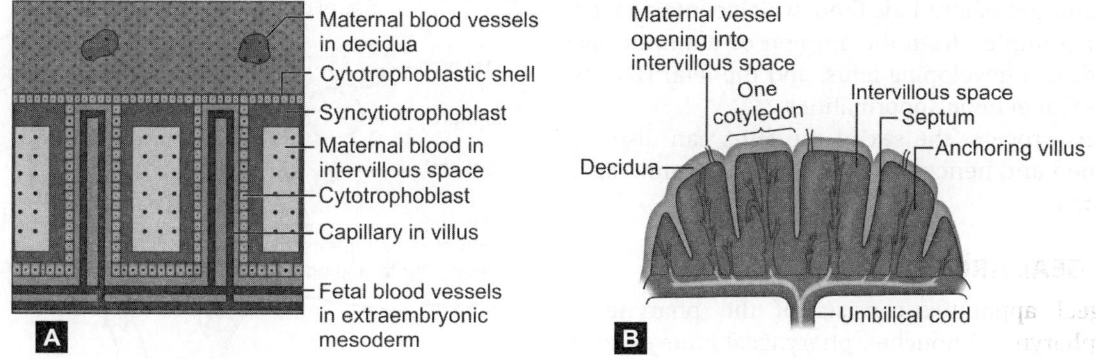

Figs 42A and B Placenta

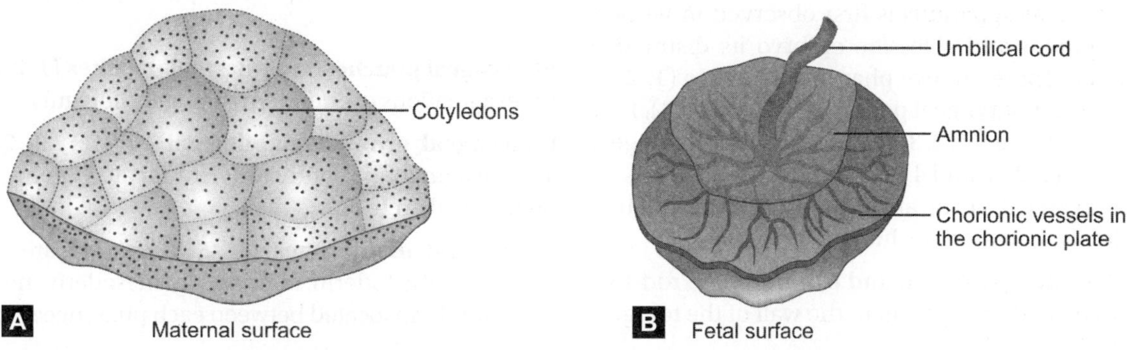

Figs 43A and B Placenta. (A) Maternal surface; (B) Fetal surface

decidual septa projects from this, which devides the maternal surface of the placenta into a number of cotyledons (Fig. 43A)

- Fetal surface—is formed by the chorion frondosum. It is covered by blood vessels, which meet at the base of the umbilical cord (Fig. 43B).

TWINS (FIGS 44A AND B)

- When a mother gives birth to two infants at the same time, they are called twins.
- Twins can either be monozygotic (identical), meaning that they develop from one zygote that splits and forms two embryos, or dizygotic (fraternal) because they develop from two separate eggs that are fertilized by two separate sperm.

MONOZYGOTIC (IDENTICAL) TWINS

Identical twins occur when a single egg is fertilized to form one zygote, which then divides into two separate embryos.

Mechanism: Regarding spontaneous or natural monozygotic twinning, a recent theory postulates that monozygotic twins are formed after a blastocyst essentially collapses, splitting the progenitor cells (those that contain the body's fundamental genetic material) in half, leaving the same genetic material divided into two on opposite sides of the embryo.

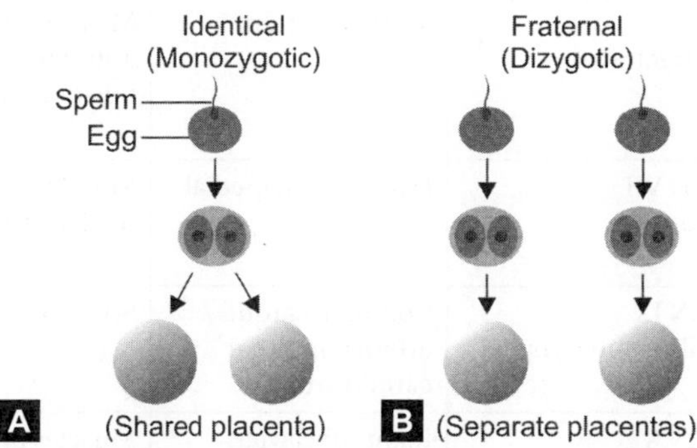

Figs 44A and B (A) Monozygotic twins; (B) Dizygotic twins

Eventually, two separate fetuses develop.

Spontaneous division of the zygote into two embryos is not considered to be a hereditary trait, but rather a spontaneous or random event.

AMNIOCENTESIS

- Amniocentesis (also referred to as amniotic fluid test or AFT) is a medical procedure used in prenatal diagnosis of chromosomal abnormalities and fetal infections.

- A small amount of amniotic fluid, which contains fetal tissues, is sampled from the amnion or amniotic sac surrounding a developing fetus, and the fetal DNA is examined for genetic abnormalities.
- Using this process, the sex of the fetus can also be determined and hence this procedure has some legal restrictions.

PHARYNGEAL ARCHES

- Pharyngeal apparatus consists of the pharyngeal arches, pharyngeal pouches, pharyngeal grooves, and pharyngeal membranes all of which contribute greatly to the formation of the head and neck (Fig. 45).
- The pharyngeal apparatus is first observed in week 4 of development and gives the embryo its distinctive appearance. There are five pharyngeal arches (1, 2, 3, 4, and 6), four pharyngeal pouches (1, 2, 3, and 4), four pharyngeal grooves (1, 2, 3, and 4), and four pharyngeal membranes (1, 2, 3, and 4).
- Pharyngeal arch 5, aortic arch 5 and pharyngeal pouch 5 completely regress in the human.

Pharyngeal arches (1, 2, 3, 4, and 6)—these are rod-like thickening of mesoderm present in the wall of the foregut.

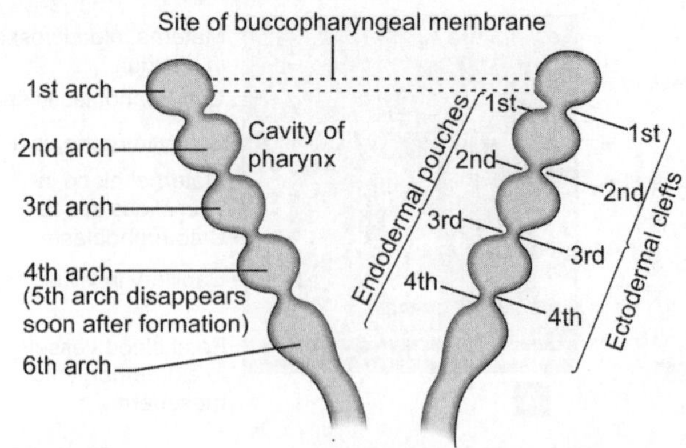

Fig. 45 Development of pharyngeal arches

Pharyngeal pouches/endodermal pouches (1, 2, 3, and 4) are evaginations of endoderm lining the foregut.

Pharyngeal grooves/ectodermal cleft (1, 2, 3, and 4) are invaginations of ectoderm located between each pharyngeal arch.

Pharyngeal membranes (1, 2, 3, and 4) are structures consisting of ectoderm, intervening (mesoderm, neural crest, and endoderm located between each pharyngeal arch.

Arch	*Nerve of arch*	*Artery*	*Muscles*	*Other derivatives*
1	CN V Trigeminal	Maxillary artery	Muscles of mastication, myelohyoid, anterior digastric, tensor veli palatini, tensor tympani	Maxilla, mandible, incus, malleus, temporal bone, palatine bone, vomer, sphenomandibular ligament
2	CN VII Facial	Hyoid and stapedial	Muscles of facial expression, posterior belly of digastric, stylohyoid, stapedius	Stapes, styloid proccss, stylohyoid ligament, lesser horn and upper body of hyoid bone
3	CN IX Glossopharyngeal	Common carotid arteries, internal carotid arteries	Stylopharyngeus	Mesoderm *Neural crest:* Greater horn and lower body of hyoid bone
4	CN X Superior laryngeal nerve	Right subclavian artery, Arch of aorta	Muscles of soft palate, muscles of pharynx	Thyroid cartilage
6	CN X Recurrent laryngeal nerve	Pulmonary arteries Ductus arteriosus	Intrinsic muscles of larynx (except cricothyroid), upper muscles of the esophagus	Cricoid cartilage

Pouch	*Derivatives*
1	Ventral part obliterated by tongue Dorsal part along with dorsal part of 2nd pouch together form epithelial lining of auditory tube and middle ear cavity (tubotympanic recess)
2	Epithelial lining of palatine tonsil crypts Tubotympanic recess
3	Inferior parathyroid gland and thymus
4	Superior parathyroid gland May contribute to thyroid gland

GENETICS

- ✧ Sex chromatin (barr body)*
- ✧ Karyotyping*
- ✧ Sex-linked inheritance*
- ✧ Klinefelter's syndrome*
- ✧ Turner's syndrome*
- ✧ Numerical abnormalities
- ✧ Down's syndrome/mongolism/trisomy 21*
- ✧ Nondisjunction
- ✧ Hemophilia

SEX CHROMATIN (BARR BODY)*

- It is a darkly stained condensed chromatin, located subjacent to the nuclear membrane of somatic cells in normal (XX) females
- It represents inactivated X chromosomes
- During interphase in females, out of two X chromosomes one become highly coiled and the other remains uncoiled (genetically active)
- The coiled, genetically inactive X chromosome is seen as heterochromatic body called sex chromatin/barr body.

Lyon's Hypothesis

- The number of barr bodies in a cell is equal to the total number of X chromosomes minus one
- It is also known as 'n-1 rule' (n-number of X chromosomes).

KARYOTYPING* (FIGS 46A AND B)

- It is a process of arranging the chromosomes of a cell in order to study the complete chromosomal complement of an individual.
- During the arrangement of chromosomes, the longest is placed at the beginning and the shortest at the end.
- The arrangement of chromosomes is known as karyotype.
- By chromosomal banding pattern, one can note certain chromosomal abnormalities such as deletion and translocation, etc.

SEX-LINKED INHERITANCE*

The genes on the X chromosome and Y chromosome is different and the genes on the sex chromosome is called sex linked.

X-linked Inheritance

- X-linked genes are exclusively to X chromosome.
  For example, the gene that codes for color vision is carried on X chromosome only. If female inherits a faulty gene, she is likely to have normal gene (because her other chromosomes are providing normal color vision)
- A female carrying the faulty gene (gene for color blindness), even though she has not color blind may pass the faulty gene on to her children and thus she is

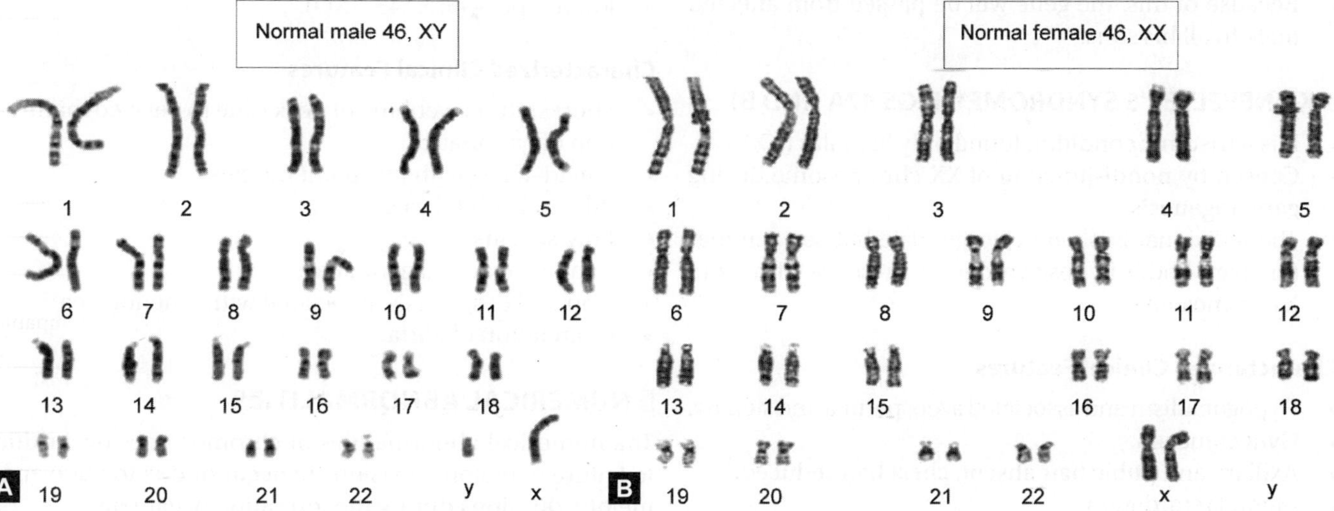

Figs 46A and B Karyotyping—male and female (normal)

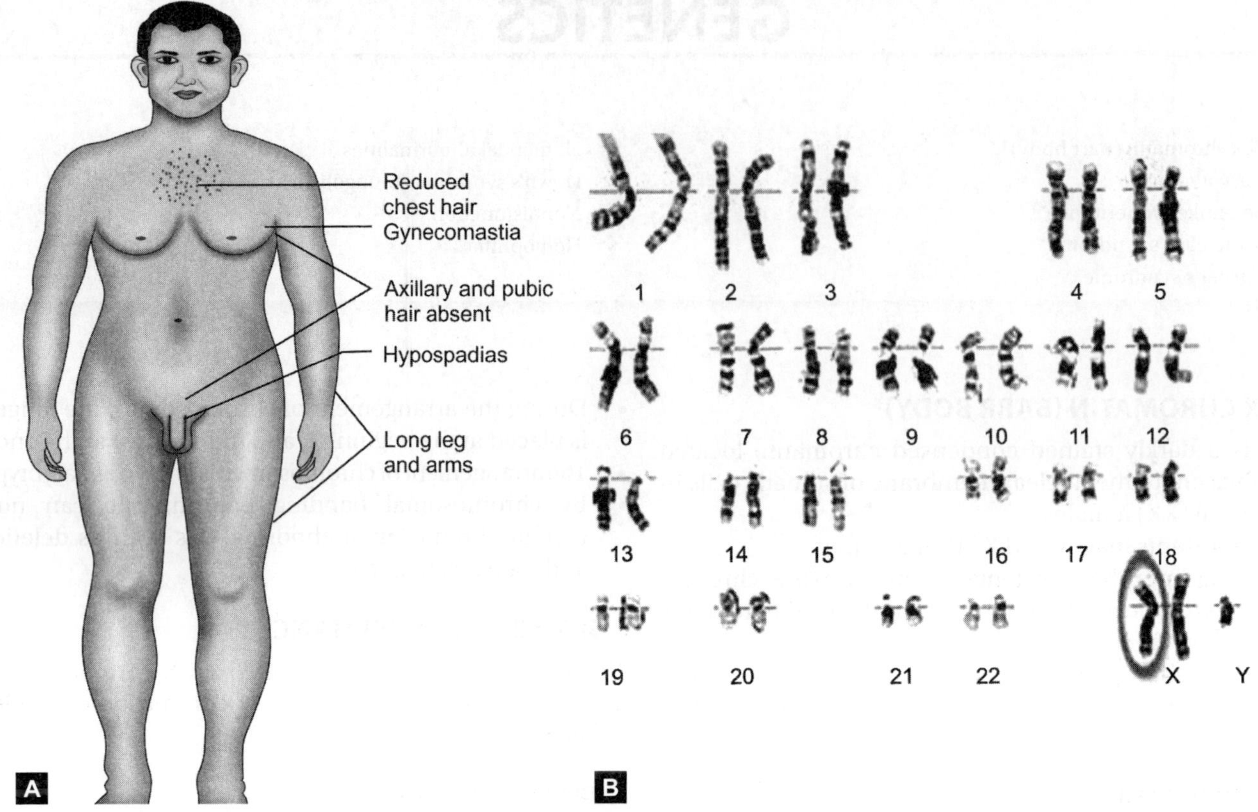

Figs 47A and B Klinefelter's syndrome

called a carrier. If the gene is faulty in male, he will be color blind because he has only one copy of that gene.

Y-linked Inheritance

- Since males have only one Y chromosome, the gene is necessarily unpaired and all the genes present on both the chromosomes will dominates.
- Because of this, the gene will be passed from affected male to all his sons.

KLINEFELTER'S SYNDROME* (FIGS 47A AND B)

- It is a trisomic condition found only in males (XXY)
- Caused by nondisjunction of XX chromosome during gametogenesis.
- The individual is phenotypically male but sex chromatin (barr body) is positive due to presence of a extra X chromosome.

Characterized Clinical Features

- Hypogonadism and associated azoospermia and sterility.
- Gynecomastia.
- Axillary and pubic hair absent, chest hair reduced.
- Mental retardation.
- Length of legs and arms are usually longer than normal.
- Increased gonadotropin level.

TURNER'S SYNDROME* (FIGS 48A AND B)

- It is a monosomic condition found only in females
- It occurs due to loss of one X chromosome, following nondisjunction of X chromosome during meiosis.
- Karyotype—45, X (45 + XO).

Characterized Clinical Features

- Short stature, webbing of neck (due to delayed maturation of lymphatics)
- Shield-chest with pin-point nipples
- Bilateral cubital valgus
- Low-set ears
- Infantile external genitalia
- Gonadal dysgenesis associated with amenorrhea
- Coarctation of aorta.

NUMERICAL ABNORMALITIES

The numerical abnormalities of chromosomes occur due to failure of meiotic divisions to occur or due to abnormal meiotic divisions during the formation of gametes.

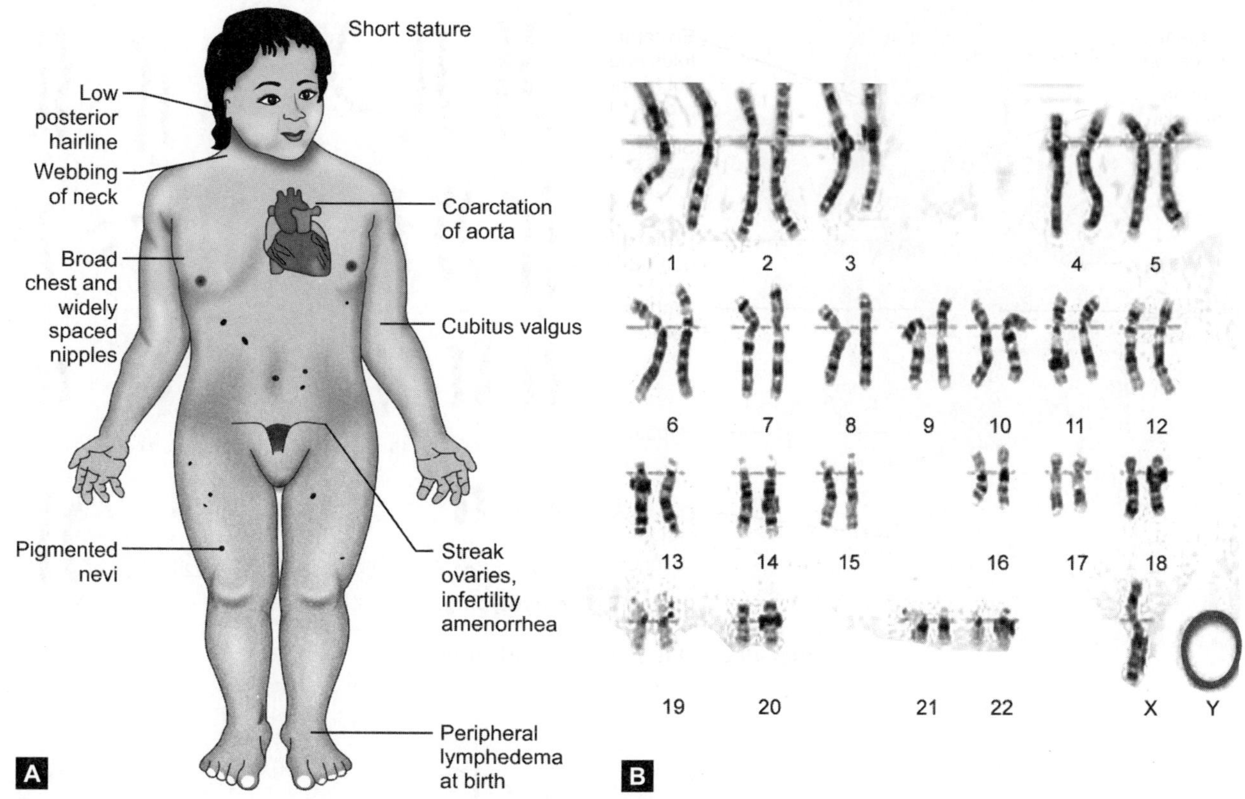

Figs 48A and B Turner's syndrome

Polyploidy

It is a condition in which chromosome number is increased in multiple of haploid (23) set of chromosomes.

- *Triploidy:* The cell contains 69 chromosomes (23 × 3)
- *Tetraploidy:* The cell contains 92 chromosomes (23 × 4).

Aneuploidy

Condition in which, chromosome number is altered by one, e.g. monosomy and trisomy occur due to nondisjunction during meiosis.

DOWN'S SYNDROME/MONGOLISM/ TRISOMY 21*

- In this, three copies of chromosome 21 (Figs 49A and B).
- This disorder is seen in majority of mangoloid babies, hence the name mongolism.

Characterized Clinical Features

- Round face with oblique palpebral fissures and inner-epicanthic folds (i.e. mongoloid facies).
- Small nose with shallow bridge, low set square ears.
- Short and broad hands with single transverse crease in the palm (simian crease) across the base of four fingers.
- Open mouth with long protruding tongue.
- Mental retardation.
- Short stature with hyperflexibility of joints.
- It is associated with low α-fetoprotein levels in amniotic fluid or maternal serum.

NONDISJUNCTION

- Failure of normal migration of chromosome during anaphase of meiosis I.
  Or, failure of migration of chromatids during meisosis II.
- It is caused by faulty spindle formation, radiation, viruses or any autoimmune disease.
- It results in the formation of abnormal gametes.
- Normally each sperm has haploid number.

HEMOPHILIA

- Due to deficiency of a clotting factor VIII.
- It occurs due to mutation of X-linked recessive gene located on the X chromosome and it is responsible for clotting factor VIII.

Characterized Clinical Features

- Excessive bleeding, mainly from gums.
- When bleeding follows trauma, it is characteristically prolonged.
- High bleeding tendency.

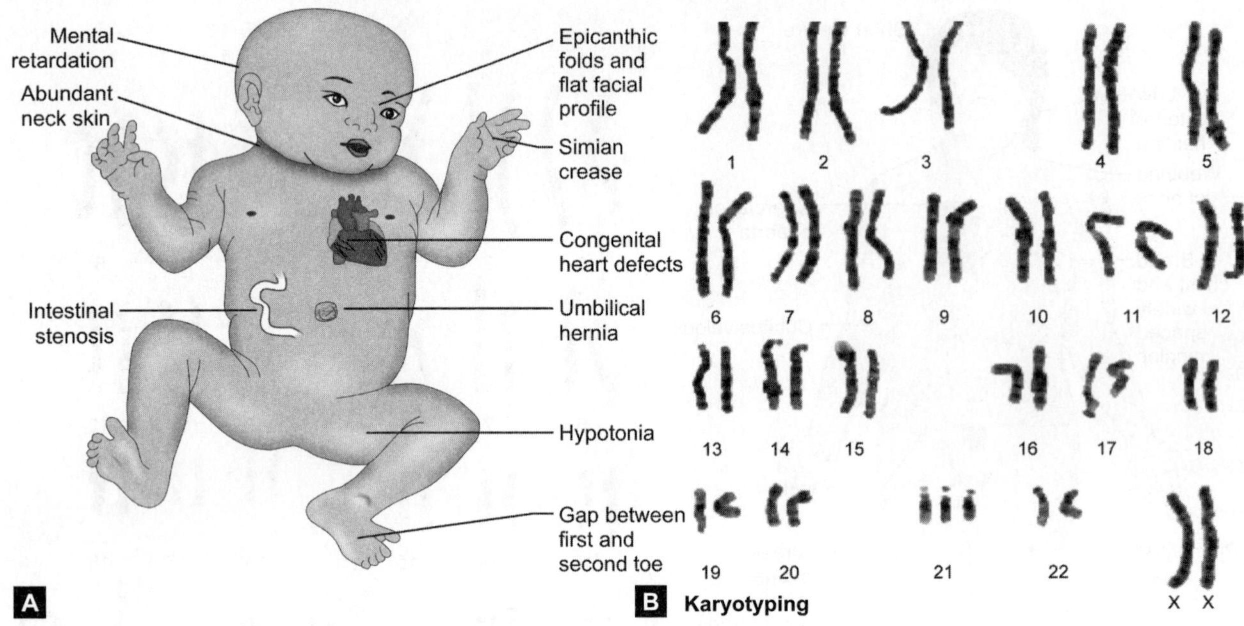

Figs 49A and B Down's syndrome

OSTEOLOGY

UPPER LIMB

CLAVICLE

Parts

- Medial end or sternal end
- Shaft
- Lateral end or acromial end (Fig. 50).

Side Determination

The side of a clavicle can be determined by:

- Holding the bone horizontally
- Flatten end is on the lateral side and the enlarged end is on the medial side
- The convexity of its medial 2/3rd and concavity of its lateral 1/3rd face forwards
- The longitudinal groove in the middle 3rd of shaft facing inferiorly.

Features and Attachments

- Only horizontally placed long bone
- First bone to start ossification and last to complete it.
- Modified long bone with membraneous ossification
- No medullary cavity.

Medial End or Sternal End

It articulates with the clavicular notch of manubrium sterni to form sternoclavicular joint (saddle, synovial joint).

Lateral End or Acromial End

It articulates with the acromion to form acromioclavicular joint (plane, synovial joint).

Shaft

It is curved and has two parts:

1. Medial 2/3rd—it is convex forwards
2. Lateral 1/3rd—it is concave forwards

Medial two-third: 4 Surfaces:

1. Anterior S—clavicular head of pectoralis major (origin)
2. Posterior S—sternohyoid (ori)
3. Superior S—clavicular head of sternocleidomastoid (ori)
4. Inferior S—subclavian groove—subclavius (ins)

Lateral one-third: It has 2 S and 2 B:

Superior S

Inferior S—conoid tubercle, trapezoid line

Anterior B—deltoid tubercle-deltoid (ori)

Posterior B—trapezius (ins).

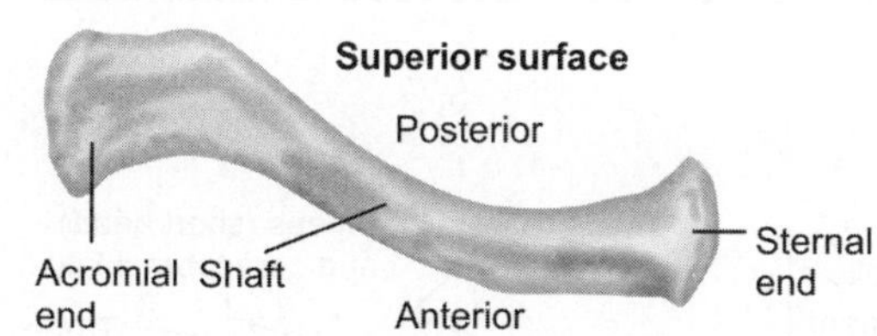

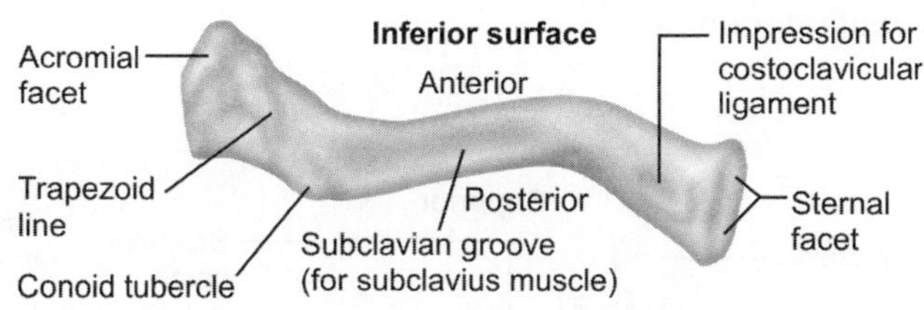

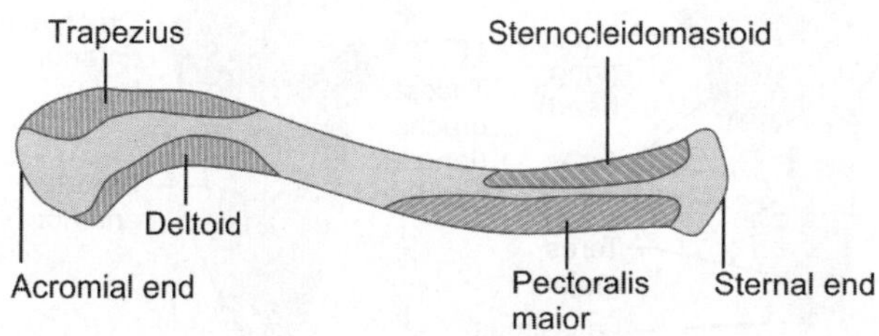

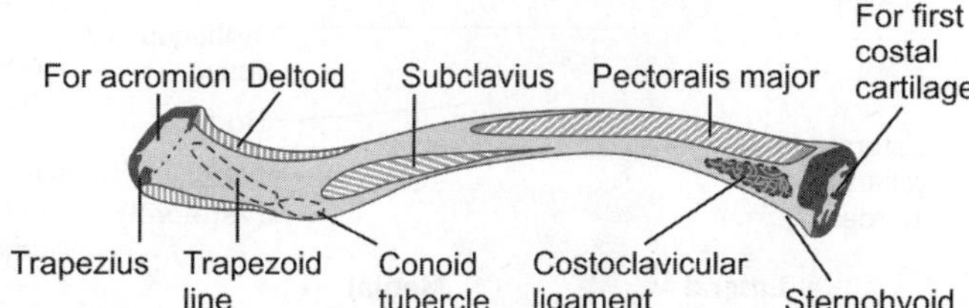

Fig. 50 Clavicle

Clinical Correlation

- *Fracture of clavicle:*
  - Most commonly fractures at the junction of lateral 1/3rd and medial 2/3rd
  - Important reasons for this particular fracture site, (i) is the weakest site, (ii) curvature of clavicle meet at this site, (iii) transmission of forces from clavicle to scapula occurs at this site.

SCAPULA

Parts (Fig. 51A)

A body and three processes:
1. Spinous processes
2. Acromion processes
3. Coracoid processes (Figs 52A and B).

Side Determination

- The glenoid cavity faces laterally, forwards and slightly upward
- Coracoid processes directed forwards
- The shelf-like spinous process is directed posteriorly.

Features and Attachments

Body—2S, 3B and 3 angles

Surfaces

Costal: Subscapular fossa (subscapularis—ori)
Dorsal: Supraspinous fossa (supraspinatus—ori) and infraspinous fossa (infraspinatus—ori)

Borders

Superior: Suprascapular nerve pass through the suprascapular foramen.

Lateral
- Infraglenoid tubercle—long head of triceps
- Upper 2/3rd—teres minor
- Lower 1/3rd—teres major
- Inferior angle—latissimus dorsi.

Medial
- Costal surface (serratus anterior-ins)
- From superior angle to root of spine (levator scapulae-ins)
- Opposite to root of spine (rhomboideus minor—ins)
- From root of spine to inferior angle (rhomboideus major—ins)

Angles

Superior: Lies over 2nd rib

Inferior: Lies over 7th rib (latissimus dorsi—ori)

Lateral: Supraglenoid tubercle—long head of biceps brachii (ori) (Fig. 51B)

Processes	*Attachments—origin*	*Attachments—insertion*
Spinous	Deltoid—lower lip of crest of spine	Upper lip of crest of spine—trapezius
Acromion	Deltoid—lateral border	Medial border—trapezius
Coracoid	• At the tip—short head of biceps brachii and coracobrachialis • Coracoacromial, coracoclavicular, coracohumeral ligament	Upper surface—pectoralis minor

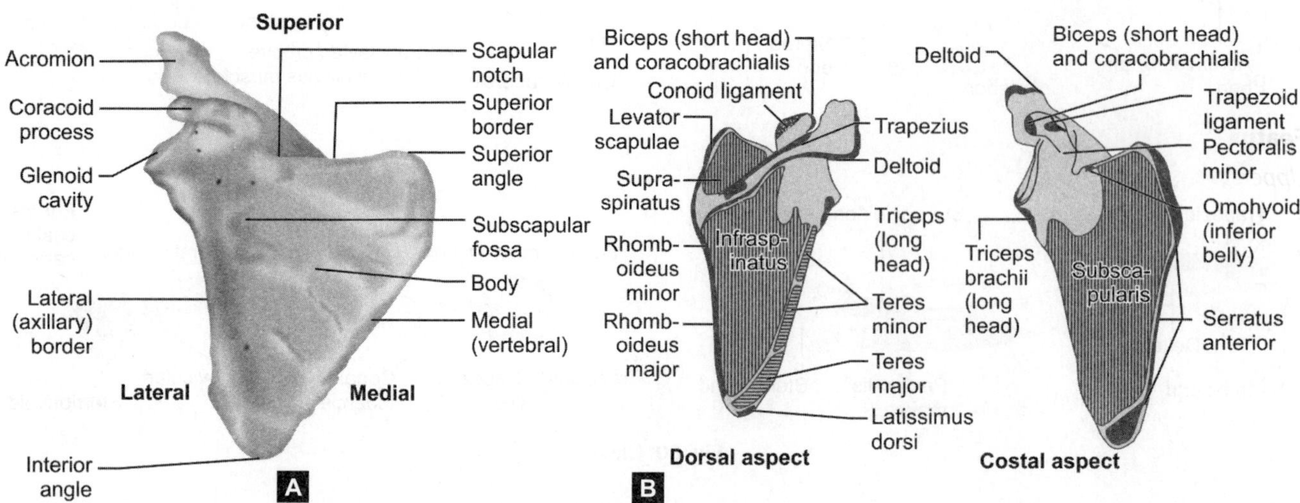

Figs 51A and B Scapula. (A) Anterior surface; (B) Muscle attachments in anterior and posterior surfaces

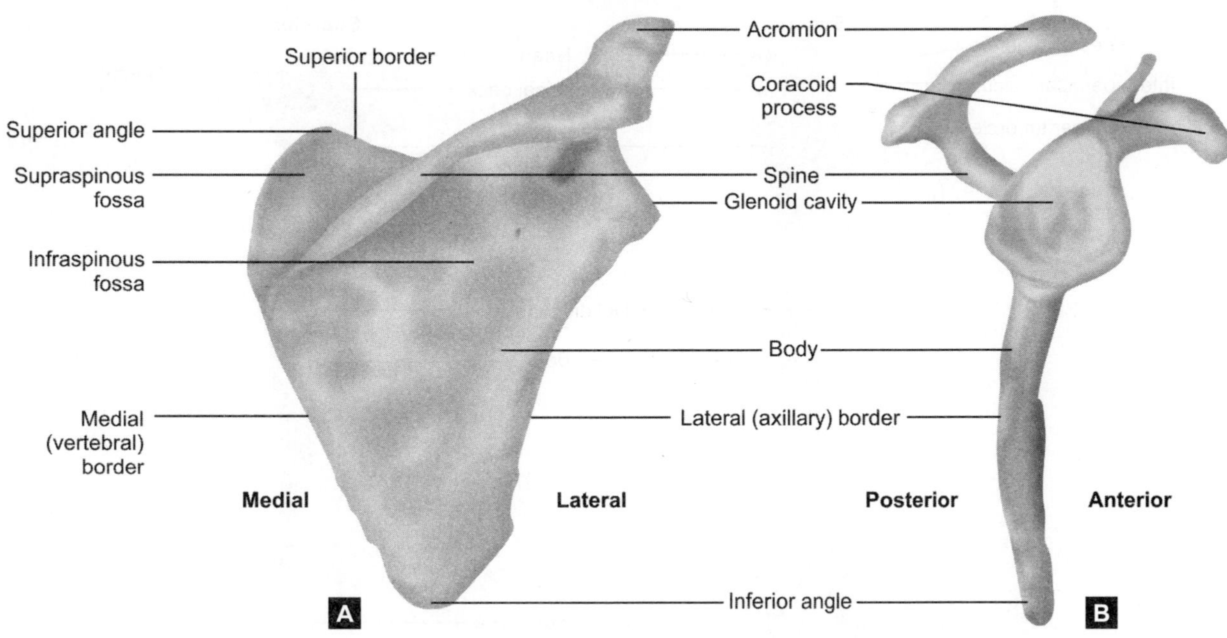

Figs 52A and B Scapula. (A) Posterior view; (B) Lateral border view

HUMERUS

Parts

- Upper end
- Shaft
- Lower end (Figs 53A and B).

Side Determination

- Hold it in vertical position
- Rounded head at the upper end faces medially, backwards and upwards
- Lesser tubercle, greater tubercle and vertical groove (intertubercular groove) at the upper end faces anteriorly.
- The olecranon fossa on the lower flattened end faces posteriorly.

Features and Attachments

Upper End

- Head
- Neck.
  - *Anatomical:* Constriction at the margin of the rounded head and provide attachment to capsular ligament except in inferomedial aspect.
  - *Surgical:* Short constriction in the upper end of the shaft, where it joins with head. Related to axillary nerve and anterior and posterior circumflex humeral artery. It is the common site of fracture.
  - *Morphological:* Junction between diaphysis and epiphysis.
- *Lesser tubercle:* Subscapularis (ins)
- *Greater tubercle:* Upper—supraspinatous, Middle—infraspinatous, Lower—teres minor mneumonic "SIT"
- *Bicipital groove/intertubercular sulcus:* Between greater and lesser tubercle and contain tendon of long head of biceps, anterior circumflex humeral artery.
- *Outer lip—pectoralis major (ins)*
  - Inner lip—teres major (ins)
  - Floor of the groove—latissimus dorsi "*lady* between 2 *majors*".

Shaft: It has three borders and three surfaces:

Borders

Anterior

Medial: Coracobrachialis (ins), supracondylar ridge—pronator teres (ori).

Lateral: Forms lateral supracondylar ridge; upper 2/3rd-brachioradialis (ori); lower 1/3rd—extensor carpi radialis longus (ECRL).

Surfaces

Anterolateral: Deltoid tuberosity—deltoid (ins)

Anteromedial: Nutrient foramen which directed towards the elbow.

Lower part—brachialis (ori)

Posterior: Radial/spiral groove lodges radial nerve and profunda brachi; on the ridge, lateral head of biceps (ori) Below spiral groove—medial head of triceps (ori).

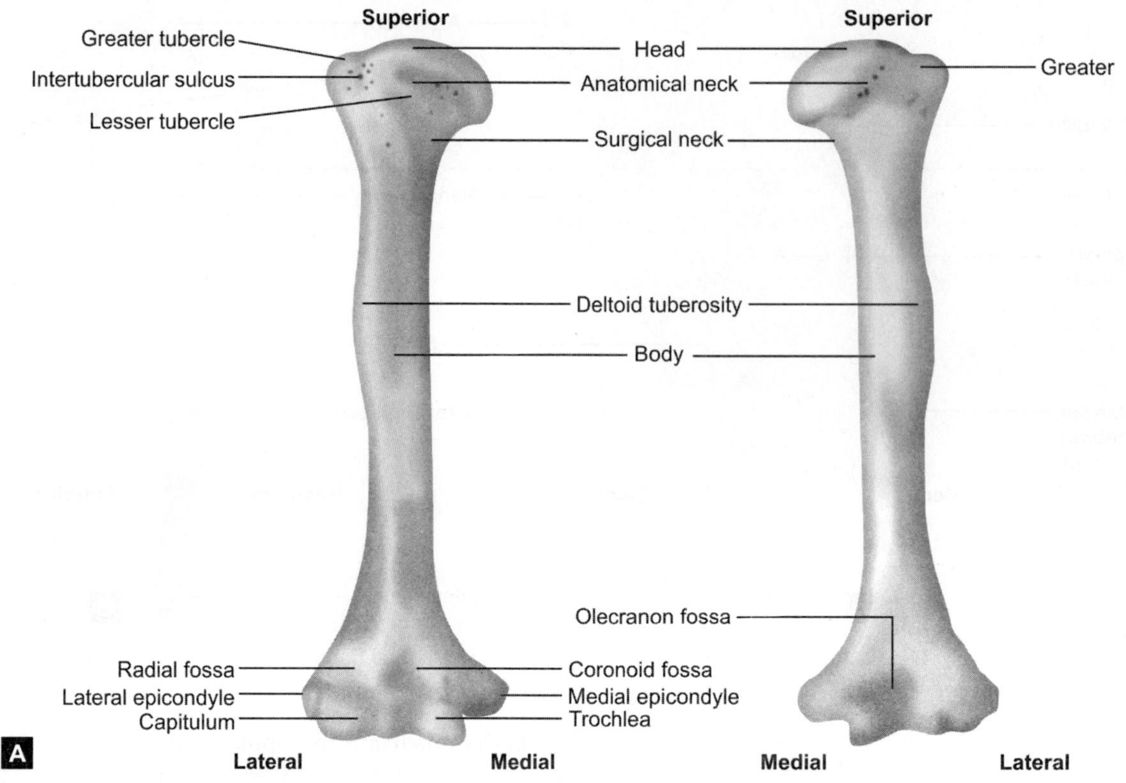

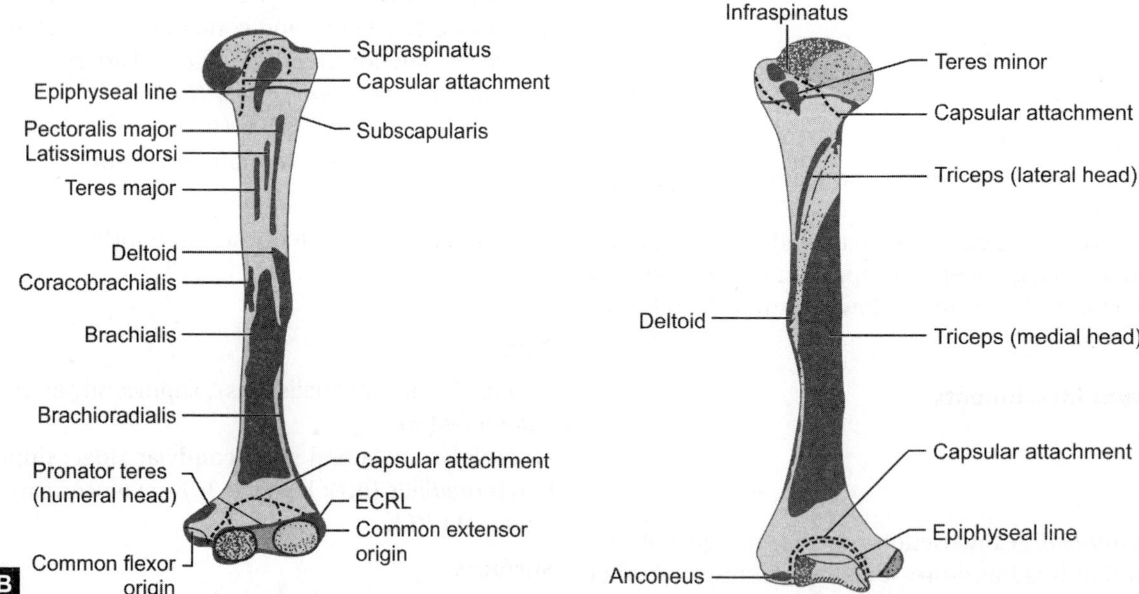

Figs 53A and B Humerus. (A) Anterior and posterior surface; (B) Muscle attachments

Lower End

Articular Part

Capitulum: Lateral rounded convex projection
Trochlea: A medial pulley shaped structure.

Nonarticular Part

Medial epicondyle: Common superficial flexor origin
Lateral epicondyle: Common superficial extensor origin, Anconeus (ori), supinator (ori)
Radial fossa: Lodge head of radius (full flexion)
Coronoid fossa: Lodges coronoid process (full flexion)
Olecranon fossa: Lodges tip of olecranon process of ulna (full extension).

Clinical Correlation

Three nerves closely related to the humerus:
1. *Ulnar nerve:* Behind the medial epicondyle.
2. *Axillary nerve:* Around the surgical neck.
3. *Radial nerve*: Radial/spiral groove.

RADIUS (FIGS 54A AND B)

Parts

- Upper end
- Shaft
- Lower end.

Side Determination

- Keep the bone vertically
- The narrow disk-shaped end (head) is directed upwards.
- The sharpest border (interosseous border) of the shaft is kept medially.
- The styloid process at the lower end is directed laterally and prominent tubercle (Listers tubercle) at the lower end faces dorsally.
- The convexity of shaft faces laterally, and concave anterior surface of shaft faces anteriorly.

Features and Attachmentsx

Upper End

- Head—articulate with capitulum, articulate medially with radial notch of ulna and is encircled by annular ligament
- Neck—supinator (ins)
- Radial tuberosity—biceps brachii (ins).

Shaft

It has three borders and three surfaces:

Borders
Anterior B: FDS (flexor digitorum superficialis)—origin
Medial (interosseous) B: Lower 3/4th—interosseous membrane (ori), pronator quadratus (ins)
Posterior B

Surfaces
Anterior S: Nutrient foramen; upper 2/3rd—FPL flexor pollicis longus (ori).
Lower 1/4th—pronator quadratus (ins).
Posterior S: APL—abductor pollicis longus (ori); EPB—extensor pollicis brevis (ori).
Lateral S: Ridge—pronator teres (ins).

Lower End

Widest part and presents five surfaces:
Lateral: Base of styloid process—brachioradialis (ins)
Medial: Bears ulnar notch for forming inferior radioulnar joint.
Inferior:
- Lateral triangular area—for articulation with scaphoid
- Medial quadrangular area—for articulation with lunate.

Posterior: Dorsal tubercle/listers tubercle—medially lodges the tendon of extensor pollicis longus (EPL). Laterally lodges the tendon of extensor carpi radialis longus (ECRL), extensor carpi radialis brevis (ECRB).
Anterior: Lower end—five surfaces are: (i) lateral; (ii) medial; (iii) inferior; (iv) posterior; (v) anterior.

Clinical Correlation

It is the weight-bearing bone of forearm; hence very important.

In fracture at the distal end of radius (Colles' fracture) the distal fragment is displaced backwards and upwards.

ULNA

Parts

- Upper end
- Shaft
- lower end (head).

Side Determination

- Keep the bone vertically
- The broad hook like end is directed upwards
- The sharp crest-like interosseous border of shaft is directed laterally
- The concavity of the hook-like upper end and the coronoid process are facing forwards.

Features and Attachments

Upper End

Two processes, two articular notches
Olecranon process: 6 Surface:
Superior: Triceps (ins)

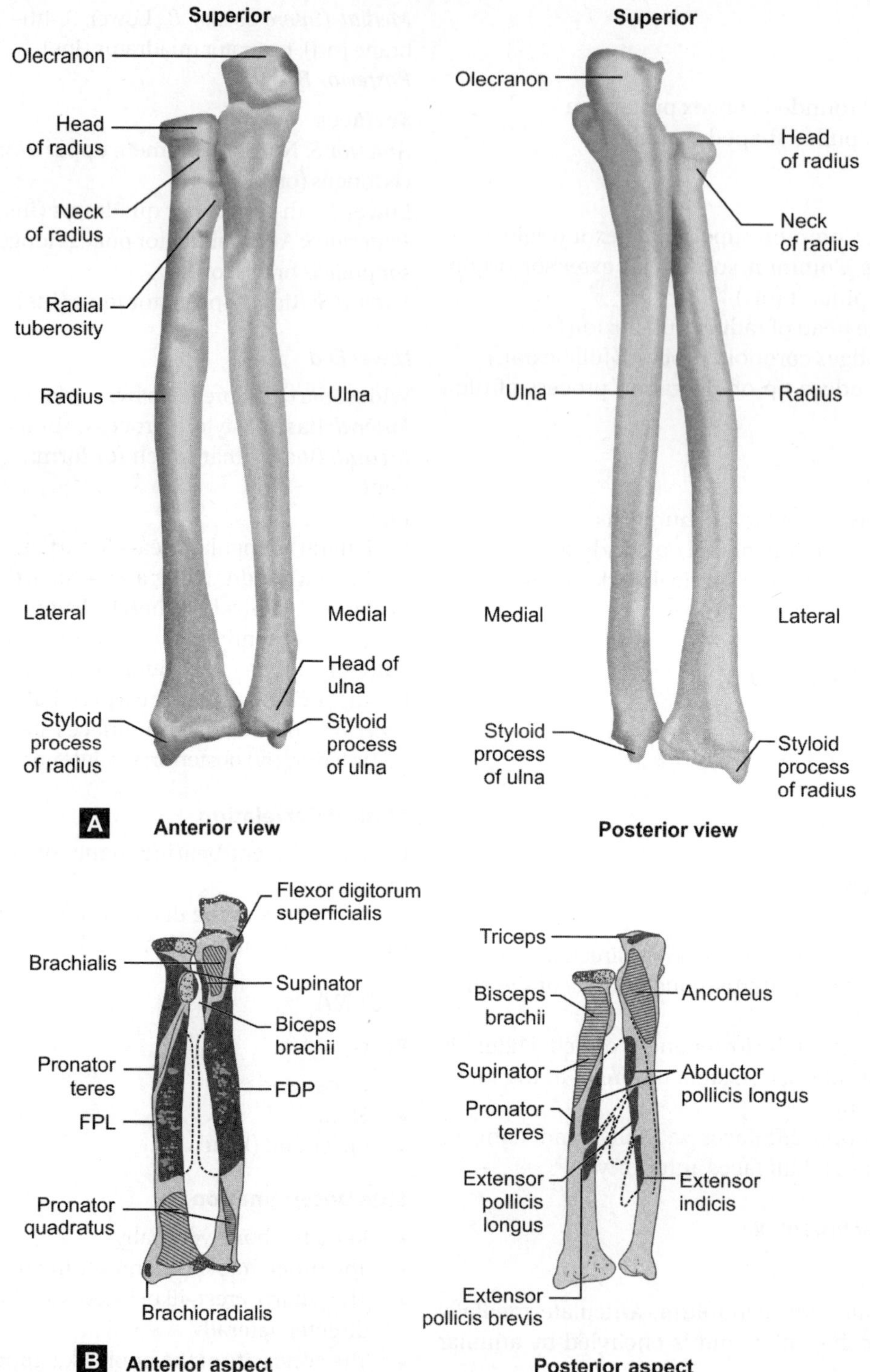

Figs 54A and B Radius and ulna. (A) Anterior and posterior surface; (B) Muscle attachments

Anterior; Posterior; Inferior; Lateral: Anconeus (ins)
Medial: FDP—flexor digitorum profundus (ori); FCU—flexor carpi ulnaris (ori).

Processes
Coronoid process: 4 Surface and 2 Borders
Superior S
Lateral S
Medial S: FDP—flexor digitorum profundus (ori)
Anterior S: Brachialis (ins)
Medial B: FDS—flexor digitorum superficialis (ori); PT—pronator teres (ori)
Lateral B: FPL—flexor pollicis longus (ori)
Notches (articular surface).

Trochlear notch: 'C' shaped (semilunar) and articulates with the trochlea of humerus.

Radial notch: Articulates with head of radius to form the superior radioulnar joint.

Shaft

3 Borders and 3 Surfaces

Borders
Lateral (interosseous): Interosseous membrane (ori).
Anterior: Upper 3/4th—FDP—flexor digitorum profundus (ori).
Posterior: FDP (ori), FCU—flexor carpi ulnaris (ori), ECU—extensor carpi ulnaris (ori).

Surfaces
Anterior: Upper 2/3rd—FDP (ori), lower 1/4th—PQ pronator quadratus (ori)
Medial: Upper 3/4th—FDP (ori)
Posterior: Above oblique line—anconeus (ins); upper-APL—abductor pollicis longus (ori); middle-EPL—extensor pollicis longus (ori); lower—extensor indicis (ori).

Lower End
Head: Presents a convex articular surface on its lateral side for articulation with the ulnar notch of radius to form inferior radioulnar joint
Styloid process: Projects downward from the posteromedial aspect of head of ulna.

Clinical Correlation

The fracture of upper 3rd of shaft of ulna with dislocation of radial head at superior radioulnar joint is called monteggia fracture dislocation.

CARPAL BONES (FIGS 55A AND B)

Wrist contains 8 carpal bones (Fig. 56).

Proximal row: Scaphoid (boat-shaped), Lunate (crescentric), Triquetral (pyramidal shaped), Pisiform (pea-shaped and articulate with triquetral at its palmar surface).

Distal row: Trapezium (quadrilateral in shape), trapezoid (shoe-shaped), capitates (largest carpal bone), hamate (wedge-shaped).

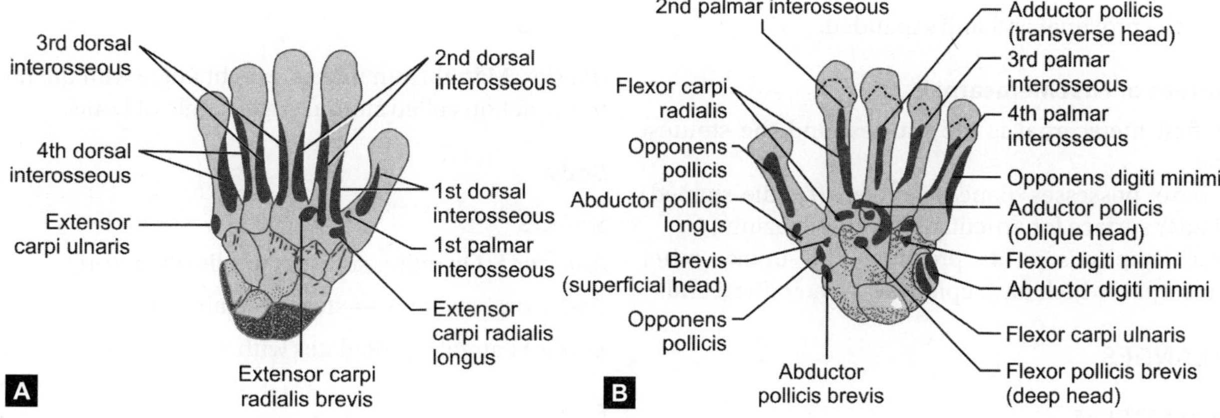

Figs 55A and B Carpals and metacarpals attachments. (A) Dorsal aspect; (B) Palmar aspect

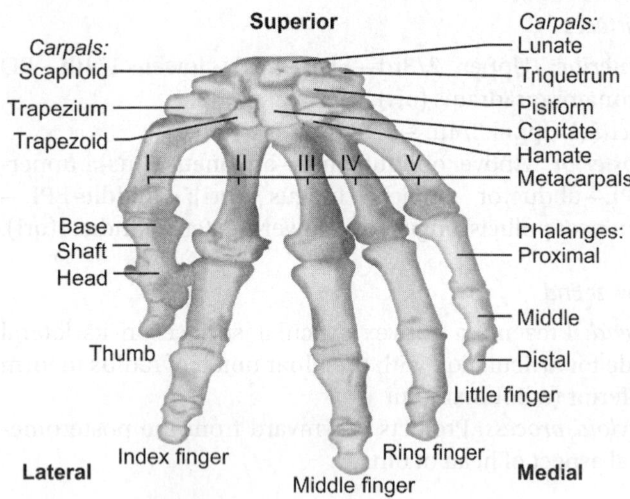

Fig. 56 Wrist bones and phalanges

Clinical Correlation

Scaphoid fracture: Fracture of scaphoid is the most common fracture and usually occurs due to fall on the outstretched hand. Clinically, it presents as the tenderness in the anatomical box.

METACARPAL BONES

Parts and Features

Head: It is at distal end and rounded.

Shaft: Extends between head and base, it is concave on palmar aspects.

Base: It is the proximal end and expanded.

Peculiarities of First Metacarpal

- The first metacarpal is the shortest and the stoutest bone.
- Its base possesses concavoconvex (saddle-shaped) articular surface for articulation with trapezium.
- It has epiphysis at its proximal end unlike other metacarpals which have epiphysis at their distal end.

PHALANGES

Parts and Features

Base: It has concave oral facet for articulation with the heads of metacarpals.

Shaft: It tapers towards head:
- Dorsal surface is convex from side to side
- Palmar surface is flat from side to side but gently concave in the long axis.

Head: The head proximal and middle phalanges are pulley shaped
- The head of distal phalanges is nonarticular and has rough horseshoe-shaped tuberosity.

THORAX

STERNUM

It is dagger-shaped, which increases slightly during inspiration and decreases during expiration.

Parts

Upper part: Manubrium sterni

Middle part: Body

Lower part: Xiphoid process.

Features and Attachments

Manubrium: Lies opposite to 3rd and 4th thoracic vertebrae.

2 Surfaces

Anterior S: Each side—sternal head of sternocleidomastoid (ori) and pectoralis major (ori)
Posterior S

4 Borders

Superior: Suprasternal notch/jugular notch.

2 Lateral

Inferior: Manubrium makes a slight angle with the body at this junction called sternal angle/angle of Louis.

Body

Surfaces

Anterior S: On either side, pectoralis major (ori).

Posterior: Lower part—sternocostalis (ori).

Border: Lateral—articulates with 2nd–7th costal cartilage.

Ends

Upper: Articulates with the manubrium at the sternal angle to form the manubriosternal joint.

Lower: Articulates with the xiphoid process to form the xiphisternal joint.

Xiphoid Process

Surfaces

Anterior S: Rectus abdominis (ins); aponeurosis of external oblique (ins).

Posteriors: Diaphragm (ori).

Lateral borders: IOA—internal oblique abdominis and transverse abdominis.

Lower end: Linea alba.

Clinical Correlation

- Site for bone marrow aspiration in adults.
- *Funnel chest (pectus excavatum):* It is an abnormal shape of thoracic cage in which chest is compressed anteroposteriorly and sternum is pushed backward
- *Pigeon chest/pectus carinatum:* It is an abnormal shape of thoracic cage in which chest is compressed side to side and sternum pushed forward and backward like a keel of a boat
- *Sternal angle:* It is an important landmark for counting ribs, check tracheal bifurcation.

RIBS

According to Features

- Typical ribs—3rd-9th
- Atypical ribs—1st, 2nd, 10th, 11th, 12th.

According to Relation with Sternum

- True ribs—1st-7th
- False ribs—8th-12th.

According to Articulation

- Vertebrosternal ribs—1st-7th
- Vertebrochondral ribs—8th-10th
- Vertebral (floating) ribs—11th and 12th.

TYPICAL RIBS

Parts

- Anterior (costal) end
- Shaft
- Posterior end.

Anatomical Position and Side Determination

- Holding it in such a way that its posterior end having head, neck and tubercle is directed posteriorly
- Its concavity faces medially and its sharp border is directed inferiorly
- Posterior end is higher and nearer the median plane than the anterior end.

Features and Attachments

Anterior End

Shaft: The costal groove present in the lower border holds: (i) intercostal vein; (ii) intercostal artery; (iii) intercostal nerve (from above downwards).

2 Borders: Superior, inferior.

2 Surfaces: External S, internal S.

Posterior end: Head, lower larger facet, upper smaller facet, neck, tubercle.

ATYPICAL RIB

1st RIB

Parts

Anterior end, shaft and posterior end.

Side Determination

- Its larger end is directed anteriorly and its smaller end is directed posteriorly
- The surface of its shaft having two grooves, is separated by a ridge is directed superiorly
- Its concave border is directed inwards and its convex border directed outwards.

Distinguishing Features

- Shortest rib
- No costal groove
- Single facet on head.

Features and Attachments

- Anterior end
- Shaft.

2 Borders: Inner—scalene tubercle—scalenus anterior (ins), Outer—serratus anterior (ori)

2 Surfaces: Superior—2 grooves, Anterior groove—lodges subclavian vein.

Posterior groove lodges the subclavian artery and lower trunk of brachial plexus.

Scalenus anterior (ins); subclavius (ins);

Inferior S

Posterior End

- *Head*
- *Neck:* The following structures form anterior relations of neck from medial to lateral side:
  - Sympathetic chain
  - First posterior intercostal vein
  - Superior intercostal artery
  - Ventral ramus of first thoracic nerve
  - Lower trunk of brachial plexus

Tubercle

LOWER LIMB

HIP BONE

Parts (Figs 57A and B)

- Ilium
- Ischium
- Pubis.

Ilium (Figs 57 and 58)

2 Ends

Upper end: Anterosuperior iliac spine—inguinal ligament, sartorius (ori)

Posterosuperior iliac spine—sacrotuberous ligament.

Iliac crest: Divided into ventral 2/3rd and dorsal 1/3rd segment

- *Ventral segment:*
  Inner lip
  Anterior 2/3rd—transverse abdominis (ori)
  Posterior 1/3rd—quadratus lumborum

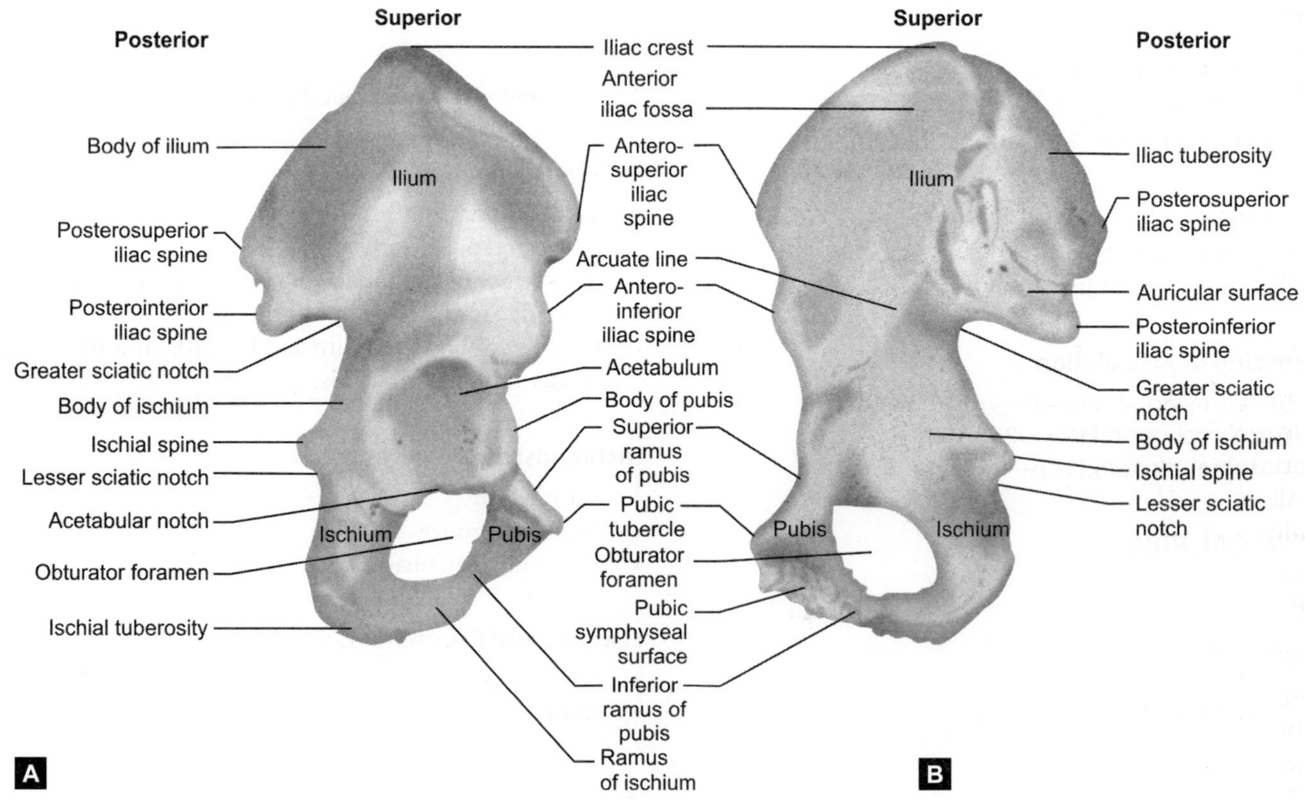

Figs 57A and B Hip bone. (A) Lateral view; (B) Medial view

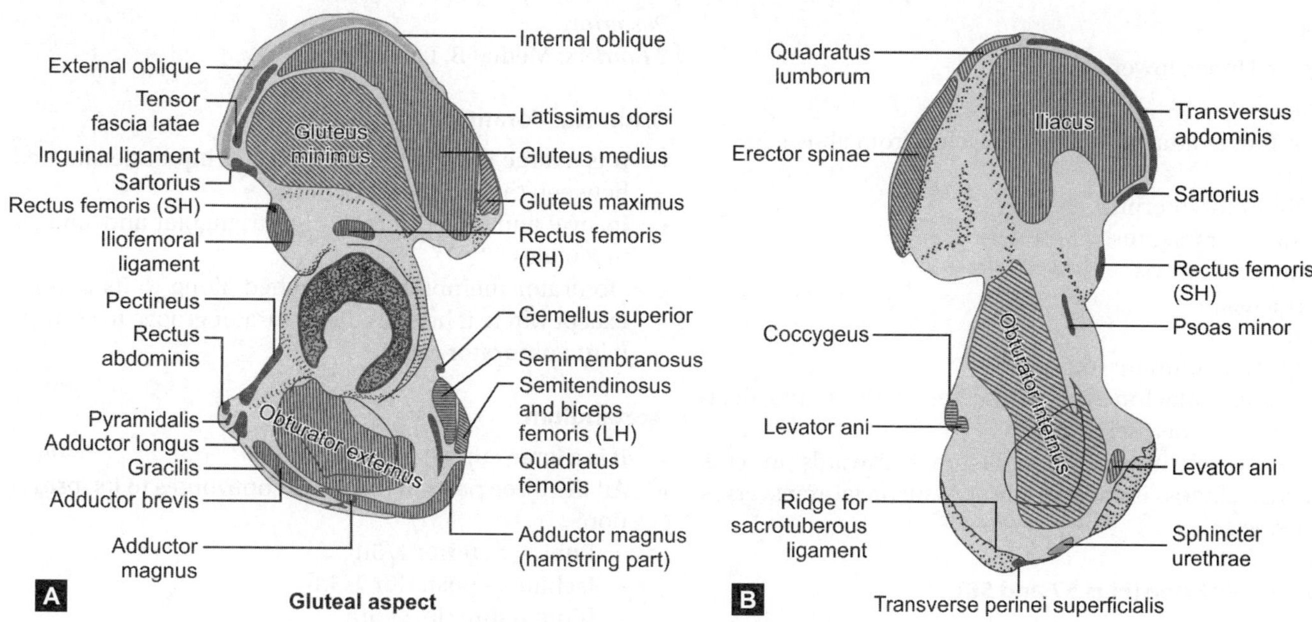

Figs 58A and B Hip bone—muscle attachments

Intermediate—internal oblique abdominis (ori)
Outer lip-tubercle of iliac crest—tensor fascia latae (ori), Lattissimus dorsi (ori), external oblique abdominis (ins)

- *Dorsal segment:* Gluteus maximus (ori).

Lower end: 3 Borders

Anterior: Anterior inferior iliac spine—straight head of rectus femoris (ori) and iliofemoral ligament (ori).

Posterior: Piriformis (ori). The dorsal aspect of ischial spine is crossed from lateral to medial side by—pudendal nerve, internal pudendal vessels, nerve to obturator internus (PIN).

Medial: Arcuate line—psoas minor (ins).

3 Surfaces

Gluteal: Divided into 4 areas by 3 gluteal line—posterior, anterior and inferior.

All are radiating from the upper margin of greater sciatic notch.

Posterior gluteal line: It meets the dorsal segment of iliac crest.

Anterior gluteal line: Meets the iliac crest.

Inferior gluteal line: Meets the anteroinferior iliac spine

- Behind the posterior gluteal line—gluteus maximus (ori)
- Between anterior and posterior gluteal line—gluteus medius (ori)
- Between anterior and inferior gluteal line—gluteus minimus (ori).

Iliac fossa: Transmits the nutrient artery.

Sacropelvic: Situated behind the medial border, on the inner side of ilium and it divided into two parts:

1. *Sacral part:*
   Iliac tuberosity: It is a rough area below and dorsal part of iliac crest.
   Auricular surface: Ear-shaped articular surface articulates with sacrum to form sacroiliac joint.
2. *Pelvic part:* Smooth and continuous with pelvic surface of the ischium—obturator internus (ori).

Ischium (Figs 57 and 58)

It is the thick posteroinferior part of hip bone and consist of body and ramus.

Body

2 Ends: Upper

Lower—ischial tuberosity—upper lateral quadrilateral area—semimembranosus (ori).

- Lower medial quadrilateral area—semitendinosus (ori) and long head of femoris (ori)
- Lower triangular area—adductor magnus (ori).

Surfaces

Femoral: Obturator internus (ori), quadratus femoris (ori)

Dorsal: Pelvic

Borders: Anterior, lateral, posterior

Lesser sciatic notch: Transmit:

- Obturator internus
- Pudendal nerve
- Nerve to obturator internus
- Internal pudendal vessels.

Ramus

Borders: Upper, lower.

Surfaces

Outer: Linear attachment to 4 muscles (from above downwards)

- Obturator internus
- Adductor magnus
- Adductor brevis
- Gracilis.

Inner:

- Upper—obturator internus
- Middle—attachment to sphincter urethrae and deep tranversus perinei muscle
- Lower—attachments from before backwards to crus penis, clitoris, ischiocavernosus, superficial transversus perinei.

Pubis/Pubic Bone (Figs 57 and 58)

It consists of three parts:

1. Body
2. Superior ramus
3. Inferior ramus.

Body

Pubic crest: It is the thickened upper border of the body of pubis

Pubic tubercle: Lateral upper border of pubic crest projects forward to form tubercle.

Surfaces: Anterior—angle between pubic crest and pubic symphysis—adductor longus (ori)

Lower part—gracilis (ori), adductor brevis (ori), obturator externus (ori)/posterior; medial (symphyseal).

Superior Ramus of Pubis

3 Borders:

Posterior: Pectineal line:

- Medial part from before backwards—lacunar ligament, reflected part of inguinal ligament, conjoint tendon, fascia transversalis
- Lateral part from behind forwards—pectineal ligament, pectineus muscle, pectineus fascia, pectoralis minor

Anterior (obturator crest); *inferior*

3 Surfaces: Pectineal—pectineus (ori); Pelvic; Obturator—obturator nerve and vessels traverse through obturator groove.

Inferior Ramus of Pubis

2 Surfaces

Anterior S: From medial to lateral—gracilis (ori), adductor brevis (ori), obturator externus (ori), adductor magnus (ori)

Posterior

2 Borders: Medial B, Lateral B

Obturator Foramen

- It is a large gap in the lower part of hip bone situated between the pubis and ischium
- Its oval and larger in males but triangular and smaller in females
- Obturator membrane is attached along to its margin except where it bridges the obturator groove to convert it into obturator canal.

Acetabulum

- It is a large cup-shaped cavity
- All the three parts of hip bone contributes to its formation:
  - Pubis—anterior 1/5th
  - Ischium—posterior 2/5th
  - Ilium—superior 2/5th
- It receives the head of femur to form the hip joint
- The acetabulum presents a horseshoe-shaped articular surface, in its periphery and nonarticular area in its central part, the acetabular fossa.
- The acetabular fossa is filled with a pad of fat.

BONY PELVIS

It is formed by two hip bones in front and on both sides, and sacrum and coccyx behind.

Pelvic Inlet (Pelvic Brim)

Posteriorly—sacral promontory

Sides—linea terminalis (anterior margin of ala of sacrum, arcuate line of ilium, iliopubic eminence, pectineal line, pubic crest)

Anteriorly—pubis symphysis

Pelvic outlet: Bounded by:

- Front—inferior pubic ligament; Behind—tip of coccyx; Anterolaterally—ischiopubic ramus
- Laterally—ischial tuberosities; Posterolaterally—sacrotuberous ligament.

Femur (Figs 59A and B)

It is the longest bone of the body.

Parts

- Upper end
- Shaft
- Lower end.

Difference between male and female pelvis		
Features	*Male*	*Female*
• Shape of inlet of pelvis	• Heart-shaped	• Transversely oval or round
• Greater sciatic notch	• Long, pointed, deep and 'U' shaped	• Wider, rounded and shallow
• Subpubic angle	• 50–70 degree, angular	• 80–100 degrees, rounded
• Ishiopubic ramus	• Everted and markedly thick	• Not everted, smooth and thin
• Ischial tuberosity	• Inverted and not so wide apart	• Everted and wider part
• Curvature of sacrum	• Sharp and uniformly concave	• Upper part is flat • Lower part is sharply curved forwards
• Sacral promontary	• More projecting inwards	• Less projecting inwards
• Auricular surface	• Extend up to 2½–3 part	• Extend up to 2–2½ pieces
• Preauricular sulcus	• Absent	

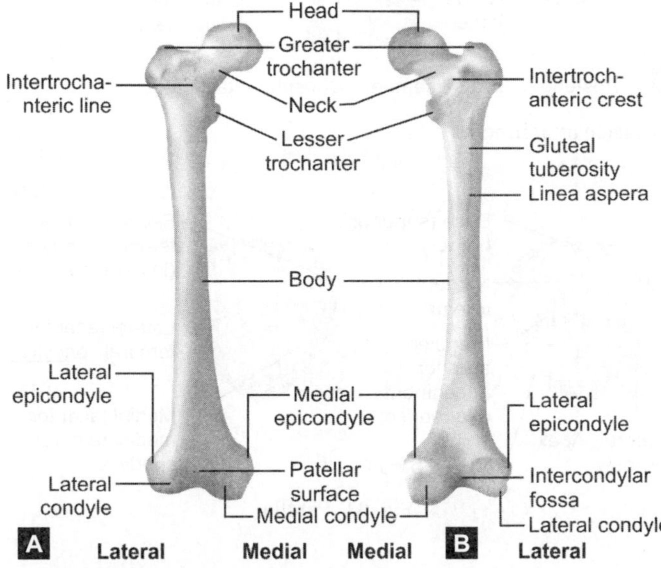

Figs 59A and B Femur. (A) Anterior view; (B) Posterior view

Side Determination

- Holding the bone vertically
- Its head faces upward, medially, and slightly forward
- Long axis of shaft directed downwards and medially with convexity of shaft facing anteriorly
- Lower surface of both the condyles are in the same horizontal plane.

Features and Attachments (Figs 60A and B)

Upper End

- *Head:* Fovea/pit-attachment of ligament of head of femur
- *Neck:*
  Intertrochanteric line: (a) Capsule of hip joint, (b) Iliofemoral ligament, (c) Vastus lateralis (ori), (d) Vastus medialis (ori)
  Intertrochanteric line: It continuous downward and medially below the lesser trochanter on the posterior aspect of femur as spiral line.
- *Greater trochanter:*
  Surfaces: Anterior—gluteus minimus (ins); Lateral-ridge—gluteus medius (ins);
  Medial: Trochanteric fossa—obturator externus (ins); Superior border—piriformis (ins)
- *Lesser trochanter:* Psoas major (ins); iliacus (ins)

Intertrochanteric crest: It presents a rounded tubercle near the middle called quadrate tubercle-quadratus femoris (ins).

Shaft

3 Borders

- Medial
- Lateral
- Posterior—linea aspera-inner lip-vastus medialis (ori), adductor longus (ins).

Linea aspera-outer lip-vastus lateralis (ori); adductor magnus (ins).

4 Surfaces

Medial, Lateral—upper 3/4th—vastus intermedius (ori),
Anterior—upper 3/4th—vastus intermedius (ori).
Upper posterior: From lateral to medial side-gluteal tuberosity-gluteus maximus (ins), adductor magnus (ins), adductor brevis (ins), pectineus (ins), iliacus (ins), vastus medialis (ins)
Lower posterior/popliteal surface: Plantaris (ori), medial head of gastrocnemius (ori)

Lower End

It is 'V' shaped.

Medial condyle: Medial epicondyle—medial head of gastrocnemius (ori); adductor tubercle—adductor magnus (ins).

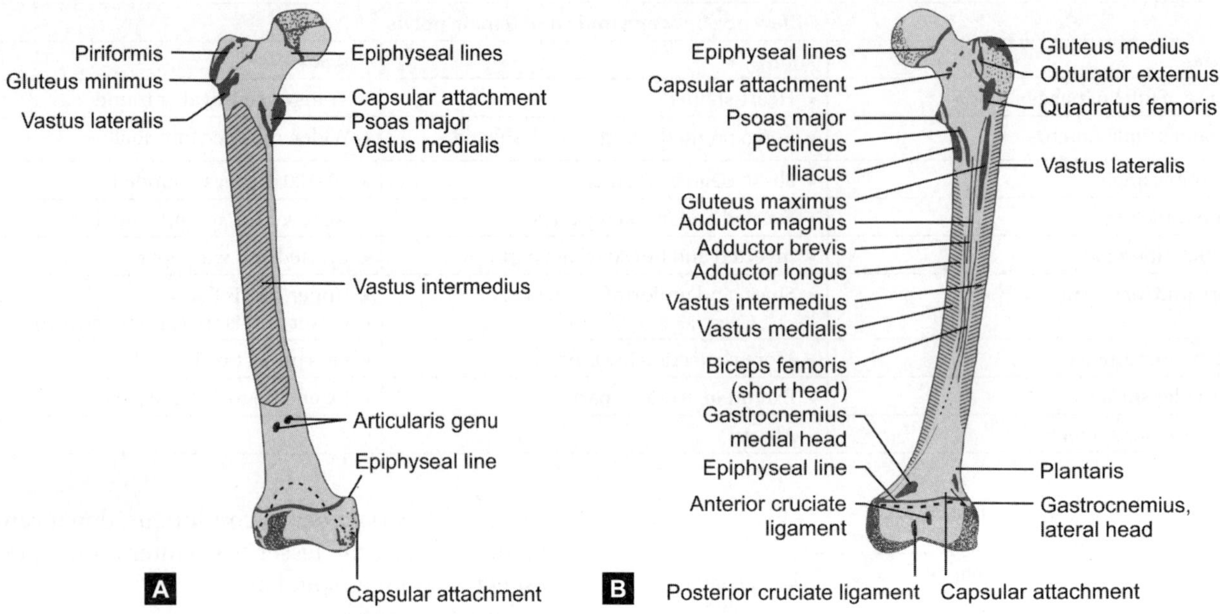

Figs 60A and B Femur—muscle attachments

Lateral condyle: Lateral epicondyle—lateral head of gastrocnemius (ori), popliteus (ori).

Intercondylar fossa: Give attachment to cruciate ligaments. *Medial wall; lateral wall*

Clinical Correlation

- The fracture of neck of femur is very common in elderly women due to osteoporotic changes in the neck.
- If the fracture affects the retinacular vessels—chief source of blood supply to the head are injured
- It will lead to delayed healing or nonunion of the fracture, or even avascular necrosis of the head of femur.

PATELLA (FIG. 61)

- It is the largest sesamoid bone, found in the tendon of quadriceps femoris.
- It is flattened and triangular bone
- Features and attachments
- Apex—ligamentum patella (ori)
- *3 Borders:*
  - *Superior*—Anterior part—rectus femoris (ins); Posterior part—vastus intermedius (ins)
  - *Lateral:* Vastus lateralis (ins)
  - *Medial:* Vastus medialis (ins)
- *2 Surfaces:* Anterior, posterior.

Clinical Correlation

- *Dislocation of patella:* It has a natural tendency to dislocate laterally due to upward and lateral pull by the quadriceps.

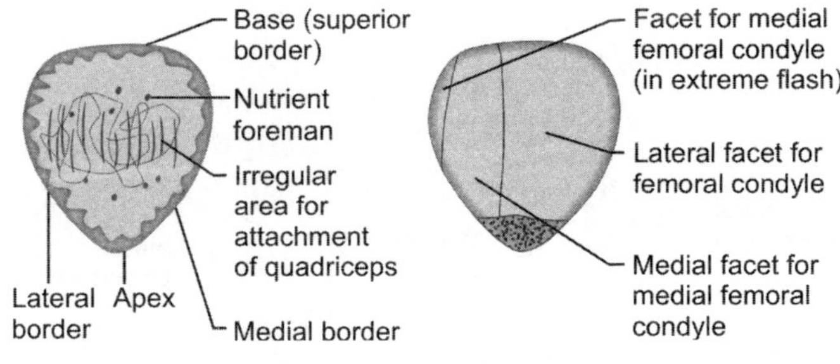

Fig. 61 Patella

- *Fracture of patella:*
  - A direct blow on the patella causes fractures it into two or more pieces
  - A sudden and forceful contraction of quadriceps femoris causes a transverse fracture of the patella.

TIBIA/SHIN BONE (FIGS 62A AND B)

Parts

Upper end, shaft, lower end.

Side Determination

- Holding the bone vertically
- Its expanded end with condyles faces upwards
- Its tibial tuberosity faces anteriorly
- Medial malleolus is on the medial side
- Superior surface of the upper end lies in a horizontal plane.

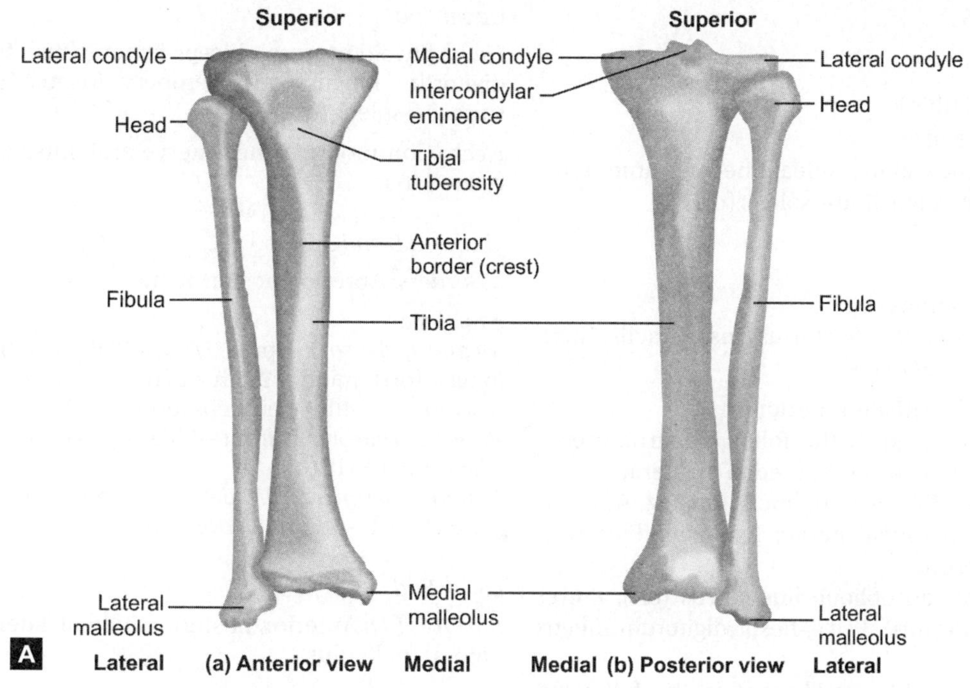

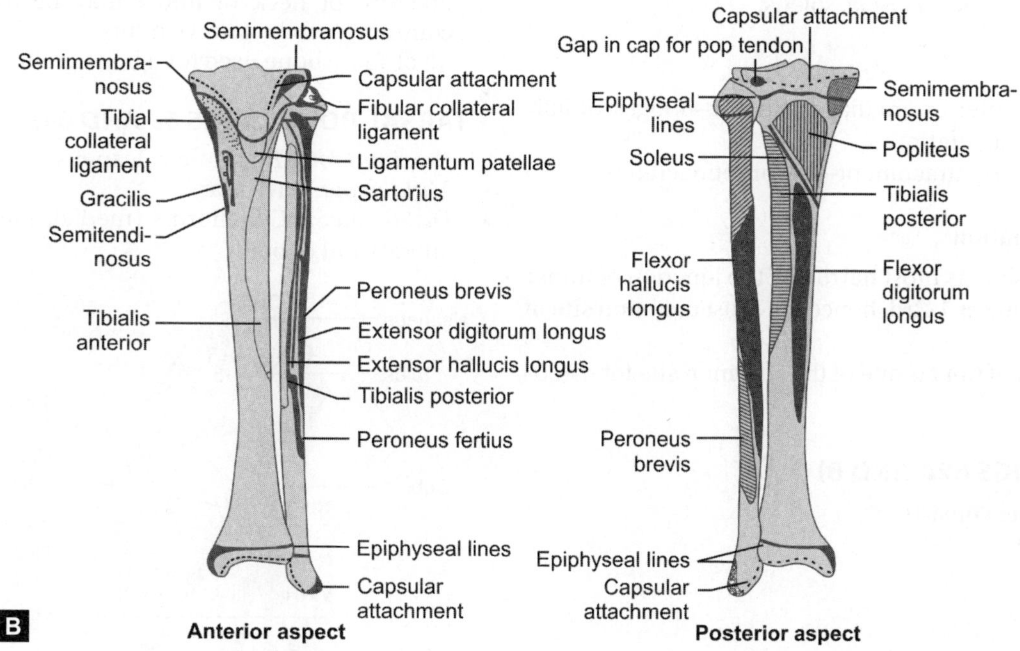

Figs 62A and B Tibia and fibula. (A) Anterior and posterior surface; (B) Muscle attachments

Upper End

- *Medial condyle:*
  Surfaces: Medial S; superior S; anterior S; posterior S—semimembranosus (ins)
- *Lateral condyle:*
  Surfaces: Anterior S, posterior S, superior S
- *Tibial tuberosity:* Ligamentum patellae (ins).

Intercondylar area: "**M**edical **C**ollege **L**ucknow, **L**ucknow **M**edical **C**ollege."

From before backwards, the intercondylar area provides attachment to 6 structures: (i) anterior horn of **M**edial menisus, (ii) anterior **C**ruciate ligament, (iii) anterior horn of **L**ateral meniscus, (iv) posterior horn of **L**ateral meniscus, (v) posterior horn of **M**edial meniscus, (vi) posterior **C**ruciate ligament.

SHAFT—3 B and 3 S

3 Borders

- Anterior (shin of tibia)
- Lateral (interosseous)
- Medial: Soleal line—above soleal line—semimembranous (ins); below soleal line—soleus (ori).

3 Surfaces

Medial: Semimembranous (ins)

From before backwards—**S**artorius (ins), **G**racilis (ins), semi**t**endinosus (ins) "SG Tins"

Lateral: Upper 2/3rd—Tibialis anterior (ori)

Lower 1/3rd is crossed by the following structures—"Tom Has A Nice Dark Pen" From medial to lateral

Tibialis anterior; **E**xtensor hallucis longus; **A**nterior tibial artery; **D**eep peroneal nerve; **E**xtensor digitorum longus; **P**eroneus tertius

Posterior: Soleal line—an oblique line soleus (ori); Lower part—tibialis posterior (ori), FDL—flexor digitorum longus (ori).

The soleal line provide attachment to the following structures—fascia covering popliteus, fascia covering soleus, deep transverse fascia, soleus.

Lower End

Surfaces (5)—anterior, medial, posterior—lodges tibialis posterior, lateral, inferior

Medial malleolus: Attachment—flexor retinaculum.

Clinical Correlation

- The tibial shaft is most narrow at the junction of upper 2/3rd and lower 1/3rd, hence the most common site of fracture
- Upper end of tibia is one of the common site for osteomyelitis.

FIBULA (FIGS 62A AND B)

It is a long bone consists of:

- Upper end
- Shaft
- Lower end.

Side Determination

- Hold it vertically
- Rounded head, directed upward
- Relatively flattened end is directed downward
- A triangular lower articular facet on its lower end faces medially
- Depression at the lower end (malleolar fossa) lies behind and below the triangular articular facet.

Upper End

Head: Styloid process—biceps femoris (ins), EDL—extensor digitorum longus (ori), peroneus longus (ori), posterior surface—soleus (ori).

Neck: Common peroneal nerve and anterior tibial artery related to it.

Shaft—3 B and 3 S

3 Borders: Anterior, posterior, medial (interosseous).

3 Surfaces

Medial (extensor): Upper 1/4th—EDL—extensor digitorum longus (ori), middle 2/4th—EHL—extensor hallucis longus (ori), lower 1/4th—peroneus tertius (ori)

Posterior (flexor): In front—tibialis posterior (ori), behind—soleus (ori), FHL (ori)

Lateral (peroneal): Upper 1/3rd peroneus longus (ori); lower 1/3rd—peroneus brevis (ori).

Lower End

Surfaces (4): Anterior, posterior, medial, lateral

Lateral malleolus.

Clinical Correlation

- Fracture of neck of fibula may be associated with common peroneal nerve injury.
- Ideal spare bone used for a bone graft.

TARSAL BONES (FIGS 63 AND 64)

- *Proximal row:* Talus and calcaneus
- *Middle row:* Navicular
- *Distal row:* 3 Cuneiforms (medial, intermediate and lateral) and cuboid.

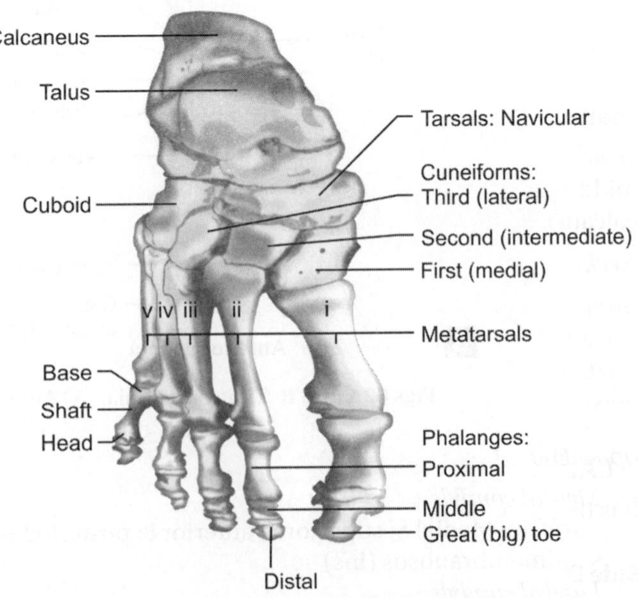

Fig. 63 Tarsal bones

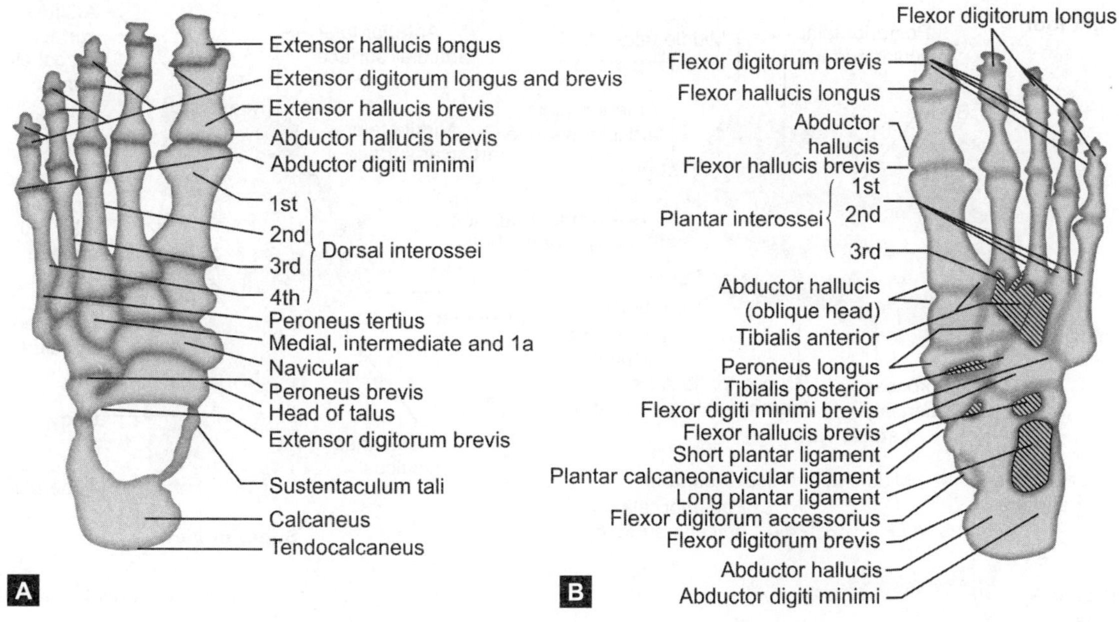

Figs 64A and B Tarsal bones—muscle attachments

TALUS

Situated in the upper surface of the anterior 2/3rd of the calcaneus, does not give attachment to any muscle.

Side Determination

- Keep it on a table top
- Its rounded head is directed forwards
- Its trochlear articular surface faces upwards
- Triangular articular surface on the side of the body faces laterally
- Comma-shaped articular surface on the side of the body is directed medially.

Features

Head: Articulation facet—posterior—art with calcaneum, middle—art with spring ligament, anterolateral art with calcaneum.
Neck: Sulcus tali.

Body: Superior articulate with tibia; Inferior articulate with calcaneum to form subtalar joint; Medial—articulate with medial malleolus; Lateral—articulate with lateral malleolus; Posterior—lodges FHL.

CALCANEUS (FIG. 65)

It is the largest and strongest bone of the foot.

Side Determination

- Holding it in the anteroposterior axis
- Its narrow end bearing concavoconvex facet faces anteriorly
- Its concave surface bearing shelf-like projection faces medially
- Surface-bearing large convex articular facet faces dorsally.

Features

Surfaces

Anterior
posterior—weight bearing during standing posture—tendocalcaneus; plantaris (ins)

Superior (dorsal):* It is divided into three areas:

1. Posterior 1/3rd (nonarticular)—preen deep to tendocalcaneus.
2. Middle 1/3rd (articular)—large oval facet—posterior facet for talus; EDB (ori).
3. Anterior 1/3rd (partly articular—for talus and partly nonarticular); a groove in front of this facet is called—sulcus calcanei; over it lies sulcus tali, and both together form sinus tarsi.

Inferior (plantar): Calcaneal tuberosity.

Lateral: Peroneal tubercle.

Medial: Sustentaculum tali: Medial surface provide attachments (from anterior to posterior): (a) spring ligament, (b) slip from tibialis posterior tendon, (c) deltoid ligament, (d) medial talocalcaneal ligament.

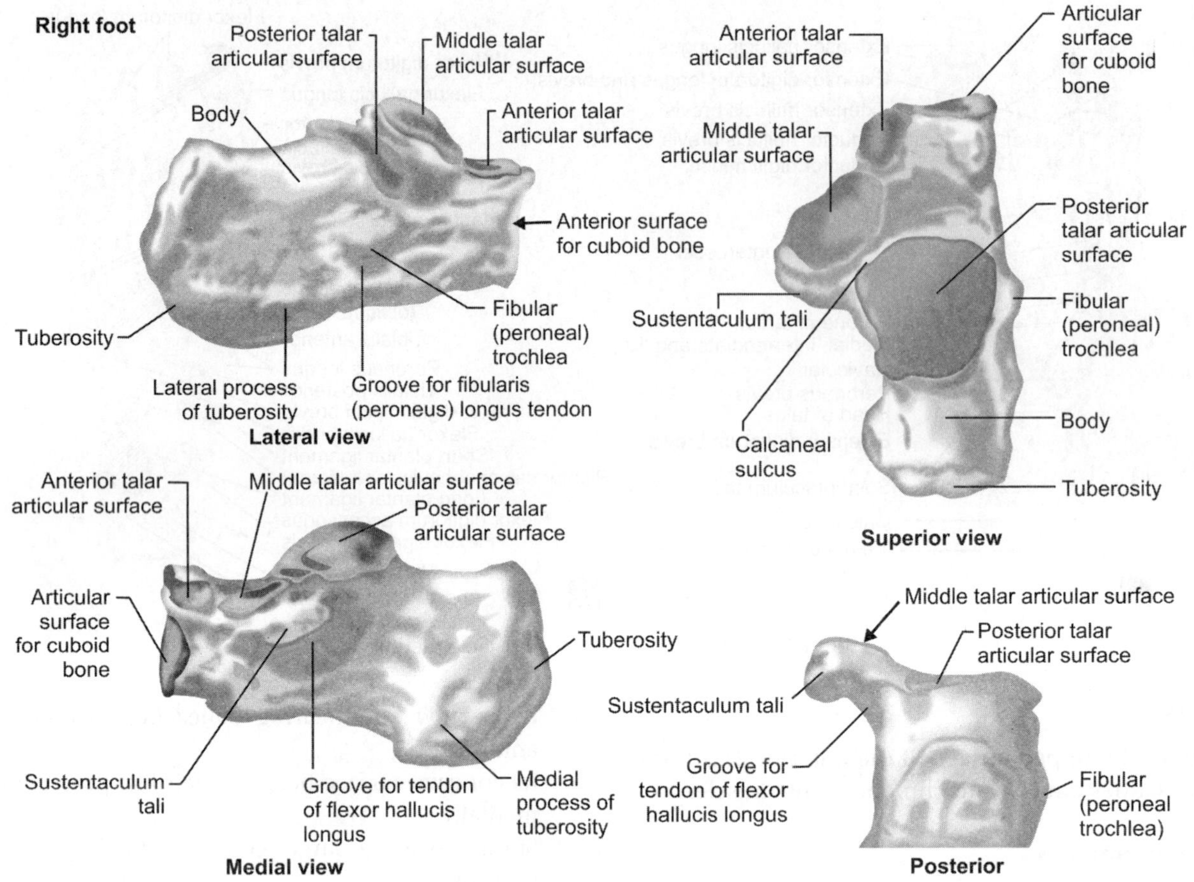

Fig. 65 Calcaneus

SKULL

Bones of the skull			
Cranial skeleton		*Facial skeleton*	
Paired bones	Unpaired bones	Paired bones	Unpaired bones
• Parietal • Temporal	• Frontal • Occipital • Sphenoid • Ethmoid	• Maxilla • Zygomatic • Nasal • Lacrimal • Palatine • Inferior nasal conchae	• Mandible • Vomer

The Exterior of Skull

Different Views

- Superior aspect (norma verticalis)
- Posterior aspect (norma occipitalis)
- Anterior aspect (norma frontalis)
- Lateral aspect (norma lateralis)
- Inferior aspect (norma basalis).

Norma Verticalis (Fig. 66A)

- *Coronal suture,* between frontal and two parietal bone
- *Sagittal suture,* between two parietal bone
- *Lambdoid suture,* between occipital and two parietal bone
- Bregma—meeting point between coronal and sagittal suture

  In fetus, it is a diamond-shaped membranous gap called anterior frontanelle.
- *Lambda*—meeting point between lamboid and sagittal sutures.

  It is the site of posterior fontanelle, which closes 2–3 months after birth.

Norma Occipitalis (Fig. 66B)

- Lambdoid suture
- *External occipital protuberance:* The most prominent point of the external occipital protuberance is called inion.
- *Superior nuchal line:* It is vertical ridge between the external occipital protuberance and posterior margin of foramen magnum.

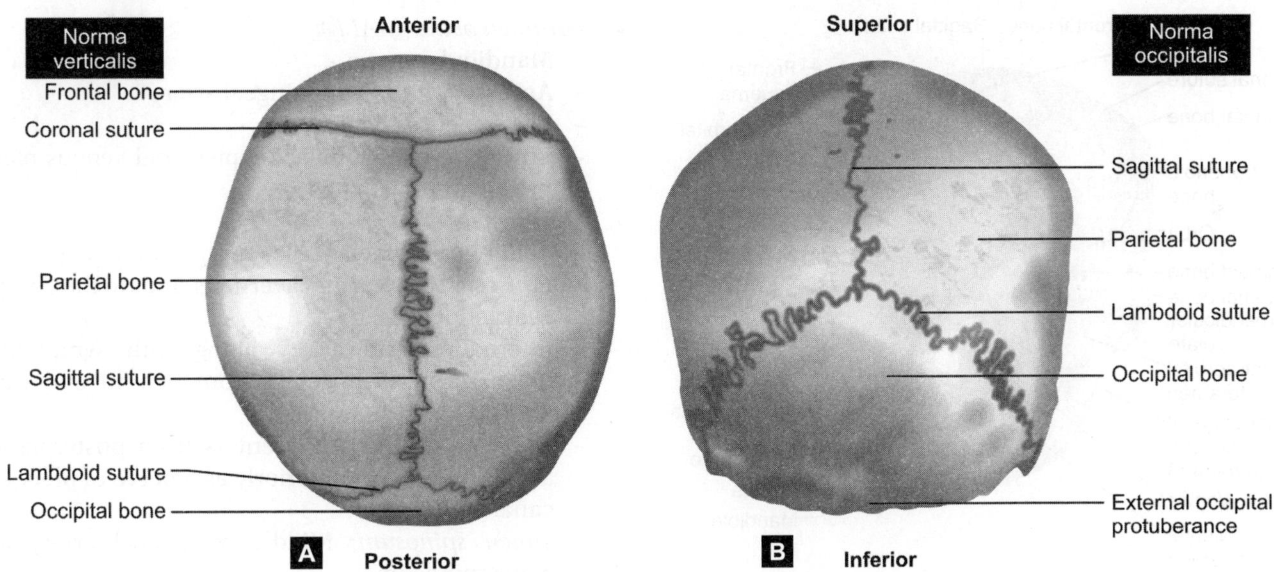

Figs 66A and B (A) Norma verticalis; (B) Norma occipitalis

- *Inferior nuchal line:* These are curved bony ridges passing laterally on each side.
- *Mastoid foramen:* Present near the occipitomastoid suture.

Norma Frontalis (Fig. 67)

It presents:

- Frontal region formed by frontal bone
- *Orbital opening:* It is quadrangular in shape and with 4 margins
  1. Supraorbital margin—formed by frontal bone
  2. Lateral orbital margin—formed by frontal process of zygomatic bone and zygomatic process of frontal bone.
  3. Infraorbital margin—formed by zygomatic bone laterally and maxilla medially
  4. Medial orbital margin—formed by the frontal bone above and anterior lacrimal crest of the maxilla below.
- Prominence of cheek formed by zygomatic bone.
- Bony external nose and anterior nasal aperture—it is formed by nasal bones and maxilla.

Norma Lateralis (Fig. 68)

- *External acoustic meatus:* It is an opening just behind zygomatic arch.
- *Asterion:* Meeting point of parietomastoid, occcipito-mastoid and lambdoid suture.
- *Temporal fossa:* It is a depression on the side of skull
- Pterion—four bones (frontal, parietal, squamous, temporal, and greater wing of sphenoid meet to form H-shaped suture
- *Infratemporal fossa:* It is a depression on the side of skull Bounded by:
  - *Medially*—lateral pterygoid plate
  - *Laterally*—ramus of mandible
- *Pterygomaxillary fissure:* It is a triangular gap between zygomatic arch and side of skull.

Norma Basalis (Fig. 69)

- Infratemporal surface of the greater wing of sphenoid—it has 4 foramina:
  1. Foramen spinosum—at the base of spine of sphenoid
  2. Foramen ovale—near the posterior end of lateral pterygoid plate
  3. Emissary sphenoid foramen (foramen of Vesalius)—between foramen ovale and scaphoid fossa
  4. Canaliculus innominatus—between foramen ovale and foramen spinosum.
- Inferior surface of the petrous temporal bone—it has an apex and is perforated by carotid canal and separated from the sphenoid by foramen lacerum.

STRUCTURES PASSING THROUGH VARIOUS FORAMINA, CANALS AND FISSURES OF THE SKULL

Norma Basalis

- *Greater palatine foramina*—greater palatine nerves and vessels
- *Pterygoid canal*—present in the pterygoid process and sphenoid process.
  - Nerve of pterygoid canal (vidians nerve)
  - Vessels of pterygoid canal

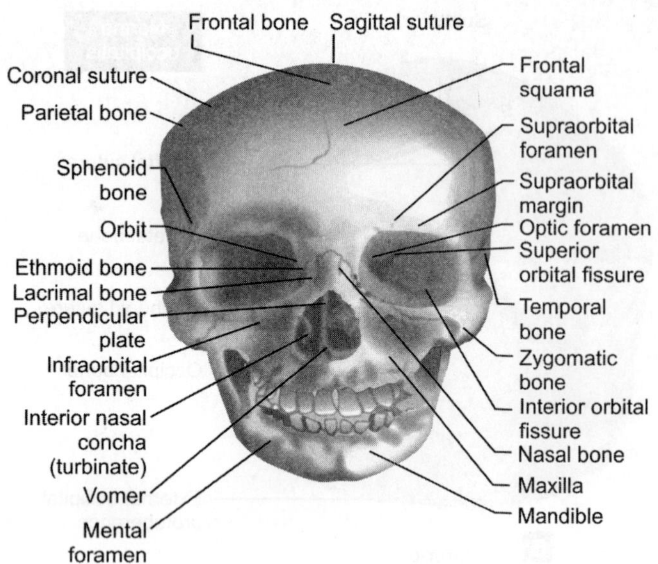

Fig. 67 Norma frontalis

- *Foramen ovale (MALE)*:
  - **M**andibular nerve
  - **A**ccessory middle meningeal artery
  - **L**esser petrosal nerve
  - **E**missary vein—connecting pterygoid venous plexus to the cavernous sinus
- *Foramen lacerum*:
  - Meningeal branch of ascending pharyngeal artery
  - *Emissary vein:* Forms cavernous sinus to the pharyngeal venous plexus
  - Internal carotid artery along with sympathetic plexus around, it enters from behind and exists above
  - Greater petrosal nerve enters from posterolateral aspect and leaves anteriorly as a nerve of pterygoid canal
- *Foramen spinosum:* Middle meningeal artery and nervous spinosum

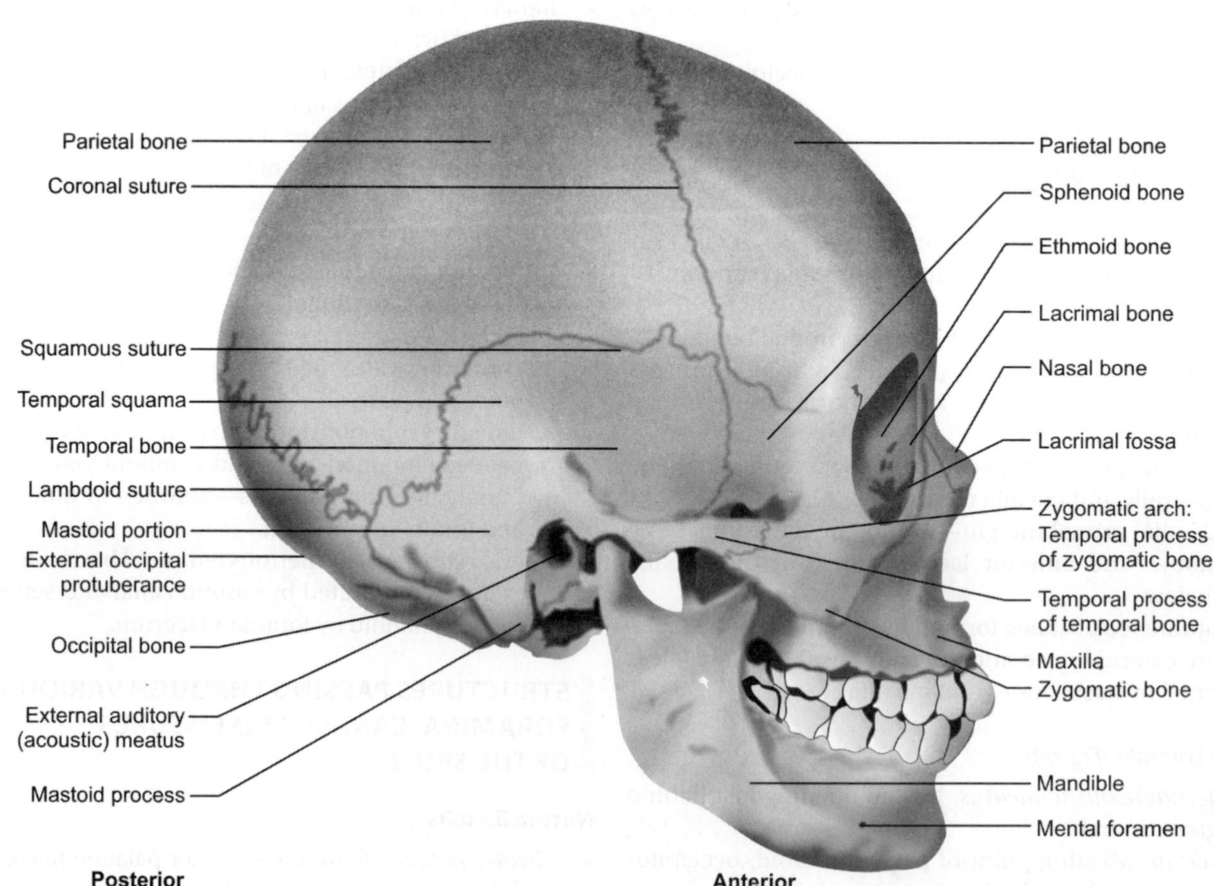

Fig. 68 Norma lateralis

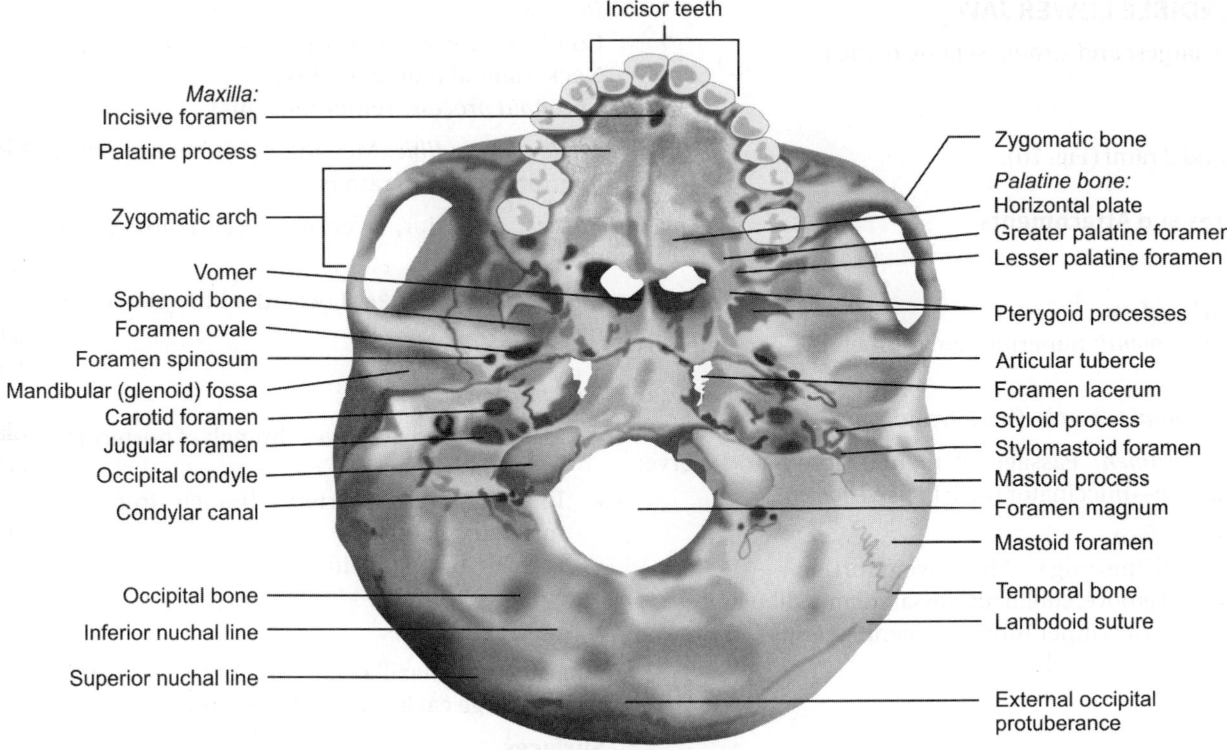

Fig. 69 Norma basalis

- *Carotid canal*: Located in inferior surface of the petrous temporal bone:
  - Internal carotid artery with sympathetic plexus around it
  - Internal carotid venous plexus connecting cavernous sinus and internal jugular vein
  - Emissary vein connecting pharyngeal venous plexus and cavernous sinus
- *Mastoid canaliculus (Arnold's canal):* Auricular branch of vagus nerve (Arnold's nerve)
- *Stylomastoid foramen:* Facial nerve and stylomastoid artery.

Norma Lateralis

- Mastoid foramen
  - Emissary vein—connecting the posterior auricular vein with transverse sinus
- Foramen magnum
- Hypoglossal canal
- Jugular foramen
- Zygomaticotemporal foramen—on the zygomatic bone
  - Zygomaticotemporal nerve and artery
- Sphenopalatine foramen—nasopalatine nerve and sphenopalatine vessels
- *Greater palatine canal*
  - Anterior, middle and posterior palatine nerves
  - Greater palatine vessels
  - Lesser palatine vessels.

Norma Verticalis

Parietal foramen: Emissary vein—connecting superficial veins of the scalp to the superior sagittal sinus.

Norma Frontalis

- Supraorbital foramen—supraorbital nerve and vessels, frontal diploic veins
- Inferior orbital fissure
  - Maxillary nerve
  - Infraorbital vessels
  - Zygomatic nerve
  - Vein connecting inferior ophthalmic vein with pterygoid venous plexus
- Infraorbital foramen—infraorbital nerve and artery and infraorbital vein
- Zygomatico-orbital foramen—zygomatic branch of maxillary nerve
- Mental foramen—mental nerve, mental artery and mental vein.

MANDIBLE LOWER JAW

It is the largest and strongest bone of the face.

Parts

Body and 2 rami (Fig. 70).

Features and Attachments

Body

External Surface
Symphysis menti: Superior genial tubercle—genioglossus (ori).

Inferior genial tubercle: Geniohyoid.

Mental foramen: Passage of mental artery and nerve; oblique line—buccinator (ori); incisive fossa.

Internal surface
Myelohyoid line/ridge—Myelohyoid (ori)
Myelohyoid groove, sublingual fossa, submandibular fossa.
Genial tubercle: Upper tubercle—genioglossus (ori); lower tubercle—geniohyoid (ori).

Ramus

2 Surfaces: Medial (internal)—Mandibular foramen, Lingula, myelohyoid groove—lodges myelohyoid nerve and vessels
Lateral (external): Masseter (ins)

4 Borders

- *Anterior:* Temporalis (ins)
- *Posterior:* Related to parotid gland
- Superior
- Inferior.

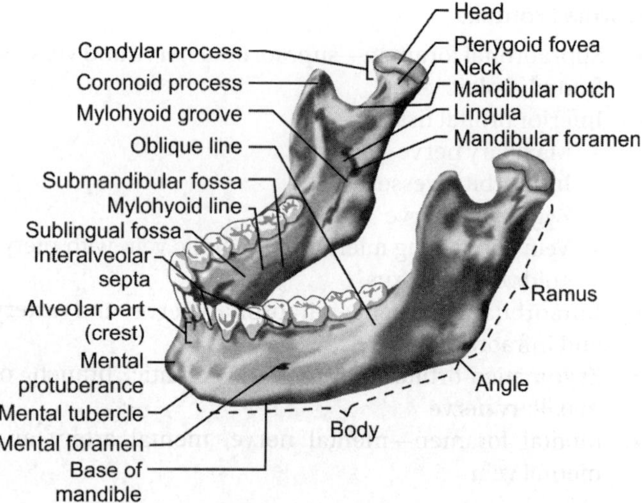

Fig. 70 Mandible

Processes
Condylar process—Pterygoid fovea—temporalis (ins)
Neck—lateral pterygoid (ins)
Coronoid process: Temporalis (ins).

Angle of mandible: Meeting point between posterior and inferior borders of ramus.

Borders: Superior; Inferior—digastric fossa-anterior belly of digastric (ori).

Mandibular foramen: Located a little above the center of ramus.

Structure Passing

- Inferior alveolar nerve—branch of posterior division of mandibular nerve
- Inferior alveolar artery—branch from 1st part of maxillary artery
- Inferior alveolar vein.

MAXILLAE

There are two maxillae and they together form upper jaw.
Body: A large cavity called maxillary sinus

Surfaces
Medial /Nasal (base): Forms lateral wall of nasal cavity.

It presents a large opening, the maxillary hiatus which lead into maxillary sinus.

Superior/Orbital: Forms major part of the floor of the orbital cavity.

Posterior/Infratemporal: Forms anterior wall of infratemporal fossa.

Anterior/facial/malar S: Forms the part of norma frontalis.

Processes: Frontal P—projects upward and articulate with the frontal bone.

Zygomatic: Extends laterally and articulates with the zygomatic bone.

Palatine: Forms greater part of hard palate.

Alveolar: Extends downwards and caries the upper teeth.

FRONTAL BONE

Parts: Squamous/vertical part: Orbital plate.

Nasal part: It presents nasal notch inferiorly and parts with nasal bone.

Orbital plate(two): Form the roof of the orbit. The two orbital plates are separated from each other by 'U'-shaped ethmoidal notch.
Superciliary arch—curved elevation above the supraorbital margin end.
Zygomatic process (two)—It joins with the frontal process of zygomatic process.

PARIETAL BONE

Parts

2 surfaces, 4 borders.

Surface

External: Superior and inferior temporal lines are present below the parietal tuberosity.

Internal: Sagittal sulcus lodges superior sagittal sinus; an impression for posterior division of middle meningeal artery; transverse sulcus—it lodges sigmoid sinus.

Borders

Superior/sagittal: Articulate with opposite parietal bone to form sagittal sinus.

Inferior/squamosal: Articulate with three bones (from anterior to posterior). Greater wing of sphenoid, squamous part of temporal bone, mastoid portion of temporal bone.

Anterior/frontal: Articulate with frontal bone.

Posterior/occipital: Articulate with occipital bone.

TEMPORAL BONE

It is an irregular pneumatic bone.

Parts

- Squamous
- Mastoid
- Petrous
- Tympanic
- Styloid process.

Squamous

Thin transparent plate of bone:

Outer surface: Forms the floor or temporal fossa. It is grooved in its center by the middle temporal artery. The zygomatic process projects laterally from the temporal surface. It joins the temporal process of the zygomatic bone to form the zygomatic arch.

Internal surface: Lies in contact with temporal lobe of brain.

Mastoid

Lies below and behind the squamous part and contains mastoid antrum. On its medial side, there is a notch called digastric notch.

Mastoid process: Lower projection that gives attachments to the muscle (before backwards), Sternocleidomastoid, semispinalis capitis, splenius capitis.

Mastoid foramen: For the passage of emissary vein, connecting sigmoid sinus and small artery from occipital artery.

External acoustic meatus: A bony canal directed anteromedially and downwards.

Tympanic part of temporal bone forms—anterior and posterior wall and floor.

Squamous temporal bone forms roof and posterior wall.

Petrous

Hardest part of the temporal bone. It has a base, apex, 3 surfaces and 3 borders. It contains middle ear and internal ear.

Trigeminal impression: Slight depression behind the apex, for trigeminal ganglion.

Arcuate eminence: It is placed posterolateral to trigeminal impression.

Tegmen tympani: Lateral to arcuate eminence.

Internal acoustic meatus: It transmits 7th and 8th cranial nerve along with labyrinthine vessels.

Groove for greater petrosal nerve; groove for lesser petrosal nerve:

Styloid process: External acoustic meatus—opens on the surface behind the mandibular fossa.

Forms about 2/3rd of external auditory meatus.

Suprameatal triangle: Also called McEwen's triangle—small depression posterior to the external acoustic meatus.

OCCIPITAL BONE

Parts

- Squamous
- Basilar
- Condylar parts (2).

Squamous

External surface: External occipital protuberance; 2 External occipital crests.

Two superior nuchal lines—trapezius, occipitofrontalis, Sternocleidomastoid (ins), two inferior nuchal lines.

Internal (Cerebral S): Internal occipital protuberance, sagittal sulcus, transverse sulcus, fossa, internal occipital crest.

Basilar: It is a wide bar of bone lies in front of the foramen magnum. Articulates with sphenoid bone.

Condylar: Situated one on each side of the foramen magnum. Medial part bears occipital condyles and lateral part bears jugular process.

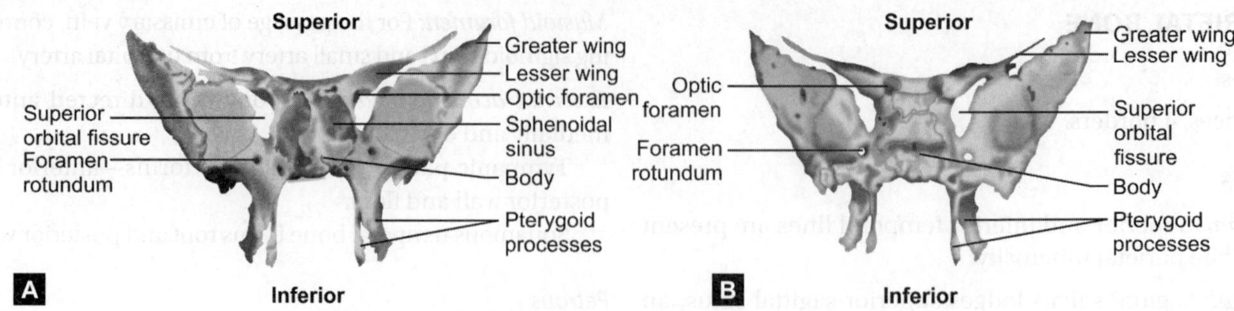

Figs 71A and B Sphenoid bone. (A) Anterior view (B) Posterior view

Condylar fossa: Depression just behind the occipital condyle.

Hypoglossal canal: In the anterior part of occipital condyle. It transmits hypoglossal nerve.

Jugular tubercle: It is the superior part of the condylar part.

SPHENOID BONE

Parts

Body, Lesser wing (2), Greater wing (2), Pterygoid process (2) (Figs 71A and B).

Body

Surfaces

Superior: Ethmoidal spine, Jugum sphenoidale, Sulcus chiasmaticus, Tuberculum sellae—it presents small conical projections called middle clinoid process.

Dorsum sellae: It presents a projection called posterior clinoid process.
Inferior: Sphenoidal rostrum, sphenoidal concha
Anterior: Sphenoidal crest
Posterior: Lateral (2)—carotid sulcus
Greater wing (2)
Pterygoid process (2)

Lesser wing (2): Arises from anterior part of the body of sphenoid by two roots. It presents a projection called anterior clinoid process.

ETHMOID BONE

Parts: Cribriform plate, Cristae galli, perpendicular plate, two labyrinths (Fig. 72).

Cranial Cavity

Floor: It is divided into three fossae:

Anterior Cranial Fossa

It lodges the frontal lobes of the cerebral hemispheres.

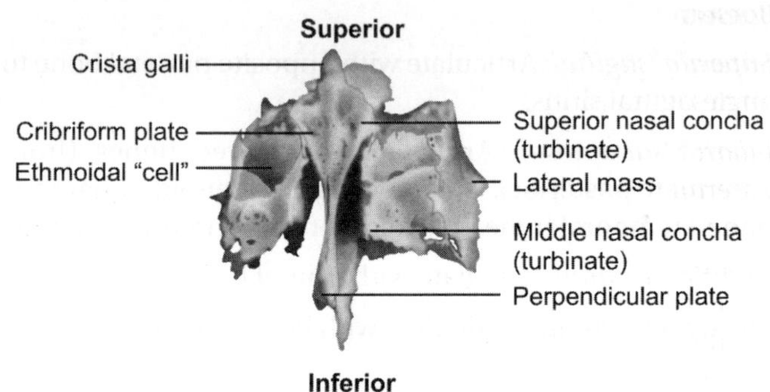

Fig. 72 Ethmoid bone

Boundaries

Anteriorly and on both the sides—frontal bone
Posteriorly—lesser wing of sphenoid on each side
Floor—anteriorly by cribriform plate of ethmoid and posteriorly by a part of the body of sphenoid
On each side—orbital plate of ethmoid

The junction between anterior and posterior borders are marked by anterior clinoid process.

Features

(a) Frontal crest, (b) Foramen cecum, (c) Crista galli, formed by perpendicular plates of ethmoid. (d) Jugum sphenoidale (on anterior part of the body of sphenoid), (e) Sieve-like cribriform plate of the ethmoid (on each side of crista galli) which separates the anterior cranial fossa from nasal cavity.

STRUCTURES PASSING THROUGH VARIOUS FORAMINA IN THE ANTERIOR CRANIAL FOSSA

- Foramen cecum—emissary vein from nasal mucosa
- Cribriform foramina—olfactory nerves surrounded by the pia and arachnoid maters

- Anterior ethmoidal foramen—anterior ethmoidal nerve and vessels
- Posterior ethmoidal foramen—posterior ethmoidal nerve and vessels.

Middle Cranial Fossa

It lodges the temporal lobe of brain and it is shaped like a butterfly.

Boundaries

Anteriorly: Posterior border of lesser wing of sphenoid

Posteriorly: Superior border of petrous temporal bone and dorsum sellae of sphenoid

Laterally: Greater wings of sphenoid and anteroinferior angle of parietal bone

Floor: Median plane—body of sphenoid

Laterally, greater wing of sphenoid + petrous temporal bone + squamous part of temporal bone

Greater wing of sphenoid—4 foramina

1. *Foramen spinosum:* It is posterior most and located at the posterior tip of the greater wing.
2. *Foramen ovale:* It is located just in front and medial to the foramen spinosum.
3. *Foramen rotundum:* It is in front and median to foramen ovale.
4. *Superior orbital fissure:* It is in front and lateral to foramen rotundum.

STRUCTURES PASSING THROUGH VARIOUS CANALS AND FORAMINA

- *Optic foramen*—Optic nerve and ophthalmic artery along with sympathetic plexus
- Superior orbital fissure: 3 parts
  1. *Structures passing through common tendinous ring:* Superior and inferior divisions of oculomotor nerve, nasociliary nerve, abducent nerve
  2. *Structures passing above and lateral to the common tendinous ring:* Trochlear nerve, frontal nerve, lacrimal nerve, lacrimal artery, superior ophthalmic vein, recurrent branch of ophthalmic artery
  3. *Structures passing below and medial to the common tendinous ring:* Inferior ophthalmic vein
- Foramen rotundum—maxillary nerve and emissary vein
- Foramen ovale-MALE
- Foramen spinosum
- Foramen lacerum
- Carotid canal.

POSTERIOR CRANIAL FOSSAE

Largest fossa: It lodges cerebellum behind and pons and medulla in front.

Boundaries

Anteriorly: Superior border of petrous temporal bone and Dorsum sellae of sphenoid

Posteriorly: Squamous part of occipital bone

On each side: Mastoid part of temporal bone and mastoid angle of parietal bone

Floor: Sloping area of sphenoid and occipital (clivus) + Foramen magnum + squamous part of temporal

Laterally: Condylar part of occipital + posterior surface of petrous temporal + mastoid part of temporal

STRUCTURES PASSING THROUGH VARIOUS CANALS AND FORAMINA

- *Internal auditory meatus:*
  - Seventh cranial (facial) nerve
  - Eighth cranial (vestibule cochlear) nerve
  - Nerves intermedius
  - Internal auditory (labyrinthine) vessels
- *Jugular foramen:*
  - Anterior part—inferior petrosal sinus
  - Middle part—9th (glossopharyngeal), 10th (vagus) and 11th (accessory) cranial nerve.
  - Posterior part—sigmoid sinus
- *Hypoglossal (anterior condylar) canal:*
  - 12th cranial (hypoglossal) nerve
  - Meningeal branch of ascending pharyngeal artery
- *Foramen magnum:* Largest foramen, divided by alar ligament

Anterior (small)—*below upwards*

- Apical ligament of dens
- Upper longitudinal band of cruciform ligament of atlas
- *Membrane tectoria:* Continuation of posterior longitudinal ligament

Posterior (large)—medulla oblongata along with meninges

Above downwards

- 2 posterior spinal arteries (right and left)
- Anterior spinal artery
- Communicating veins between internal and basilar venous plexus.

Below upwards

- 2 vertebral arteries (right and left) surrounded by sympathetic plexus
- Spinal roots of two accessory nerves (right and left).

VERTEBRAE

Difference between vertebrae (Figs 73 to 76).

	Cervical	*Thoracic*	*Lumbar*
Body			
• Shape	Transversely oval	Heart-shaped	Kidney-shaped
• Facet on body	Absent	Present	Absent
Transverse process	Short, thin, horizontal	Long, thick downwards	Thin, intermediate in size
Foramen transversarium	Present	Absent	Absent
Facet	Absent	Present	Absent
Spinous process	Short, bifid and horizontally backwards	Long, triangular and obliquely downwards	Intermediate in size Quadrangular horizontally backwards
Vertebral foramen	Large, triangular	Small, round	Intermediate, triangular
Superior articular process	Upward and backward	Forwards	Backward
Inferior articular process	Downward and forwards	Backward	Forwards and laterally
Superior vertebral notch	Deep	Shallow	Shallow
Inferior vertebral notch	Deep	Deep	Deep
Movements			
Flexion and extension	More	Little	More
Lateral flexion	Possible	Very little	Possible
Rotation	Very little	More	Very little

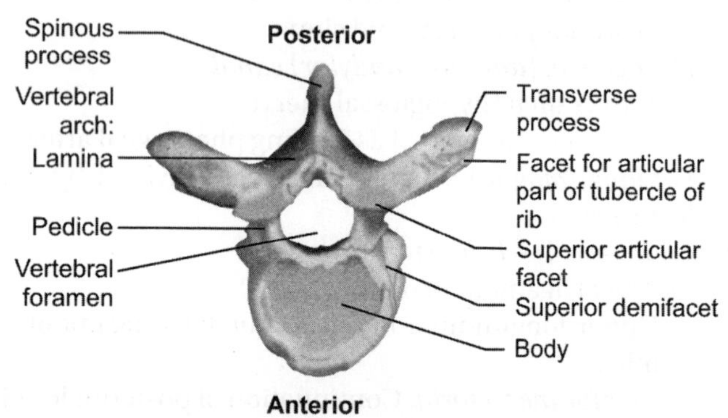

Fig. 73 Typical thoracic vertebrae

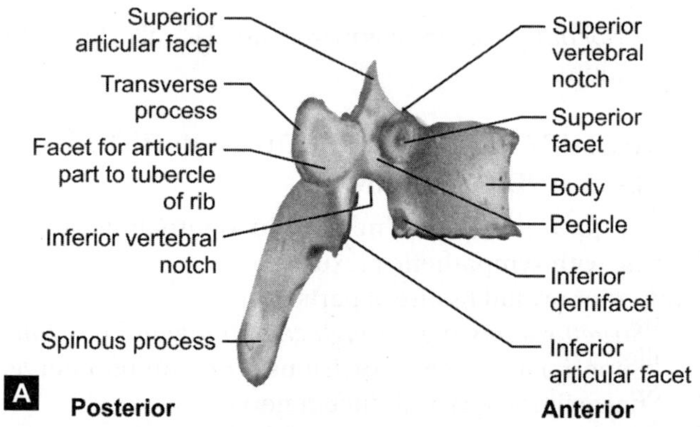

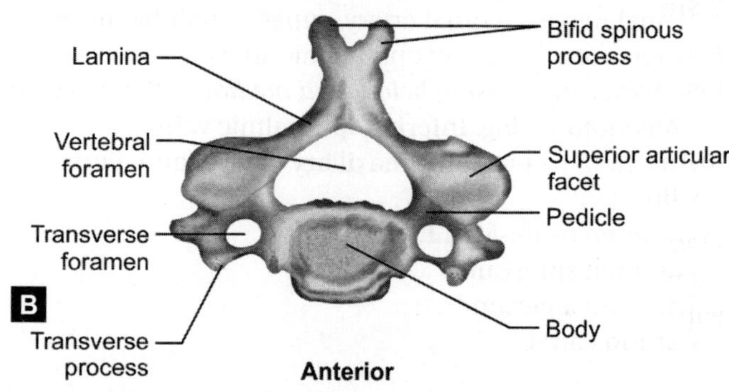

Figs 74A and B Typical cervical vertebrae. (A) Right lateral view; (B) Superior view

SACRUM (FIGS 77A AND B)

Formed by the fusion of 5 sacral vertebrae:

Apex: Formed by the inferior surface of the 5th sacral vertebrae. It has an oval facet for articulate with coccyx to form the sacrococcygeal joint.

Base: Directed upward and forward. Formed by the superior surface of the first sacral vertebrae.

Anterior Border-Sacral Promontory

- *Body:* Body of 1st sacral fuses with 5th lumbar vertebrae

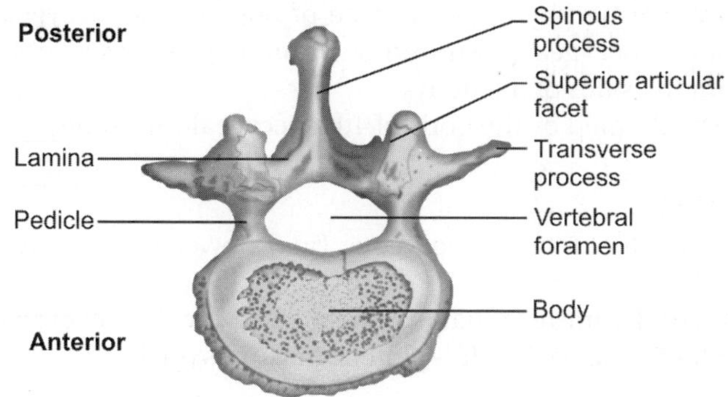

Fig. 75 Lumbar vertebrae (Superior view)

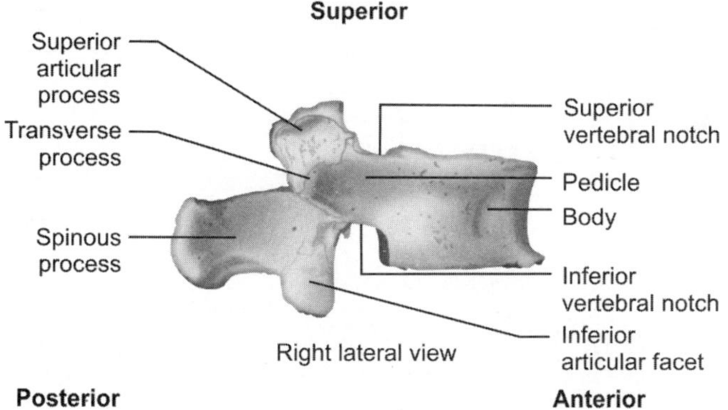

Fig. 76 Lumbar vertebrae (right lateral view)

- *Vertebral foramen:* Triangular in shape. Lying behind the body and leads to sacral canal
- *Pedicle:* Short and directed backward and laterally
- *Laminae:* Quite oblique
- *Transverse process:* They fuse with corresponding costal transverse element to form alae of sacrum, lateral part—iliacus (ori)
- *Spinous process:* Forms the first spinous tubercle
- *Superior articular facet:* Prominent and projects upwards.

3 Surfaces

Pelvic S: Four transverse ridges that indicate the line of fusion of 5 sacral vertebrae.

Median sacral vessels and sympathetic trunk are related to this surface.

Bodies of middle 3 sacral vertebrae—piriformis (ori).

Dorsals: Rough, irregular and convex. The lamina of 5th sacral vertebrae fail to join be hind, forming a U-shaped gap called sacral hiatus.

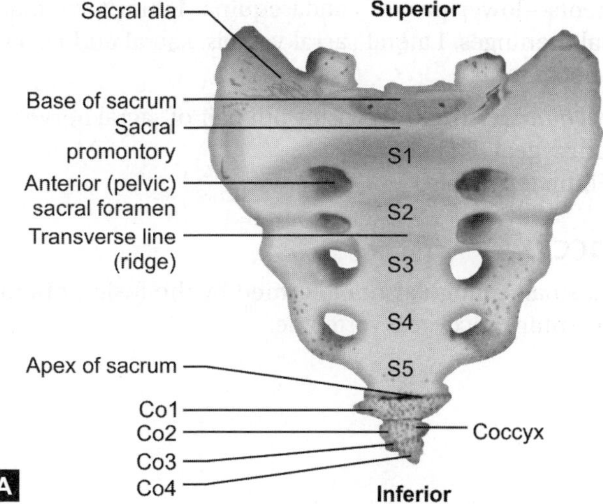

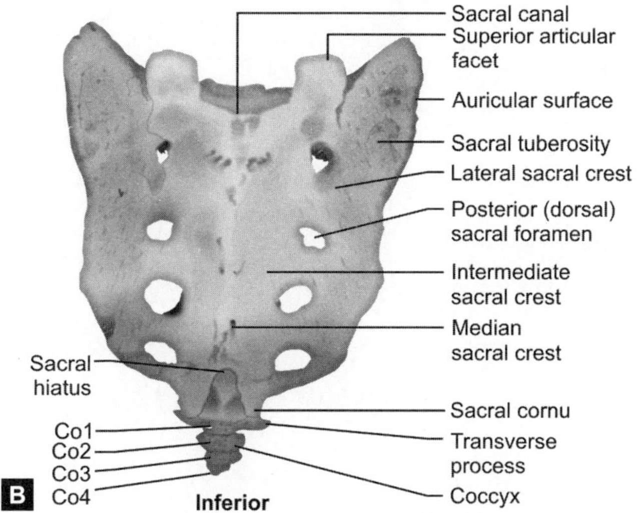

Figs 77A and B Sacrum and coccyx. (A) Anterior view; (B) Posterior view

'U' shaped area—erector spinae area enclosed by it—multifidus.

Lateral (2): Wide above and narrow below. Upper wider part bears an inverted L-shaped auricular surface anteriorly and a deeply pitted area posteriorly.

From behind forwards—gluteus maximus, sacrotuberous ligament, sacrospinous ligament, coccygeus

SACRAL CANAL

- Formed by the superimposed vertebral foramina of the sacral vertebrae.
- Lower end opens at sacral hiatus.

Contents—lower part of cauda equina, Filum terminale, Spinal meninges, Lateral sacral vessels, sacral and coccygeal nerve roots.

Sacral hiatus: Structure passing 5th pair of sacral nerves

- Coccygeal (C1) nerves
- Filum terminale.

COCCYX

It is a small triangular bone formed by the fusion of four rudimentary coccygeal vertebrae.

Base: Formed by upper surface of body of 1st coccygeal bone. Coccygeal cornu-bony prominences arises from both the sides of the body.

Apex: Formed by the body of 4th coccygeal vertebrae.

Surfaces

Pelvic: Upper two—coccygeus (ins), lower two—levator ani (ins)

Dorsal: Filum terminale is attached to the 1st coccygeal vertebra; On each side—gluteus maximus (ori).

RADIOLOGY

STANDARD VIEWS OF A RADIOGRAPH

- *Anteroposterior view:*
  - It is taken with the X-ray tube anterior to the subject and the film posteriorly placed
  - Posterior structures are better visualized in this view
- *Posteroanterior view:*
  - In this, X-ray tube placed posteriorly and the film anteriorly.
  - Anteriorly placed structures are more clearly visualized.
  - The more commonly taken X-ray of chest is PA view.
- *Lateral view:*
  - Right lateral view—when the film is in contact with the right side of the subject.
  - Left lateral view—when the film is kept against the left side of the subject.
- *Oblique view:* The subject stands in front of upright film cassette holder and is then turned 45 degree oblique (right/left).

Types of Radiographs

- *Plain radiographs:* When X-rays are allowed to pass through the subject without the use of any medium the translucent portions appear black on the developed X-ray plate, whereas the dense area absorbs the X-rays in varying degrees resulting in different shades of white
- *Contrast radiographs:* When X-rays are taken after filling a cavity or space with a contrast medium in order to visualize the lumen of the viscus or extent of the cavity.

The contrast media are of two types:

1. *Opaque:* Barium sulfate for the gastrointestinal tract, iodine compounds for the urinary tract.
2. *Translucent:* Air or oxygen for ventricles of brain.

UPPER LIMB

Plain radiography is mainly required.

Shoulder Joint (Fig. 78A)

View: Anteroposterior

Type: Ball and socket

Articulating surfaces—glenoid cavity and head of humerus.

Identify: Acromion, acromioclavicular joint, anatomical neck of humerus, clavicle, coronoid tubercle, coracoid process, glenoid cavity, greater tuberosity of humerus, head of humerus.

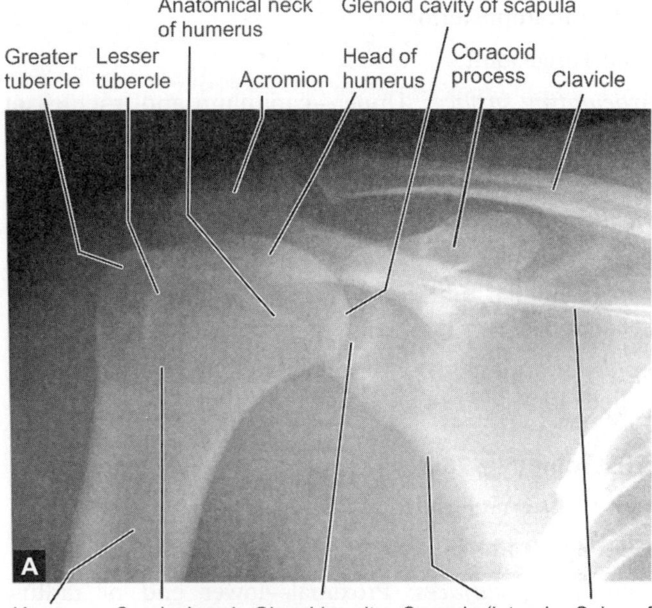

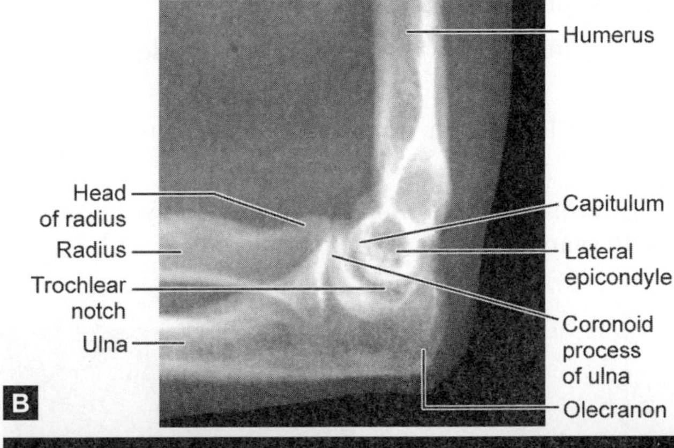

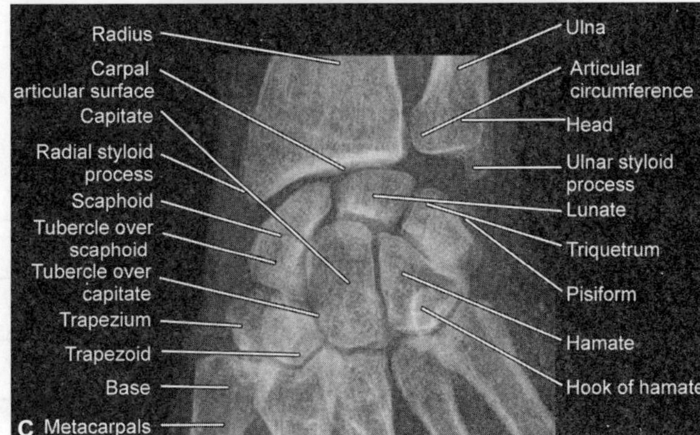

Figs 78A to C (A) Shoulder joint; (B) Elbow joint; (C) Wrist joint

Applied: Most common site of dislocation—inferiorly (disproportionate area of articulating surfaces and laxity of capsule; endangers axillary nerve).

Elbow Joint (Fig. 78B)

View: Anteroposterior

Type: Hinge joint

Articulating surfaces: Upper—capitulum and trochlea of humerus.

Lower: Head of radius, and trochlear notch of humerus.

Identify: AP view: Medial and lateral epicondyle, olecranon process, trochlea.

Lateral: Radial tuberosity, olecranon, coronoid process, epicondyles.

Applied: Student's elbow (miner's elbow), tennis elbow, pulled elbow.

Wrist Joint (Fig. 78C)

View: Posteroanterior

Type: Ellipsoid

Articulating surfaces: Proximal—lower end of radius, articulating disc of inferior—radioulnar joints.

Distal: Scaphoid, lunate, triquetral.

Identify: Proximal row—scaphoid, lunate, triquetral, and pisiform.

Distal row: Trapezium, trapezoid, capitate, hamate.

Applied

- Pisiform—age determination (present > 8 years, absent < 12 years).
- Colle's fracture, Smith's fracture
- Scaphoid—avascular necrosis.

First Carpometacarpal Joint

View: Posteroanterior

Type: Saddle

Articulating surfaces: Trapezium, base of 1st metacarpal.

Applied: Only carpometacarpal joint having separate joint cavity.

LOWER LIMB

Hip Joint (Fig. 79)

View: Anteroposterior

Type: Ball and socket (multiaxial)

Articulating surfaces: Acetabulum of hip bone and head of femur.

Identify: Greater trochanter, acetabulum, head of femur, lesser trochanter, Shoemaker's line, Bryant's triangle Shenton's line—the line of the upper margin of the obturator foramen following the same curves as that of the under surface of the neck and medial side of the shaft of the femur.

Applied-congenital dislocation: Here upper margin of the acetabulum is developmentally deficient.

Perthes disease: Characterized by destruction and flattening of the head of femur.

Knee Joint (Figs 80A and B)

View: Anteroposterior (taken in full extension).

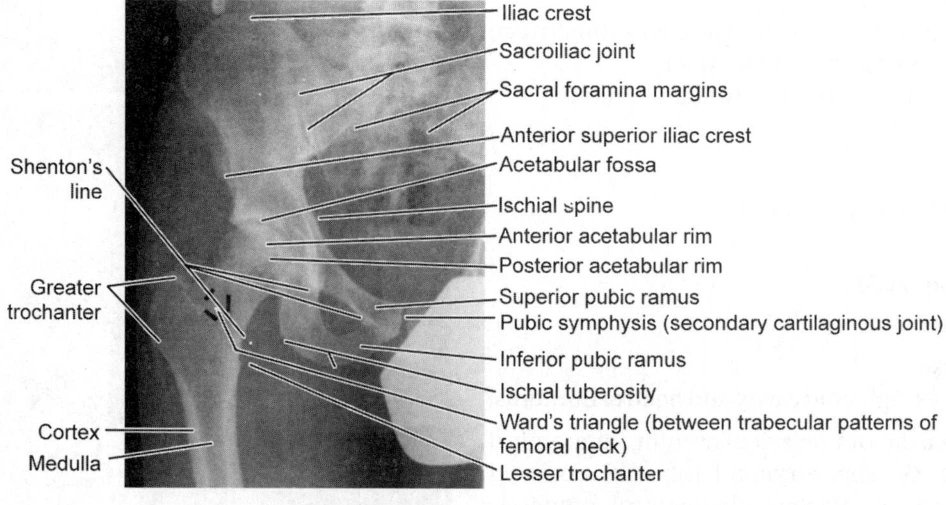

Fig. 79 Hip joint—anteroposterior view

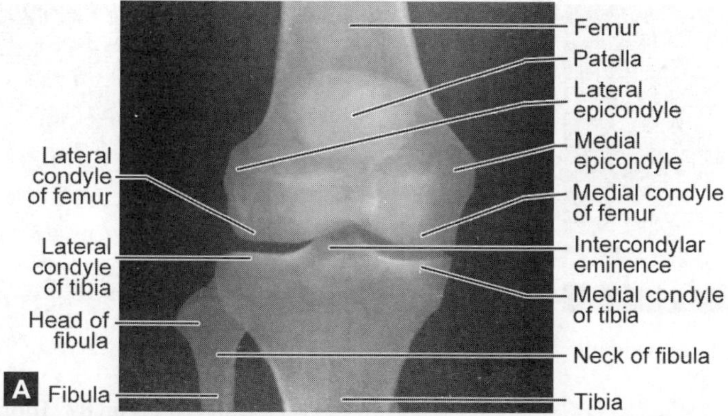

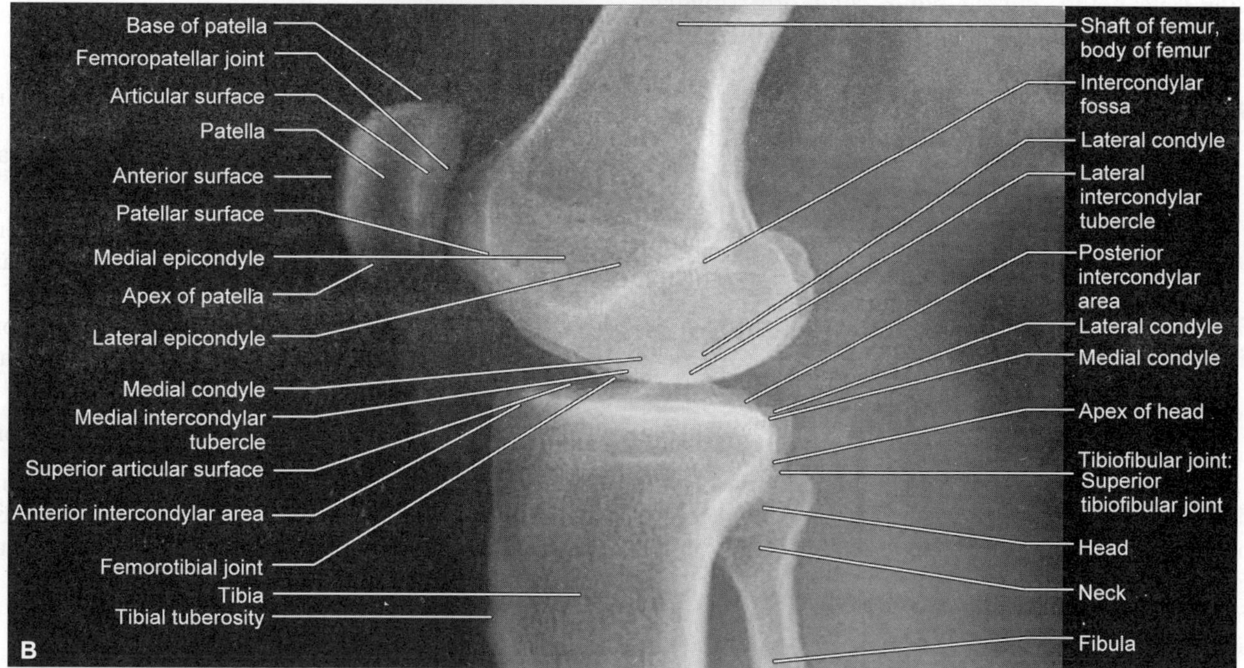

Figs 80A and B Knee joint. (A) AP view; (B) Lateral view

Lateral (partially flexed and its lateral aspect placed next to film)

Type: Modified hinge joint

Articulating surfaces: Condyles of tibia, condyles of femur and patella.

Identify: Condyles, head and styloid process of fibula, intercondylar eminence of tibia, intercondylar notch of femur, patella.

Applied: Baker's cyst is a central swelling occurs due to osteoarthritis of the knee joint.

Ankle Joint (Fig. 81)

View: Anteroposterior and lateral (in this lateral malleolus is on the film)

Type: Hinge

Articulating surfaces: Lower end of tibia and fibula and talus.

Identify: Lower end of tibia, fibula, talus.

Applied: Dislocation of the ankle—accompanied by fracture of one of the malleoli.

Acute sprains of medial and lateral ankles.

Subtalar Joint

View: Anteroposterior

Type: Plane synovial

Articulating surfaces: Inferior surface of talus, superior surface of calcaneum.

Foot

View: Anteroposterior and lateral

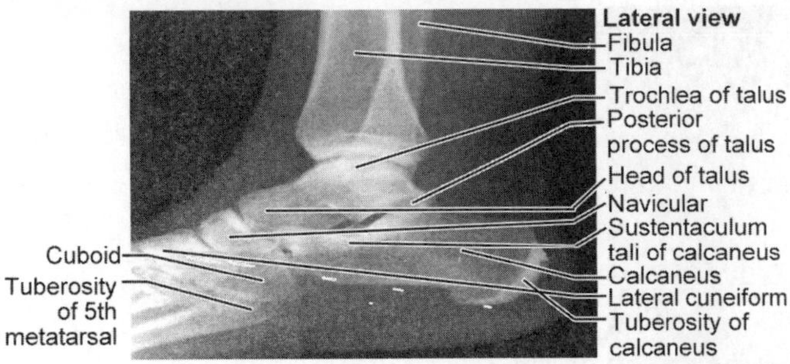

Fig. 81 Ankle—lateral view

Identify: Calcaneum, cuboid bone, cuneiform (medial, lateral and intermediate) intertarsal joint spaces, metatarsals, navicular, phalange, talus, tarsal bones.

Applied: Mallet toe, hammer toe, claw toe.

THORAX

View: Posteroanterior (Fig. 82)

Identify: Apex of heart

- Cardiovascular shadow (due to heart and great vessels).
- Breast shadow (appear as homogeneous, opacities limited below by a crescentic margin.
- *Cardiophrenic angle:* Right and left are formed where the domes, covered by the diaphragmatic pleura, meet the lateral walls of the thorax.
- *Diaphragm:* Convex upwards and consisting of two domes—right, left and they are separated in the center by the shadow of the heart.
- Fundus of stomach.
- *Hilar shadow:* It appears as two thin paintbrush-like shadows. The images of hila consist of vascular bronchial and lymphoglandular components.
- *Lung fields:* The translucency of the lung parenchyma is due to the presence of air in the alveoli and bronchi.
- *Ribs:* The lungs are striped by the projections of the overlying ribs.
- Arch of aorta.
- *Aortic knuckle:* Arch of aorta seen as a projection at upper left margin of cardiac shadow.

View: Right or left lateral view.

Identify: Cardiac shadows:

- Cupola of diaphragm
- Descending aorta
- Inferior angles of the scapulae
- Lung field
- Esophagus
- Retrosternal and retrocardiac space
- Sternum
- Thoracic vertebrae
- Trachea.

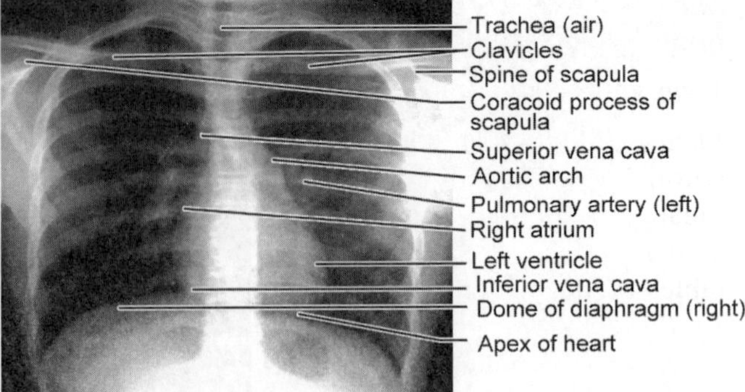

Fig. 82 Thorax—PA view

Bronchogram

It is used to visualize the bronchial tree and is an important aid for diagnosis and localization of lung disease.

Right bronchus: Shorter, broad, direct communication with trachea.

Left bronchus: Narrower, longer and obliquely placed.

Aortogram: Helps to identify branches of aorta.

Mammogram: To detect abnormalities of breast.

HEAD AND NECK

View: Anteroposterior

Identify: Coronal suture, greater wing of sphenoid, lambdoid suture, lesser wing of sphenoid, mandibular condyles, mastoid process, nasal fossa, orbits, petrous temporal, sagittal suture (Figs 83 and 84).

Frontal sinus: Appears as translucent areas above and between the orbits.

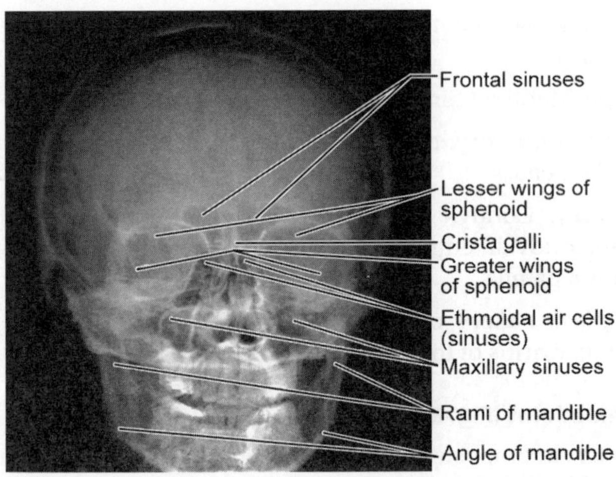

Fig. 83 Anteroposterior (AP) view

Maxillary sinus: Lies adjacent to the inferior margin of the orbit and petrous temporal shadow is superimposed.

View: Lateral

Identify: Anterior clinoid process, anterior cranial fossa, coronal suture, external ear, external and internal auditory meatus, frontal sinus, hard palate and teeth, lambdoid suture, middle meningeal groove, orbit, outer and inner tables, pineal body, posterior clinoid process

- *Pituitary fossa:* Round/oval depressions resting on the sphenoidal air sinus
- *Pineal body:* A small shadow above and behind the external auditory meatus
- *Mastoid air cells:* Appear as honeycomb translucencies lying behind the rig of external auditory meatus
- *Sphenoidal sinus:* Translucent areas below and anterior to the hypophyseal fossa
- *Transverse sinus:* Appears as translucent curved bandlike shadow about 1 cm wide behind the petrous temporal areas.

Frontal sinus
Hypophyseal fossa (sella turcica)
Greater wing of sphenoid
Coronal suture
Sphenoidal sinus
Lambdoid suture
Condyle of mandible
Mastoid air cells
Palatine process of maxilla
Maxillary sinus
Coronoid process of mandible
Dens of axis (C2 vertebra)
Anterior arch of atlas (C1 vertebra)

Fig. 84 Skull—lateral view

VERTEBRAL COLUMN (FIGS 85A AND B)

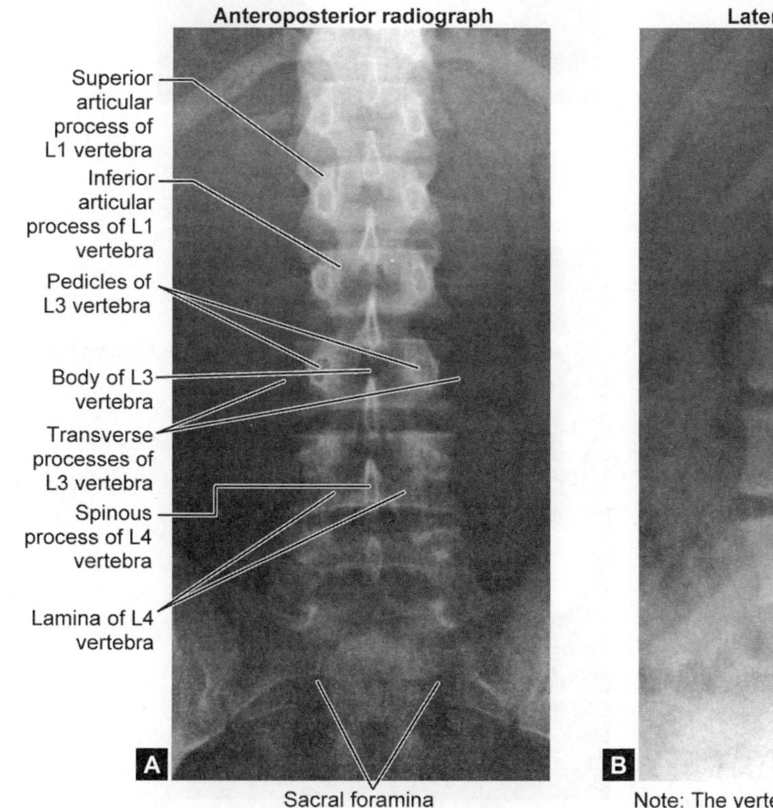

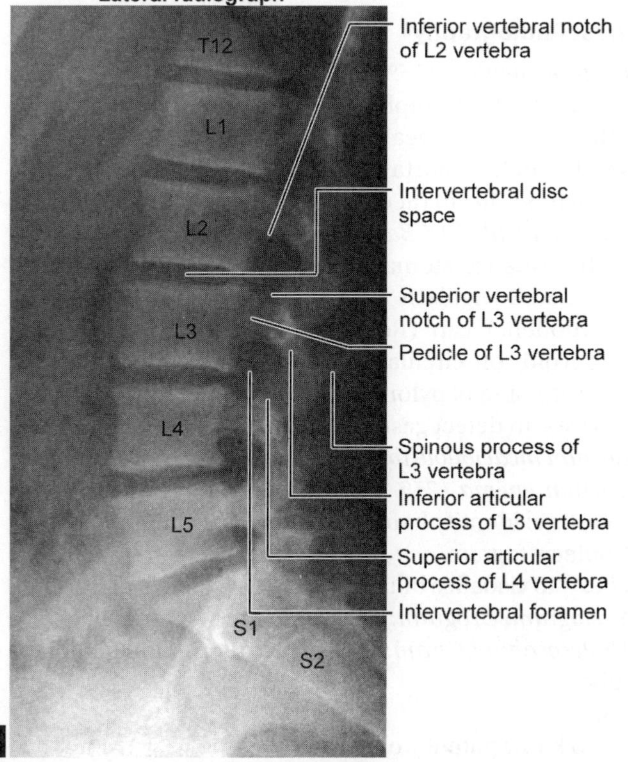

Figs 85A and B (A) Vertebral column—AP view; (B) Vertebral column—Central view

ABDOMEN

Plain X-ray Radiography

The X-ray of the abdomen is called 'KUB Film' because it is usually employed for the examination of the urinary tract and the letter symbolize 'Kidney, Ureters and Bladder'.

Bony Structures

- Coccyx
- Iliac crest
- Lower ribs
- Lumbar vertebrae
- Sacral foramina
- Sacroiliac joints
- Pubic symphysis.

Soft Tissues

- Alimentary canal
- Kidney
- Liver
- Psoas muscle
- Spleen.

Uses: To detect stones in kidney, ureter and bladder.

Contrast Radiography

- *Barium swallow (75% Ba) (Fig. 86):* Helps to identify constrictions of esophagus—15 cm from incisor tooth (pharyngoesophageal junction), 22.5 cm from (crossed by arch of aorta), 27.5 cm from (crossed by left bronchus), 40 cm (at opening in the diaphragm)
- *Barium meal (50% Ba) (Fig. 87)*
  - To visualize stomach, first part of diaphragm and incisura angularis
  - Duodenal cap (Reason—first part of duodenum devoid of circular mucus fold kept patent by protrusion of pylorus)
  - Use—to detect gastric tumor, peptic ulcer
- *Barium meal follow through:* To visualize small intestine
- *Barium enema (25% Ba) (Fig. 88):* To examine large intestine; identify haustrations and sacculation
- Cholecystogram
  Uses—to visualize biliary apparatus to detect gallstones
- *Pyelogram/Urogram:* To visualize urinary tract
- *Hysterosalpingogram:* To visualize uterus and fallopian tube.
  Uses:
  - To know patency of uterus
  - Study shape and size of uterus and fallopian tube
  - Detect anomalies of female genital tract

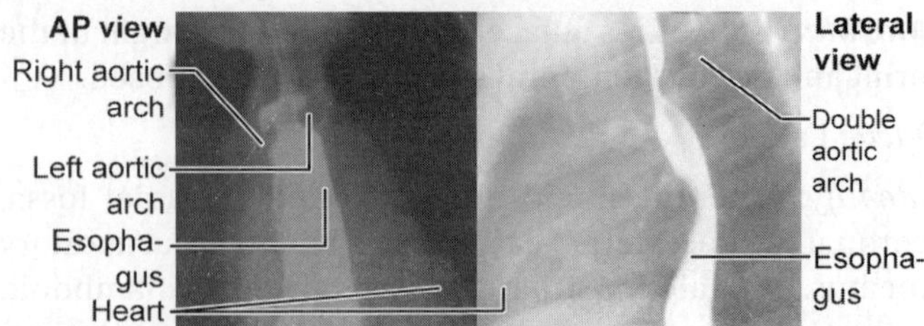

Fig. 86 Double aortic arch barium swallow shows impingement of the vascular malformation upon the esophagus both posteriorly and bilaterally. The impingement upon the trachea as well can result in tracheomalacia

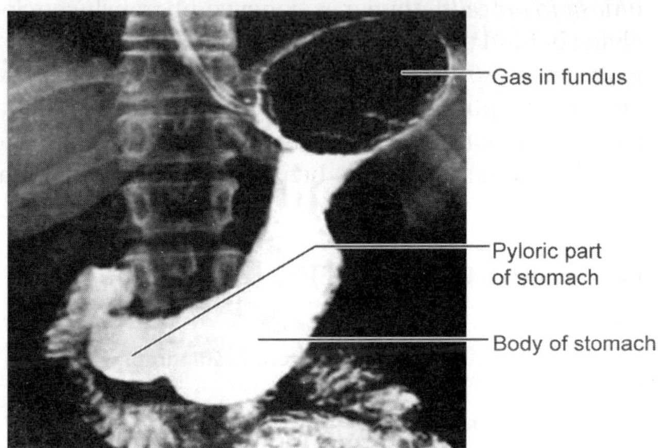

Fig. 87 Barium meal

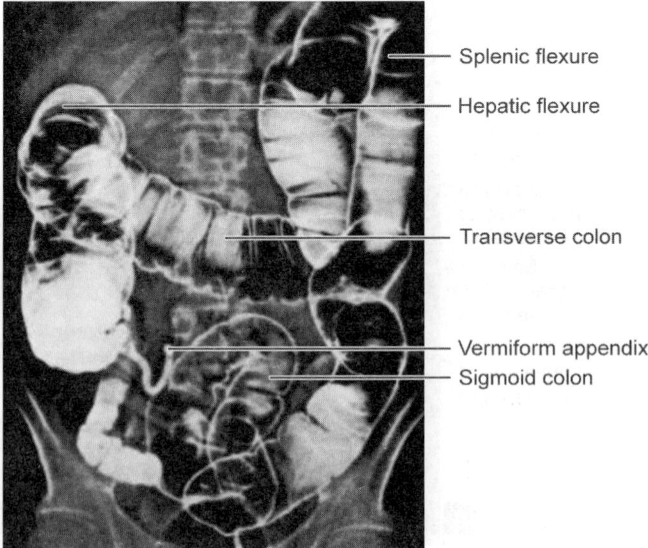

Fig. 88 Barium enema

Computed Tomography

- It allows 360° rotation of X-ray tube.
- A thin fan-shaped X-ray beam penetrates the body and produces a cross-sectional view of tissue within it.
- By revolving the X-ray tube around the body, CT machine views thin "slices" of the body from many angles. Hundreds of crystal chip detectors move in an arc with the X-ray tube. The detectors on the opposite side of the tube record what the scanner sees and deliver their information into a digital computer which compares the many views to make a single 3D video image.
- It has a profound use in lesions of the brain and spinal cord.
- It is a noninvasive and quick method to evaluate patients with brain, spinal cord and vertebral column lesions.
- Hematomas, infective lesions of the brain, cerebrovascular accidents whether due to infarct or hemorrhage can be differentiated easily.
- Ventricular system enlargement or displacement can be easily recognized.
- The lesion of the vertebral column-like infectious tumors, congenital abnormalities in the craniovertebral region, disc prolapse, spondylosis can be clearly seen.
- CT images have number of advantages over conventional chest radiographs, for example, the absence of confusing superimposition of structures and superior contrast resolution.
- Enlargement of lymph and spleen can be visualized clearly.

Magnetic Resonance Imaging (MRI)

- Instead of X-rays, a combination of radiowaves and a strong magnetic fields are used in this revolutionary technique.
- The tissues having higher water density appear brightest with MRI, since it focuses on the behavior of hydrogen atoms in water molecules.
- It can distinguish the brain's white matter and water rich gray matter.
- Teeth and bones which contain little water do not appear at all in MRI, enabling doctors to see tissues surrounded by bone such as the spinal cord.
- It is being increasingly used for imaging heart and great vessels, as it can distinguish between tissues better than CT scanning and can identify structures containing flowing blood.
- It has limitations in calcified structures because they contain very small amount of water.

SURFACE MARKING

UPPER LIMB

- *Axillary Artery*
  - The arm is held at the right angles to the trunk and palm is directed upwards.
  - Point A—midpoint of clavicle.
  - Point B—on the medial side of arm just in front of posterior axillary fold.
  - Join A and B by a straight line.
- *Brachial Artery*
  - Point B
  - Point C—1 cm below the midpoint of the elbow joint on its anterior aspect.
  - Join B and C by a straight line.
- *Radial Artery*
  - Point C
  - Point D—in front of wrist, medial to styloid process of radius.
  - Point E—in the anatomical snuff box.
  - Join C, D and E
- *Ulnar Artery*
  - Point C
  - Point F—A point at the junction of the upper 1/3rd with the lower 2/3rd of the forearm near its medial border.
  - Point G—at the lateral edge of pisiform.
  - Join C, F and G.
- *Superficial Palmar Arch*
  - Point G
  - Point H—hook of hamate.
  - Point I—at the center of palm at the level of distal border of extended thumb.
  - Point J—at the distal border of thenar eminence in line with cleft between index and middle finger.
  - Join G, H, I and J
- *Deep Palmar Arch*
  - Lies 1 cm proximal to superficial palmar arch
  - Point A—Proximal end of 1st intermetacarpal space
  - Point B—Distally to hook of hamate.
  - Join A and B by a horizontal line.
- *Flexor Retinaculum*
  - Point A—Mark the hook of hamate
  - Point B—Mark the crest of trapezium
  - Point C—Put a point on the pisiform bone.
  - Point D—Put a mark on the tubercle of scaphoid.
  - Join A, B, C and D
- *Pisiform Bone:* It is felt at medial border of the base of hypothenar eminence.
- *Hook of Hamate:* It is marked by a point at the medial border of hypothenar eminence distal to pisiform.
- *Crest of Trapezium:* It is recognized by applying deep pressure over thenar muscles.
- *Tubercle of Scaphoid:* It is situated at the base of the thenar eminence and it is felt below the lower border of radius.
- *Spine of Third Thoracic Vertebra:* Spine of scapula meets medial border.
- *Spine of Seventh Thoracic Vertebra:* Inferior angle of scapula.

THORAX

Pleura

Apex (Cervical Pleura)

- Point A—medial 1/3rd of clavicle
- Point B—sternoclavicular joint
- Point C—between point A and B but 3.5 cm above clavicle.
- Join A, B, C.

Right Costomediastinal Reflection

- Point B
- Point D—midpoint of sterna angle
- Point E—xiphisternal joint
- Join B, D, E.

Left Costomediastinal Joint

- Point B
- Point D
- Point F—in the midline at the level of left 4th costal cartilage
- Point G—little lateral to point F
- Point E
- Join B, D, F, G and E.

Costodiaphragmatic Reflection

- Compare it with inferior border of lung
- Point E
- Point H—where midclavicular line cuts 8th rib
- Point I—where midclavicular lines cut 10th rib
- Point J—2 cm lateral to the upper border of 12th thoracic spine
- Join E, H, I and J.

Lungs

Apex

Point A—2.5 cm above the medial 1/3rd of the clavicle.
Point B—sternoclavicular joint
Join A and B by a convex line facing upwards.

Anterior Border

Right Lung
- Point B
- Point C—midpoint of sternal angle
- Point D—6th right intercostals junction
- Join B, C and D.

Left Lung
- Point B
- Point C
- Point E—left 4th sternocostal junction
- Point F—little lateral to the point E
- Point G—2.5 cm lateral to left margin of sternum on 6th costal cartilage.
  Join B, C, E, F and G.

Inferior Border
- Point D
- Point G
- Point H—where midclavicular line cuts 6th rib
- Point I—where midaxillary line cuts the 8th rib
- Point J—2 cm lateral to spine of the 10th thoracic vertebrae
- Right lung—join D, H, I, J
- Left lung—join G, H, I, J.

Posterior Border
- Point A—2.5 cm lateral to the 7th cervical spine.
- Point B—2.5 cm lateral on the 10th thoracic spine.
- A vertical line joining the two points represents the posterior border of the lung.

Heart

Apex (Apex Beat)

Left 5ft intercostal space slightly medial to the midclavicular line or about 9 cm from the midline.

Right Border
- Point A—1.2 cm lateral to the margin of right 3rd costal cartilage
- Point B—3.7 cm lateral to the median plane in the right 4th ICS
- Point C—end of right 6th costal cartilage
- Join A, B, C with a slight convexity to the right.

Lower Border
- Point A
- Point D—xiphisternal junction
- Point E—apex beat
- Join A, D and E.

Left Border
- Point E
- Point F—1.2 cm from the sternal margin on the lower border of 2nd costal cartilage
- Join E and F with a left convexity.

Upper Border
Join the Point A and F.

Pulmonary Orifice

Lies partly behind the upper border of the left 3rd costal cartilage and partly behind the sternum. It is represented by a horizontal line 2.5 cm long.

Aortic Orifice

Lies below and a little to the right of pulmonary orifice. It corresponds to a line 2.5 cm long drawn from the medial end of the left 3rd intercostal space downwards and to the right.

Mitral Orifice

Lies behind the left half of the sternum opposite the 4th costal cartilage and can be represented by a line 3.0 cm long passing downwards and to the right.

Tricuspid Orifice

It can be represented by a line 4 cm long commencing in the median plane opposite the 4th costal cartilage and passing downwards and slightly to the right.

HEAD, NECK AND BRAIN

Parotid Duct
- Point A—lower border of conchae of ear.
- Point B—midway between ala of nose and red margin upper lip.
- Middle 3rd of line AB represents parotid duct.

Parotid Gland

Anterior Border
- Point C—upper border of mandibular condyle.
- Point D—little above the center of masseter muscle.
- Point E—2 cm below and behind the angle of mandible.
- Join C, D and E.

Posterior Border
- Point E
- Point F—apex of mastoid process
- Join E and F.

Upper Border

- Point C
- Point F
- Curved line below external auditory meatus across the lobule of the ear.
- Join C and F.

Thyroid Gland

Lobes

- Extend upto—middle of the thyroid cartilage, below to the cartilage.
- Laterally—extends and overlapped by anterior border of sternocleidomastoid.
- Upper pole is pointed.
- Lower pole is broad and rounded.

Isthmus

- Marked by two transverse parallel lines (each 1.2 cm long) on the trachea.
- Upper line is 1.2 cm below the cricoid cartilage.
- Lower line is 2.5 cm below the cricoid cartilage.

Common Carotid Artery

- Point A—sternoclavicular joint.
- Point B—on the anterior border of sternocleidomastoid at the level of upper border of thyroid cartilage.
- Join A and B.

Internal Carotid Artery

- Point B
- Point C—on the posterior border of mandibular condyle.
- Join B and C.

Facial Artery

- Point A—at anterior inferior border of masseter muscle.
- Point B—1.2 cm lateral to angle of mouth.
- Point C—medial angle of eye.
- Join A, B and C which curves forward almost to the ala of nose.

Middle Meningeal Artery

Trunk

- Point A—just in front of preauricular point.
- Point B—2 cm above middle of zygomatic arch.
- Join A and B.

Anterior Division

- Point C—pterion.
- Point D—middle point of vertex.
- Join C, D and B.
- Line BC is with slight anterior convexity upwards and backwards.

Posterior Division

- Point E—on upper limit of attachment of auricle.
- Point F—lambda.
- Join H and I.

Internal Jugular Vein

- Point A—on the neck medial to lobule of ear.
- Point B—medial end of clavicle.
- Join A and B.

Transverse Sinus

Marked by two parallel lines, 1.2 cm apart:

- First point—at the inion.
- Other point—at the mastoid process.

Central Sulcus

- Point A—1.2 cm behind the midpoint between nasion and inion.
- Point B—5 cm above the preauricular point.
- Join A and B by a curved line.

LOWER LIMB

Femoral Artery

- Point A—midpoint between the anterior superior iliac spine and pubic symphysis (midinguinal point).
- Point B—adductor tubercle (just above medial epicondyle of femur).
  Upper 2/3rd of line represents artery.

Sciatic Nerve

- Point A—2.5 cm lateral to the midpoint between posterior superior iliac spine and ischial tuberosity.
- Point B—middle of line joining the ischial tuberosity and apex of the greater trochanter.
- Point C—upper angle of the popliteal fossa or midpoint between upper 2/3rd and lower 1/3rd of back of the thigh.
- Join A, B and C.

Popliteal Artery

- Point A—midpoint of 'middle and lower one-third' of the thigh. 2.5 cm medial to the midline on the back of thigh.
- Point B—midpoint between 2 femoral condyles.
- Point C—on the midline on the back of leg at the level of tibial tuberosity.
- Join A, B and C.

Anterior Tibial Artery

- Point A—2.5 cm below the medial side of head of the fibula.
- Point B—midway between the two malleoli.
- Join A and B.

Dorsalis Pedis Artery

- Point A—midpoint of two malleoli.
- Point B—proximal end of the 1st intermetatarsal space.
- Join A and B.

Flexor Retinaculum

- Point A—medial malleolus
- Point B—calcaneum
- Draw a 2.5 cm broadband passing downwards and backwards by connecting the point A and B.

ABDOMEN AND PELVIS

Sagittal Planes

Median Vertical Plane

- Point A—suprasternal notch
- Point B—pubic symphysis
- Line joining A and B.

Lateral Vertical Plane

- Point C—midway between anterior superior iliac spine and pubic symphysis.
- Point D—middle of clavicle (midway between suprasterna notch and acromioclavicular joint).
- Join C and D.

Transverse Planes

Transpyloric Planes/Addison's Plane

It lies at the lower border of L1:

- Point E—midway between A and B.
- Point F—tip of 9th costal cartilage.
- Join C and D.

Subcostal Plane

- Draw transverse line below 10th rib. It lies on upper border of L3.
- Transtubercular plane.
- Draw transverse line at the level of tubercle on iliac crest. It lies on the upper border of L5.

Liver

Upper Border

- Point A—little below right nipple.
- Point B—xiphisternal joint.
- Point C—little below and medial to the left nipple.
- Join A and B. Also B and C by convex lines (AB is more convex).

Right Border

- Point D—1 cm just below the tip of right 10th costal cartilage.
- Draw convex line by connecting A and D.

Lower Border

- Point E—tip of right 9th costal cartilage.
- Point F—on the transpyloric plane in the midline.
- Point G—tip of 8th left costal cartilage.
- Join D, E, F, G, and C.

Gallbladder

The fundus of the gallbladder is marked at the right angle between the right costal margin and outer border of rectus abdominis (linea semilunaris).

Kidney

The kidney marked within Morris'parallelogram, which is drawn in the following way:

- Two horizontal lines, one through T11 and other through L3 spines.
- Two vertical lines, one 25 cm and other 9 cm from the median plane.
- Hilum lies 5 cm from the transpyloric plane.
- Upper pole lies 4–5 cm from the midline.
- Lower plane lies 6–7 cm from the midline (at the umbilical plane on the right side and at the subcostal plane in the left side).

Ureter

Posterior Surface Marking

- Point A—4 cm from median plane at the level of lower border of L1.
- Point B—posterior superior iliac spine.
- Join A and B.

Appendix

- Appendicular orifice—2 cm below the ileocecal orifice.
- Appendix is marked by two parallel lines 1 cm apart and 7–10 cm long extending from the appendicular orifice, usually upwards behind the cecum.

Spleen

- Marked on left side of back.
- Long axis—corresponds to 10th rib.
- Upper border—corresponds to upper border of 9th rib.
- Lower border—corresponds to lower border of 11th rib.
- Medial end—4–5 cm from the midline.
- Lateral end on the midaxillary line.

Cecum

- Marked in the right iliac fossa.
- 6 cm long and 7.5 cm broad and its axis directed downwards and slightly medially.

SYSTEMIC EMBRYOLOGY

HEAD AND NECK

- Development of face*
- Development of upper lip and anomalies
- Development of palate and anomalies
- Tongue development and nerve supply
- Thyroid—development and anomalies.

Face* (Fig. 89)

- It develops around the stomatodeum
- In the early 5th week of IUL, the stomatodeum is deepened by the development of 5 processes:
  - (i) Frontonasal process above (The mesoderm covering the developing forebrain proliferates and forms a downward projection).
  - (ii) and (iii) right and left maxillary process arising from the first mandibular arch, lateral to the stomatodeum.
  - (iv) and (v) right and left mandibular processes arising caudally from the first arch.

Nasal placodes: These are formed just above the stomatodeum.

Formed by the ectoderm overlying the frontonasal process.

Nasal pits: The placodes soon sink below the surface to form the nasal pits.

Medial and lateral nasal processes: The medial and lateral edges of each pit are raised above the surface to form the medial and lateral nasal processes respectively.

Development of Upper Lip*

- The right and left nasal pits come close together.
- Each maxillary process now grows medially and fuses first with lateral nasal processes and then with medial nasal processes.
- Medial and lateral nasal processes also fuse with each other.
- In this way, external nares are formed.
- *Philtrum:* The mesodermal basis of the median part of the lip.
  It is formed from the frontonasal process.
- The mesodermals of the lateral part is formed from the maxillary process.
- The overlying skin of upper lip is derived from the ectoderm covering the maxillary process.
- Muscles of the face are derived from the mesoderm of the second branchial arch and are supplied by the facial nerve.

Development of Lower Lip

The mandibular process of two sides grow towards each other and fuse in the midline to form the lower lip.

Development of Nose

- Initially the external nasal apertures are widely separated each other due to intervening median nasal processes.
- Gradually, these apertures come closer as the median nasal processes become thinner.

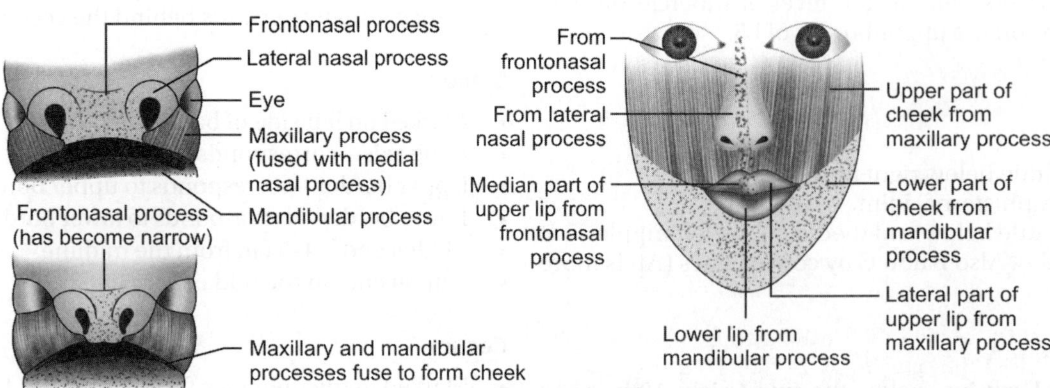

Fig. 89 Development of face

- The nasal septum develops from the thinned out median nasal process.
- Deepened nasal pits are called nasal sacs, which are separated from the stomatodeum by bucconasal membrane.
- This membrane soon breaks so that nasal sacs communicate with the stomatodeum by an opening called posterior nasal aperture.
- During the formation of the secondary palate, the lower edge of nasal septum fuses with the medial edges of the palatal processes.
- Thus oral cavity is completely shut off from the nasal cavity and the posterior nasal apertures shift backward to open into the nasopharynx.
- The lateral nasal processes form the lateral wall of the nose.

Developmental Anomalies of the Face

- *Harelip*—the upper lip of the hare normally has a cleft. Hence, the term harelip is used for defects of the lip (Fig. 90A).
- *Oblique facial cleft*—Nonfusion of the maxillary and lateral nasal processes gives rise to a cleft running from the medial angle of the eye to the mouth.

  The nasolacrimal duct is not formed (Fig. 90B).
- *Lateral facial cleft*—lack of fusion in one side.
- *Bilateral facial cleft*—lack of fusion in both sides.

Development of Palate*

- It is formed from three components (Figs 91A to E):
  - *Two palatal process:* Formed as a plate-like shelf which grows medially from each maxillary process.
  - *Primitive palate:* Formed from the frontonasal process.
- The definitive palate is formed by the fusion of these three embryonic components by a Y-shaped suture.
- The fusion takes place in anteroposterior direction.
- Membranous ossification occurs in the anterior part of the palate to give rise to the hard palate.
- Ossification does not extend into the most posterior portion which remains as the soft palate.

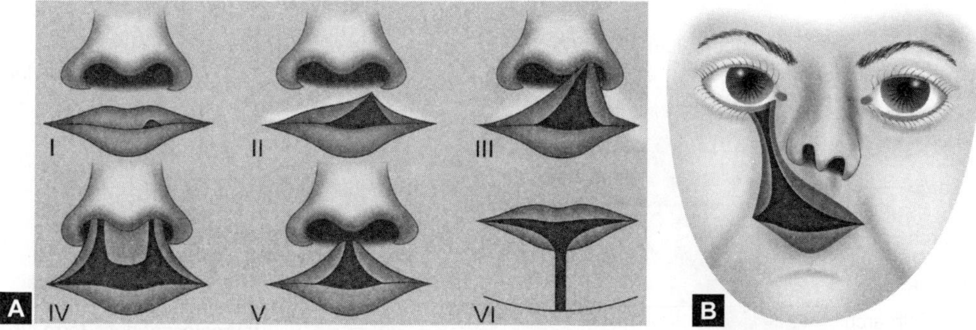

Figs 90A and B (A) Varieties of harelip; (B) Oblique facial cleft

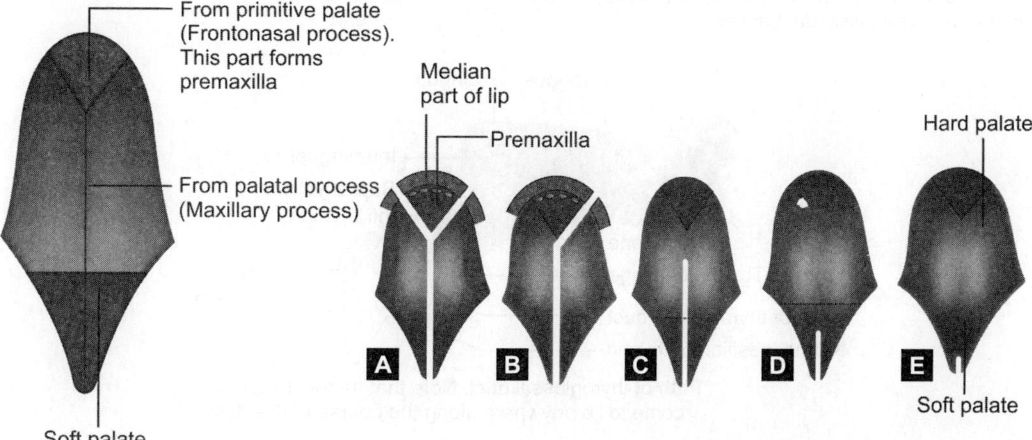

Figs 91A to E Varieties of cleft palate. (A) Complete nonfusion, giving rise to a Y-shaped cleft, accompanied by (bilateral harelip); (B) The left maxillary process has fused with the premaxilla, but not with right maxillary process. The cleft is accompanied by (unilateral harelip); (C) Midline cleft extending into the hard palate; (D) Cleft of soft palate; (E) Bified uvula

- The part of the palate derived from the frontonasal process forms the premaxilla, which carries the incisor teeth.

*Cleft Palate**

Defective fusion of the various components of the palate gives rise to the clefts in the palate:
- Cleft of the palate that extends to its anterior end is associated with harelip.
- Clefts of the palate result in anomalous communication between the mouth and the nose.

Thyroid Gland* (Fig. 92)

- It develops mainly from the thyroglossal duct.
- The medial ends of two mandibular (first) arches are separated by a midline swelling called tuberculum impar.
- Immediately behind the tuberculum, the epithelium of the floor of the pharynx shows a thickening in the midline. This region is soon depressed below the surface to form a diverticulum called thyroglossal duct.
- The site of origin of diverticulum shows a depression called foramen cecum. The diverticulum grows down in the midline into the neck.
- Its tip bifurcates and gives rise to two lobes of the gland.

Anomalies

- *Lingual:* Under the mucosa of the tongue
- *Intralingual:* Embedded in the muscular substance of the tongue
- *Suprahyoid:* In the neck, above the hyoid bone
- *Infrahyoid:* Below the hyoid bone, above its normal position
- *Intrathoracic:* Entire or part of it lies in the thorax.

Tongue* (Figs 93 and 94)

- Tongue develops from the floor of the developing mouth.
- The medial most part of the mandibular arch proliferates to form lingual swellings.
- The lingual swellings are separated by tuberculum impar in the midline.
- Behind the tuberculum impar foramen cecum is formed.

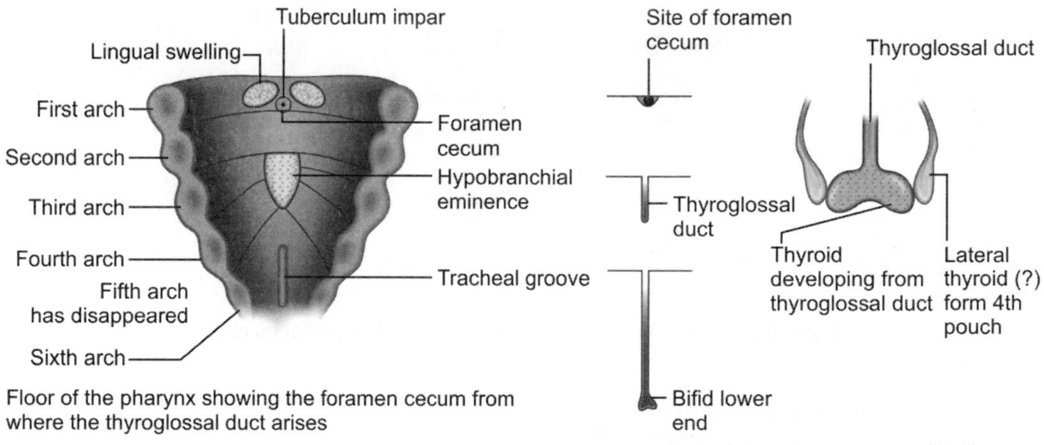

Floor of the pharynx showing the foramen cecum from where the thyroglossal duct arises

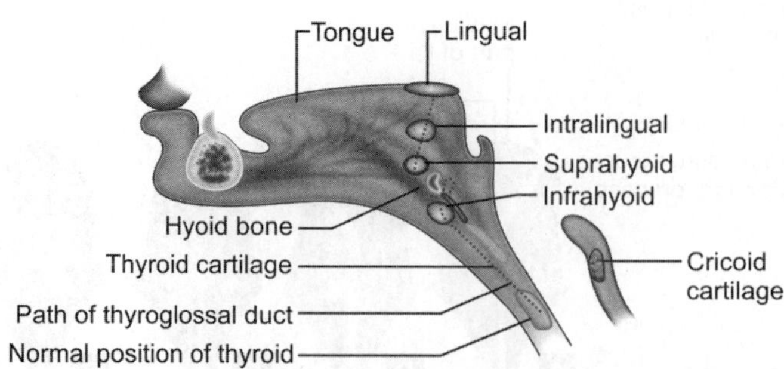

Path of thyroglossal duct. Note that thyroid tissue may come to lie anywhere along the course of this duct

Fig. 92 Development of thyroid gland

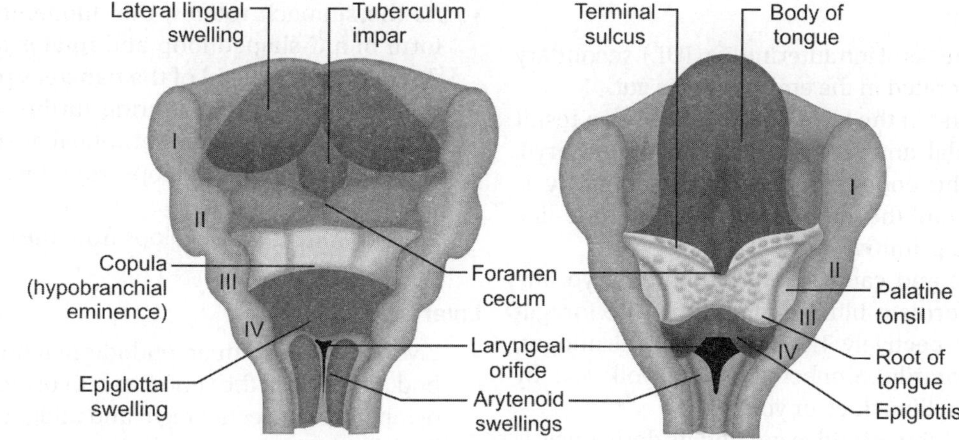

Fig. 93 Development of tongue–I

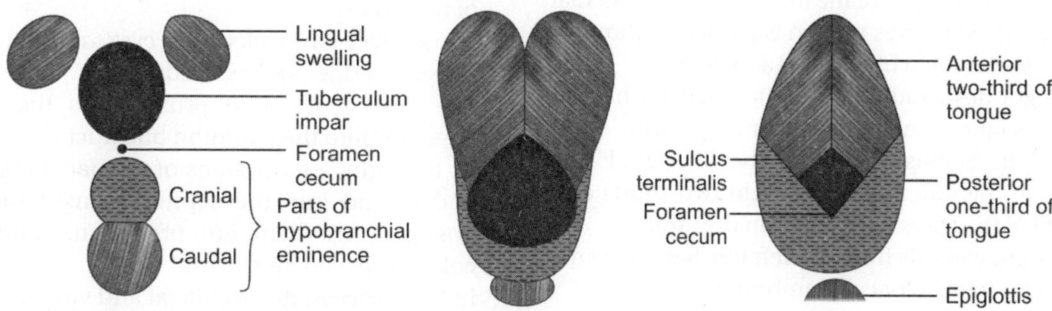

Fig. 94 Development of tongue–II

- Another midline swelling called hypobranchial eminence is formed in relation to medial ends of 2nd, 3rd and 4th arches.
- The eminence subdivides into the cranial part called copula, related to the 2nd and 3rd arch and the caudal part related to the 4th arch.
- Anterior 2/3rd is formed by fusion of the tuberculum impar and the two swellings. Posterior 1/3rd is formed from the copula.
- In this situation, 2nd arch mesoderm gets buried below the surface. The 3rd arch mesoderm grows over it to fuse with the mesoderm of 1st arch.
- Posterior most part of the tongue is developed from the 4th arch
- The musculature of tongue is developed from the occipital myotomes.

Nerve Supply

Anterior 2/3rd—General sensation-lingual branch of trigeminal nerve

Taste sensation—Chordae tympani branch of facial nerve

Posterior 1/3rd—General sensation } Glossopharyngeal nerve
Taste sensation

Posterior most part—superior pharyngeal nerve

Anomalies

Macroglossia: Too large tongue

Microglossia: Too small tongue

Aglossia: Absence of tongue

Tongue-tie/ankyloglossia: Apical part of the tongue anchored to the floor of the mouth by an overdeveloped frenulum.

ABDOMEN AND PELVIS

- Liver—development
- Pancreas—development and anomalies*
- Kidney—development and anomalies*
- Urinary bladder—development and anomalies
- Development of uterus*.

Alimentary System

- At the end of 3 weeks of intrauterine life (IUL), secondary yolk sac incorporated in the embryo as the gut.
- Endoderm is first in the form of a flat sheet, as a result of cephalocaudal and lateral folding of the embryo, a portion of the endoderm-lined yolk sac cavity is incorporated into the embryo to form a tube-like structure called primitive gut.
- In the cephalic and caudal parts of the embryo, the primitive gut forms a blind-ending tube, the foregut and hindgut, respectively. The middle part, the midgut, remains temporarily connected to the yolk sac by means of the vitelline duct, or yolk stalk.
- Development of the primitive gut and its derivatives is usually discussed under four sections:
  1. The pharyngeal gut or pharynx, extends from the buccopharyngeal membrane to the trachea-bronchial diverticulum; since this section is particularly important for development of the head and neck.
  2. The foregut lies caudal to the pharyngeal tube and extends as far caudally as the liver outgrowth.
  3. The midgut begins caudal to the liver bud and extends to the junction of the right two-thirds and left third of the transverse colon in the adult.
  4. The hindgut extends from the left third of the transverse colon to the cloacal membrane.

Duodenum

- The terminal part of the foregut and the cephalic part of the midgut form the duodenum.
- As the stomach rotates, the duodenum takes on the form of a C-shaped loop and rotates to the right. The duodenum and head of the pancreas press against the dorsal body wall and during further development it becomes fixed in a retroperitoneal position.
- *Upper duodenum:* Develops from the caudal most part of the foregut.
- *Lower duodenum:* Develops from the cranial most part of the midgut.

Liver

- Liver develops from an endodermal bud called hepatic bud. Arises from the ventral aspect of the gut, at the point of junction between foregut and midgut (Figs 95A to E).
- Bud divides into two parts. The larger cranial *part called pars hepatica*, which invades the septum transversum and rapidly enlarges to give rise to right and left lobes of the liver.
- The smaller part called *pars cystica*, which gives rise to the gallbladder and cystic duct.
- The part of the bud proximal to the pars cystica develops into the common bile duct.
- As the right, left divisions of the pars hepatica enlarge and extend into the septum transversum, the cells arising from them are broken up into interlacing columns called hepatic trabeculae.
- In this process, the umbilical and vitelline veins which line the septum transversum are broken up to form the sinusoids of the liver. Sinusoids are also formed from the mesenchyme of the septum transversum.

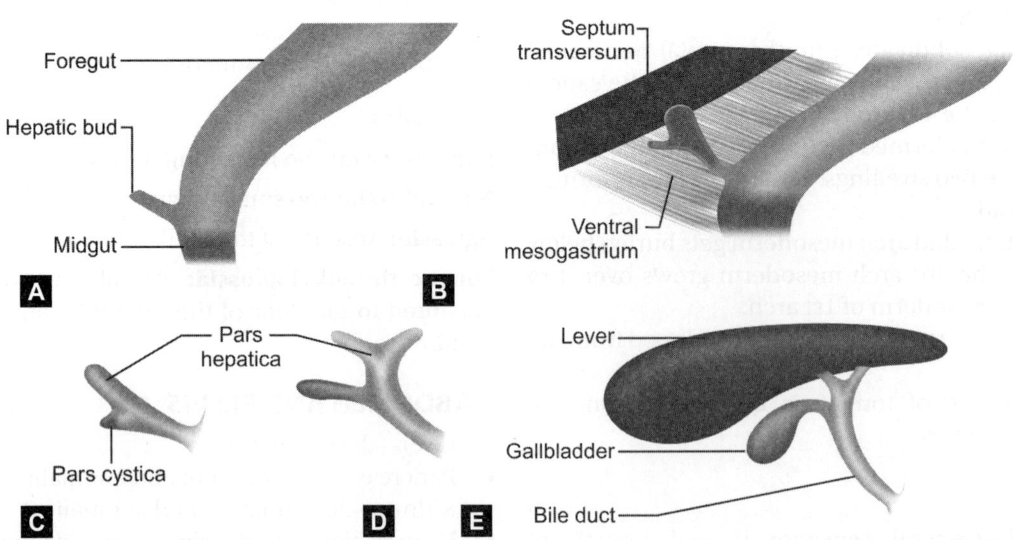

Figs 95A to E Development of the biliary apparatus. (A) Hepatic bud arises from the gut at the junction of foregut and midgut; (B) It grows forwards the septum transversum through the ventral mesogastrium; (C to E) The buds divide into pars hepatica (that forms the liver) and the pars cystica (that forms the gallbladder). The part of the hepatic bud proximal to its division forms the bile duct

- This portion of the septum, which consists of densely packed mesoderm, will form the central tendon of the diaphragm. The surface of the liver that is in contact with the future diaphragm is never covered by peritoneum; it is the bare area of the liver.

Pancreas*

- It develops from two endodermal buds:
  1. *Ventral bud:* Arises in close relation to the hepatic bud in the inferior angle between it and the duodenum
  2. *Dorsal bud:* Arises from the dorsal aspect of the gut.
- When the duodenal loop falls to the right, the ventral bud comes to point to the right and the dorsal bud to the left (Figs 96A to D).
- As a result of differential growth of the wall of the gut, attachment of the ventral bud also shifts to the left side.
- The two buds fuse to form one single mass.
- The ventral bud gives rise to the lower part of the head and the uncinate process of the pancreas.
- The dorsal bud gives rise to upper part of head, body and tail.

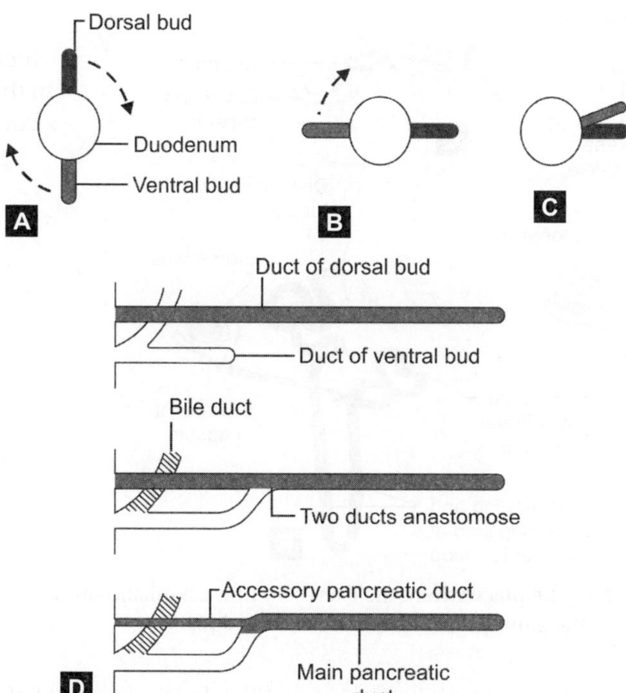

Figs 96A to D Development of pancreas: Changes in the relative position of pancreatic buds. (A) Initial position in which the ventral and dorsal buds lie in the direction indicated by their names; (B) Position after duodenal loop falls to the left; (C) The attachment of the ventral bud moves to the left and the two buds now lie close together; (D) Development in series

- Main pancreatic duct is formed, in which distal part is formed by the duct of dorsal bud and its proximal part formed by the duct of ventral bud.
- The accessory pancreatic duct is formed from the duct of dorsal bud between the anastomosis and the duodenum.

Anomalies

Pancreatic Abnormalities

Occasionally, however, the right portion of the ventral bud migrates along its normal route, but the left migrates in the opposite direction. In this manner, the duodenum is surrounded by pancreatic tissue, and an annular pancreas is formed. The malformation, sometimes, constricts the duodenum and causes complete obstruction.

Accessory pancreatic tissue may be anywhere from the distal end of the esophagus to the tip of the primary intestinal loop. Most frequently, it lies in the mucosa of the stomach and in Meckel's diverticulum, where it may show all of the histological characteristics of the pancreas itself.

Urogenital System

Functionally, the urogenital system can be divided into two entirely different components: the urinary system and the genital system.

Urinary System

*Kidney**

3 parts—pronephros, mesonephros, and metanephros (Figs 97A to C)

Pronephros: At the beginning of the fourth week, the pronephros is represented by 7 to 10 solid cell groups in the cervical region. These groups form vestigial excretory units, nephrotomes that regress before more caudal ones are formed. By the end of the 4th week, all indications of the pronephric system have disappeared.

Mesonephros: The mesonephros and mesonephric ducts are derived from intermediate mesoderm from upper thoracic to upper lumbar (L3) segments. Early in the 4th week of development, during regression of the pronephric system, the first excretory tubules of the mesonephros appear. They lengthen rapidly, form an S-shaped loop, and acquire a tuft of capillaries that will form a glomerulus at their medial extremity. Around the glomerulus the tubules form Bowman's capsule, and together these structures constitute a renal corpuscle. Laterally, the tubule enters the longitudinal collecting duct known as the mesonephric or Wolffian duct.

By the end of the second month, the majority have disappeared. In the male, a few of the caudal tubules and

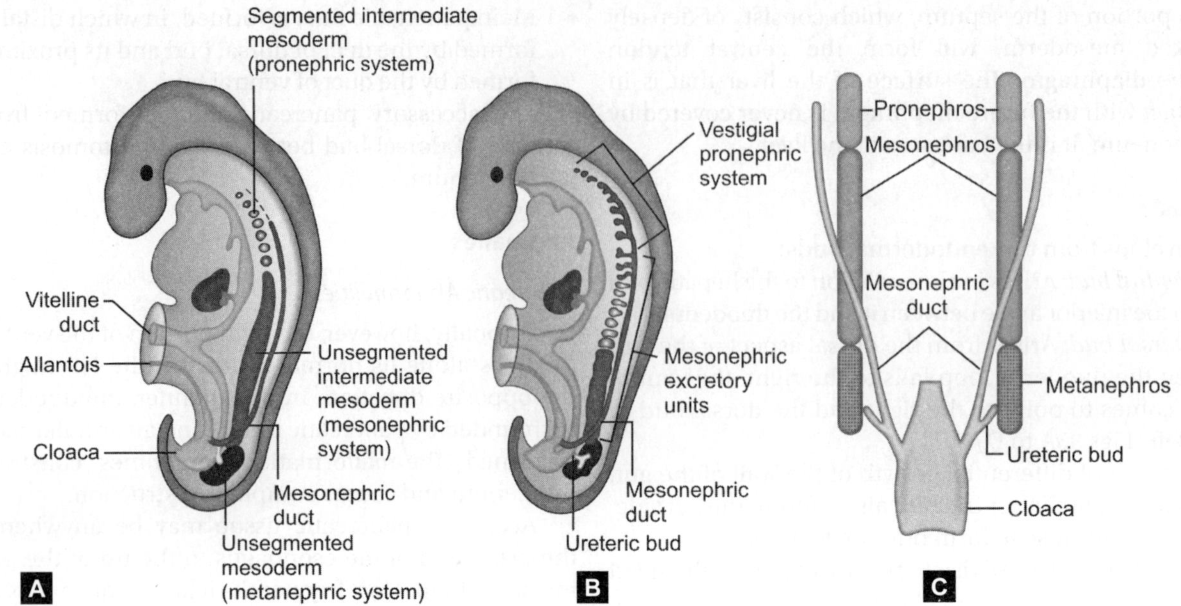

Figs 97A to C Development of kidney

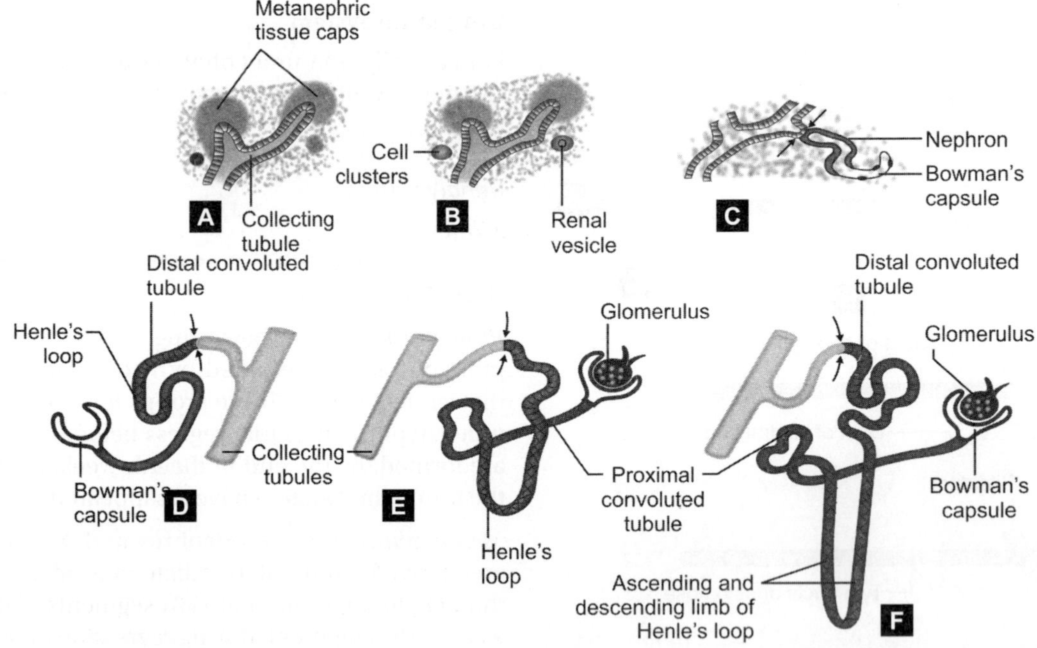

Figs 98A to F Development of a metanephric excretory unit. Arrows, the place where the excretory unit establishes and with the collecting system, allowing flow of urine from the glomerulus into the collecting ducts

the mesonephric duct persist and participate in formation of the genital system, but they disappear in the female.

Metanephros (the Definitive Kidney) (Figs 98A to F): The third urinary organ, the metanephros, or permanent kidney, appears in the fifth week. Its excretory units develop from metanephric mesoderm in the same manner as in the mesonephric system. The development of the duct system differs from that of the other kidney systems.

Collecting system: Collecting ducts of the permanent kidney develop from the *ureteric bud*, an outgrowth of the mesonephric duct close to its entrance to the cloaca. Subsequently, the bud dilates, forming the primitive renal pelvis, and splits into cranial and caudal portions, the future major calyces.

The ureteric bud gives rise to the ureter, the renal pelvis, the major and minor calyces, and approximately 1 to 3 million collecting tubules.

Clinical Correlates

Anomalies

- *Horseshoe kidney:* Lower poles of the two kidneys may be fused. It does not ascend higher than the level of inferior mesenteric artery.
- *Pancake kidney:* Two kidneys may form one mass.
- *Lobulated kidney:* Lobulations of the kidney may persist.
- *Congenital polycystic kidney:* Forms numerous cysts.

Urinary Bladder*

During the 4th to 7th weeks of development, the cloaca divides into the urogenital sinus anteriorly and the anal canal posteriorly. The urorectal septum is a layer of mesoderm between the primitive anal canal and the urogenital sinus. The tip of the septum will form the perineal body.
Three portions:

1. The *upper* and largest part is the urinary bladder. Initially, the bladder is continuous with the allantois, but when the lumen of the allantois is obliterated, a thick fibrous cord, the urachus, remains and connects the apex of the bladder with the umbilicus.
   In the adult, it is known as the median umbilical ligament.
2. *Pelvic* part of the urogenital sinus which in the male gives rise to the prostatic and membranous parts of the urethra.
3. *Phallic* part of the urogenital sinus.

The mucous membrane of the urinary bladder developed as follows:

- Entire mucosa, except the internal trigone develops from the endoderm of vesicourethral part of cloaca.
- The apex of the bladder is derived from the absorbed proximal part of the allantois diverticulum. Distal part obliterates to form urachus.
- The internal trigone is derived from the mesoderm by incorporation of caudal part of mesonephric duct. The mesonephric ducts open into the pelvic part of urogenital sinus and the common excretory ducts blend with the dorsal wall of the vesicourethral part of cloaca.

Consequently, the ureters, initially outgrowths from the mesonephric ducts, enter the bladder separately those of the mesonephric ducts move close together to enter the prostatic urethra and in the male become the ejaculatory ducts.

Since both the mesonephric ducts and ureters originate in the mesoderm, the mucosa of the bladder formed by incorporation of the ducts (the trigone of the bladder) is also mesodermal.

With time the mesodermal lining of the trigone is replaced by endodermal epithelium, so that finally the inside of the bladder is completely lined with endodermal epithelium.

Ureter

The ureter derived from the part of the ureteric bud that lies between the pelvis of the kidney and the vesicourethral canal.

Anomalies

- Duplication of ureter
- Instead of opening into the urinary bladder, ureter may end in the prostatic urethra, ductus deferens, seminal vesicle or rectum in the male and the urethra, vagina, etc. in the female.
- Blind ureter—ureter not connected to the kidney
- Hydroureter—ureter dilated.

Genital System

*Genital Ducts**

Mesonephric ducts: These ducts extend caudally from the mesonephric tubules to the dorsal wall of the pelvic part of urogenital sinus through the urorectal septum.

Derivatives of Mesonephric Ducts and Tubules

In males: Mesonephric tubules—superior aberrant ductules, efferent ductules of testis mesonephric duct—ureter, canal of epididymis, ductus deferens, ejaculatory ducts.

In females: Mesonephric tubules-regress and mesonephric duct—duct of epoophoron (duct of Gartner).

Paramesonephric duct: These are duct developed in either sex in the 6th week as a longitudinal groove-like invagination of coelomic epithelium on the lateral side of the mesonephric duct. The margins of the duct fuse to form the duct (Fig. 99).

Derivatives of Paramesonephric Ducts

In males, appendix of testis, utricle of prostate
In females, uterine tubes, uterus, upper vagina.

Uterus*

- The caudal part of paramesonephric ducts fuse in the midline to form uterovaginal canal.

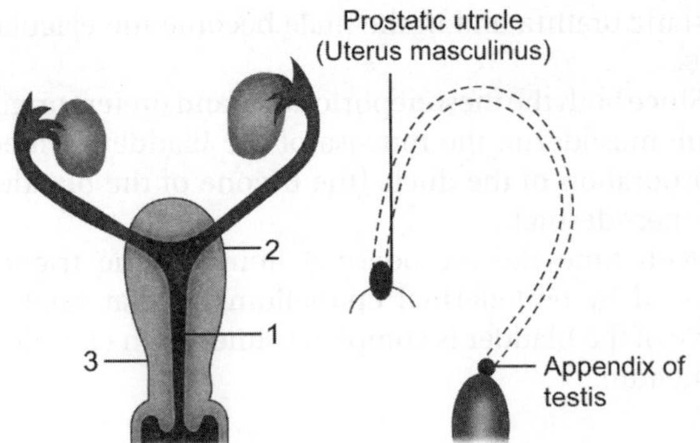

Fig. 99 Fate of paramesonephric test

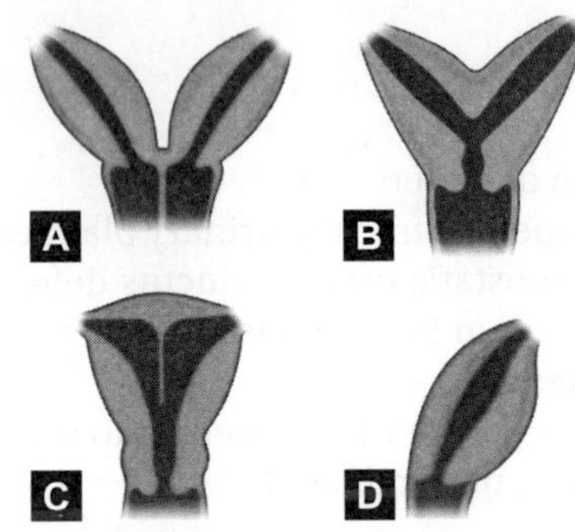

Figs 100A to D Anomalies of the uterus. (A) Duplication of uterus and vagina; (B) Bicornuate uterus; (C) Septum in uterus; (D) Unicornuate uterus

- Its caudal end comes in contact with the dorsal wall of the definitive urogenital sinus.
- The epithelium of the uterus develops from the utero-vaginal canal.
- The myometrium is derived from surrounding mesoderm.
- As the thickness of the myometrium increases, the unfused part of the two paramesonephric ducts come to be partially embedded within its substances and the fundus is formed.
- The uterine tubes developed from the unfused part of the paramesonephric duct.

Anomalies (Figs 100A to D)

- Didelphys—double uterus, double cervix and double vagina
- Bicornis bicollis—double uterus, double cervix and a single vagina
- Septate uterus—uterus with a septum
- Arcuate uterus—fundus of the uterus is concave
- Unicornuate uterus—one half of the uterus may be absent
- Atresia of vagina
- Atresia of cervix.

Descent of Testis*

- During fetal life, the testis gradually descend to the scrotum
- 2nd month—begins
- 3rd month—reaches iliac fossa
- 4th-6th month—at the site of deep inguinal ring
- 7th month—pass through the inguinal canal
- End of 8th month—normally in the scrotum.

Structure	*Male derivative*	*Female derivative*
Gonad	Testis	Ovary
Sex cords	Sertoli cells Seminiferous tubules	Granulosa cells
Primordial germ cells	Spermatozoa	Ova
Paramesonephric duct	Appendix of testis Utricle of prostate	Uterine tube, uterus Upper vagina
Mesonephric duct	Appendix of epididymis, Epididymis, Ductus deferens, Ejaculatory duct Seminal vesicle	Appendix of ovary Gartner's duct
Mesonephric tubules	Vasa efferentia Paradidymis	Epoophoron Paroophoron
Genital tubercle	Penis	Clitoris
Genital swellings	Scrotum	Labia majora
Urethral folds	Floor of penile urethra	Labia minora

THORAX

- Development of heart
  - Right atrium
  - Interatrial septum
- Development of aortic arches
- Fetal circulation.

Heart

- The heart arises in the 3rd week, in the form of two capillaries which differentiate in a cephalocaudal direction, and fuse with each other to form the endothelial heart tube (Fig. 101).
- This tube has a series of dilatations.
  - Bulbus cordis (most distally and lies at the arterial end of the heart)
    Distal 1/3: Truncus arteriosus—forms ascending aorta (continuous with the aortic sac and with the right and left pharyngeal arch arteries and it further continues with right and left dorsal aorta)
    Middle 1/3: Conus—forms outflow tracts of right and left ventricle
    Proximal 1/3: Forms primitive right ventricle (trabeculated part)

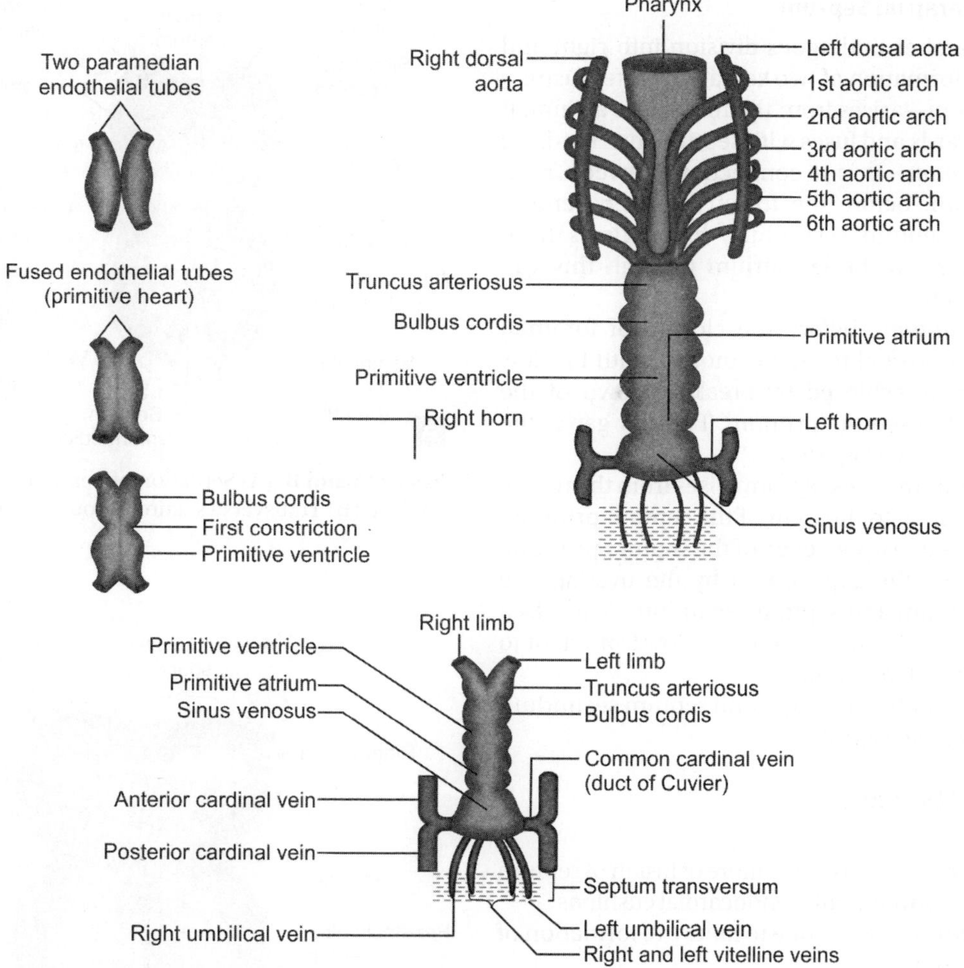

Fig. 101 Stages of developing heart tube

- Ventricle—forms primitive left ventricle (trabeculated part)
- Atrium—forms primitive atrium. It is partitioned to form right and left atria
- Sinus venosus (it lies in the venous end of the heart)

- It has a body and right and left horns.
- Body is absorbed into right atria and forms smooth part of right atrium.
- One vitelline vein (from the yolk sac), one umbilical vein (from the placenta), and one common cardinal vein (from the body wall) join each horn of the sinus venosus.
- Left horn of sinus venosus retrogresses. The remnant forms part of coronary sinus.
- Right horn of sinus venosus is absorbed into the right atrium.
- Right common cardinal vein forms part of superior vena cava.
- Right umbilical vein disappears.
- Right vitelline vein forms part of inferior vena cava.

Bending of heart tube-initially, the tube runs straight from the venous to the arterial end.

Formation of Atria*

- The sinus venosus and the primitive atrial chamber are at first connected by a wide opening.
- Finally, the opening becomes narrow and shifts to the right.
- The slit has right and left margins called the right and left venous valves.
- Cranially, these two fuses to form a structure called the septum spurium.
- The atrioventricular canal divides into right and left halves.
- Two thickenings, atrioventricular cushions appear on its dorsal and ventral valves. They grow towards each other and fuse.
- The fused septum forms the septum intermedium.

Formation of Interatrial Septum*

- The atrial chamber undergoes division into right and left halves by formation of two septa (that later fuse).
- *Septum primum*—arises from the roof of the atrium. It grows downwards and fuses with septum intermedium
- *Foramen primum*—it is a connection between right and left atrium, before the fusion between septum primum and septum secundum, blood flows from the right atrium to the left atrium through this gap (Figs 102A and B).
- *Foramen secundum*—before the closure of foramen primum, it is essential to create another path for flow of blood. This is achieved by breaking down of the upper part of the septum primum. The new gap is the foramen secundum (Fig. 103).
- Septum secundum—this septum arises from the roof of the atrial chamber, to the right of the septum primum, which overlaps free upper edge of the septum primum.
- Foramen ovale—the gap formed by the overlapping of septum primum and septum secundum, it acts as a valvular aperture that allows blood to flow from right to left, but not from left to right.

After birth, the septum primum and septum secundum fuse to form interatrial septum.

Interatrial Septal Defects

About 3 types:

1. *Ostium primum defect*—due to failure of fusion of septum primum with atrioventricular endocardial cushions.
2. *Ostium secundum defect*—due to failure of formation of septum secundum.
3. *Patent foramen ovale*—foramen ovale persists even after birth.

Aortic Arches*

- Before the folding of the embryo, two primitive aortae lie between the notochord and dorsal wall of yolk sac.
- The aorta have 3 parts, namely, ventral aortae, first aortic arches and dorsal aortae.
- Cephalic to truncus arteriosus, the ventral aorta fuses to form aortic sac, which bifurcates into the right and left limbs, connected to the dorsal aorta by the first aortic arches.
- Successive arterial arches appear in the second to sixth pharyngeal arches, each being connected ventrally to the right or left horn of aortic sac and dorsally to the dorsal aortae.
- In the early stage, there are six arterial arches but later 1st, 2nd, and 5th arches disappear (Figs 104A and B).

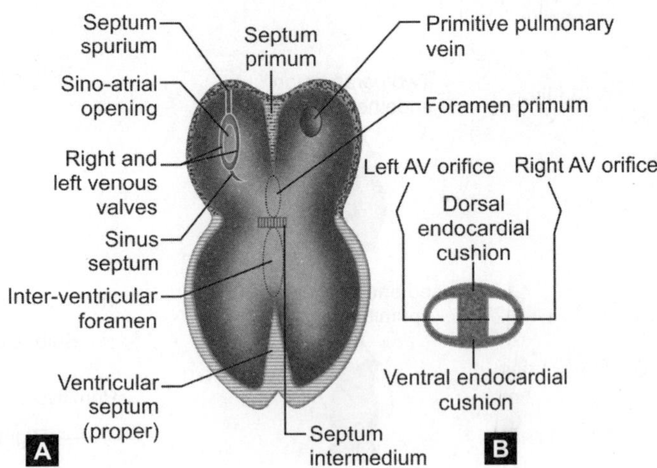

Figs 102A and B (A) Septation of heart; formation of foramen primum; (B) Transverse section through atrioventricular canal

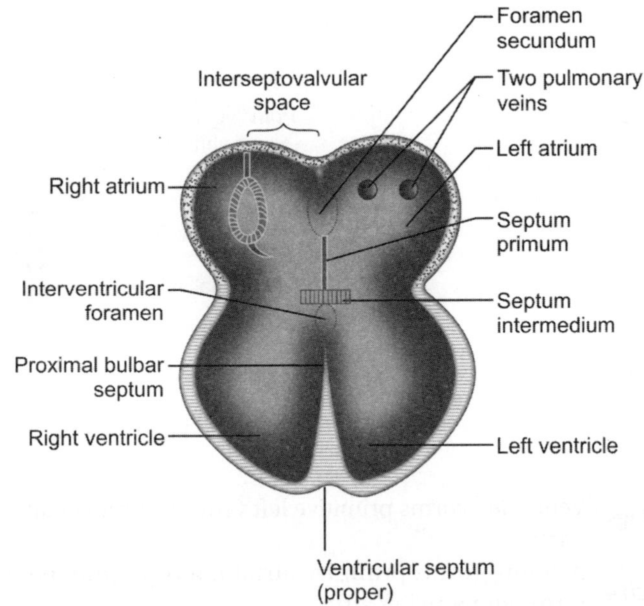

Fig. 103 Septation of heart; formation of foramen secundum

Arches 1 and 2

The first and second arches disappear early.

Arch 3

The third aortic arch constitutes the commencement of the internal carotid artery, and is therefore, named the carotid arch.

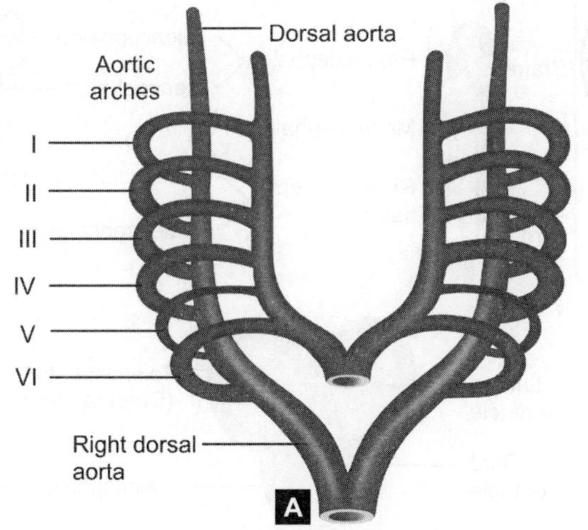

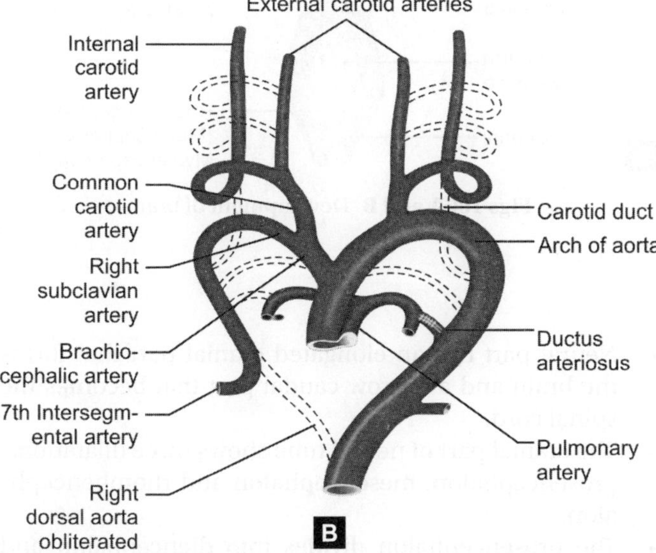

Figs 104A and B (A) Arches of aorta; (B) Formation of aorta

Arch 4

The fourth right arch forms the right subclavian as far as the origin of its internal mammary branch; while the fourth left arch constitutes the arch of the aorta between the origin of the left carotid artery and the termination of the ductus arteriosus.

Arch 5

The fifth arch disappears on both sides.

Arch 6

The proximal part of the sixth right arch persists as the proximal part of the right pulmonary artery while the distal section degenerates.

The sixth left arch gives off the left pulmonary artery and forms the ductus arteriosus; this duct remains pervious during the whole of fetal life, but then closes within the first few days after birth due to increased O_2 concentration.

Adult derivatives	*Embryological structures*
• Ascending aorta	• Truncus arteriosus
• Arch of aorta	• Aortic sac, left horn of aortic sac and left 4th arch artery
• Descending aorta	• Left dorsal aorta and fused dorsal aorta
• Brachiocephalic artery	• Right horn of aortic sac
• Right subclavian artery	• Right 4th arch artery and 7th cervical intersegmental artery
• Left subclavian artery	• Left 7th cervical intersegmental artery
• Common carotid artery	• Proximal part of 3rd arch artery
• Internal carotid artery	• Distal part of 3rd arch artery and cervical part of dorsal aorta.
• External carotid artery	• As a bud from 3rd arch artery
• Pulmonary trunk	• Truncus arteriosus
• Pulmonary artery	• Part of 6th arch artery
• Ductus arteriosus	• Part of left 6th arch artery between lung and aorta

Fetal Circulation*

The fetal blood charged with nutritive material and oxygen, leaves the placenta to enter the left umbilical vein, which traverses the umbilical cord to end in the remaining branch of portal vein (Fig. 105).

Most of the blood brought in the right atrium by inferior vena cava is shunted through foramen ovale into left atrium, thereby short-circuiting pulmonary circuit. It then passes through the left ventricle into the ascending aorta and aortic arch and by their branches, it is distributed to the heart, head, neck and upper limb. The blood from head, neck and upper limb returns to the right atrium through superior vena cava (Flow chart 3).

From right atrium, it passes to right ventricle and then into pulmonary trunk. From here most of the blood is short circuited to the aorta by ductus arteriosus, that connects the left pulmonary artery to the aortic arch just beyond the origin of left subclavian artery.

Remnants after the closure of fetal circulatory structures	
Fetal structures	*Adult remnants*
• Ductus venosus	• Ligamentum venosum
• Foramen ovale	• Fossa ovalis
• Ductus arteriosus	• Ligamentum arteriosum
• Right and left umbilical arteries	• Medial umbilical ligament
• Left umbilical vein	• Ligamentum teres hepatis

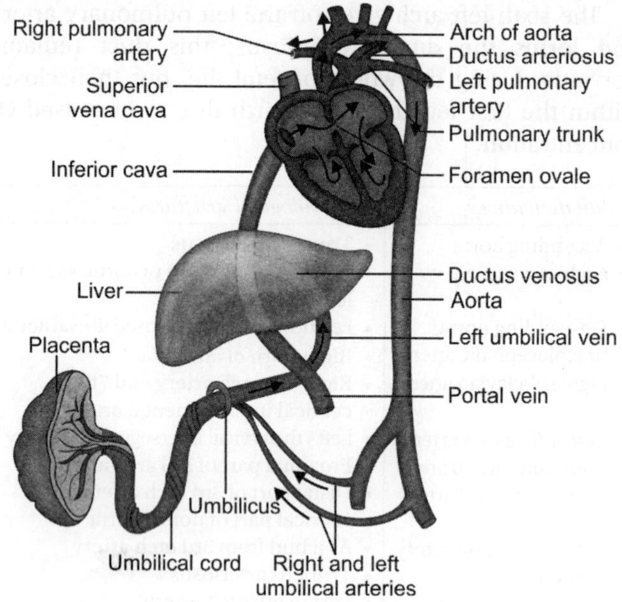

Fig. 105 Fetal circulation

Flow chart 3 Fetal circulation

Umbilical arteries → Placenta (organ of oxygenation in fetus) → Umbilical vein (left) → Portal vein → Through ductus venosus (liver bypassed) → Inferior vena cava → Right atrium

Right atrium → Right ventricle → Pulmonary trunk → Through ductus arteriosus (lungs bypassed) → Descending aorta → Umbilical arteries

Right atrium → Through foramen ovale → Left atrium → Ascending aorta → Descending aorta

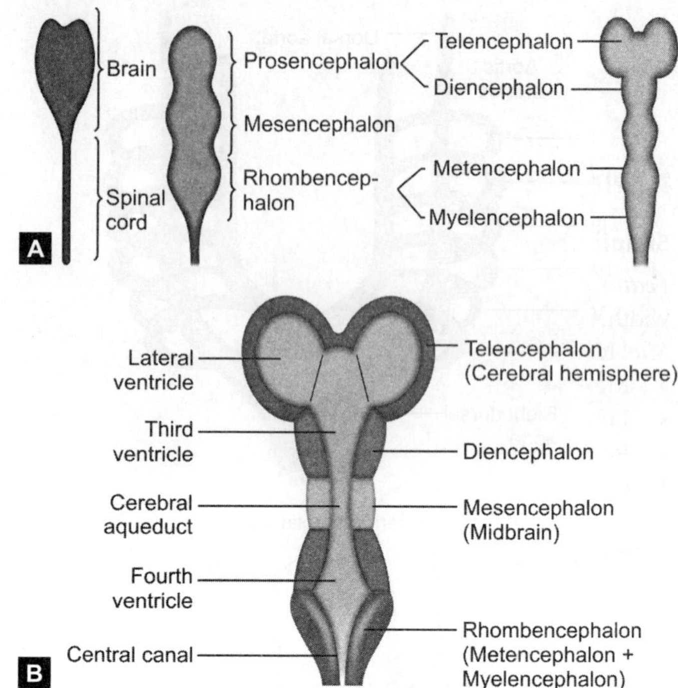

Figs 106A and B Development of brain

Brain

- Ectoderm overlying the notochord becomes thickened to form the neural plate (Figs 106A and B).
- Neural plate is converted into neural groove, and then to neural tube.
- Neural part has an elongated cranial part that forms the brain and a narrow caudal part that becomes the spinal cord.
- The cranial part of neural tube shows three dilatations, prosencephalon, mesencephalon and rhombencephalon.
- The prosencephalon divides into diencephalon and telencephalon.
- The rhombencephalon divides into metencephalon and myelencephalon.
- The telencephalon forms most of the cerebral hemisphere including the corpus stratum. Lateral ventricle is the cavity of the telencephalon.
- The diencephalon forms the thalamus, hypothalamus and related structures. Its cavity is the 3rd ventricle.
- The mesencephalon forms the midbrain. Its cavity forms the cerebral aqueduct.
- The metencephalon forms the pons. It also forms the cerebellum.
- The myelencephalon forms the medulla oblongata.
- The 4th ventricle is the cavity of rhombencephalon.

HISTOLOGY

EPITHELIUM

Simple Squamous Epithelium

Features: Cells are flattened, height is very little compared to width. Centrally placed nuclei.
Site: Endothelium (lining of blood vessels)
- Mesothelium (lining of body cavities)
- Lung alveolus
- Parietal layer of Bowman's capsule

Function: Active transport by pinocytosis.

Simple Cuboidal Epithelium

Features: Cells have same length as width.
Site: Thyroid follicles
- Kidney tubule
- Pigmented layers of retina
- Germinal layers of retina

Function: Secretion.

Simple Columnar Epithelium

Features: Cells are cylindrical in shape and tall in appearance with oval nucleus (height of cells is greater than width).

Simple Columnar Nonciliated Epithelium

Features: Absence of cilia over free surface.
Site: Lining of stomach
- Intestine
- Gallbladder.

Function: Absorption, secretion.

Simple Columnar Ciliated Epithelium

Features: Cells have cilia over its free surface. Cytoplasm is finely granular and an oval nucleus is placed in the basal portion.
Site: Uterine tube, respiratory tract, uterus.
Function: Transport, secretion.

Pseudostratified Columnar Epithelium

Features: Nuclei of cells are at different levels.

Epithelium is ciliated (e.g. trachea, large bronchi) or nonciliated and may contain goblet cells.
Site: Nonciliated epithelium found in the large excretory duct.

Auditory tube and male urethra
Function: Protection of underlying tissue.

Stratified Squamous Nonkeratinized Epithelium

Features:
- Basal layer—may be columnar/cuboidal in shape.
- Intermediate cells—irregularly polyhedral in shape become increasingly flattened as they move towards superficial layer.
- Superficial layer—thin squamous cell.

Site: Epithelium lining oral cavity
Tongue, esophagus, vagina, anal canal
Function: Protection of deeper tissue.

Stratified Squamous Keratinized Epithelium

Features: Superficial cells become dead, dehydrated and non-nucleated like scales and these dead cells become hard (cornified). These cells contain a substance called keratin.
Site: Epithelium of the skin (epidermis)
Function: Protection
- Prevent absorption of water
- Keratin prevents dehydration of underlying tissue.

Stratified Cuboidal Epithelium

Features: Consists of 2 or more layers of cells and superficial layer is cuboidal in shape.
Site: Ducts of sweat glands.
Functions: Protection and limited absorption.

Stratified Columnar Epithelium

Features: Two or more layers of cells and superficial layer is columnar.
Site: Epithelium lining large ducts of some glands
Fornix of conjunctiva and urethra
Function: Protection.

Transitional Epithelium/Urothelium

When relaxed	Many layers of cells are seen
When stretched	Only 3 or 4 layers are seen

Superficial cell	Large and dome-shaped giving characteristic wavy border to the luminal surface.
Intermediate	Polyhedral/pear-shaped cells
Basal cells	Columnar in shape

Site: Epithelium lining urinary tract, renal pelvis, calyces, ureter.
Function: Effective barrier prevents absorption of toxic substances from urine.

CONNECTIVE TISSUE

Fibers—Collagen

Features: Composed of protein called collagen.
- They do not branch.
- Fibers are strong, inelastic but flexible in nature.
- Run in wavy nature.
- Each collagen fiber consists of small parallel fibers.
- They are synthesized by fibroblast.

Elastic

- They are composed of a protein called elastin.
- Synthesized by fibroblast and smooth muscle cell.
- Fibers are singly and not in bundles, branch and anastomose with each other.

Reticular

- Very thin immature fibers.
- Structurally symmetrical to collagen fibers.
- Composed of collagen type III.
- Form supportive framework of lymphoid organs and glands.

Loose Areolar Connective Tissue

Features: Few loosely arranged collagen and elastic tissue:
- Large number of connective tissue cells.
- Large amount of ground substance and that consist of hyaluronic acid and chondroitin sulfate.

Site: Lies beneath the epithelium of lamina propria.
Surrounds blood vessels, nerves, viscera, muscle, etc.
Function: Provides support to the epithelium.
Acts as packing material around various structures.

Adipose Tissue

Features: Empty space in each fat cell giving a honeycomb appearance (empty space is due to dissolution of lipid droplet)
- Thin rim of cytoplasm
- Eccentrically placed flattened nuclei (signet ring appearance)
- Lobules separated by septa.

Site: Present in superficial fascia, deep to skin, bone marrow, mesentery, etc.
Function: Serves as energy reserve
- Supports and protects structures, which it surrounds.
- Prevents heat loss through skin.

Reticular Connective Tissue (Special Stain)

Features: Network of reticular fibers and reticular cells
- Cells tend to be star-shaped with radiating processes
- Reticular fibers are stained brown to black with silver salts

Site: Spleen, lymph node, liver, bone marrow, etc.
Function: Provides structural supports to various organs.

Elastic Tissue (Special Stain)

Features: They are stained brown to black.
Fibroblasts and ground substances are present in small spaces intervening between fibers.
Site: Tunica media of large artery.
Function: Provides elasticity to the tissue.

Dense Regular Connective Tissue

Features: Bundles of parallel collagen fibers.
- Rows of tendon cells/fibrocytes between the fiber bundle
- Less amount of ground substance.

Site: Present in tendon and aponeurosis of muscle and ligament.
Function: They provide great resistance to pulling force and are flexible.

Dense Irregular Connective Tissue

Features: Compactly packed irregular bundles of collagen fibers
- Thin elastic fibers are also present.
- Less number of cells is seen.

Site: Dermis of skin, dura mater, epimysium, pericardium, periosteum.
Function: Provide strength to the tissue.

Cartilage

Hyaline Cartilage

Features: Glassy nature—homogeneous basophilic matrix (because collagen fibrils present in the matrix have the same refractive index as that of the ground substance)
- Deeply stained (more basophilic) matrix surrounding the cells in the lacunae forming the capsular or territorial matrix and less basophilic interterritorial matrix/interstitial matrix.
- Isogenous groups (cell nests) of chondrocytes
- Perichondrium covering the cartilage

Sites: Fetal skeleton, ends of adult bone, nose, costal cartilage, trachea, bronchi and larynx
Epiphyseal plate made up of hyaline cartilage.
Function: Provides smooth surface for movements at joints.
- Provides support.

Elastic Cartilage

Features: Have all the features of hyaline cartilage except for the presence of elastic fibers in the matrix (nonhomogeneous)
- Closely packed chondrocytes with eccentric nuclei
- Perichondrium covering the cartilage.

Site: Pinna of ear, epiglottis, arytenoids, corniculate and cuneiform cartilages of larynx, external auditory meatus, auditory tube.
Function: Provide shape, support and elasticity to the organ.

Fibrocartilage

Features: Dense bundles of collagen (type I) fibers.
- Chain of chondrocytes (of similar size) between the collagen bundles
- Absence of perichondrium.

Site: Inter-vertebral disc
- Pubic symphysis
- Manubriosternal joint.

Function: Capable of resisting compressive and shear forces.

BONE

Compact Bone (Cross Section)

Features: Haversian system with Haversian canals and concentric lamellae of bone matrix.
- Interstitial lamellae and circumferential lamellae are present.
- Lacunae containing osteocytes and radiating canaliculi.
- Volkmann's canals are present.
  (Refer: General Anatomy—Bone)

COMPACT BONE (LONGITUDINAL SECTION)

Features: Haversian canals and Volkmann's canals are present.
Lamellae and lacunae are seen parallel to Haversian canal.

MUSCULAR TISSUE

Skeletal Muscle

Features: Long cylindrical fibers without branching.
- Many flat peripheral nuclei are present.
- Cross-striations showing dark A bands and light I bands.
- Endomysium separating muscle fibers.
- Perimysium separating the fascicle.
- Epimysium covering the muscle.
  For example, triceps, biceps, adductor muscles.

Function: Contraction, under voluntary control; quick, forceful contraction.

Smooth Muscle

Features: LS of smooth muscle fibers are spindle-shaped cells with tapering end.
- Nucleus is elongated and centrally placed.
- No striations.

Location: Gastrointestinal tracts, walls of blood vessels urinary bladder, ureter, uterus.
Function: Contraction, under involuntary control
Continuous, rhythmic contraction.

Cardiac Muscle

Features: Cross-striations with dark A bands and light I bands (less prominent).
- Short, branching fibers
- Single, oval centrally placed nucleus
- Presence of intercalated disc.

Function: Contraction, under involuntary control; slow, sustained contraction.

LYMPHOID TISSUE

Thymus

Features: Many lobules of lymphoid tissue having outer cortex and inner medulla.

Cortex	*Medulla*
Densely packed lymphocytes	Loosely packed lymphocytes
Few pale stained macrophages	Postcapillary venules
Epithelial reticular cell	Presence of eosinophilic—Hassall's corpuscles

- Hassall's corpuscles—have a central core of degenerated epithelial cells, which form a pink staining hyaline mass.
- Darkly stained cortex and lightly stained medulla in each lobule.

Lymph Node

Features: Presence of lymphatic nodules in the cortex.
- Thin capsule that surrounds the lymph node
- Dense paracortex between cortex and medulla
- Darkly stained cortex and lightly stained medulla
- Medullary cords and sinuses in the medulla
- Subcapsular sinus
- Lightly stained germinal center (secondary nodule), made of large lymphocytes.

Function: It serves as a filter of lymph.
- The foreign bodies are presented to lymphocytes
- Production of both T and B lymphocytes
- B lymphocytes are mature to form plasma cells.

Spleen

Features: Thick capsule.
- Trabeculae cut at different planes carrying trabecular blood vessels.
- Darkly stained round areas, the white pulp is distributed randomly among the red pulp.

- Each nodule of white pulp has an eccentrically placed arteriole (arteriole placed eccentrically at the margin of germinal center).
- White pulp showing germinal center, marginal zone, periarterial lymphatic sheat around the central artery.
- Red pulp containing splenic cords and sinusoids.

Function: Filtration of blood
- Immune response against antigens
- Site for production of T and B lymphocytes
- Formation of blood cell during fetal life.

Tonsil

Features: Crypts lined by stratified squamous epithelium.
- Subepithelial lymphatic nodules which may show germinal centers.
- Mucous glands are present.
- Epithelium extends into the substance of tonsil in the form of tonsillar crypts.
  For example, palatine tonsil.

Function: Production of lymphocytes
- Immunological response against antigens.

NERVOUS TISSUE

Peripheral Nerve

Features: Darkly stained axon surrounded by a lightly stained myelin sheath.
- Bundles of nerve fibers
- Endoneurium—separating each nerve fiber
- Perineurium—connective tissue sheath around each fascicule
- Epineurium—covering entire nerve.

Optic Nerve

Features: Presence of central vessels of retina.
- Bundles of myelinated nerve fibers are present
- Dura mater—outer-most covering
- Arachnoid mater—it is separated from dura mater by subdural space
- Piamater—it is separated from arachnoid by subarachnoid space.

Motor Ganglion/Sympathetic Ganglion

Features: Small scattered, angular multipolar neurons of uniform size.
- Multipolar neurons are scattered among nerve fibers
- The eccentrically placed euchromatic nucleus with its prominent nucleolus
- Poorly defined satellite cells.

Sensory Ganglion/Spinal Ganglion

Feature: Groups of rounded pseudo-unipolar neurons with varying size.
- Well-defined cuboidal satellite cells forming a cellular capsule around the cell body.
- The darkly stained round nuclei of cell body forms a ring around the neuron.
- Epineurium, forming the capsule of the ganglion.

Cerebral Cortex

Features: It has 6 layers:
1. *Molecular layer/plexiform layer:* It is the most superficial, well-defined layer consists of nerve fibers and horizontal cells of Cajal.
2. *External granular layer:* Contains large number of stellate cells and small pyramidal cells.
3. *External pyramidal layer:* Mainly made of medium sized pyramidal cells and few stellate cells and cells of Martinotti.
4. *Internal granular layer:* Composed of closely packed stellate cells and horizontally oriented white fiber band called outer band of Baillarger.
5. *Internal pyramidal layer/ganglionic layer:* Consists of large pyramidal cells and few stellate cells and cells of Martinotti intermixed with many nerve fibers.
6. *Multiform layer/layer of polymorphic cells:* It is the deepest layer and it contains predominantly fusiform cell and few stellate cells and cells of Martinotti.

Under the microscope, the molecular layer deep to piamater can be easily identified.

Cerebellar Cortex

Features: It has 3 layers:
1. *Molecular layer:* Lightly stained superficial thick layer and it contains few stellate cells and basket cells.
2. *Purkinje cell layer:* Purkinje cells are large flask-shaped neurons and arranged in a single row.
3. *Granular layer:* Stained deeply with hematoxylin because it is densely packed with very small granule neurons. Branching white mater in the center of each folium.

INTEGUMENTARY SYSTEM

Thick/Glabrous Skin

Features: Thick epidermis made up of keratinized stratified squamous epithelium.
- It has 5 layers—(i) Stratum corneum, (ii) stratum lucidum, (iii) stratum granulosum, (iv) stratum spinosum, (v) stratum basale.
- Absence of hair follicles and sebaceous glands
- Presence of sweat glands in the deeper parts of dermis
- Hypodermis is infiltrated with adipose tissue
  (for more details about the layers of dermis (Refer to General Anatomy, page 26)

Thin/Hairy Skin

Features: Thin epidermis made up of keratinized stratified squamous epithelium: It has all the layers of thick skin except stratum lucidium.

Dermis contains:

- Hair follicle enclosing the root of hairs
- Sebaceous glands, which opens into the hair follicle
- Arrector pili muscle; a band of smooth muscle extending from the hair follicle to the dermis
- Sweat glands in the deeper parts of dermis.

BLOOD VESSELS

Large/Elastic Artery

For example, aorta, carotid artery, subclavian artery.

Features:

- *Tunica intima:* Includes endothelium and well-developed subendothelial tissue. Poorly defined fenestrated internal elastic lamina.
- *Tunica media:* 40–70 layers of fenestrated elastic lamina arranged circularly.
- *Tunica adventitia:* Composed of fibroelastic connective tissue with vasa vasorum.

Medium Sized/Muscular Artery

For example, radial artery, ulnar artery.

Features:

- *Tunica intima:* Well-developed internal elastic lamina and no subendothelial tissue.
- *Tunica media:* Smooth muscle cells arranged circularly.
- *Tunica adventitia:* More elastic fibers.

Large Vein

Features:

- *Tunica intima:* Well-developed layer, formed by endothelial and subendothelial tissue
- *Tunica media:* Absent
- *Tunica adventitia:* Well-developed and is the thickest coat. Which is formed by longitudinal fibers of smooth muscle.

Medium-sized Vein

Features: Large collapsed vein.

- *Tunica intima:* Endothelium supported by subendothelium and no internal elastic lamina
- *Tunica media:* Few circularly arranged smooth muscle fibers and less elastic fibers
- *Tunica adventitia:* Fibroelastic connective tissue carrying vasa vasorum.

RESPIRATORY SYSTEM

Trachea

Features:

- *Mucosa:*
  - *Epithelium:* Thick and is formed of pseudostratified ciliated columnar epithelium with goblet cells
  - *Lamina propria:* Fibroelastic connective tissue in which the elastic fibers are longitudinally oriented.
- *Submucosa:* Mixed glands (tracheal glands)
- *Cartilage and smooth muscle layer:* C-shaped hyaline cartilage
- Adventitia.

Lungs

Features:

- Pulmonary alveoli giving honeycomb appearance in sections.
- Simple squamous epithelium lining the alveoli.
- *Alveolar ducts:* Squamous epithelial lining supported by smooth muscle fiber.
- *Respiratory bronchiole:* Lined by ciliated cuboidal epithelium, with Clara cells replacing goblet cells.
- *Terminal bronchiole:* Thick, smooth muscle layer and absence of glands and cartilage in its wall.

GLANDS

Serous Gland

Features: Darkly stained serous acini with narrow lumen.

- Round, centrally placed nucleus in the serous cells
- Well-developed duct system (intercalated, interlobular, intralobular)
- Secrete thin watery material, rich in enzymes.

Site: Parotid gland.

Mucous Gland

Features: Lightly stained mucous acini/tubule with large lumen.

- Flat peripheral nuclei in the mucous cell.
- Poorly developed duct system (interlobular)
- Secretes thick viscous material for protection and lubrication.

Site: Sublingual gland.

Mixed Gland

Features: Darkly stained serous and lightly stained mucous acini.

- Serous demilune (crescent shaped path of serous cell)
- Moderately developed duct system
- Secretes watery and viscous material from both acini.

Site: Submandibular gland.

DIGESTIVE SYSTEM

Tongue (Filiform and Fungiform Papilla)

- *Filiform papilla:* Conical shaped and lined partly by keratinized stratified squamous epithelium. No taste buds are found in them.
- *Fungiform papilla:* Round mushroom shaped and lined by stratified nonkeratinized squamous epithelium. Taste buds may be seen on the top surface. They have rounded summits and narrower bases.
- Below the lamina propria, the skeletal muscles are running in different direction.

Tongue Circumvallate Papilla

Features: Inverted cone-shaped sunken papilla.
- Deep sulcus or furrow around the papilla
- Papilla lined by stratified squamous epithelium
- Lightly stained taste buds are seen on the lateral wall
- von Ebner's (serous) gland
- Skeletal muscle running in different directions
- Arranged in a row just anterior to sulcus terminalis.

GASTROINTESTINAL TRACT

General Plan

- *Mucosa:*
  - Epithelium
  - Lamina propria—made of connective tissue containing glands and lymphoid accumulations.
  - Muscularis mucosa—made of smooth muscle, inner circular and outer longitudinal.
- *Submucosa:* Consists of fibroelastic connective tissue:
  - Contains Meissner's nerve plexus
  - May contain glands (esophagus and duodenum)
- *Muscularis externa:*
  - Two-muscle layer—inner circular and outer longitudinal
  - Contains Auerbach's nerve plexus.
- *Adventitia/Serosa:*
  - Adventitia consists of only loose connective tissue without peritoneum
  - Serosa consists of peritoneum.

Esophagus

- *Mucosa:*
  - *Epithelium:* Stratified squamous nonkeratinized
  - *Lamina propria:* Contains esophageal cardiac glands in the lower part of esophagus
  - *Muscularis mucosa:* Single longitudinal layer of smooth muscle
- *Submucosa:* Contains esophageal glands (compound tubule-alveolar mucus glands)
- *Muscularis externa:* Thick
  - Upper 1/3rd → Only skeletal muscle
  - Middle 1/3rd → Both skeletal and smooth muscle
  - Lower 1/3rd → Only smooth muscle
- *Adventitia:* Same as GIT.

Stomach—Fundus

- *Mucosa:*
  - Epithelium—shallow gastric pits lined by simple columnar epithelium
  - Lamina propria—long tubular fundic glands
    - Chief/zymogenic cell (small cuboidal cells with basophilic cytoplasm) and parietal cells (large pyramidal cells with acidophilic cytoplasm) in the fundic glands
- Submucosa
- *Muscularis externa:* Three layers of smooth muscle (inner oblique, middle circular, outer longitudinal)
- Serosa.

Stomach—Pylorus

- *Mucosa:*
  - Epithelium—deep gastric pits lined by simple columnar epithelium
  - Lamina propria—pyloric glands (mucous)
- Submucosa
- *Muscularis externa:* Middle circular layer thickens to form pyloric sphincter
- Serosa.

SMALL INTESTINE

Mucosa:
- *Epithelium:* It is made up of simple columnar absorptive epithelium with goblet cells.
  - The epithelium and the underlying lamina propria shows finger-like invaginations called intestinal villi.
  - Thick glycocalyx overlies the epithelium, which helps in the adsorption of pancreatic enzymes.
  - Epithelium shows tubular invaginations from the base of the villi into the lamina propria known as crypts of Lieberkuhn (simple tubular intestinal glands) and these crypts are lined by columnar epithelium and goblet cells.
- *Lamina propria:* It is the connective tissue that contains fibroblasts, mast cells, plasma cells, lymphocytes + crypts of Lieberkuhn + lacteals + capillary loops. (other structures are same as the general plan of GIT)

Duodenum

Mucosa:
- *Epithelium:* Short leaf-like intestinal villi lined by simple columnar epithelium with a few goblet cells

- *Submucosa:* Brunner's gland/duodenal glands (compound tubule alveolar glands—they are lined by columnar cells having flattened basal nuclei).

  They open in the bottom of the crypts and secrete thin alkaline mucus to neutralize acid chime and to protect duodenal mucosa from autodigestion.

  (Other structures are same as the general plan of GIT)

Jejunum

- *Mucosa:* Long club-shaped intestinal villi lined by simple columnar epithelium with goblet cells (more than that of duodenum) larger and more numerous circular folds.
- *Submucosa:* Absence of Brunner's gland and Payer's patches (other structures are same as the general plan of GIT).

Ileum

- *Mucosa:* Short slender finger-like intestinal villi lined by simple columnar epithelium with numerous goblet cells.
- *Submucosa:* Payer's patches (lymphoid aggregations) are present (other structures are same as the general plan of GIT).

LARGE INTESTINE

Vermiform Appendix

Mucosa:

- *Epithelium:* Few crypts of Lieberkuhn lined by simple columnar epithelium with goblet cells
  - Absence of intestinal villi
  - Small angular lumen compared to the thick wall
- *Lamina propria:* Lymphatic nodules

  (Other structures are same as the general plan of GIT)

Large Intestine/Colon

- *Mucosa:*
  - *Epithelium:* Presence of more crypts of Lieberkuhn with large number of goblet cells without intestinal villi
  - Lamina propria
  - *Muscularis mucosa:* Well-defined
- Submucosa
- *Muscularis externa:* Outer longitudinal layer thickened to form ribbon-like bands (3 in number) called taenia coli.
- *Serosa:* Presence of fat-filled peritoneal pockets called appendices epiploicae.

Pancreas

- Pancreatic lobules are separated by interlobular connective tissue septae containing blood vessels
- Darkly stained serous acini
- Lightly stained islets of Langerhans
- Beta cells—small basophilic cells in the center
- Alpha cell—large acidophilic cells at periphery.

Liver

- Liver lobules are hexagonal in shape and the lobules are not delineated by interlobular connective tissue septa, the shape can be defined by drawing imaginary lines connecting the portal triads present at the angles of the lobules.
- Each portal tract (portal triad contains branches of portal veins, hepatic artery, bile duct.
- Central vein in the center of the lobule and radiating plates of hepatocytes (darkly stained) separated by sinusoids (lightly stained).

Gallbladder

- *Mucosa:* Lined by simple tall columnar epithelium which is thrown into fold:
  - Presence of microvilli gives a brush border appearance.
  - Muscularis mucosa and submucosa are absent.
- *Fibromuscular layer:* Composed of circularly arranged smooth muscle fiber.
- *Serosa/Adventitia:* Both are present.

URINARY SYSTEM

Kidney

Features: Darkly stained cortex

- Large round renal/malpighian corpuscle (glomerulus + Bowman's capsule)
- Darkly stained proximal convoluted tubule (PCT)
- Lightly stained distal convoluted tubule (DCT)
- PCTs are lined by cuboidal epithelium with brush border (microvilli)
- Presence of brush border makes the lumen of the PCT smaller
- DCTs are lined by cuboidal epithelium without brush border and which makes the lumen larger.

Lightly stained medulla:

- Loop of Henle, lined by simple squamous epithelium.
- Collecting tubule, lined by simple cuboidal epithelium.
- Papillary duct, lined by simple squamous epithelium.
- Vasa recta, lined by endothelium
- Large amount of interstitial connective tissue.

Ureter

- *Mucosa:*
  - *Epithelium:* Transitional epithelium
  - *Lamina propria:* Rich in elastic fibers

  The mucosa is thrown into longitudinal folds which give a star-shaped appearance to the lumen.
- *Muscle coat:* Smooth muscles arranged as inner longitudinal and outer circular.
- *Adventitia:* Fibroelastic connective tissue carrying blood vessels, nerves and lymphatics.

Urinary Bladder

Mucosa: Composed of transitional epithelial lining and underlying lamina propria.

Muscle coat: Thickest coat and is made of smooth muscle fiber in bundle separated by connective tissue.

Internally and externally fibers are longitudinal
Middle-thicker layers of circular fibers.

Serosa/adventitia: Forms the outer most coats.

MALE REPRODUCTIVE TISSUE

Testis

- *Tunica albuginea:* Thick collagenous connective tissue capsule at the periphery.
- *Tunica vasculosa:* Vascular
- The seminiferous tubules are embedded in the interstitial connective tissue
- Interstitial cells of Leydig (large acidophilic cells) are seen on the interstitium and blood vessels
- In the seminiferous tubule, spermatogenic cells forming a stratified epithelium. The arrangement of cells from basement membrane to lumen:
  - Spermatogonia
  - Spermatocytes
  - Spermatids
  - Sperms
- Tall columnar sertoli cells with triangular or oval nucleus are found attached to the base of seminiferous tubule
- The sperms are attached to the cytoplasm of sertoli cells.

Epididymis

- *Features:*
  - Connective tissue capsule at the periphery
  - Sections of ductus epididymis, which are lined by pseudostratified columnar epithelium with stereo-cilia
  - Circularly arranged smooth muscle fibers around each ductus
  - Clumps of spermatozoa in the lumen.

Vas Deferens/Ductus Deferens

- *Mucosa:* Pseudostratified columnar epithelium with stereo-cilia
- *Muscular layer:* Smooth muscle fibers are arranged into inner longitudinal, middle circular, and outer longitudinal
- *Adventitia:* Fibromuscular connective tissue carrying blood vessels and nerves
  - Small stellate lumen and clumps of sperms in the lumen.

Prostate Gland

- Large irregular prostatic alveoli lined by pseudostratified columnar epithelium
- Prostatic concretions or corpora amylacea (condensed secretions
- Fibromuscular stroma made of fibrous tissue intermixed with smooth muscle fibers and the prostatic urethra lined by transitional epithelium.

Penis

- Paired corpora cavernosa
- Single corpus spongiosum traversed by penile urethra (lined by stratified columnar epithelium)
- Thick fibrous tunica albuginea.

FEMALE REPRODUCTIVE SYSTEM

Ovary

Peripheral cortex: Ovarian follicles are embedded in the cellular stroma

- *Primordial follicles:* Primary oocyte surrounded by squamous follicular cells
- *Primary follicle:* Containing primary oocyte surrounded by cuboidal follicular cells
- *Graafian follicle:* Containing secondary oocyte and surrounded by corona radiata.
- Externally the follicles are covered by theca folliculi
- Antrum folliculi is lined by membrane granulosa
- Eccentrically placed secondary oocyte surrounded by cumulus oophorus.
- Atretic follicle
- *Corpus luteum:*
  - Granulosa lutein cells—large pale staining cells with vesicular nuclei found at the deeper part of the corpus luteum
  - Theca lutein cells—smaller and found at the periphery.

Fallopian Tube

- *Mucosa:* Highly folded and lined by simple columnar ciliated epithelium

- *Muscle layer:* It is made of smooth muscle; inner circular and outer longitudinal.
- *Serosa:* Mesothelium supported by connective tissue.

Uterus

- *Mucosa/Endometrium:*
  - *Epithelium:* Simple columnar epithelium
  - *Lamina propria:* Contains blood vessels and simple tubular uterine glands.
- *Muscle layer/Myometrium:* The fibers in the inner and outer layers are arranged longitudinally and the middle layer is very thick and is circularly arranged.
- *Serosa/Perimetrium:* Mesothelial lining (simple squamous epithelium) supported by connective tissue rich in blood vessels and elastic fibers.

Uterus—Proliferative Phase

- Thickness of endometrium—2–3 mm
- Simple columnar epithelium
- Few, simple straight tubular uterine glands with narrow lumen
- Highly cellular and nonedematous stroma
- Spiral arteries do not reach the superficial part of the endometrium.

Uterus—Secretory Phase

- Thickness of endometrium—4–6 mm
- Hypertrophied columnar epithelium
- More, highly tortuous glands with dilated lumen
- Highly vascular and edematous
- Spiral arteries reach the superficial part of the endometrium.

MAMMARY GLAND

- Each gland consists of 15–20 breast lobes (tubule alveolar gland) and these lobes are separated by interlobular septa.
- From each lobe, lactiferous ducts are arising and it forms lactiferous sinus and ultimately opens into the nipple.

Nonlactating Mammary Gland

- More connective tissue and adipose tissue.
- Less glandular tissue.
- Interlobular connective tissue septum is thick.
- Under-developed alveoli represented by cords of cells.
- Extensive branching of duct system.

Lactating Mammary Gland

- Less connective tissue and adipose tissue.
- More glandular tissue.
- Interlobular connective tissue septum is thin.
- Compactly packed, well-developed alveoli with distended lumen containing milk.
- Extensively branching alveoli form the lobule. Ducts are few.
- Simple cuboidal epithelium lining the alveoli.

Placenta

- Villi cut in different planes.
- Large stem villi and small terminal villi reflecting the extensive branching nature of villi.
- The villi are separated by intervillous space and it contains maternal blood.
- The villi area lined by syncytiotrophoblast and at places the nuclei are aggregated to form syncytial knots.
- Blood vessels are predominantly seen in the central core of large stem villi.

Umbilical Cord

- Two arteries (thick wall with narrow lumen) and one vein (thin wall with wide lumen)
- Umbilical vessels are embedded in a mass of gelatinous mucoid connective tissue (Wharton's jelly)
- Amniotic epithelium (simple cuboidal epithelium).

ENDOCRINE GLANDS

Thyroid and Parathyroid

Features: Thyroid follicles are lined by simple cuboidal epithelium.

- Thyroid follicles are filled with colloid (thyroglobulin).
- Parafollicular cells or clear cells between thyroid follicles (sometimes within the follicles).

Parathyroid: Small basophilic chief cells in large number

- Large eosinophilic oxyphil cells in small number
- These cells are arranged in clusters or anastomosing cords between sinusoidal capillaries.

Adrenal/Suprarenal Gland

Features: Peripheral cortex (darkly stained).

- Zona glomerulosa—columnar cells are arranged in the form of rounded clusters
- Zona fascicularis—polyhedral cells are arranged in the form of fascicles or columns
- Zona reticularis—small dark acidophilic cells are arranged in the form of anastomosing cords.
  - Central medulla (lightly stained)
  - Composed of chromaffin cells and sympathetic ganglion.

Pituitary Gland

Features: Main 3 parts:

1. *Pars distalis:* Containing chromophobes (light cells) and chromophils (dark cells). They are arranged as cords/clusters in between the sinusoidal capillaries: Two type of chromophils: (i) acidophil, (ii) basophil.
2. *Pars intermedia:* Separated from pars distalis by hypophyseal cleft.
3. *Pars nervosa:* Containing unmyelinated nerve fibers arising from hypothalamic nuclei and pituicytes.

SPECIAL SENSES

Cornea

Features: Five layers, from superficial to deep

1. *Corneal epithelium:* Stratified squamous epithelium.
2. *Bowman's membrane:* Homogeneous acellular layer.
3. *Substantia propria:* Several layers of collagen fibrils with fibroblast in between them.
4. *Descemet's membrane:* Homogeneous acellular layer.
5. *Endothelium:* Simple squamous or simple cuboidal epithelium.

Retina

Features: Made of 10 layers:

1. Pigment epithelium—simple cuboidal.
2. Layer of rods and cones.
3. External limiting membrane.
4. Outer nuclear layer.
5. Outer plexiform layer.
6. Inner nuclear layer.
7. Inner plexiform layer.
8. Ganglionic cell layer.
9. Nerve fiber layer.
10. Internal limiting membrane.

HISTOLOGY DIAGRAMS

EPITHELIUM (FIGS 107 TO 111)

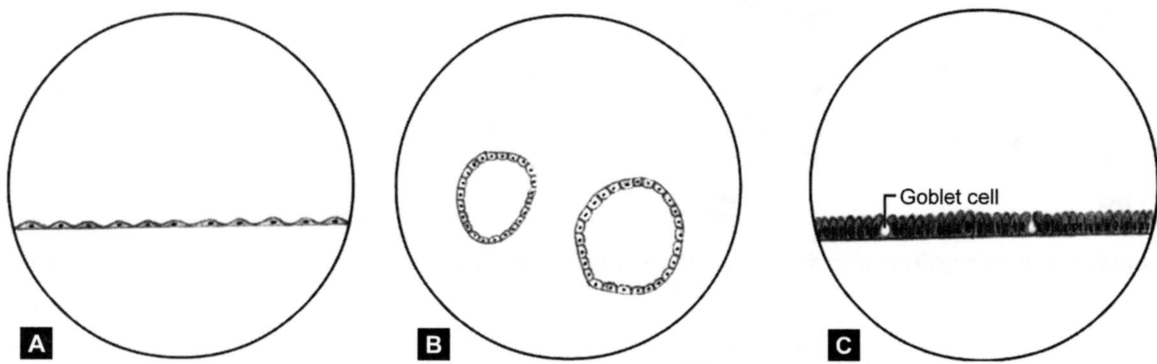

Figs 107A to C (A) Simple squamous epithelium; (B) Simple cuboidal epithelium; (C) Simple columnar epithelium (*For color version, see Plate 1*)

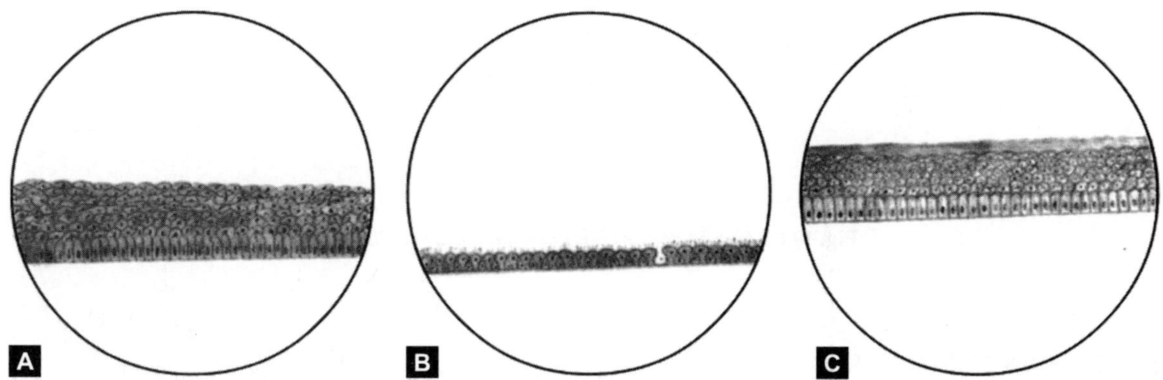

Figs 108A to C (A) Pseudostratified epithelium; (B) Stratified squamous non-keratinized epithelium; (C) Stratified squamous keratinized epithelium (*For color version, see Plate 2*)

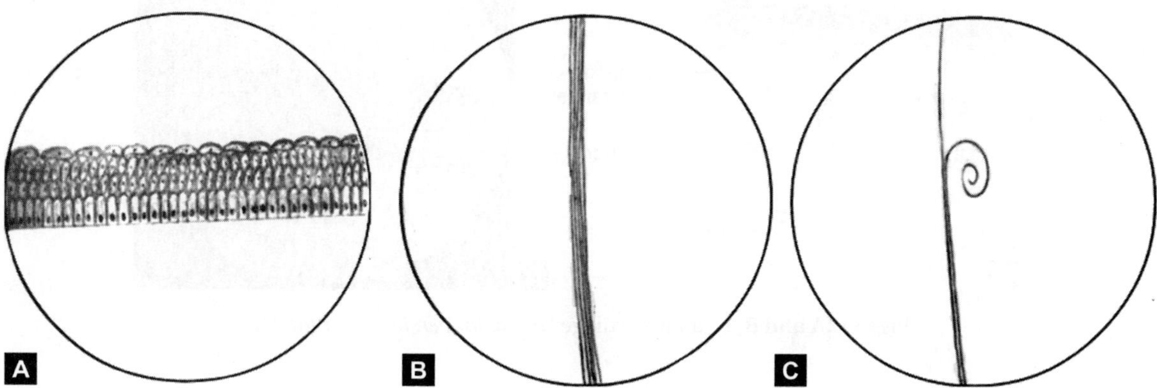

Figs 109A to C (A) Transitional epithelium; (B) Collagen fiber; (C) Elastin fiber (*For color version, see Plate 2*)

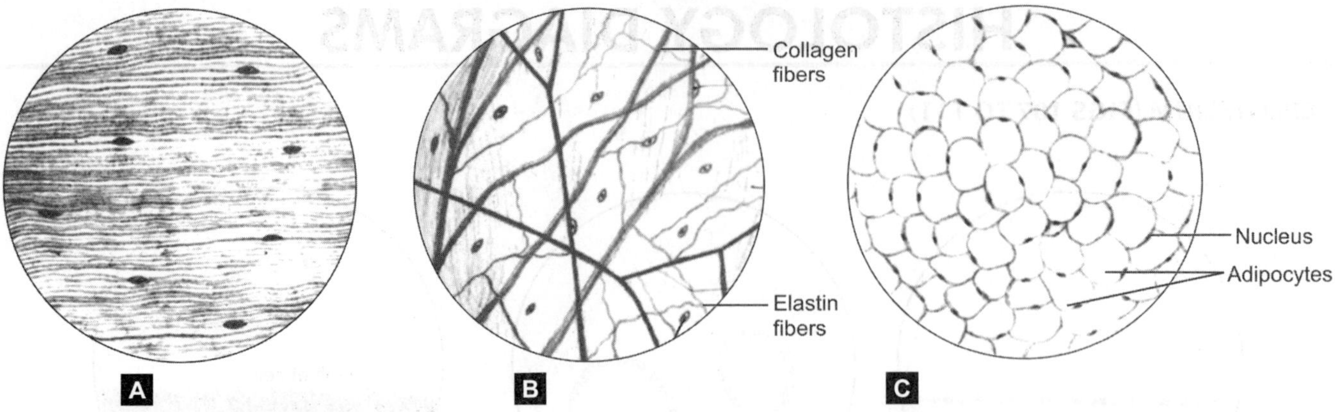

Figs 110A to C (A) Dense regular connective tissue; (B) Loose connective tissue; (C) Adipose tissue (*For color version, see Plate 2*)

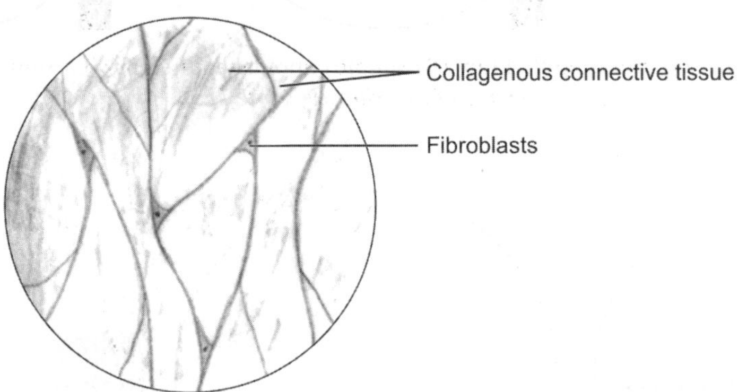

Fig. 111 Mucoid tissue (*For color version, see Plate 3*)

CARTILAGE (FIGS 112 TO 114)

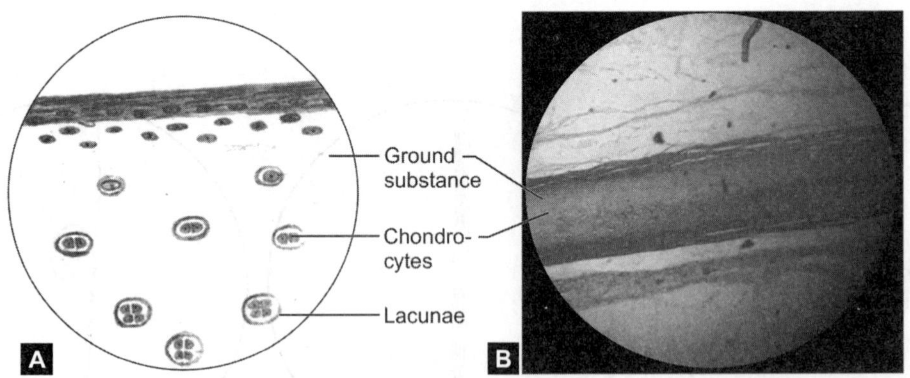

Figs 112A and B Hyaline cartilage (*For color version, see Plate 3*)

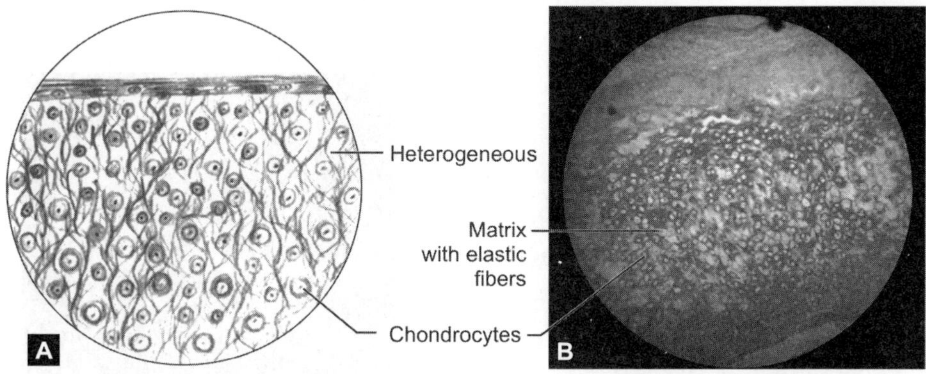

Figs 113A and B Elastic cartilage (*For color version, see Plate 3*)

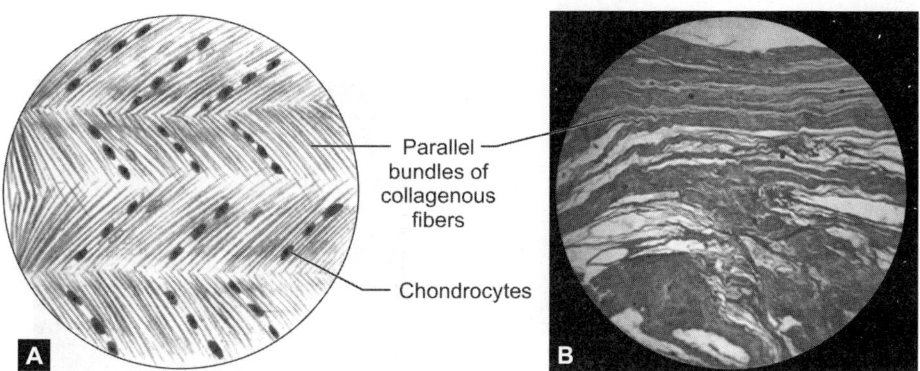

Figs 114A and B Fibrocartilage (*For color version, see Plate 4*)

BONE (FIGS 115A AND B)

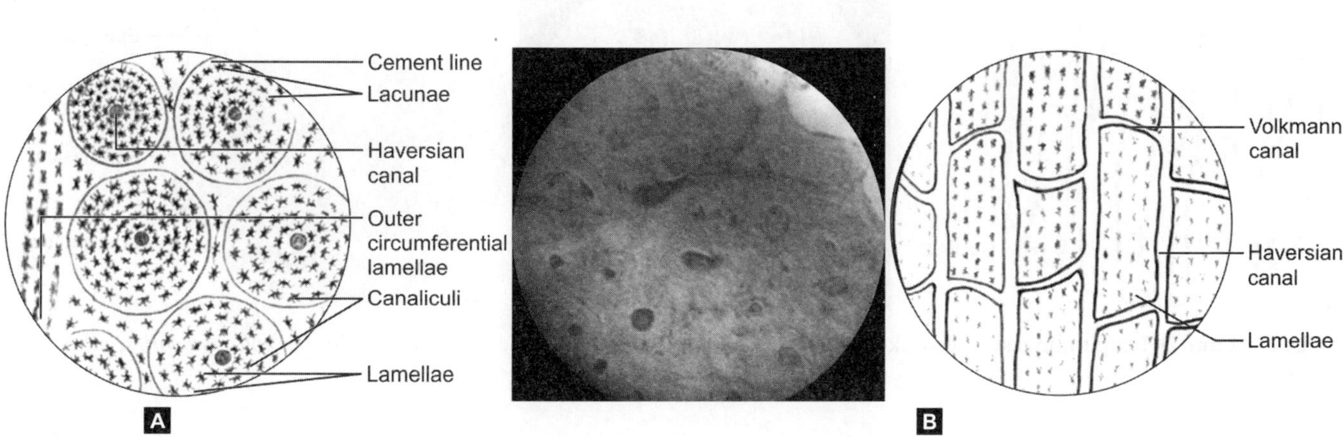

Figs 115A and B (A) Transverse section of bone; (B) Longitudinal section of bone (*For color version, see Plate 4*)

MUSCULAR TISSUE (FIGS 116 TO 118)

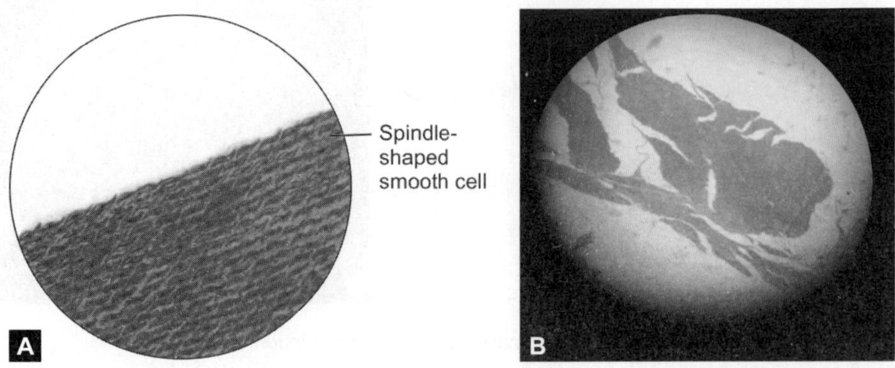

Figs 116A and B Smooth muscle (*For color version, see Plate 4*)

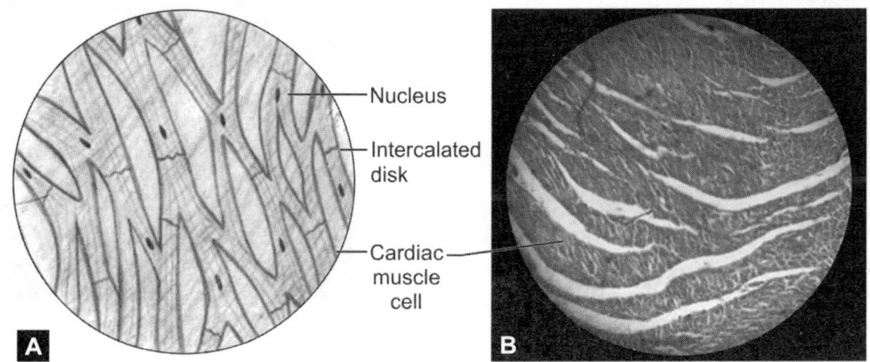

Figs 117A and B Cardiac muscle (*For color version, see Plate 5*)

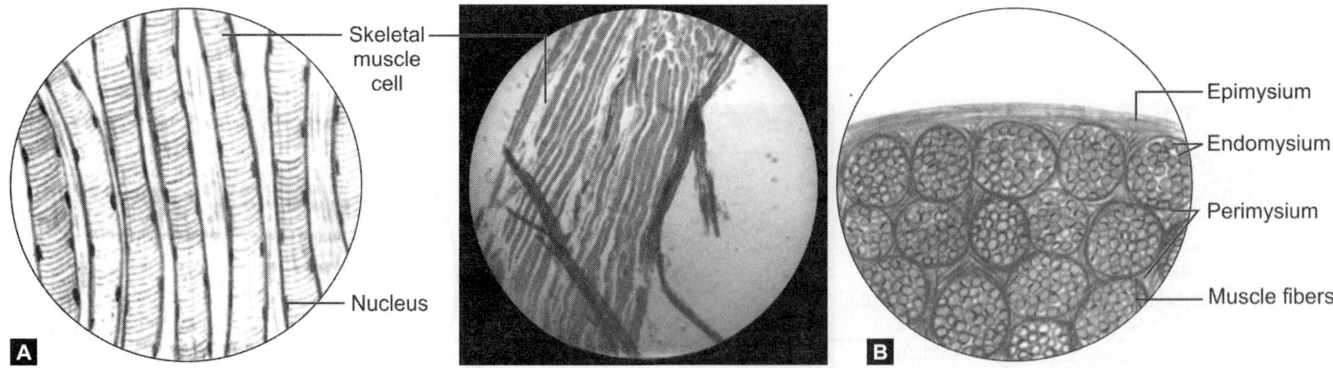

Figs 118A and B Longitudinal section of skeletal muscle; (B) Transverse section of skeletal muscle (*For color version, see Plate 5*)

LYMPHOID TISSUE (FIGS 119 TO 122)

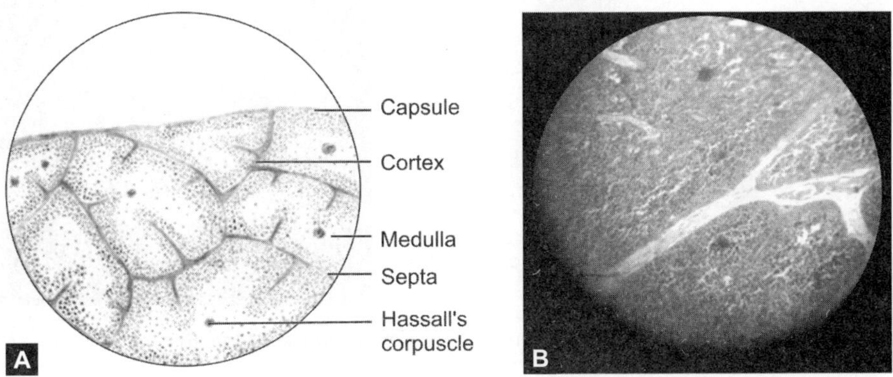

Figs 119A and B Thymus (*For color version, see Plate 5*)

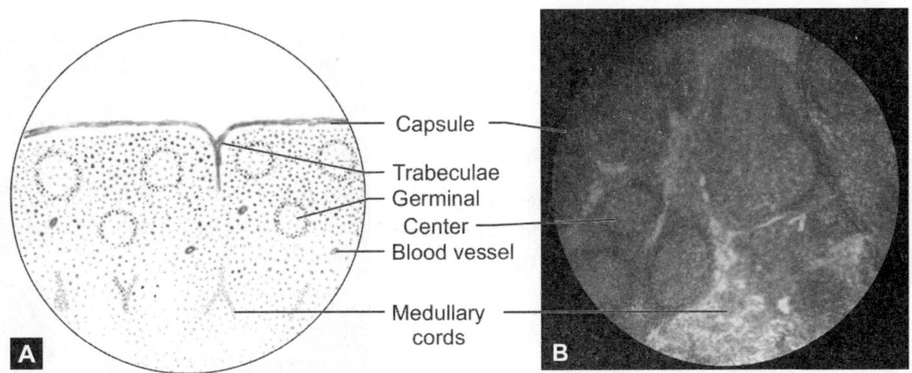

Figs 120A and B Lymph node (*For color version, see Plate 6*)

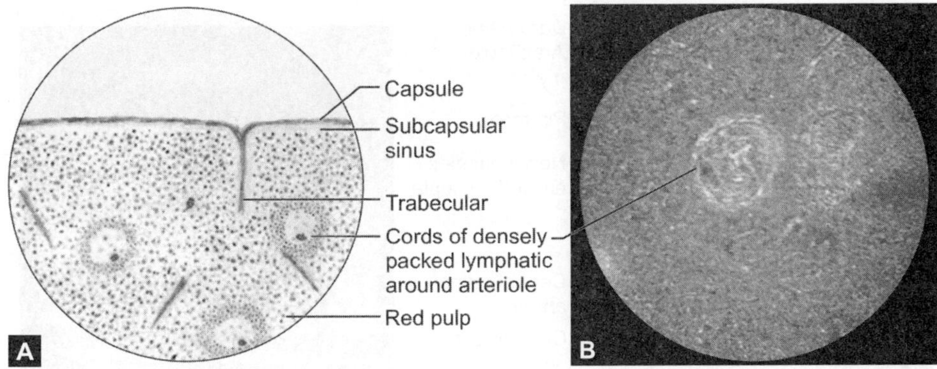

Figs 121A and B Spleen (*For color version, see Plate 6*)

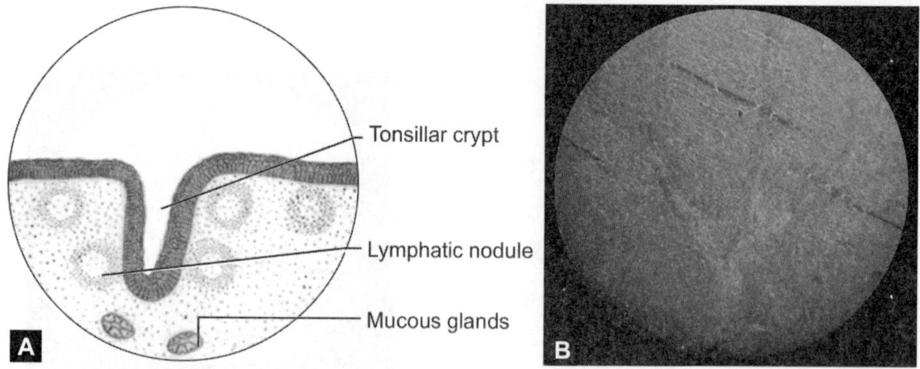

Figs 122A and B Tonsil (*For color version, see Plate 6*)

NERVOUS TISSUE (FIGS 123 TO 129)

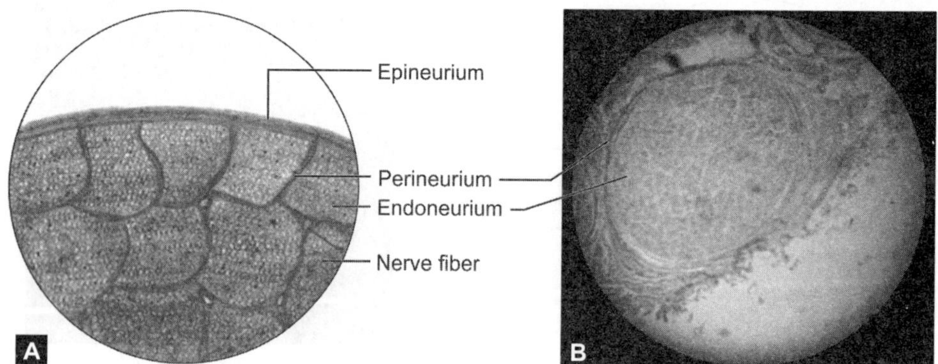

Figs 123A and B Peripheral nerve (*For color version, see Plate 7*)

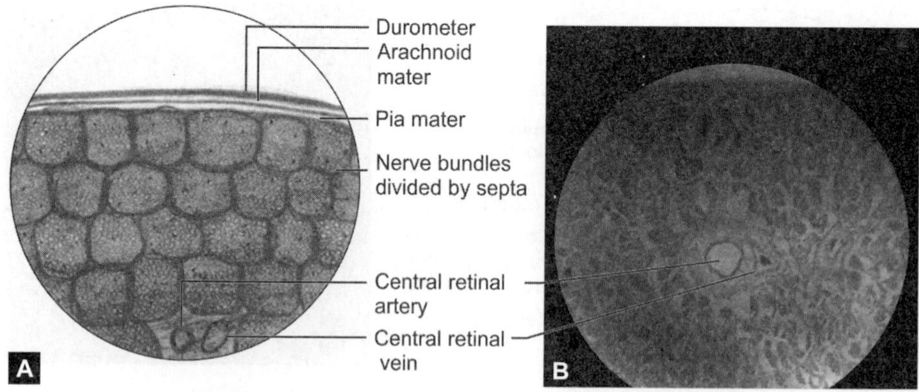

Figs 124A and B Optic nerve (*For color version, see Plate 7*)

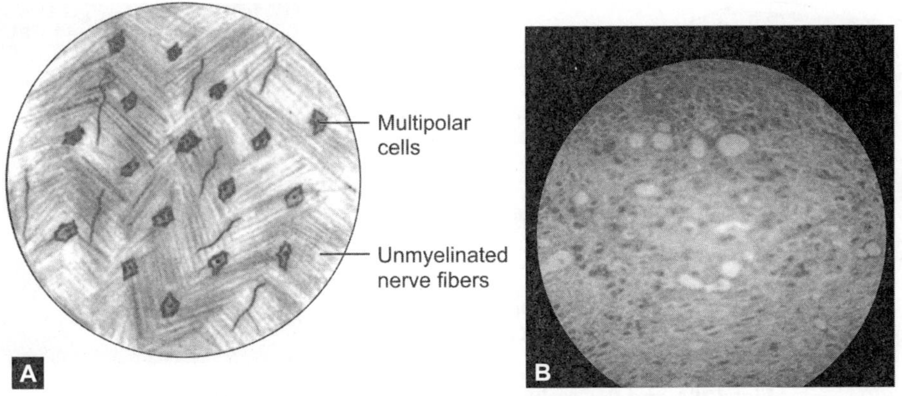

Figs 125A and B Sympathetic (Autonomic ganglion) (*For color version, see Plate 7*)

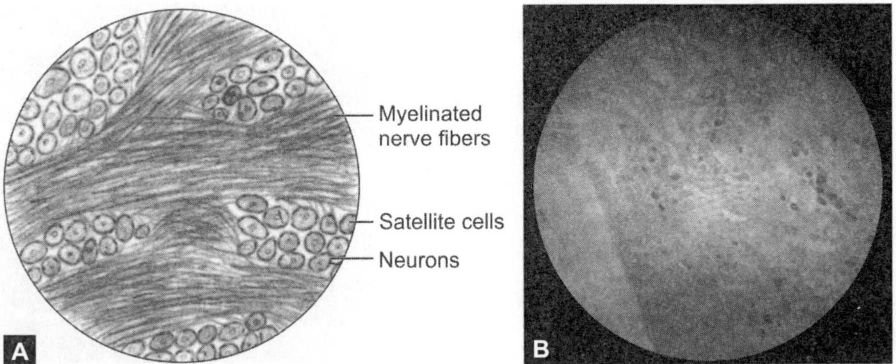

Figs 126A and B Dorsal root (Sensory) ganglion (*For color version, see Plate 8*)

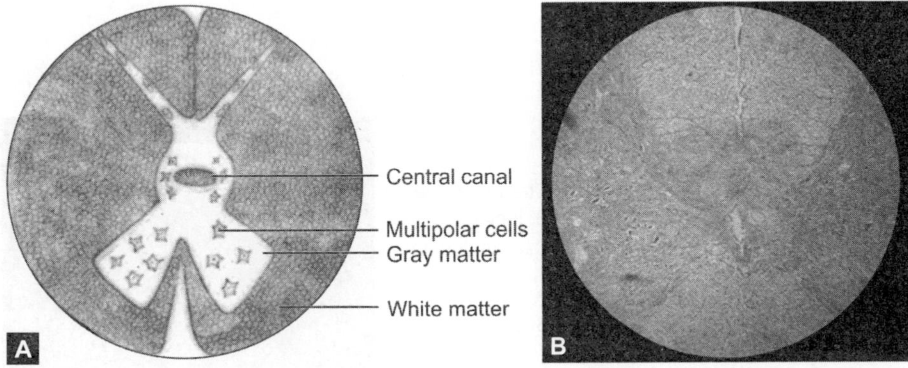

Figs 127A and B Spinal cord (*For color version, see Plate 8*)

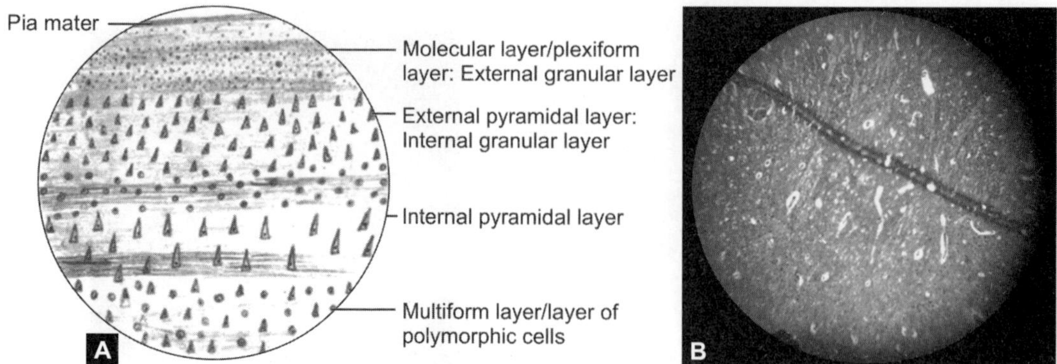

Figs 128A and B Cerebral cortex (*For color version, see Plate 8*)

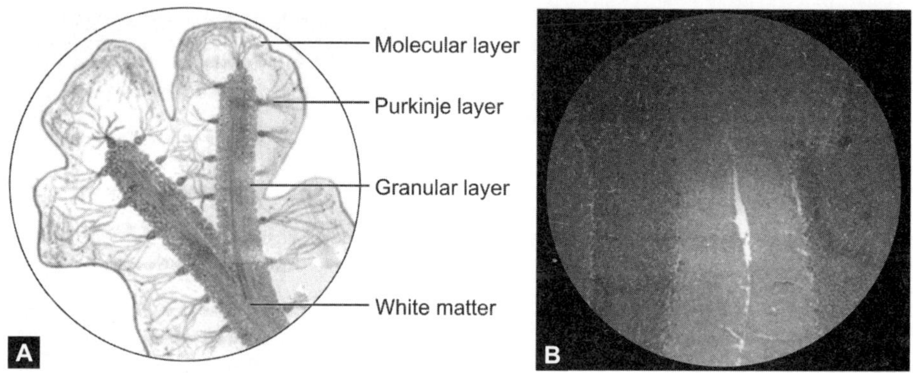

Figs 129A and B Cerebellum (*For color version, see Plate 9*)

SKIN (FIGS 130 AND 131)

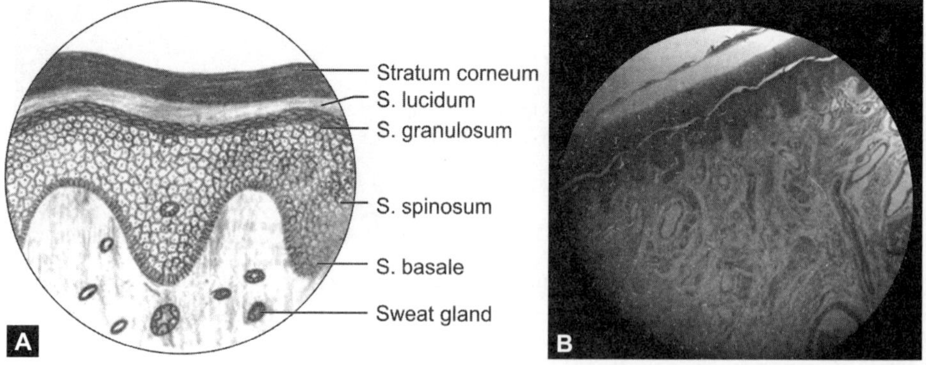

Figs 130A and B Thick skin (*For color version, see Plate 9*)

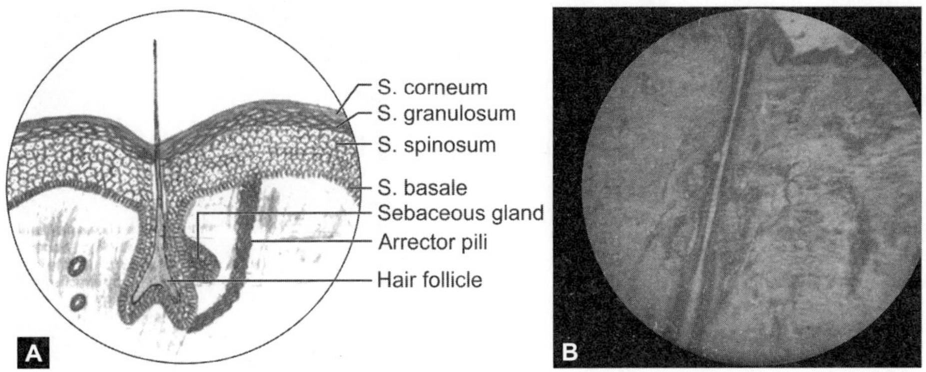

Figs 131A and B Thin skin (*For color version, see Plate 9*)

BLOOD VESSELS (FIGS 132 TO 135)

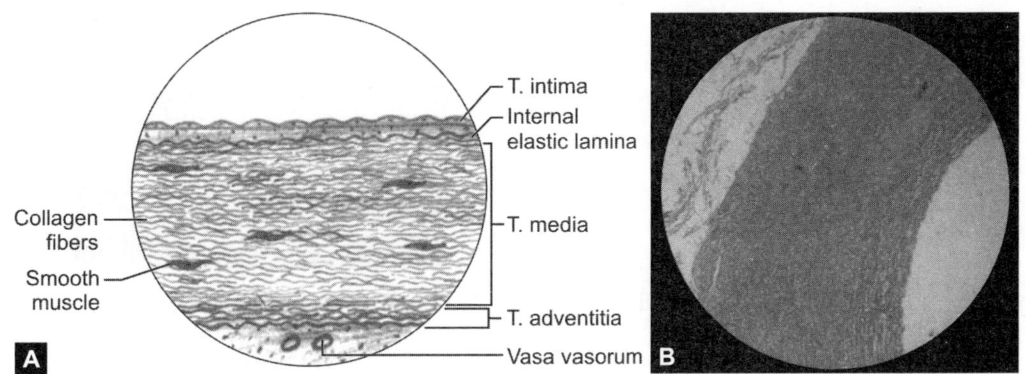

Figs 132A and B Large/elastic artery (*For color version, see Plate 10*)

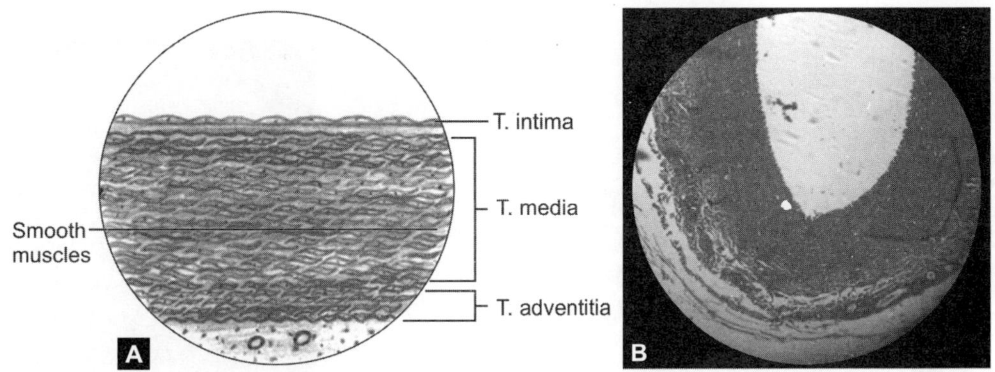

Figs 133A and B Medium sized/muscular artery (*For color version, see Plate 10*)

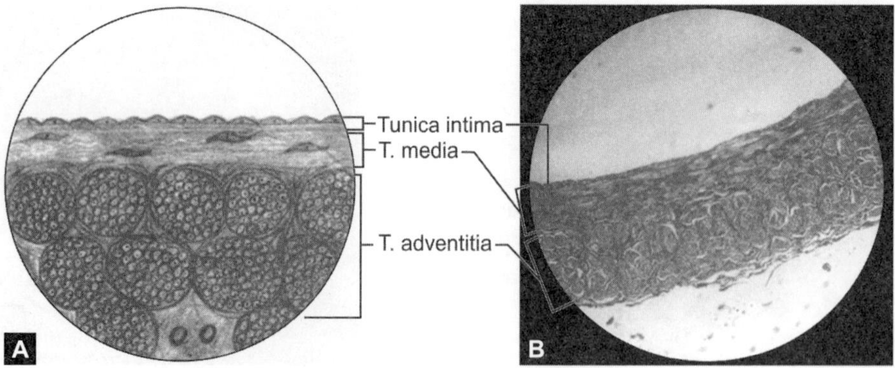

Figs 134A and B Large vein (*For color version, see Plate 10*)

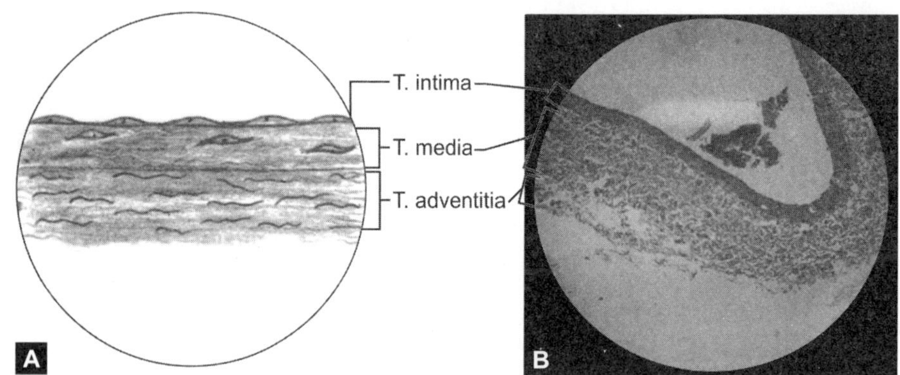

Figs 135A and B Medium-sized vein (*For color version, see Plate 11*)

RESPIRATORY SYSTEM (FIGS 136 AND 137)

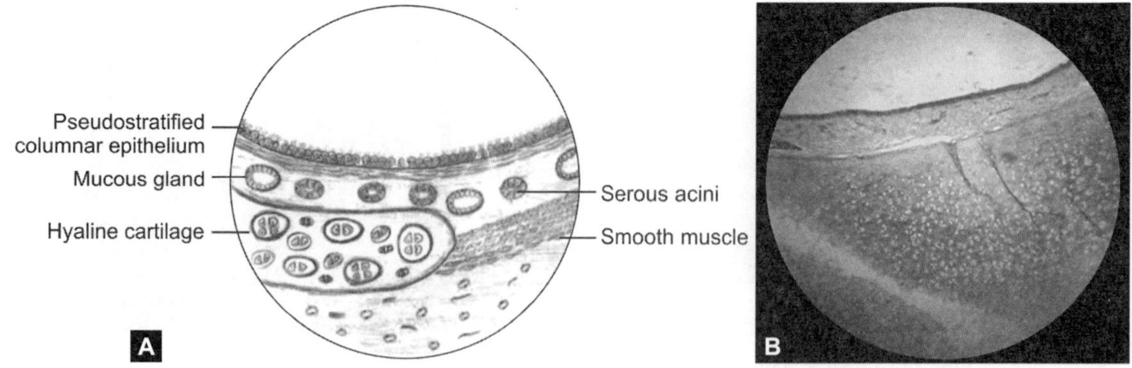

Figs 136A and B Trachea (*For color version, see Plate 11*)

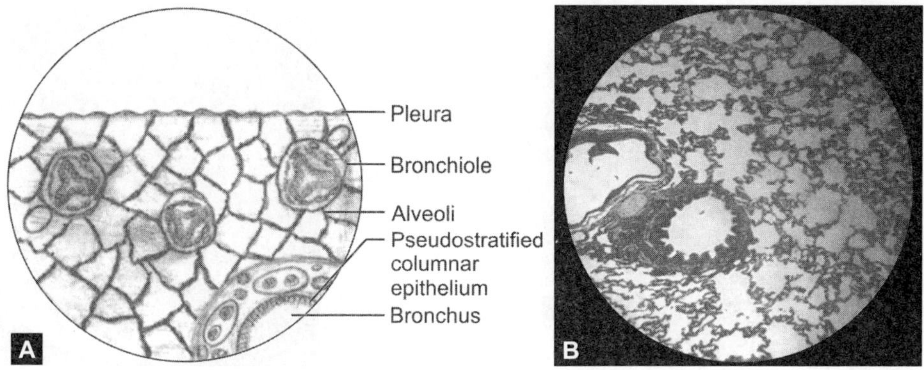

Figs 137A and B Lungs (*For color version, see Plate 11*)

GLANDS (FIGS 138 TO 140)

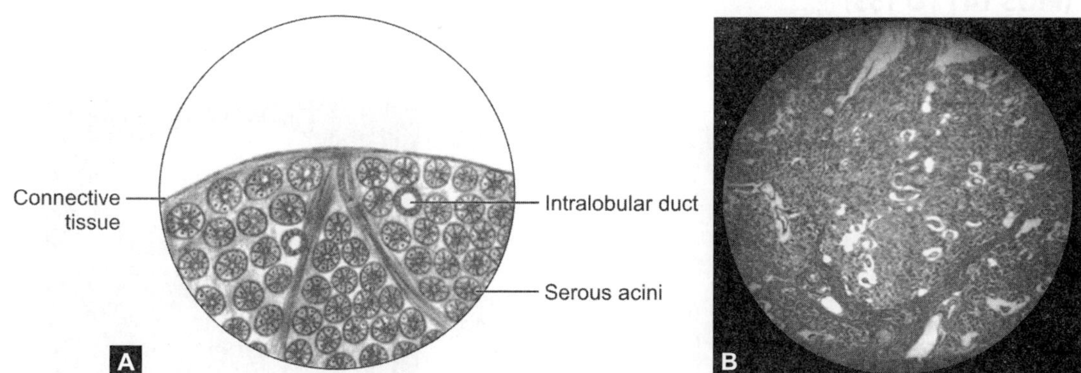

Figs 138A and B Serous salivary gland—parotid gland (*For color version, see Plate 12*)

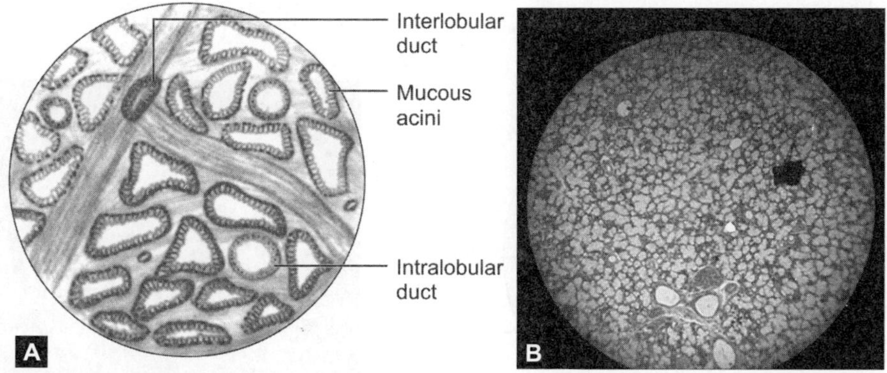

Figs 139A and B Mucous salivary gland—sublingual gland (*For color version, see Plate 12*)

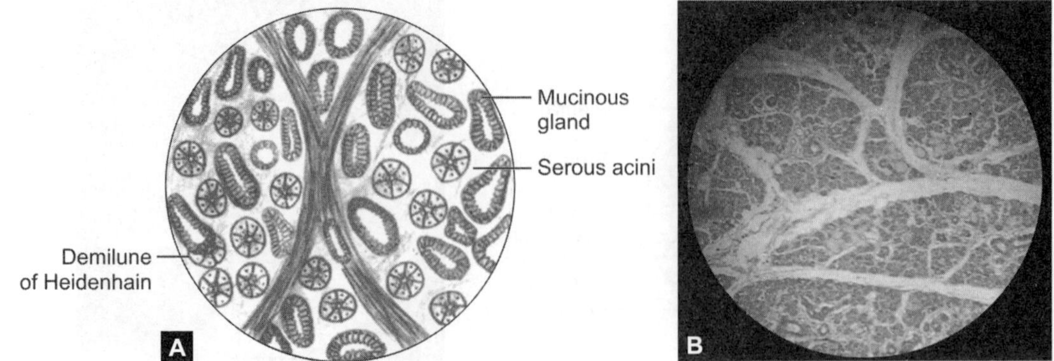

Figs 140A and B Mixed salivary gland—submandibular gland (*For color version, see Plate 12*)

TONGUE (FIGS 141 TO 153)

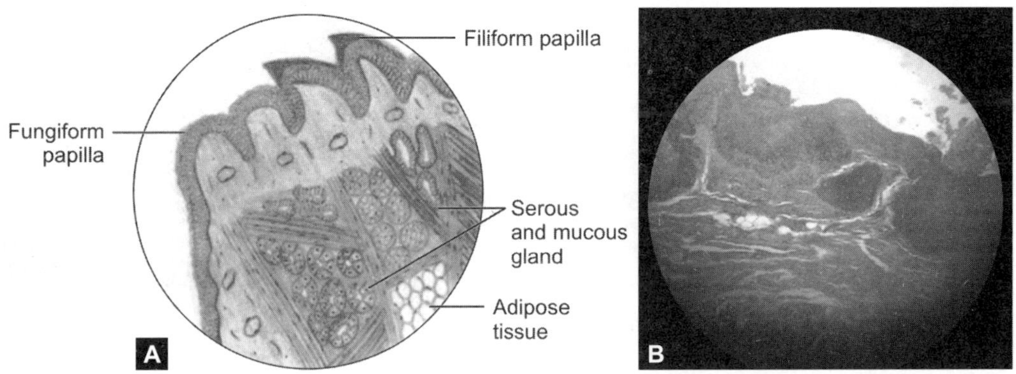

Figs 141A and B Filliform and fungiform papillae (*For color version, see Plate 13*)

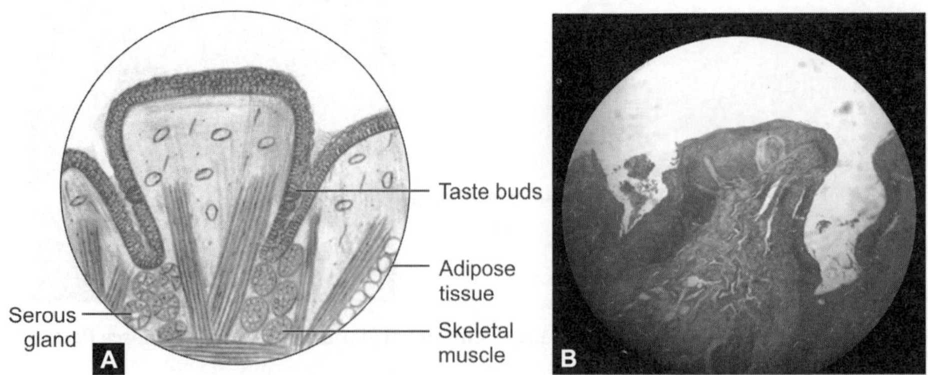

Figs 142A and B Circumvallate papillae (*For color version, see Plate 13*)

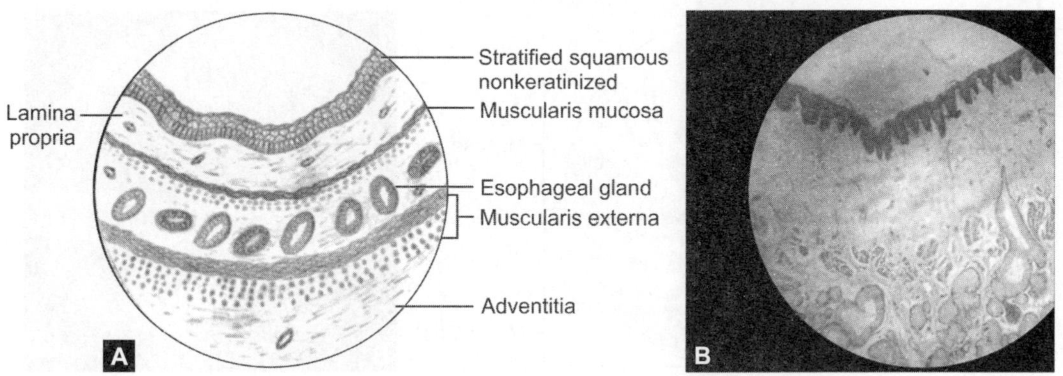

Figs 143A and B Esophagus (*For color version, see Plate 13*)

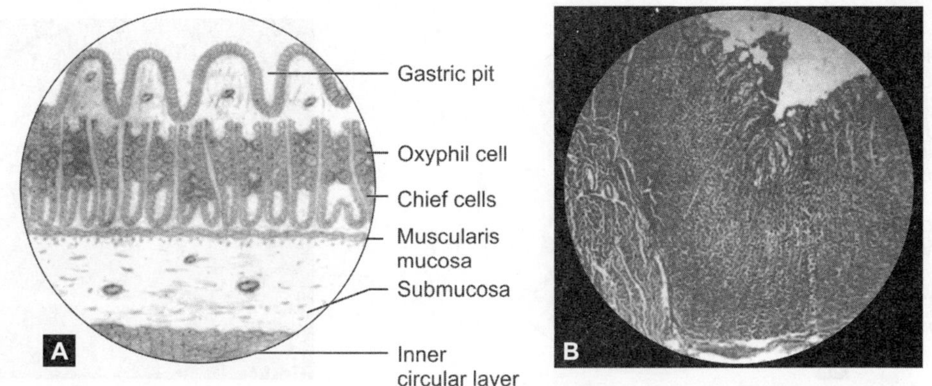

Figs 144A and B Stomach—fundus (*For color version, see Plate 14*)

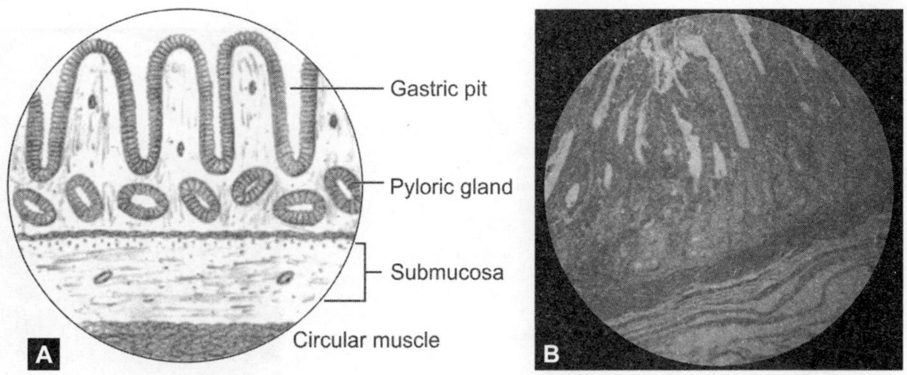

Figs 145A and B Stomach—pylorus (*For color version, see Plate 14*)

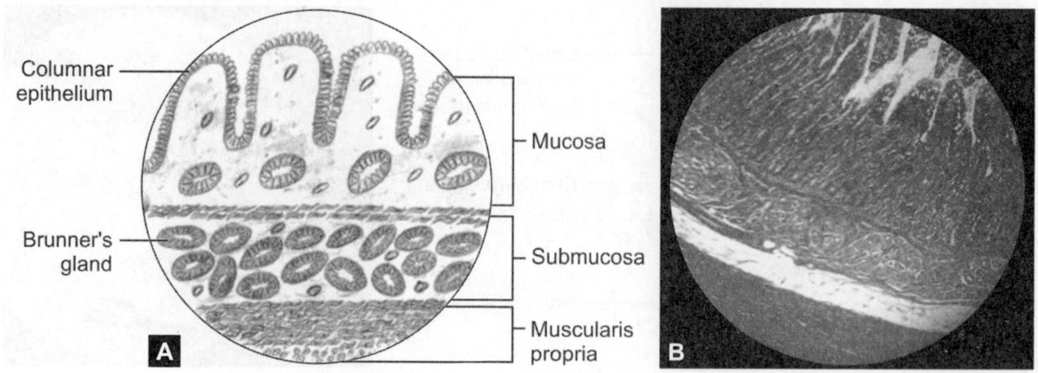

Figs 146A and B Duodenum (*For color version, see Plate 14*)

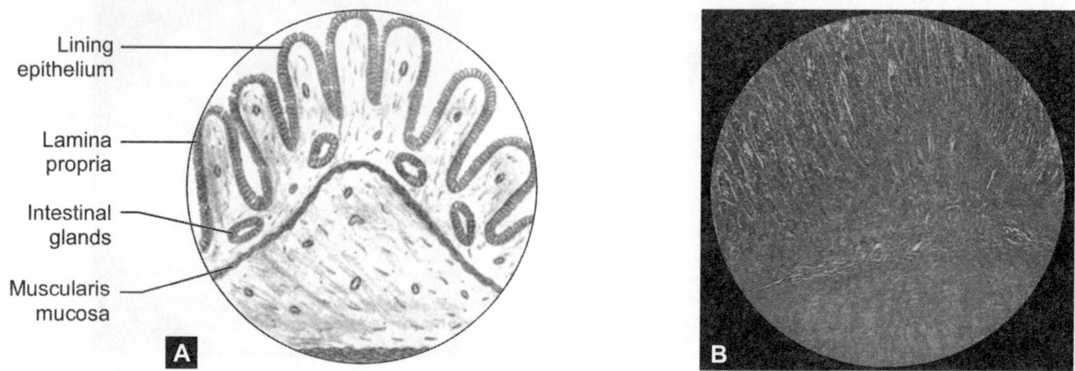

Figs 147A and B Jejunum (*For color version, see Plate 15*)

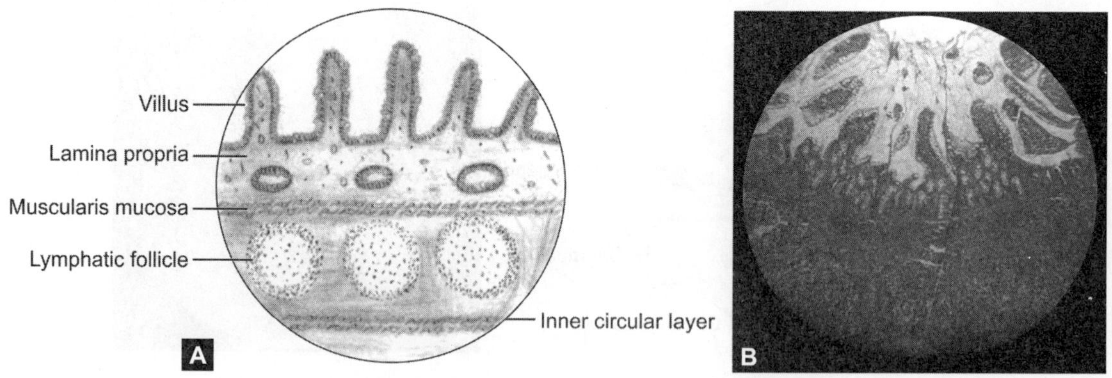

Figs 148A and B Ileum (*For color version, see Plate 15*)

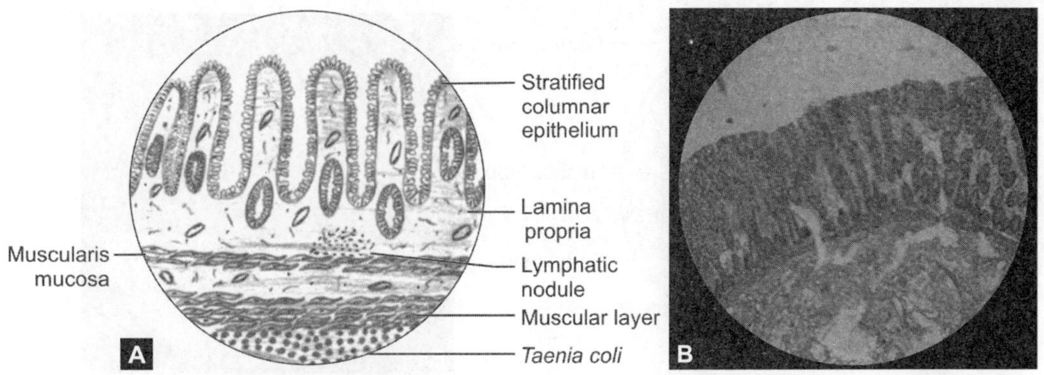

Figs 149A and B Large intestine (*For color version, see Plate 15*)

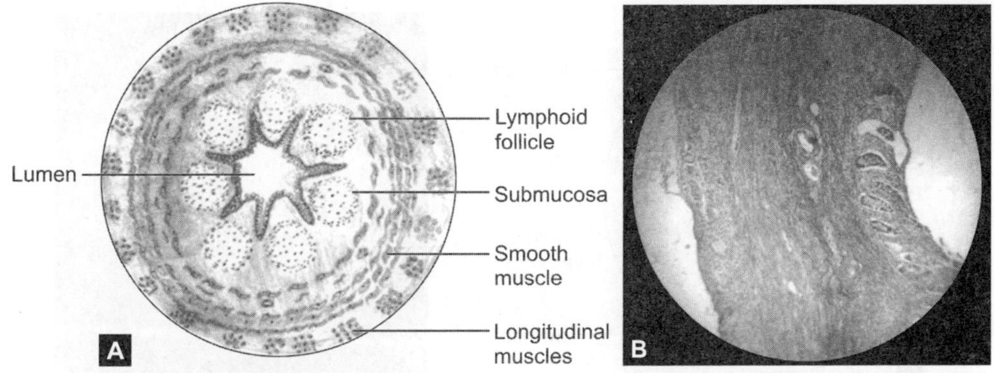

Figs 150A and B Vermiform appendix (*For color version, see Plate 16*)

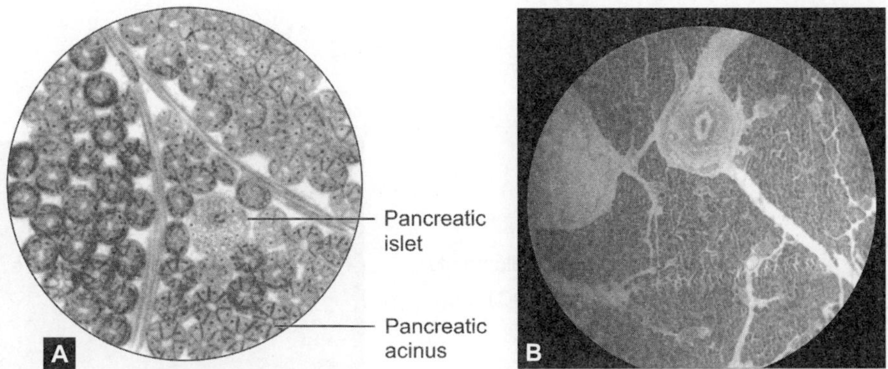

Figs 151A and B Pancreas (*For color version, see Plate 16*)

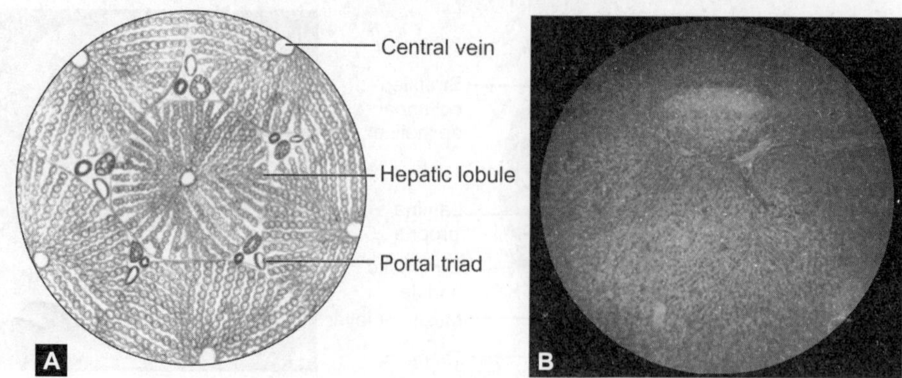

Figs 152A and B Liver (*For color version, see Plate 16*)

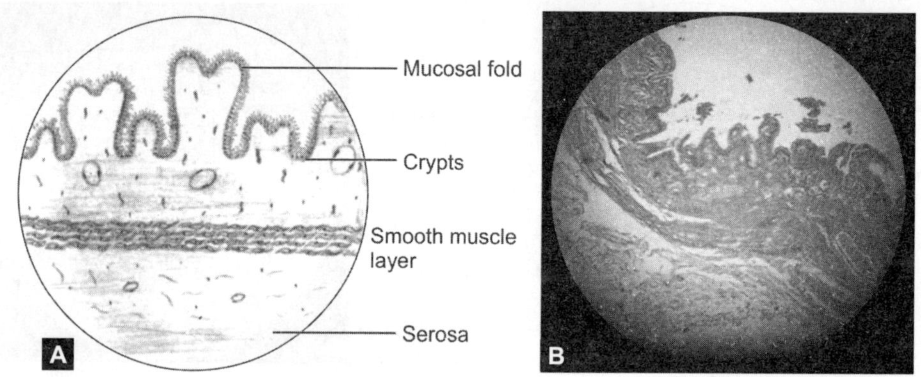

Figs 153A and B Gallbladder (*For color version, see Plate 17*)

URINARY SYSTEM (FOGS 154 TO 156)

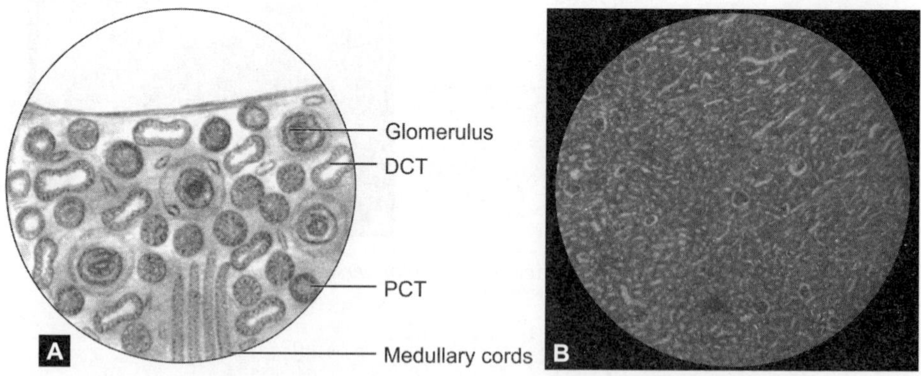

Figs 154A and B Kidney (*For color version, see Plate 17*)

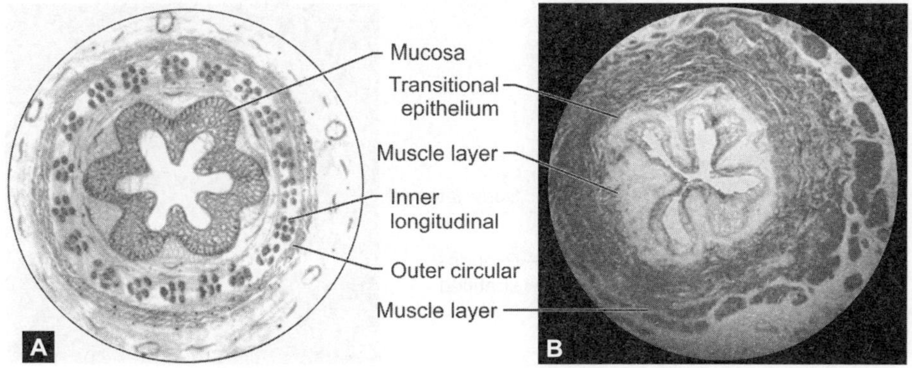

Figs 155A and B Ureter (*For color version, see Plate 17*)

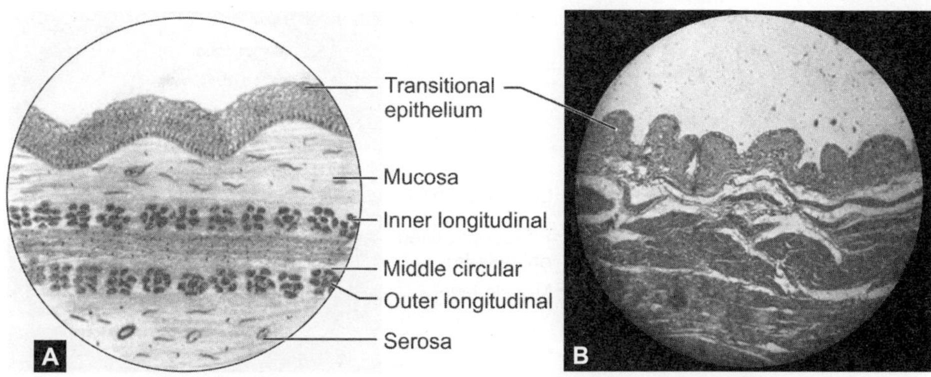

Figs 156A and B Urinary bladder (*For color version, see Plate 18*)

MALE REPRODUCTIVE SYSTEM (FIGS 157 TO 160)

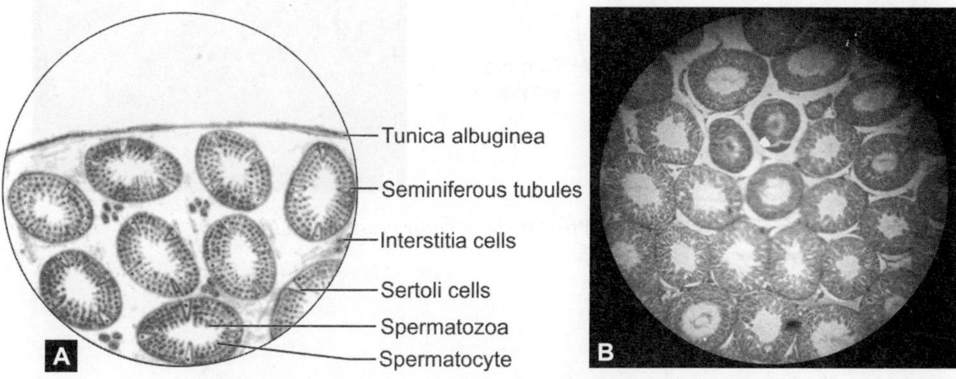

Figs 157A and B Testis (*For color version, see Plate 18*)

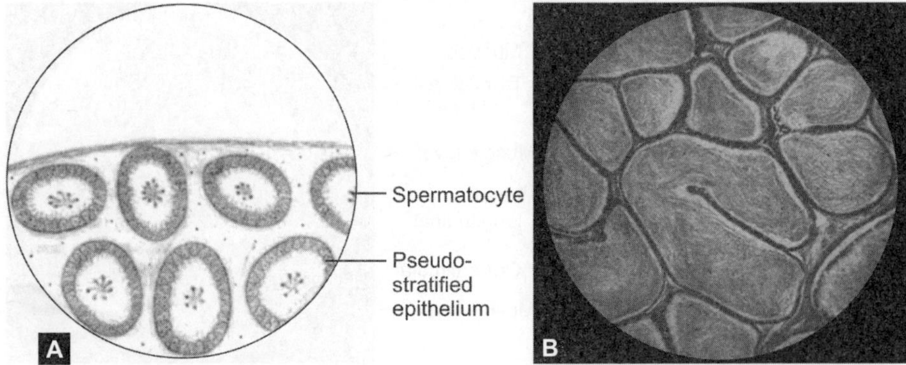

Figs 158A and B Epididymis (*For color version, see Plate 18*)

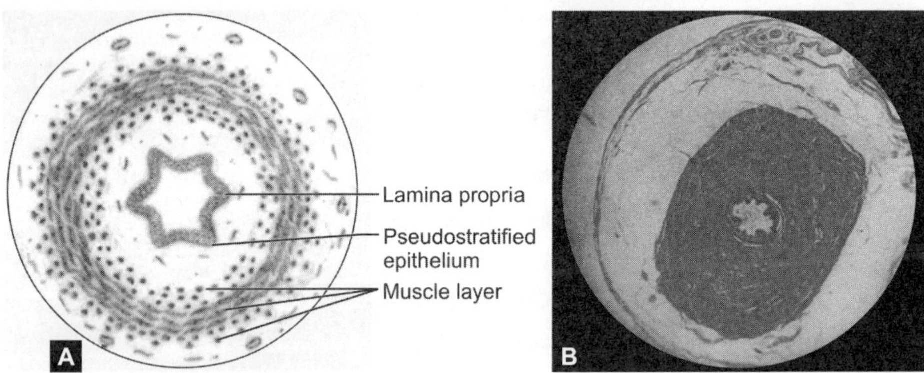

Figs 159A and B Ductus deferens (*For color version, see Plate 19*)

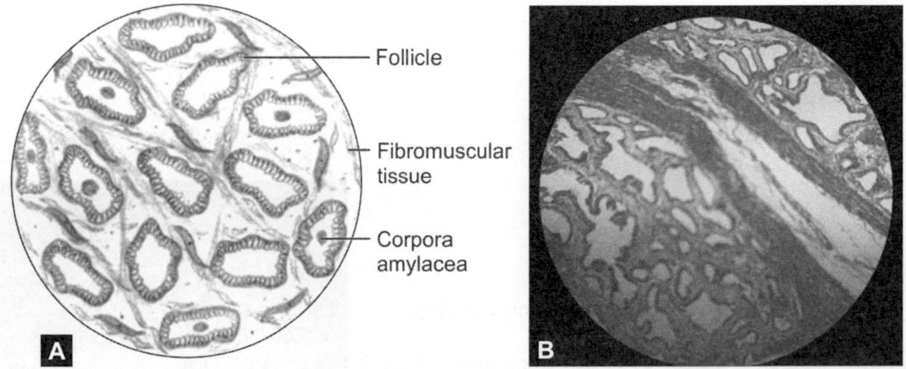

Figs 160A and B Prostate (*For color version, see Plate 19*)

FEMALE REPRODUCTIVE SYSTEM (FIGS 161 TO 164)

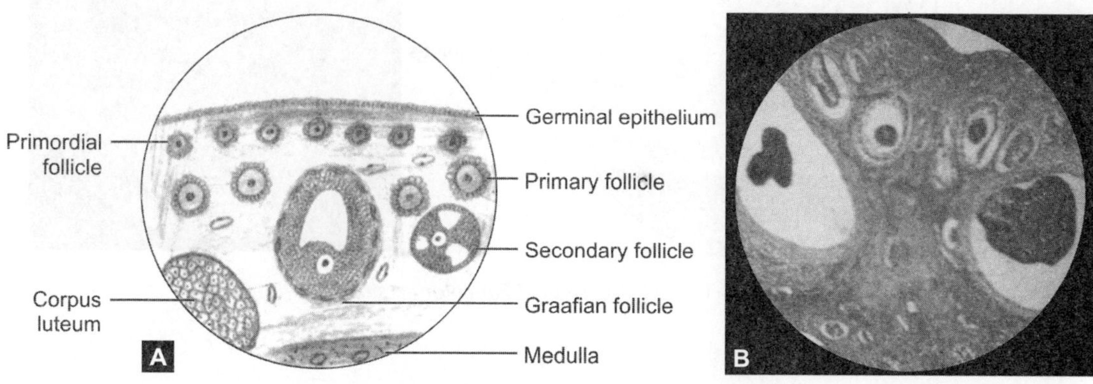

Figs 161A and B Ovary (*For color version, see Plate 19*)

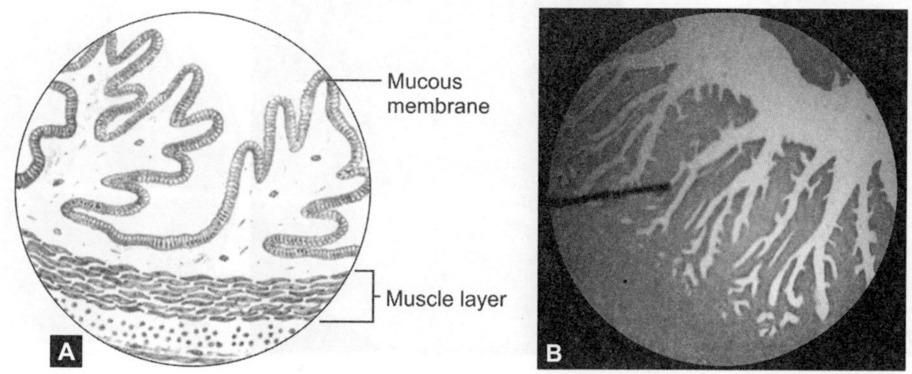

Figs 162A and B Fallopian tube (*For color version, see Plate 20*)

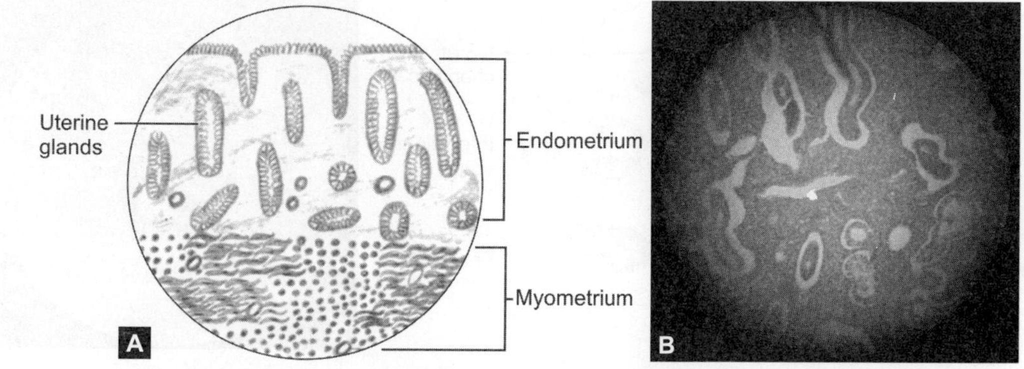

Figs 163A and B Uterus—proliferative (*For color version, see Plate 20*)

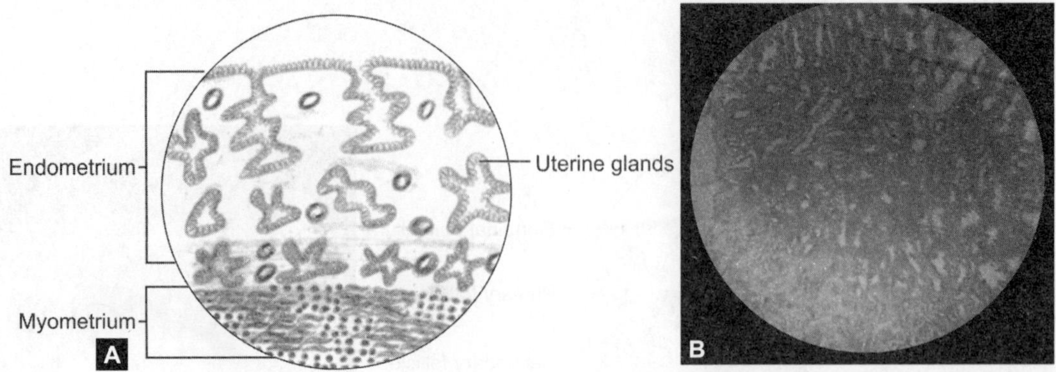

Figs 164A and B Uterus—secretory (*For color version, see Plate 20*)

MAMMARY GLAND (FIGS 165 TO 167)

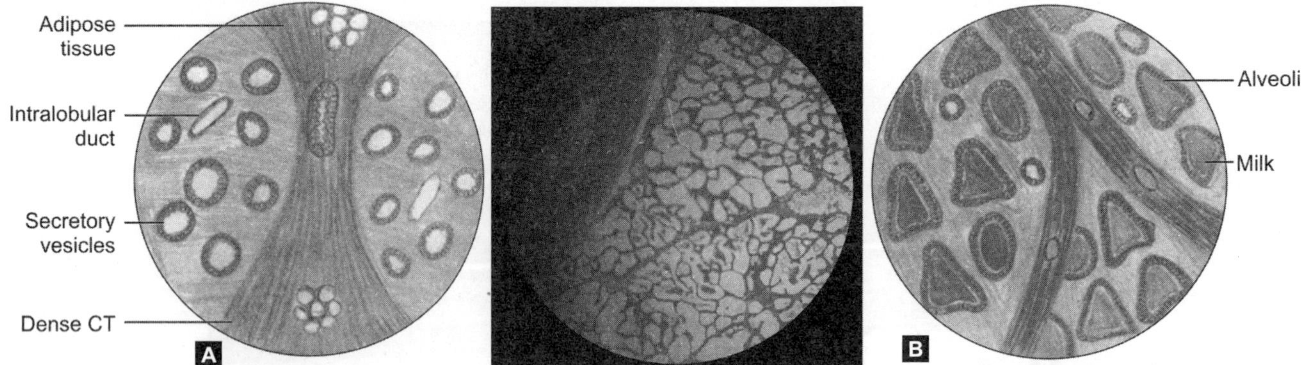

Figs 165A and B (A) Inactive mammary gland; (B) Active mammary gland (*For color version, see Plate 21*)

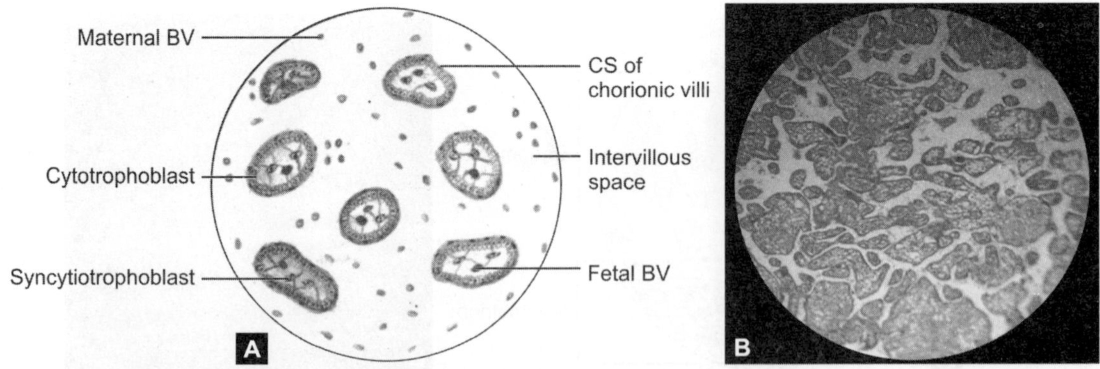

Figs 166A and B Placenta (*For color version, see Plate 21*)

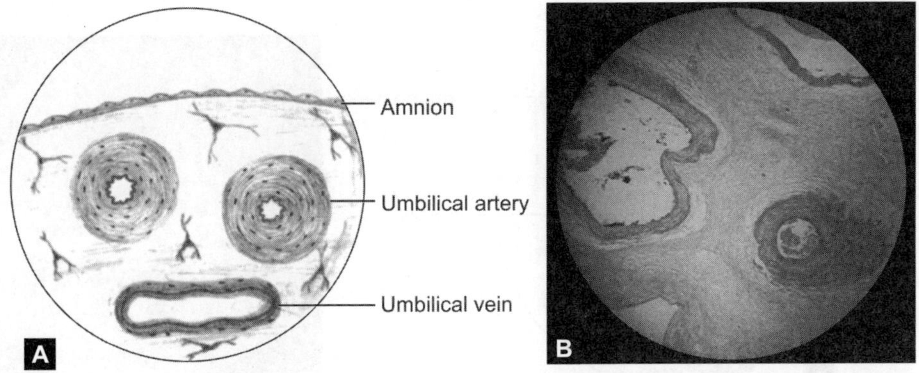

Figs 167A and B Umbilical cord (*For color version, see Plate 21*)

ENDOCRINE GLANDS (FIGS 168 TO 170)

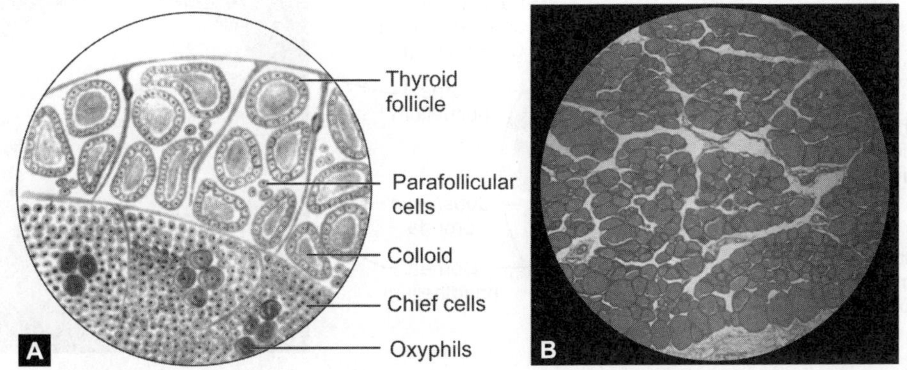

Figs 168A and B Thyroid and parathyroid glands (*For color version, see Plate 22*)

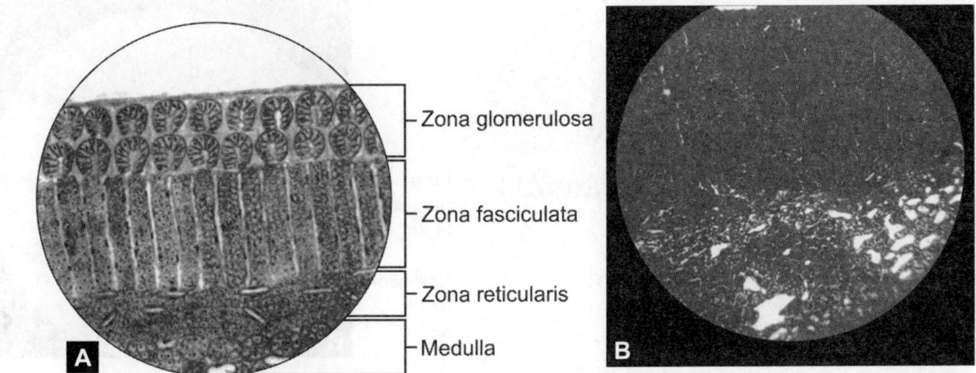

Figs 169A and B Suprarenal gland (*For color version, see Plate 22*)

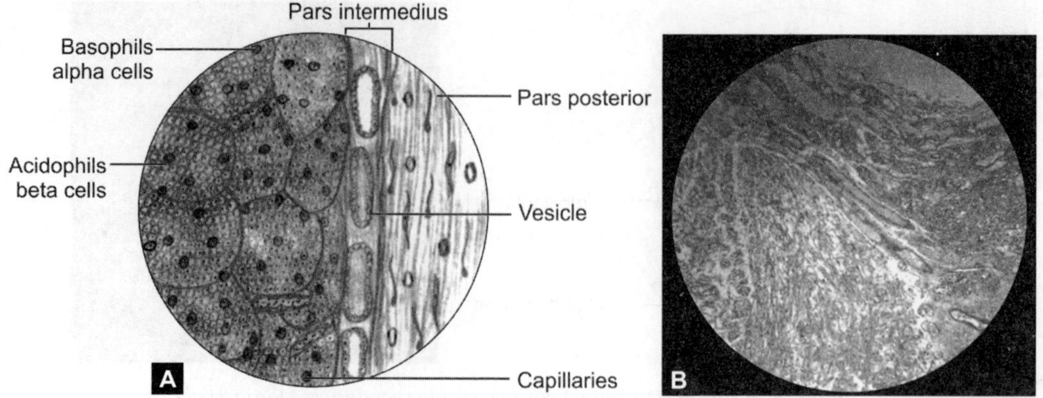

Figs 170A and B Pituitary gland (*For color version, see Plate 22*)

SPECIAL SENSES (FIGS 171 AND 172)

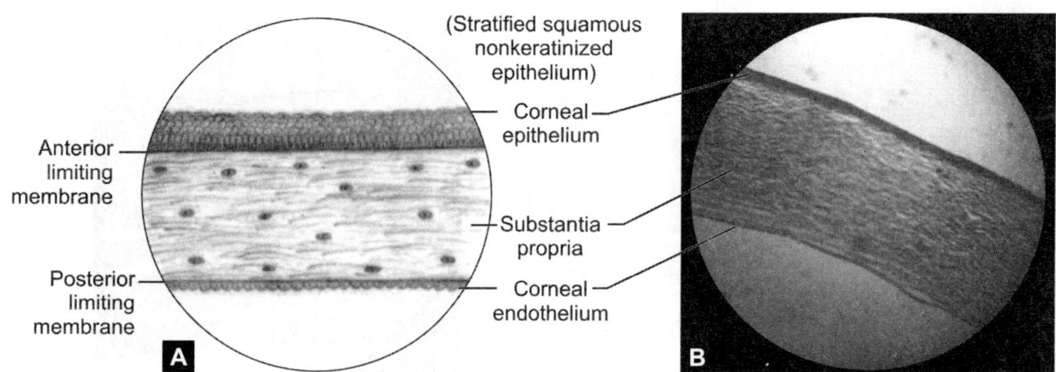

Figs 171A and B Cornea (*For color version, see Plate 23*)

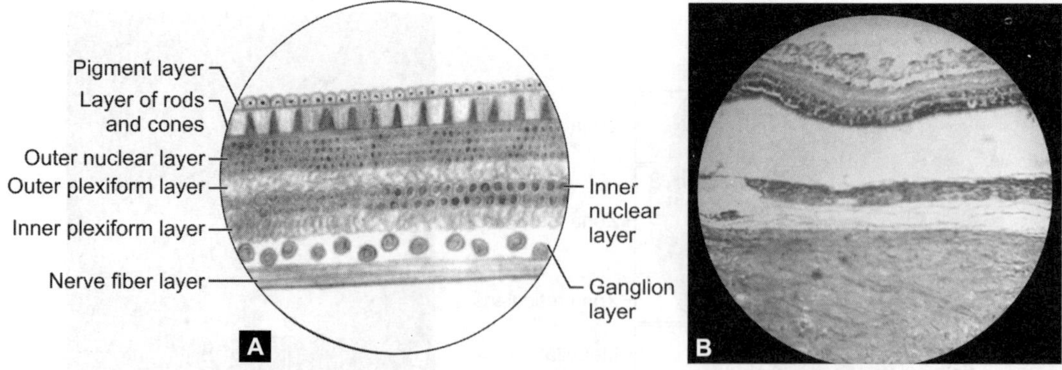

Figs 172A and B Retina (*For color version, see Plate 23*)

GROSS SPOTTERS

UPPER LIMB

- Axillary artery
- Brachial artery
- Cephalic vein
- Median cubital vein
- Axillary nerve
- Radial nerve
- Ulnar nerve
- Median nerve
- Musculocutaneous nerve
- Pectoralis major
- Biceps
- Adductor pollicis
- Brachialis
- Quadrangular spaces
- Upper triangular space
- Lower triangular space
- Deltoid
- Anatomical snuff box
- Flexor retinaculum
- Extensor retinaculum
- Palmar aponeurosis
- Superficial palmar arch
- Deep palmar arch
- Interosseous membrane
- Anconeus
- Palmaris longus
- Triceps
- Pronator quadratus
- Lumbricals
- Interossei
- Serratus anterior
- Anterior-interosseous nerve
- Supinator

LOWER LIMB

- Great saphenous vein
- Femoral artery
- Profunda femoris artery
- Popliteal artery
- Dorsalis pedis artery
- Obturator nerve
- Femoral nerve
- Sciatic nerve
- Common peroneal nerve
- Tibial nerve
- Deep peroneal nerve
- Adductor magnus
- Gluteus maximus, medius, minimus
- Flexor digitorum accessories
- Gastrocnemius
- Soleus
- Sartorius
- Popliteus
- Peroneus longus
- Iliotibial tract
- Femoral sheath
- Femoral canal
- Adductor canal
- Tendocalcaneus
- Retinacula
- Dorsum of foot
- Sole of foot
- Ligaments of knee joint

THORAX

- Cervical pleura
- Parietal pleura
- Pulmonary ligament
- Lungs
- Root of lung
- Trachea
- Right atrium
- Interatrial septum
- Heart
- Arch of aorta
- Coronary arteries
- Azygos vein
- Thoracic duct
- Superior vena cava

HEAD AND NECK

- External jugular vein
- Ansa cervicalis
- Digastrics
- Internal jugular vein
- External carotid artery
- Mylohyoid
- Sternocleidomastoid
- Vagus nerve
- Hypoglossal nerve
- Submandibular gland
- Trachea
- Cricothyroid

- Posterior cricoarytenoid
- Orbicularis oculi
- Orbicularis oris
- Buccinators
- Facial artery
- Facial vein
- Parotid gland
- Parotid duct
- Muscles of mastication
- Middle meningeal artery
- Cornea
- Eye lens
- Retina
- Nasal septum
- Paranasal air sinus
- Lateral wall of nasopharynx
- Tongue
- Soft palate
- Auditory tube
- Vocal fold
- Scalp
- Mandibular nerve
- Lingual nerve

BRAIN

- Spinal cord
- Filum terminale
- Ligamentum denticulatum
- Cauda equina
- Medulla
- Pons
- Cerebellum
- Superior colliculus
- Inferior colliculus
- Fourth ventricle
- Thalamus
- Third ventricle
- Central sulci
- Lateral sulci
- Calcarine sulcus
- Corpus callosum
- Circle of Willis
- Tentorium cerebelli
- Falx cerebri
- Internal capsule

ABDOMEN

- Inguinal canal
- Stomach
- Greater omentum
- Duodenum
- Liver
- Porta hepatis
- Ligamentum teres
- Gallbladder
- Portal vein
- Falciform ligament
- Spleen
- Kidney
- Ureter
- Testis
- Vas deferens
- Spermatic cord
- Scrotum
- Uterus
- Internal iliac artery
- Rectus sheath
- Diaphragm
- Vermiform appendix
- Pancreas
- Renal pelvis
- Trigone of bladder
- Prostate
- Ovary
- Fallopian tube
- Umbilical cord
- Colon
- Celiac trunk

CLINICAL QUESTIONS

1. A 50-year-old woman came to the hospital with complaints like inability to close her right eye tightly, accumulation of food in the vestibule of mouth during eating, on the right side and inability to puff out her cheek properly. On examination, it was found that there was loss of wrinkles on forehead on right side, dribbling of saliva from right corner of her mouth. The case was diagnosed to be Bell's palsy. Based on your knowledge in anatomy answer the following questions:
   (a) Name the nerve affected in this case and give the probable site of the involvement of the nerve causing the above complaints.
   (b) Mention the origin and course of the nerve up to the face.
   (c) Name the branches of the nerve on the face.
   (d) Name the muscle groups supplied by this nerve and give two common characteristics of the above nerve.
   (e) Give reasons for the presenting complaints (NK-609).

Ans. Refer to 'Facial Nerve'.

2. A 65-year-old man came to the hospital with difficulty in passing urine and increased frequency of micturition during night time. His condition was diagnosed as benign enlargement of prostate. With your knowledge of anatomy, answer the following questions:
   (a) Name the lobe of the prostate which is usually involved in this condition.
   (b) Briefly describe its coverings, lobes, venous and lymphatic drainage.
   (c) Mention the types of gland found in the prostate with the help of a diagram.
   (d) Name the part of the urethra passing through it. Give its internal features (NK-763).

Ans. Refer to 'Middle Lobe'.

3. A patient suffering from leprosy came with complaints of weakness in the right hand. On examination it was found that there was sensory loss of medial one and hail fingers and medial side of palmar and dorsal aspects of hand. The patient has a difficulty in holding the card between thumb and index finger:
   (a) Name the nerve affected in this case.
   (b) Describe the course and branches of this nerve.
   (c) Explain the inability of the patient to hold the card between thumb and index finger (NK-176).

Ans. Refer to 'Ulnar Nerve'.

4. A 60-year-old man while rushing to catch a train in the railway station felt severe chest pain with profuse sweating and tingling sensation along the medial aspect of his left arm. He was soon taken to the hospital where an ECG showed irregularities. His blood pressure dropped dramatically and he lapsed into deep coma and died several minutes later. Postmortem study revealed total obstruction of left coronary artery and near complete obstruction of the right coronary artery. Answer the following questions:
   (a) Explain how a coronary artery disease produces retrosternal chest pain, tingling sensation along the medial side of his left arm and increased sweeting.
   (b) Briefly describe the origin, course and areas of distribution of the coronary arteries.
   (c) What is meant by left artery dominance?
   (d) Obstruction to which coronary artery is more likely to produce irregularities in hearts rhythm and why?
   (e) Mention the sites where the branches of LCA and RCA anastomose; what is the functional significance of these anastomosis (NK-262).

Ans. Refer to 'Blood supply of heart'.

5. A young man had an injury in the lower end of the right arm during a fall on the ground. He had complaints of numbness of the front and back of ring and little fingers and later showed abnormal position of these fingers. X-ray of right arm revealed fracture of lower end of right humerus. Based on your knowledge in anatomy answer the following questions:
   (a) Name the nerve that may be injured in this case causing the complaints.
   (b) Name the part of humerus to which the nerve is closely related.
   (c) Give the root value and origin of that nerve.
   (d) Give the course and distribution of the nerve.
   (e) Name the deformity of the hand and give the anatomical reason for that (NK-176).

Ans. Refer to 'Ulnar Nerve'.

6. A 50-year-old man had complaints of abdominal pain immediately after food, vomiting and passing blood in the stool. Chronic gastric ulcer was diagnosed in this case after clinical examination and investigations. Answer the following questions:
   (a) Name the parts of stomach.
   (b) Give the nerve supply and arterial supply of stomach.
   (c) Name the different glands present in the mucosa and their secretions.
   (d) Name the common site of the gastric ulcer and give the anatomical reason for this.

(e) Mention 2 investigations usually done in this case (NK- 666).

Ans. Refer to 'Stomach'.

7. A 25-year-old lady presented with abdominal pain. On examination, urine pregnancy test was positive and ultrasonography showed gestational sac in the uterine tube. With your knowledge, answer the following questions:
   (a) Name the clinical condition probably affecting in this case.
   (b) Give the length of the uterine tube.
   (c) Name its parts.
   (d) Mention its blood supply.
   (e) Give its microscopic structure with the help of a diagram (NK-769).

Ans. Refer to 'Ectopic Pregnancy'.

8. A 25-year-old lady had the complaints of swelling in the front of her neck. On examination, a solitary nodular swelling was found in the midline of neck. The swelling was moving with swallowing. Answer the following questions:
   (a) Name the gland that causes the swelling.
   (b) Give its parts and closely related structures.
   (c) Mention its arterial supply.
   (d) Add a note on its development.
   (e) Give the reason for the movement of the swelling with swallowing (NK-338).

Ans. Refer to 'Thyroid gland'.

9. A man came to the hospital with complaints of a swelling over the back of head after receiving a severe blow. On examination, the skin over the swelling was intact. The swelling was fluctuant and limited to the area occupied by the underlying bone hematoma of the scalp was diagnosed. Answer the following questions:
   (a) Give the extent of scalp.
   (b) State the details of the different layers.
   (c) Name the layer containing the blood clots in the above case.
   (d) Which is the dangerous layer of scalp and why is it called so?
   (e) Give the arterial supply of scalp (NK-320).

Ans. Refer to 'Scalp'.

10. A 55-year-old woman with children had complaints of something descending down into the pelvis and low backache. On vaginal examination, it was seen that the external opening of cervix was found at the vaginal orifice. Answer the following questions:
   (a) Name the organ that is affected and mention the probable condition affecting the organ.
   (b) Name the parts of the organ and state its normal position.
   (c) Name the supports of the organ.
   (d) Give the blood supply of the organ.
   (e) Mention the common causes that lead to the present condition in the above case (NK-770)

Ans. Refer to 'Uterine Prolapse'.

11. A 50-year-old woman had a complaint of a swelling in the right groin. On examination, the swelling was found to be below and lateral to the pubic tubercle. It was also found that the swelling increased in size during coughing. The swelling was diagnosed as herniation of the abdominal contents. Answer the following questions:
   (a) Name the canal through which the herniation occurred and give the normal contents of the canal.
   (b) Give the boundaries of the upper opening of the canal to abdomen and the clinical significance of the medial boundary.
   (c) Give the anatomical reason for the common occurrence of this herniation in females.
   (d) Name the structures lying in the compartments lateral to the canal.
   (e) Give the formation of this sheath (NK-845).

Ans. Refer to 'Femoral Hernia'.

12. A man had complaints of fever, breathlessness and chest pain on right side. The pain was aggravated by respiratory movements. On examination, a rubbing sound could be heard with stethoscope during respiration. X-ray chest was advised. Answer the following questions:
   (a) Name the structure affected in this case and name the organ covered by it.
   (b) Give the parts of the structure giving their nerve supply.
   (c) Name the cavity it bounds and its recess.
   (d) Give the applied importance of this recess.
   (e) Name the structures from superficial to deep, a needle has to traverse to collect the fluid filled in the cavity (NK-216).

Ans. Refer to 'Pleura (pleural effusion)'.

13. During a football game a 20-year-old player was knocked by another player on the lateral aspect of the knee. He felt severe pain on the right knee and was unable to extend his right knee joint. Answer the following questions:
   (a) Name the most probable structures of knee joint that can be injured in this case.
   (b) Write briefly about the intra-articular structures of the knee joint.
   (c) Name the movements of the knee joints.
   (d) What is meant by unlocking of the knee joint and name the muscle producing it?

Ans. Medial meniscus Bucket handle tear.

14. A 55-year-old man experienced gripping chest pain on physical exertion. The pain was radiating to the inner side of left arm and was found to be relieved on rest. Answer the following questions: Angina
   (a) Name the organ affected in this case.
   (b) Give the most common cause leading to the symptoms presented by the man.
   (c) Name the arteries and their branches supplying the organ.
   (d) Give its venous drainage.
   (e) Name the investigations to be done in this case.

Ans. Refer to 'Heart-blood supply'.

15. In a man, hospitalized for three weeks after a motor bike accident, it was noticed that his left arm was medially rotated and adducted while the forearm was pronated and extended. An area of sensory loss was also noticed along the lateral side of left upper arm. Answer the following questions:
   (a) Name the deformed position of his left upper limb.
   (b) Give the probable sites of lesion of the nerve plexus to produce this deformity.
   (c) Name the nerves at this point of lesion.
   (d) Name the muscles paralyzed to produce this deformity and give their nerve supply.
   (e) Give reasons for the sensory loss of area mentioned above.

Ans. Refer to 'Erb's Palsy'.

DIAGRAMS (FIGS 173 TO 243)

These are commonly asked diagrams.

UPPER LIMB

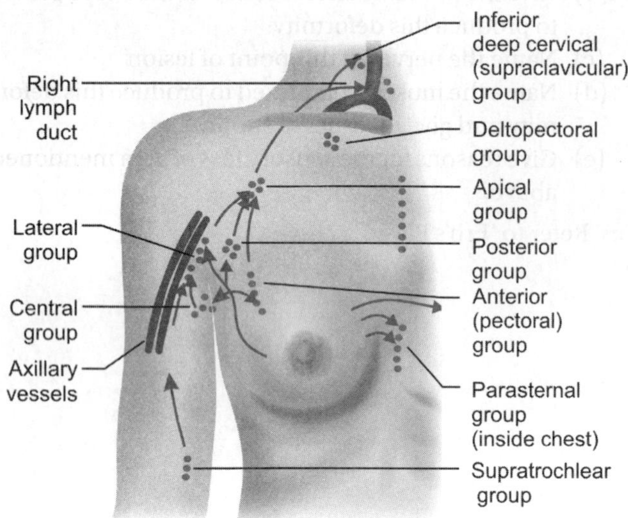

Fig. 173 The lymph nodes of the axilla and the lymphatic drainage of the breast

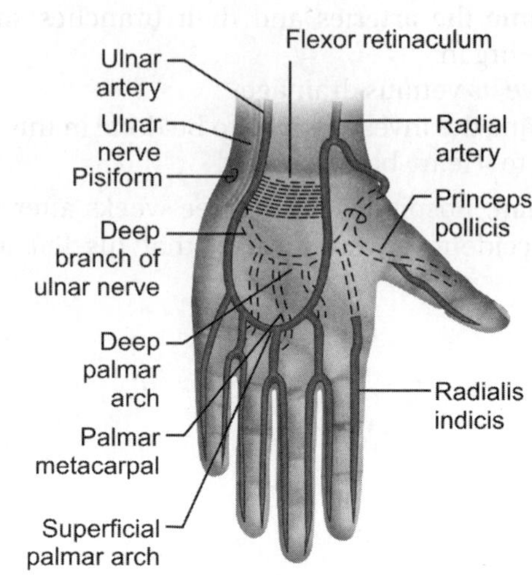

Fig. 174 Superficial palmar arch

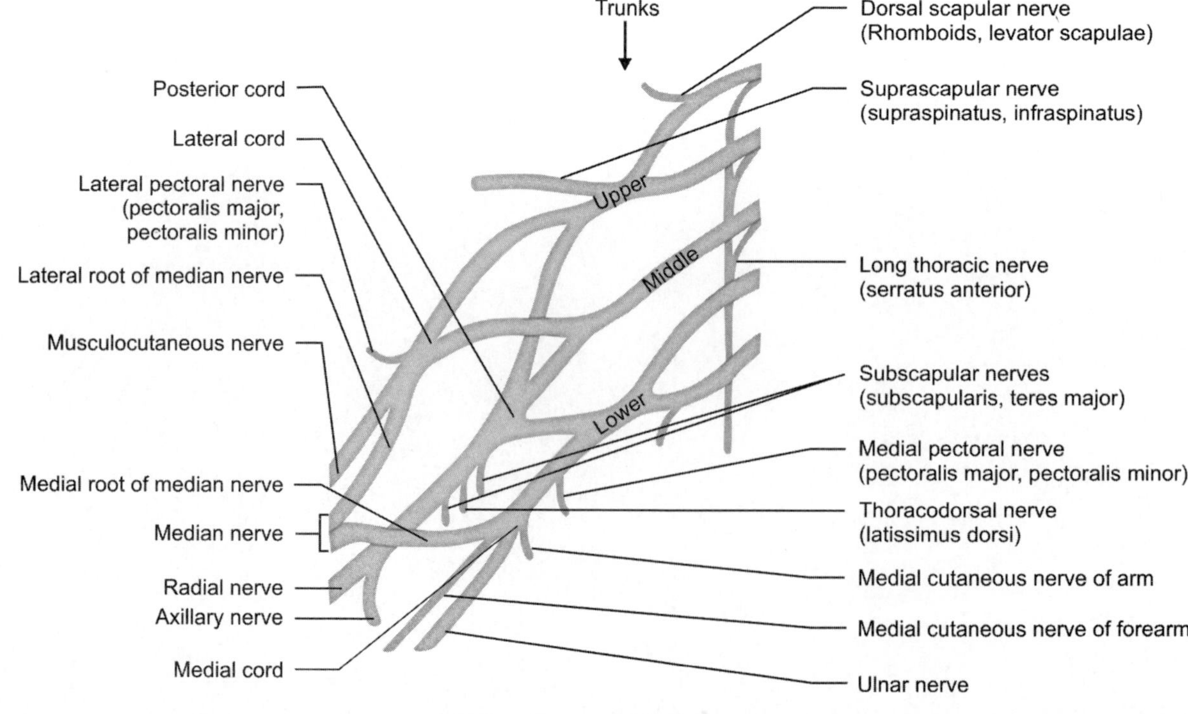

Fig. 175 Brachial plexus

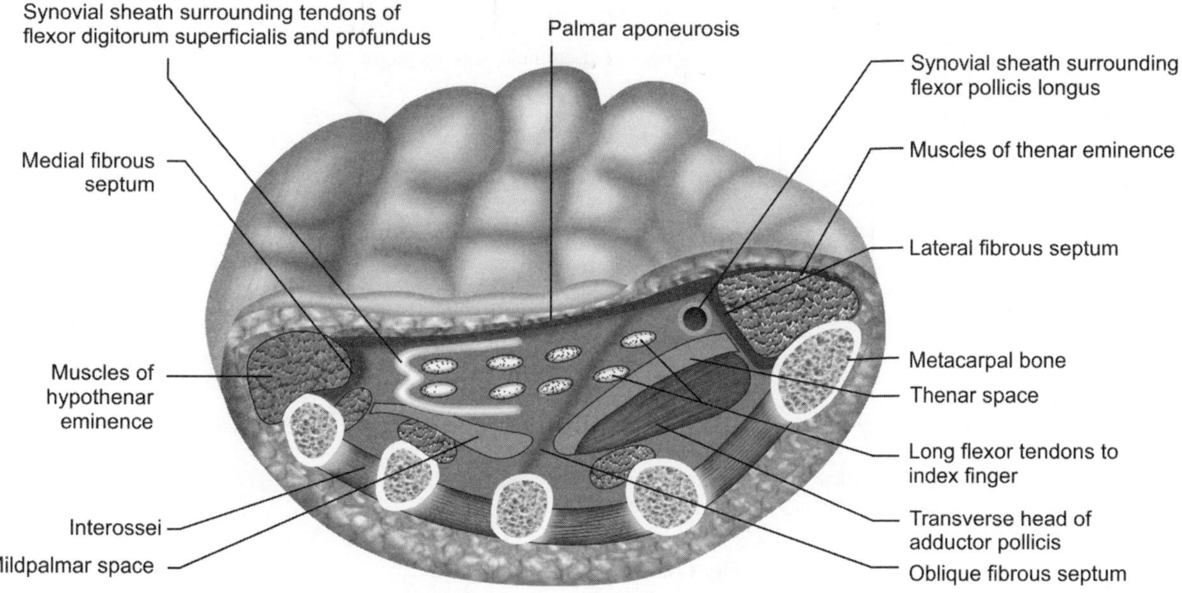

Fig. 176 Cross section through hand

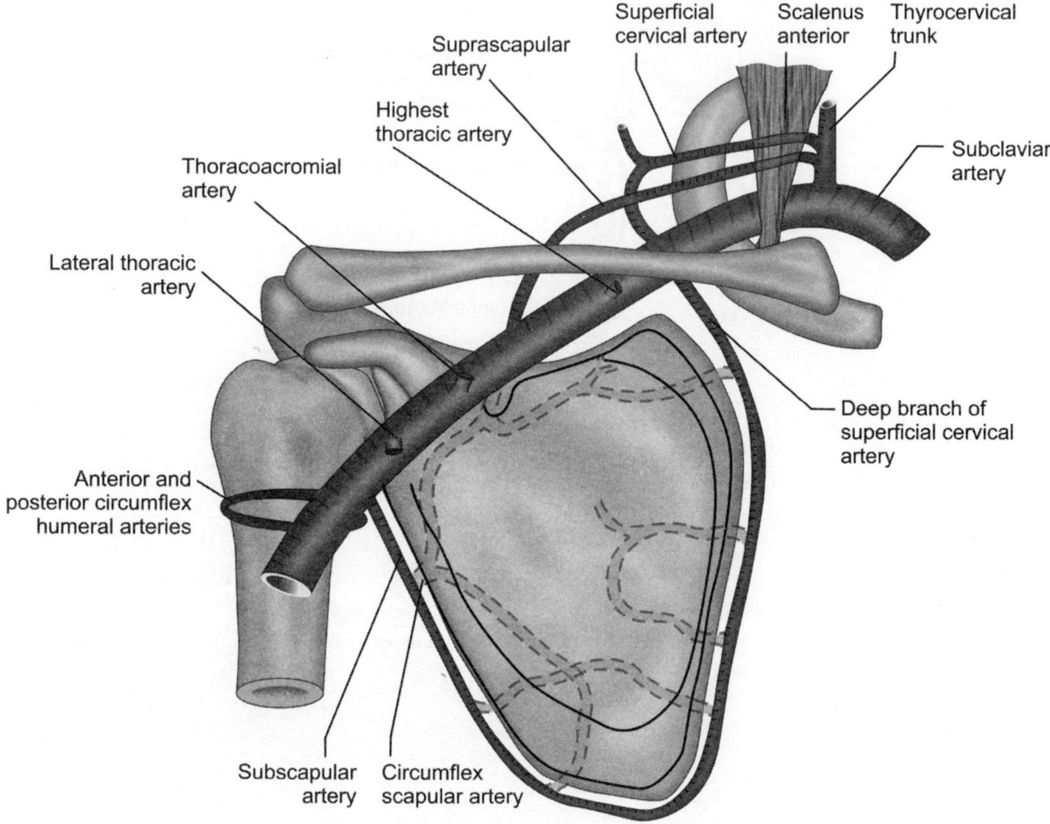

Fig. 177 Anastomosis around scapula

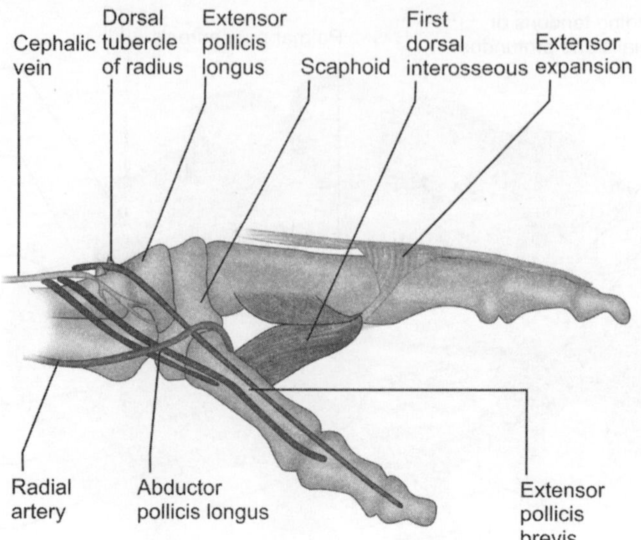

Fig. 178 Anatomical snuff box

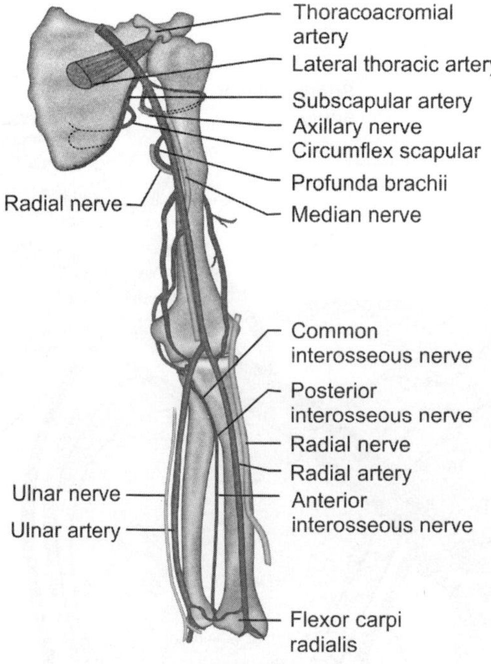

Fig. 179 Course of brachial artery

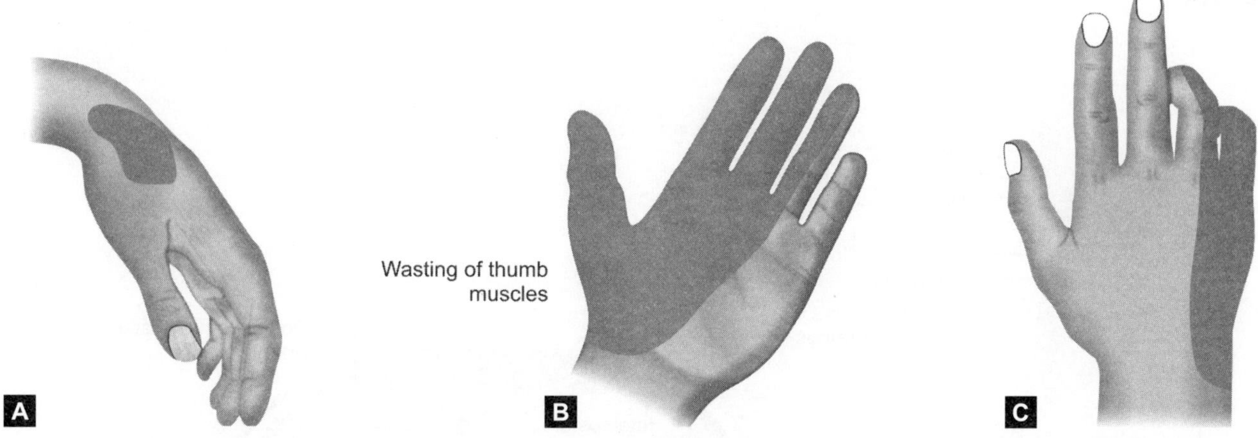

Figs 180A to C Common nerve palsies. (A) Radial nerve palsy; (B) Median nerve palsy; (C) Ulnar nerve palsy

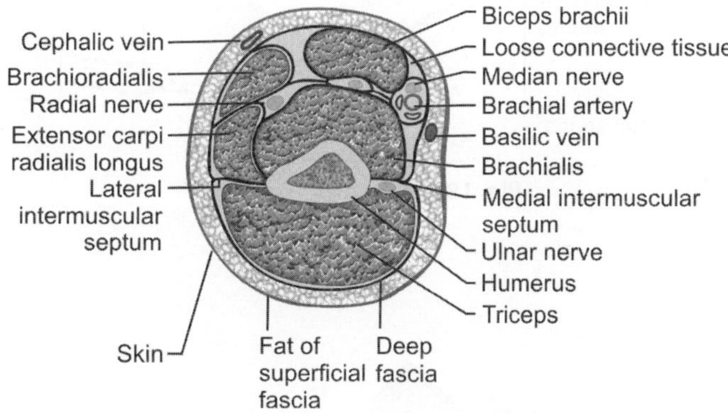

Fig. 181 Cross section through arm

THORAX

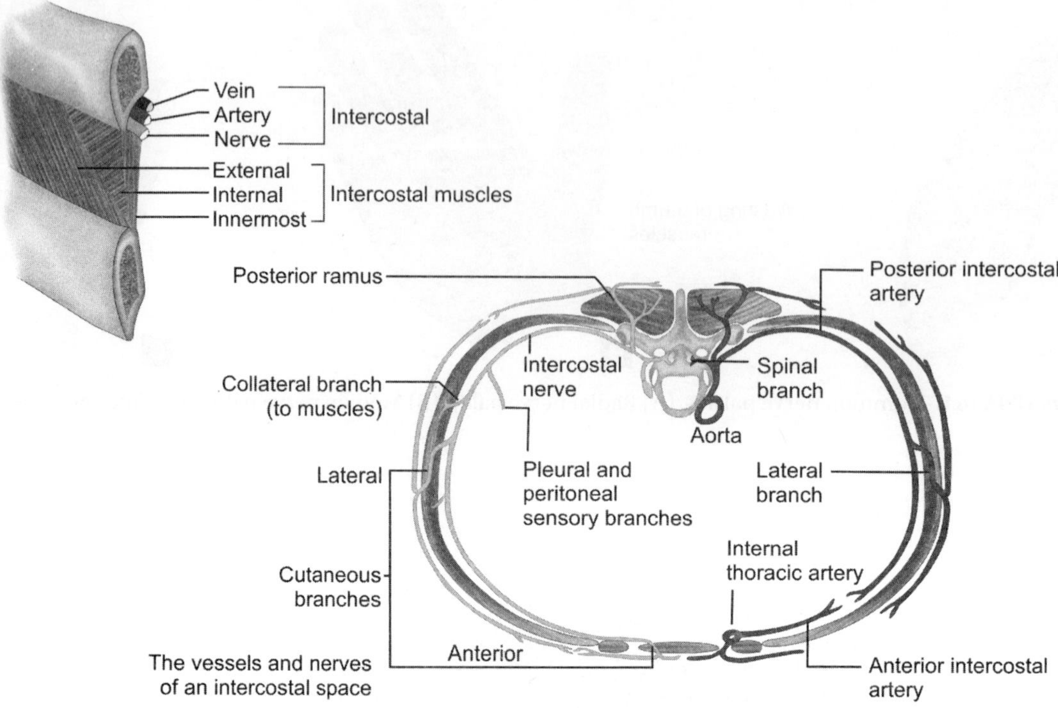

Fig. 182 Intercostal space

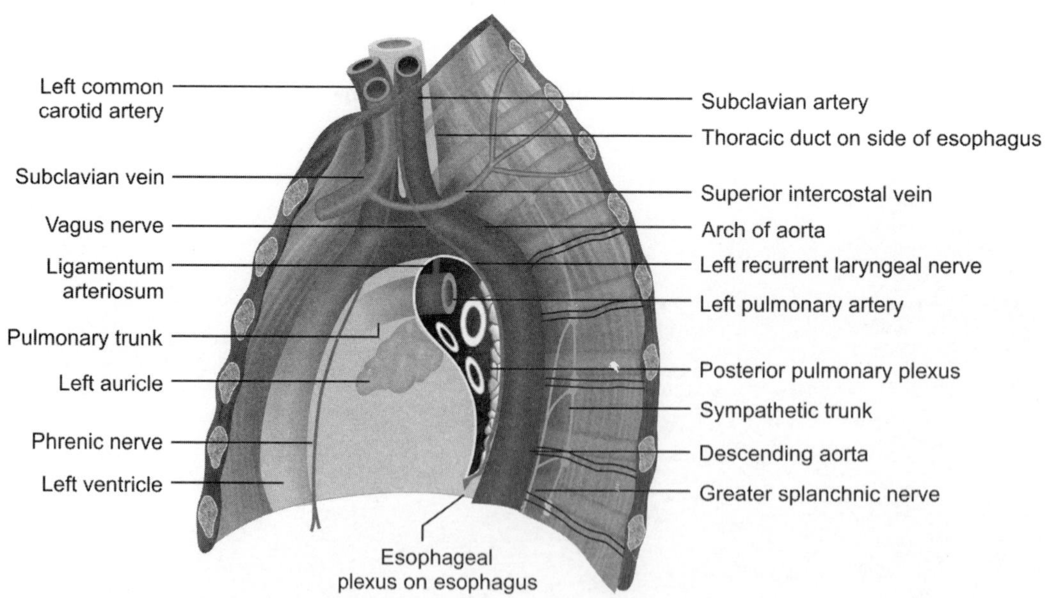

Fig. 183 Left side of mediastinum

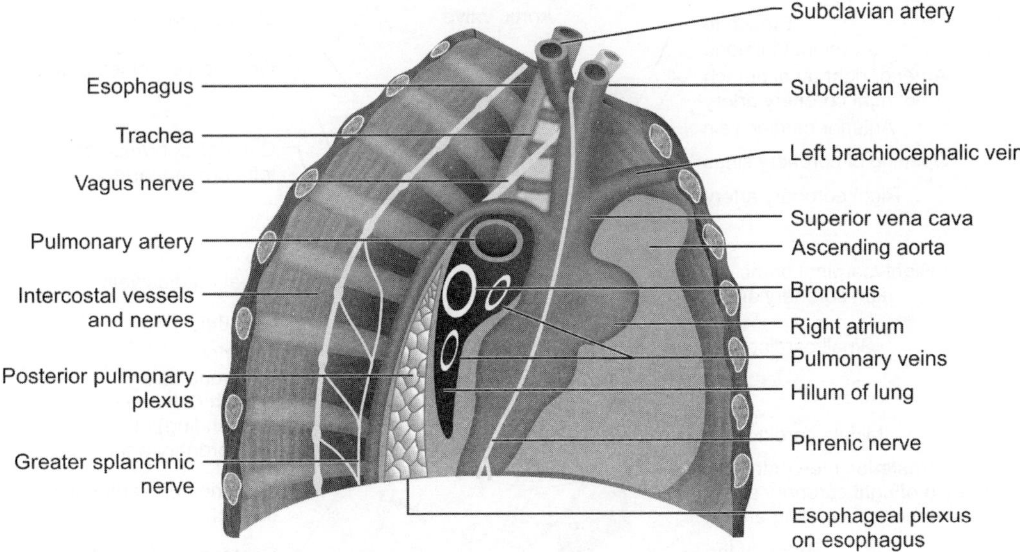

Fig. 184 Right side of mediastinum

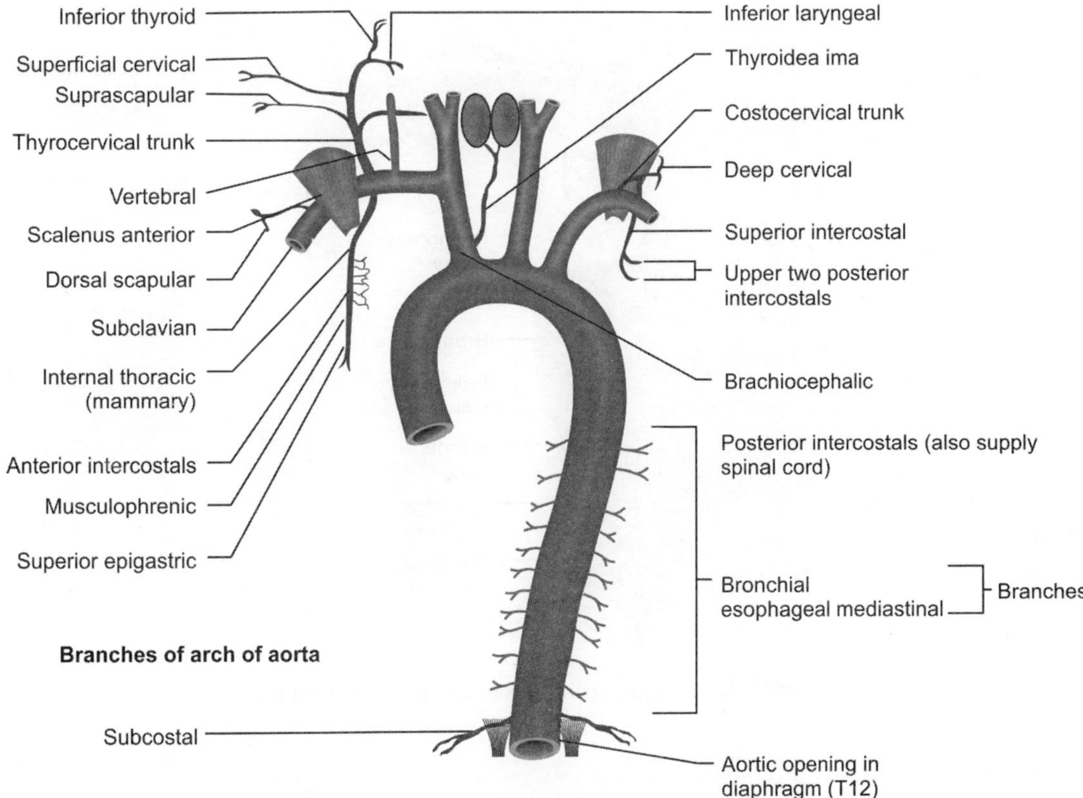

Fig. 185 The branches of the arch and the descending thoracic aorta

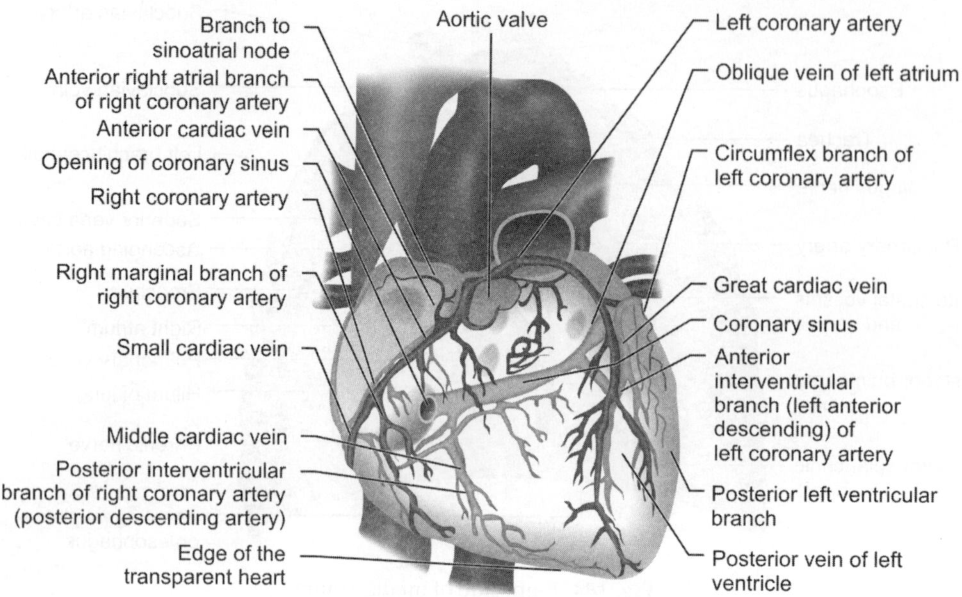

Fig. 186 Coronary arteries and cardiac veins

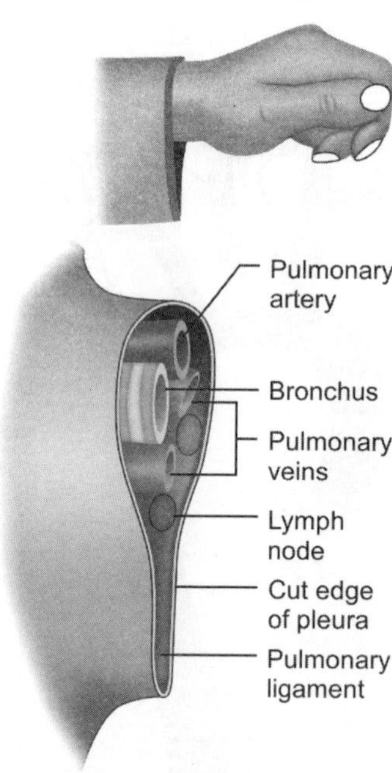

Fig. 187 The principal structures in the hilum of the lung

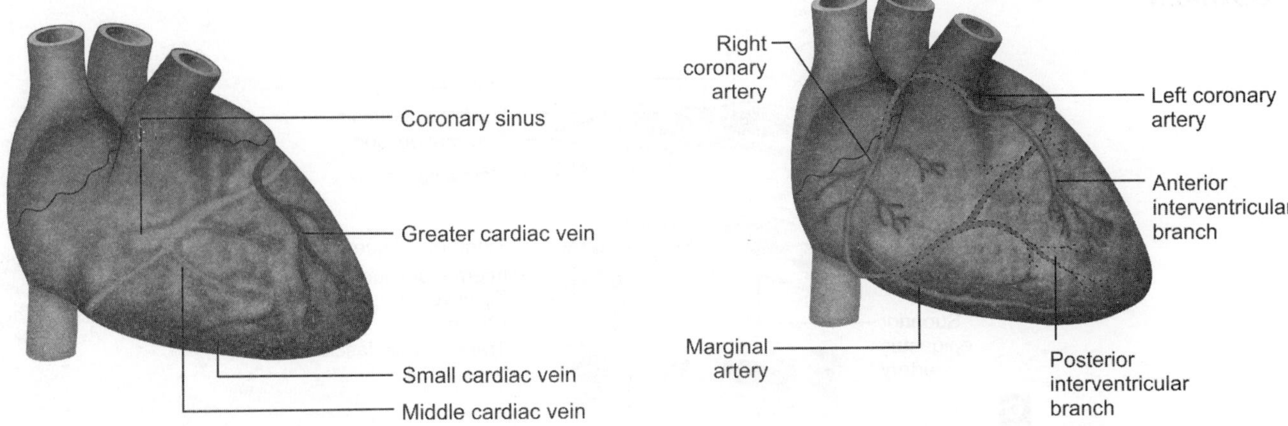

Fig. 188 The venous drainage of the heart

Fig. 189 The coronary arteries variations are common

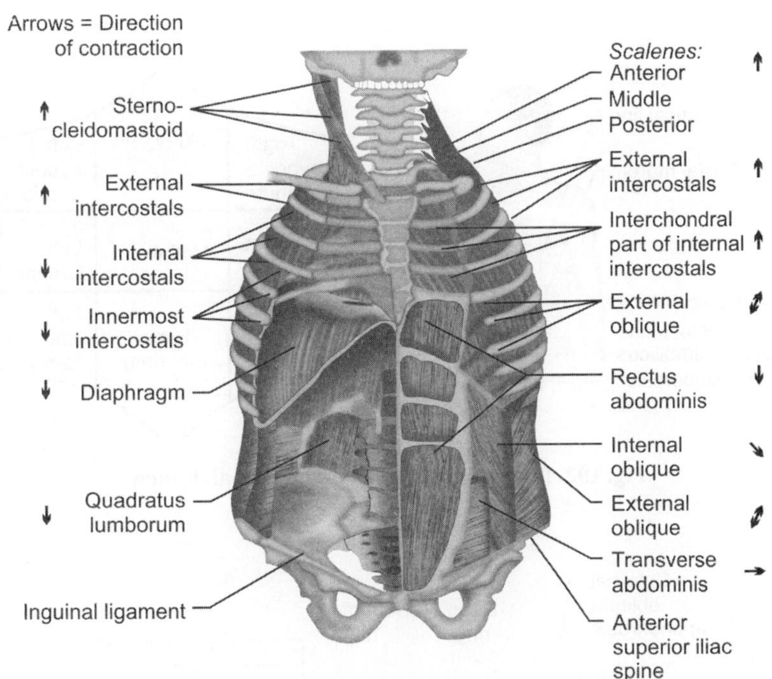

Fig. 190 Muscles of respiration

ABDOMEN

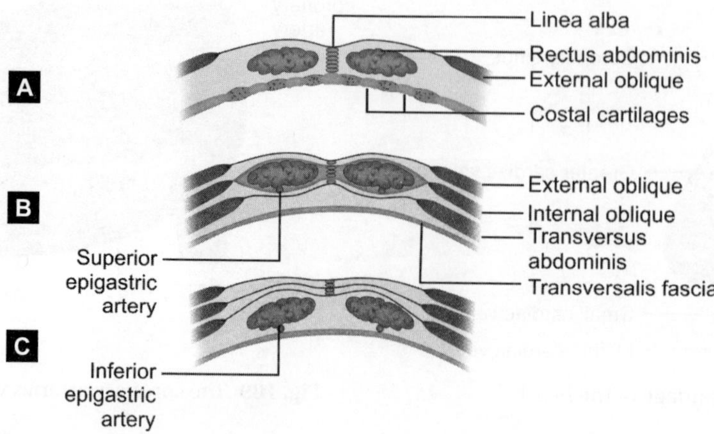

Figs 191A to C Transverse sections through the rectus sheath. (A) Above the costal margin; (B) Above the umbilicus; (C) Above the pubic symphysis

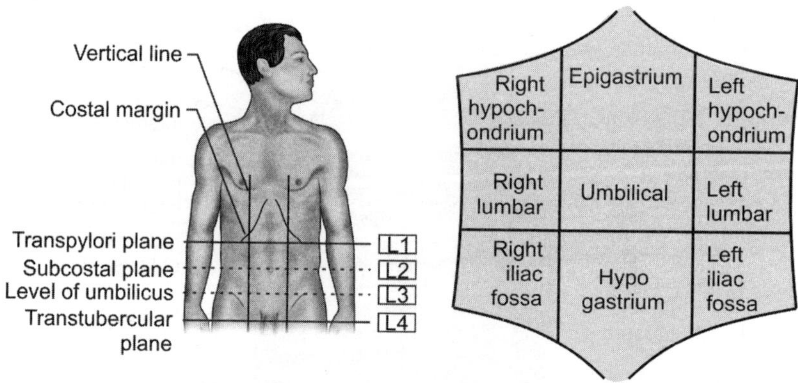

Fig. 192 Imaginary planes of margins of abdomen

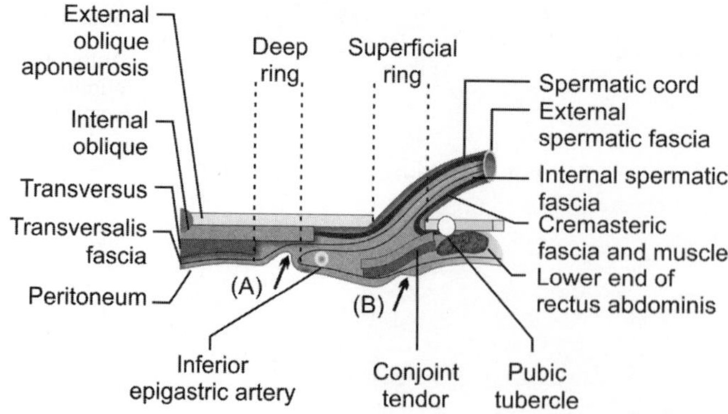

Fig. 193 A horizontal section through the inguinal canal (diagrammatic). (A) and (B) show the sites of indirect and direct herniae respectively

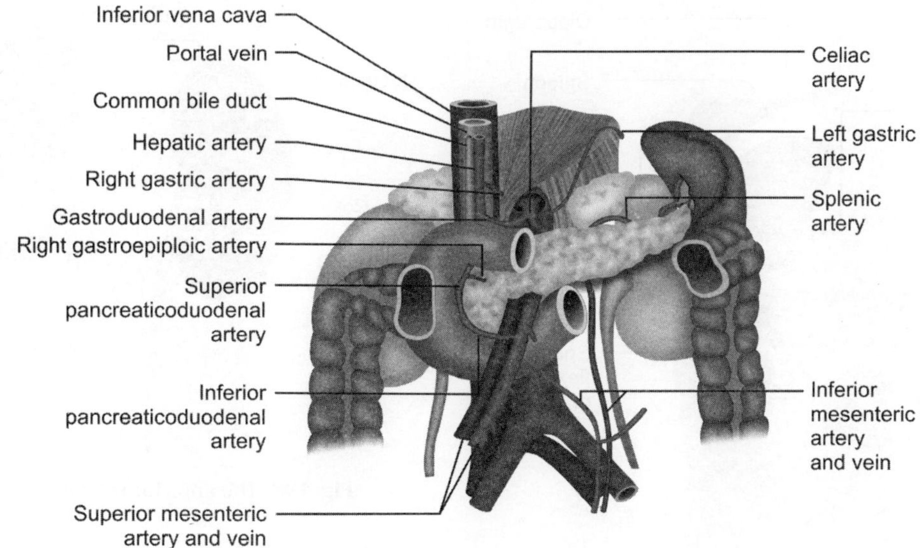

Fig. 194 The relations of the pancreas

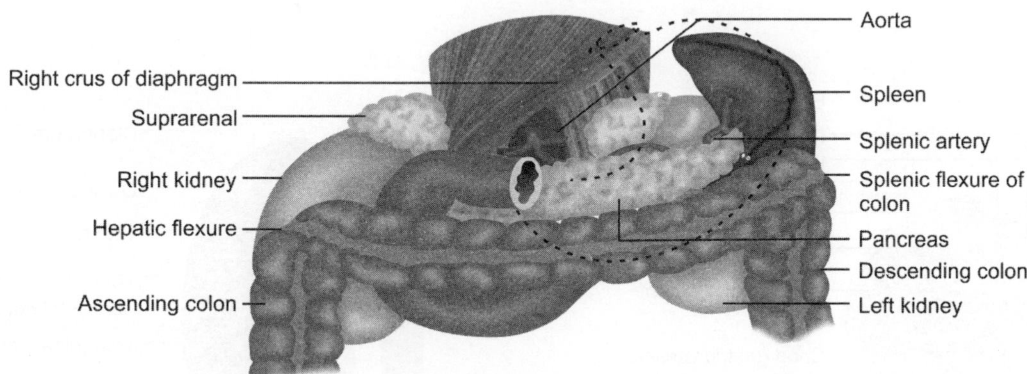

Fig. 195 Stomach bed

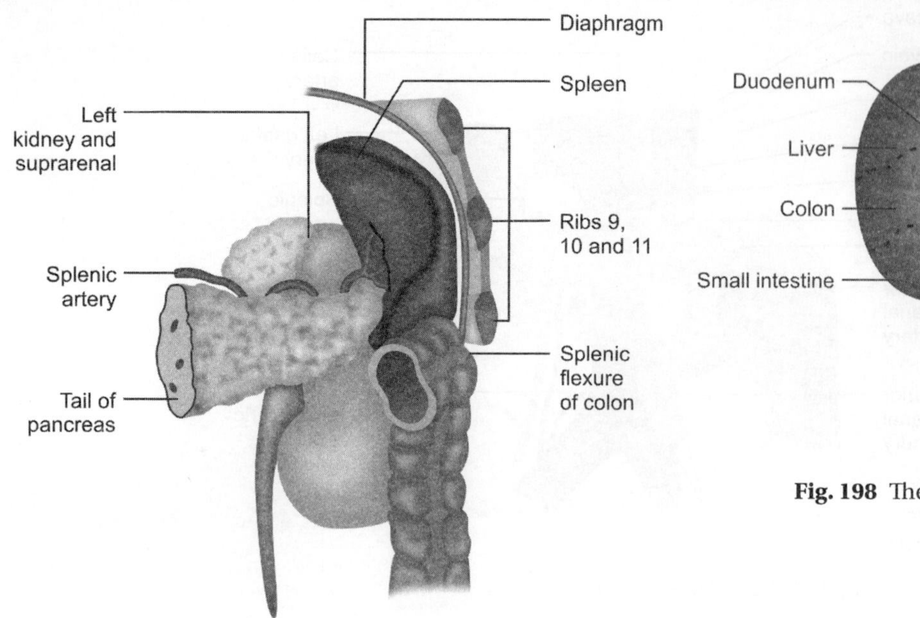

Fig. 196 The relations of the spleen

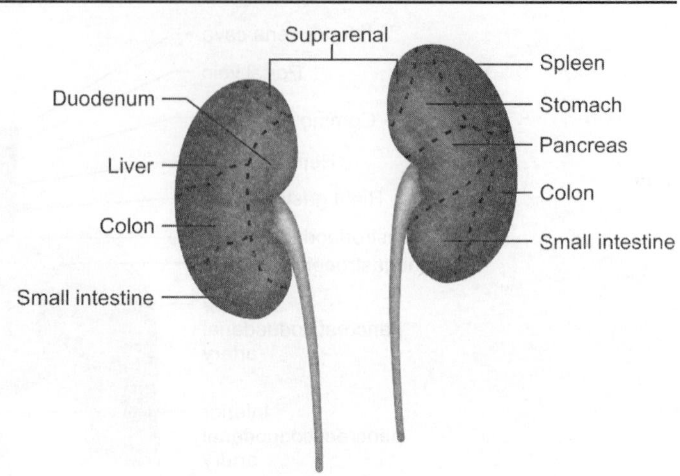

Fig. 198 The anterior relations of the kidneys

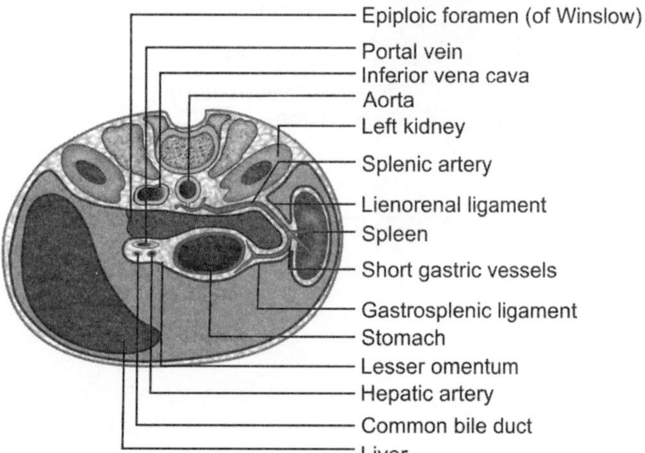

Fig. 197 A horizontal section through the abdomen

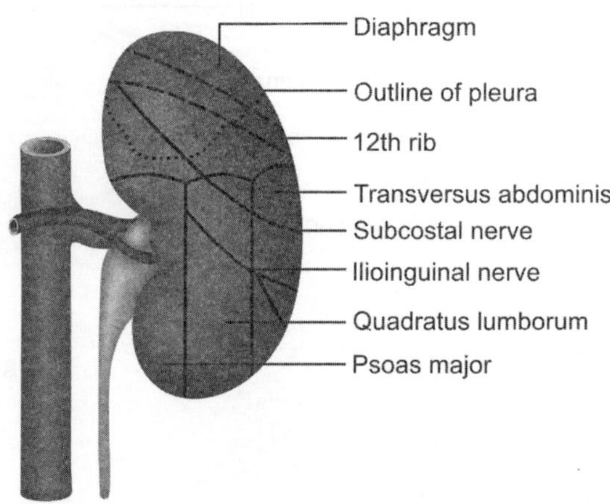

Fig. 199 The posterior relations of the kidneys

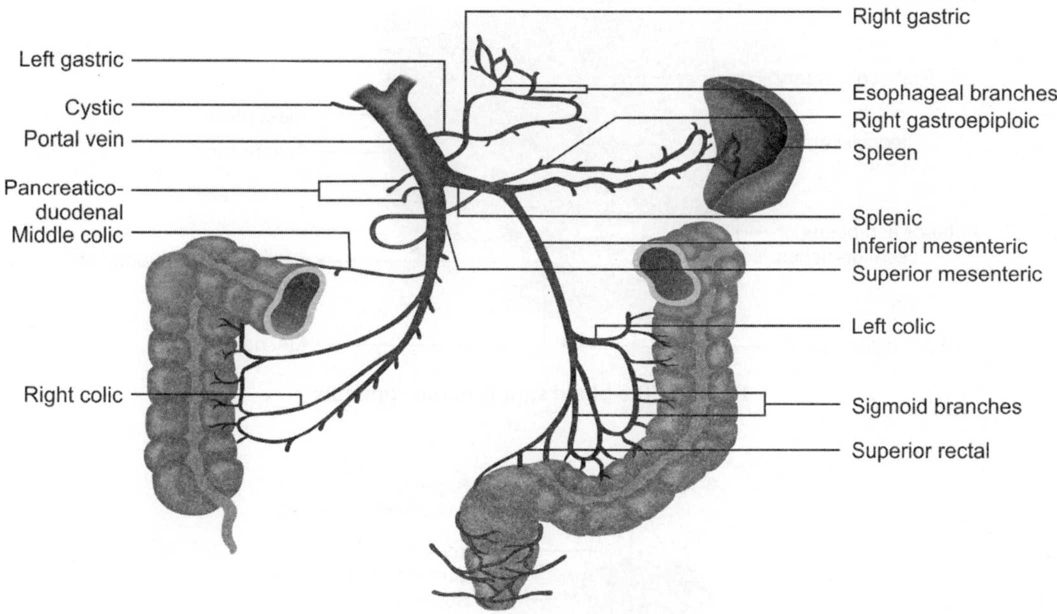

Fig. 200 The portal system. Note the anastomoses with the systemic system (orange) in the esophagus and the anal canal

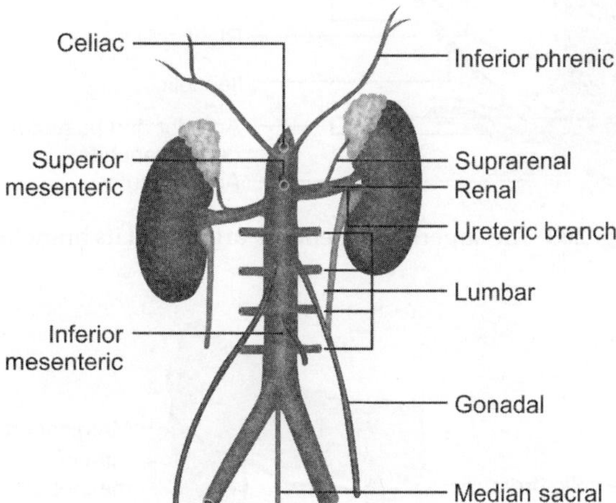

Fig. 201 The abdominal aorta and its branches

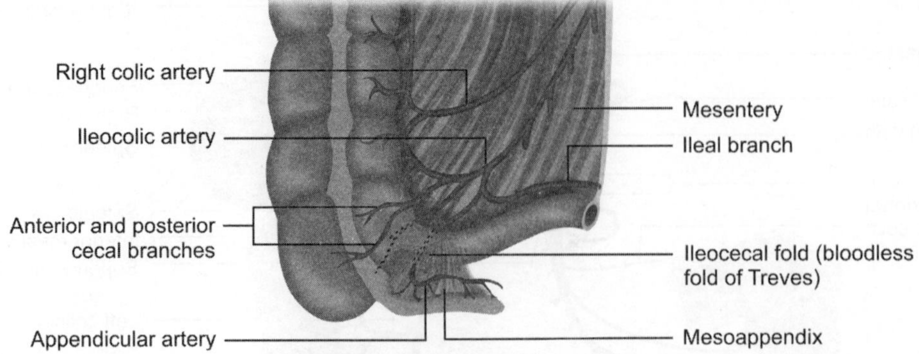

Fig. 202 The blood supply of the appendix

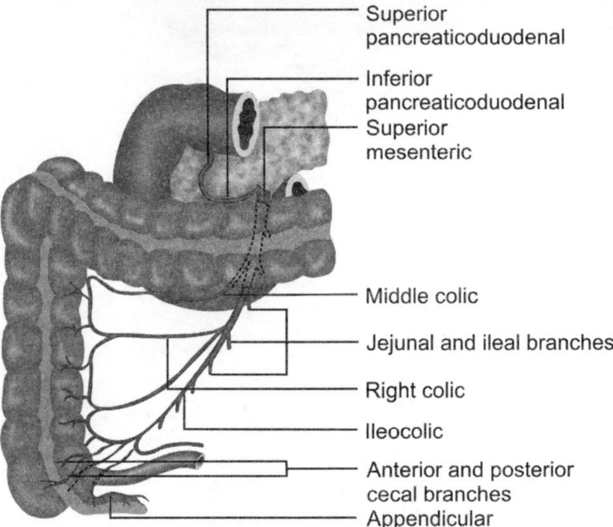

Fig. 203 The superior mesenteric artery and its branches

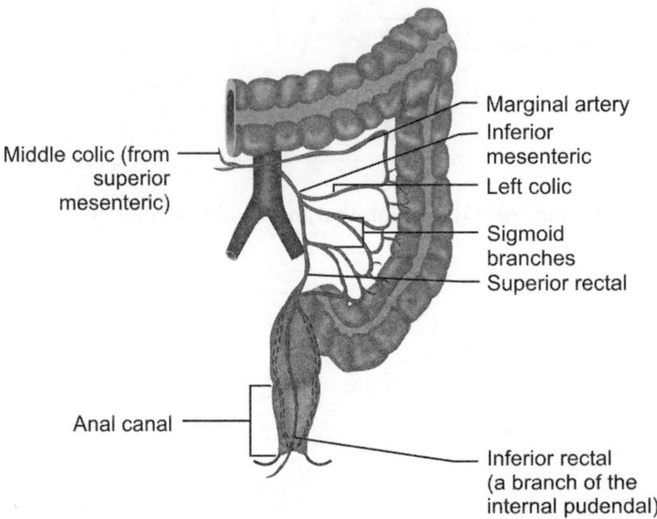

Fig. 204 The inferior mesenteric artery and its branches

HEAD AND NECK

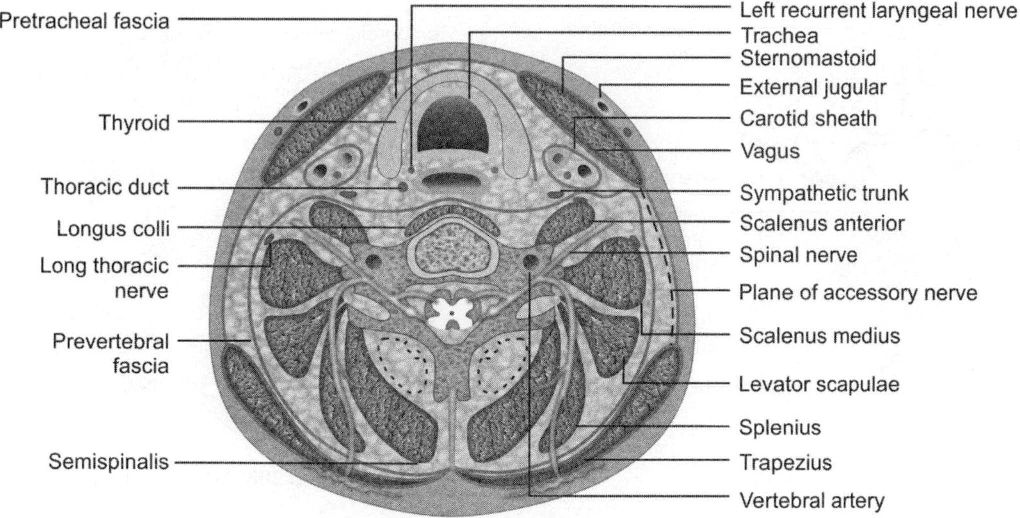

Fig. 205 Cross section through neck

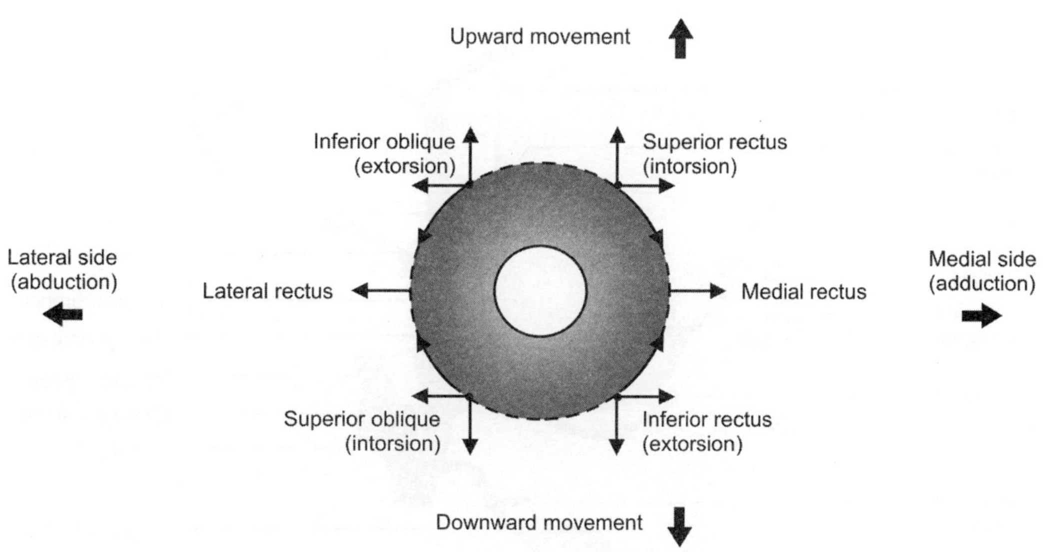

Fig. 206 Muscles used in eyeball movements

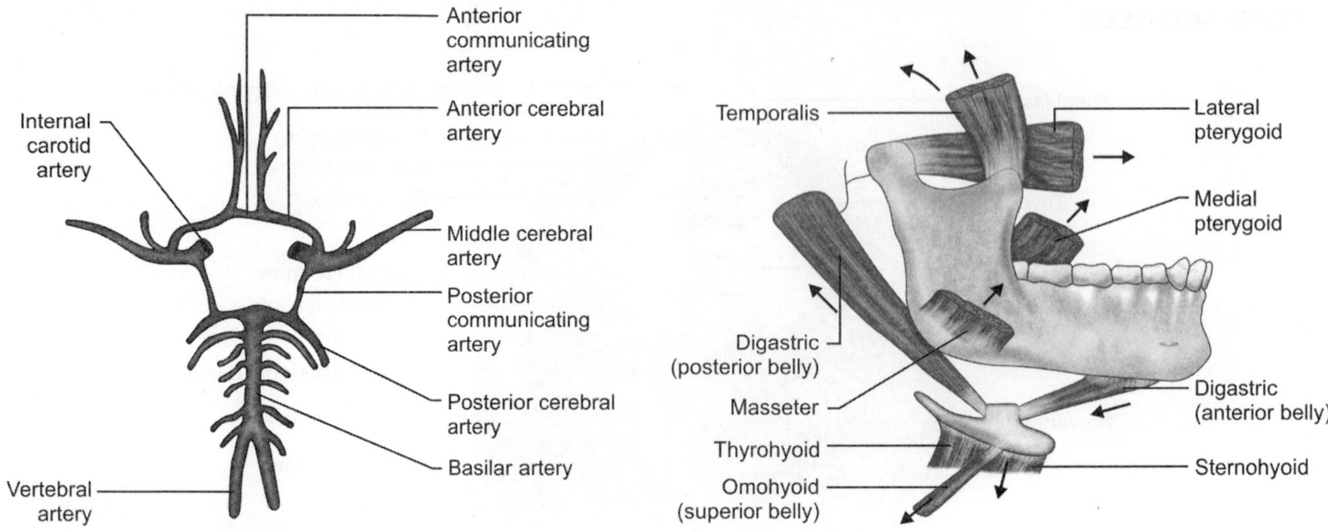

Fig. 207 Circle of Willis

Fig. 208 Muscles of mastication

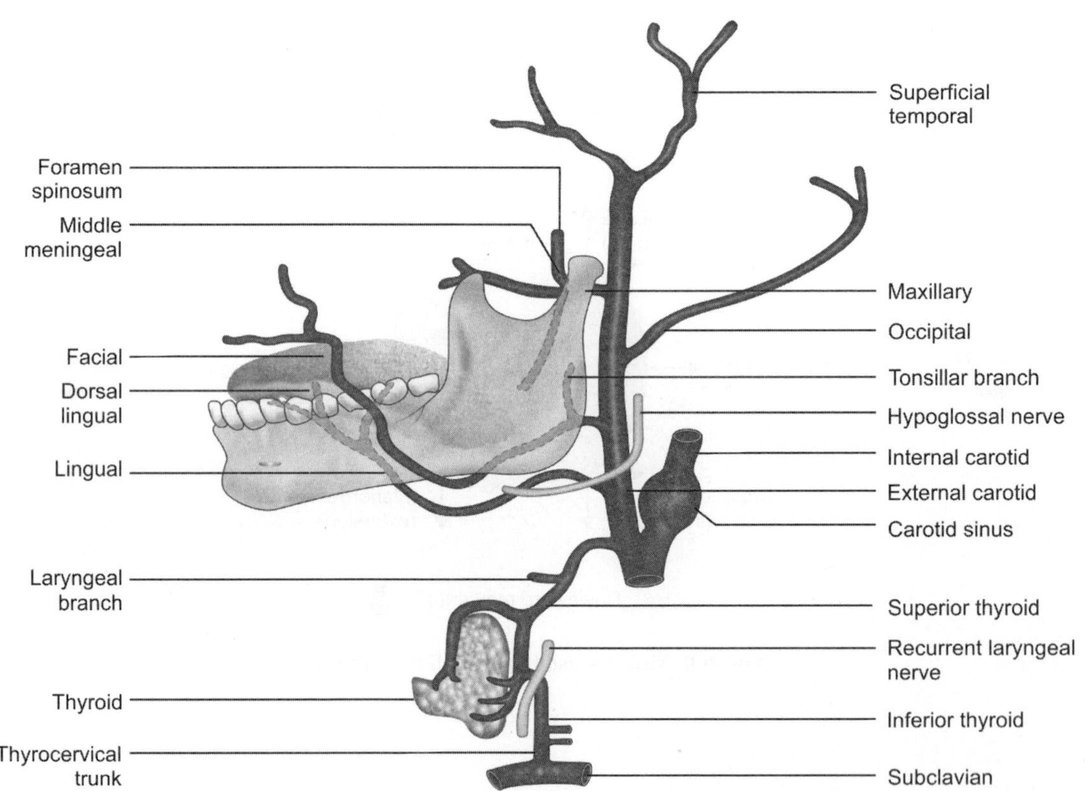

Fig. 209 The course and main branches of the external carotid artery

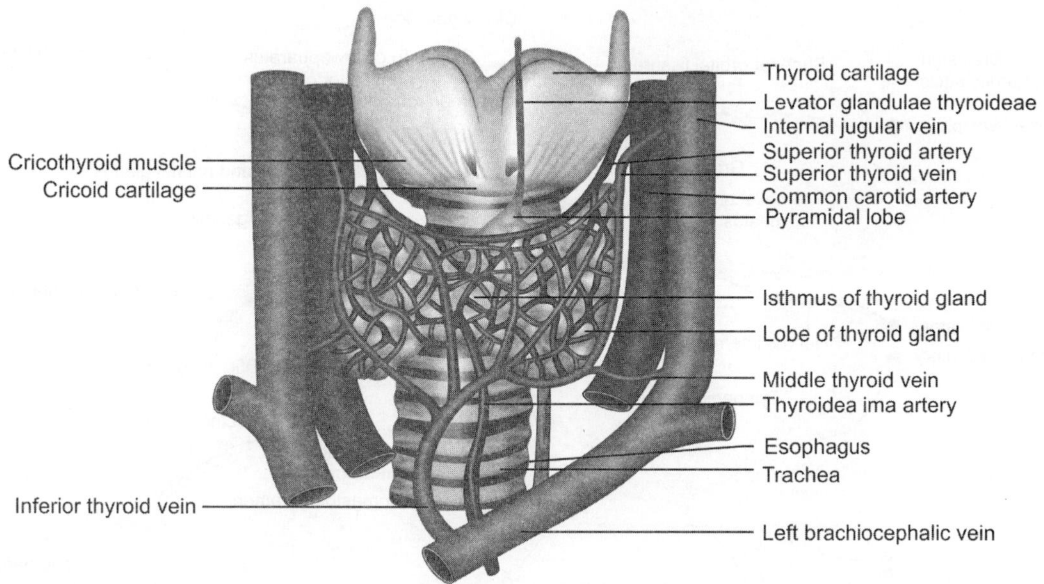

Fig. 210 Blood supply of thyroid gland

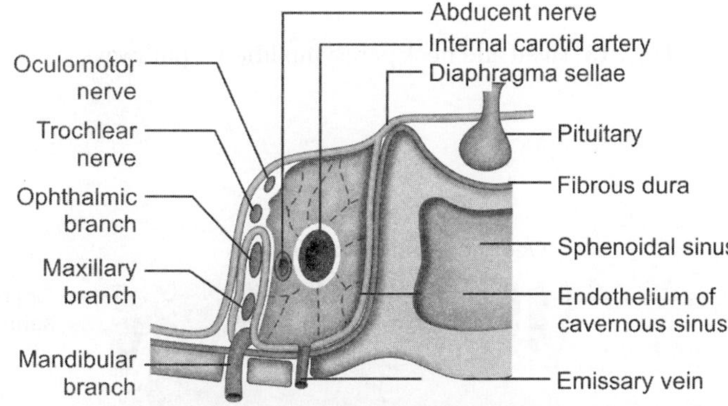

Fig. 211 A cross-section through the cavernous sinus

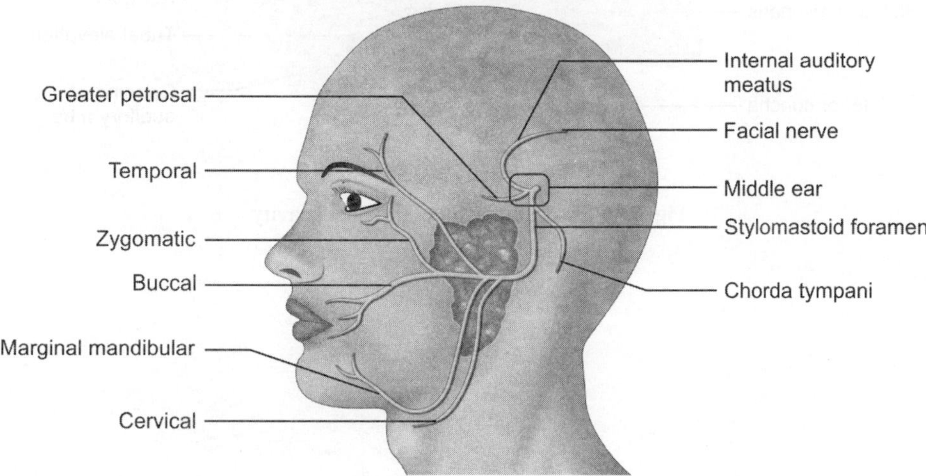

Fig. 212 The course of the facial nerve

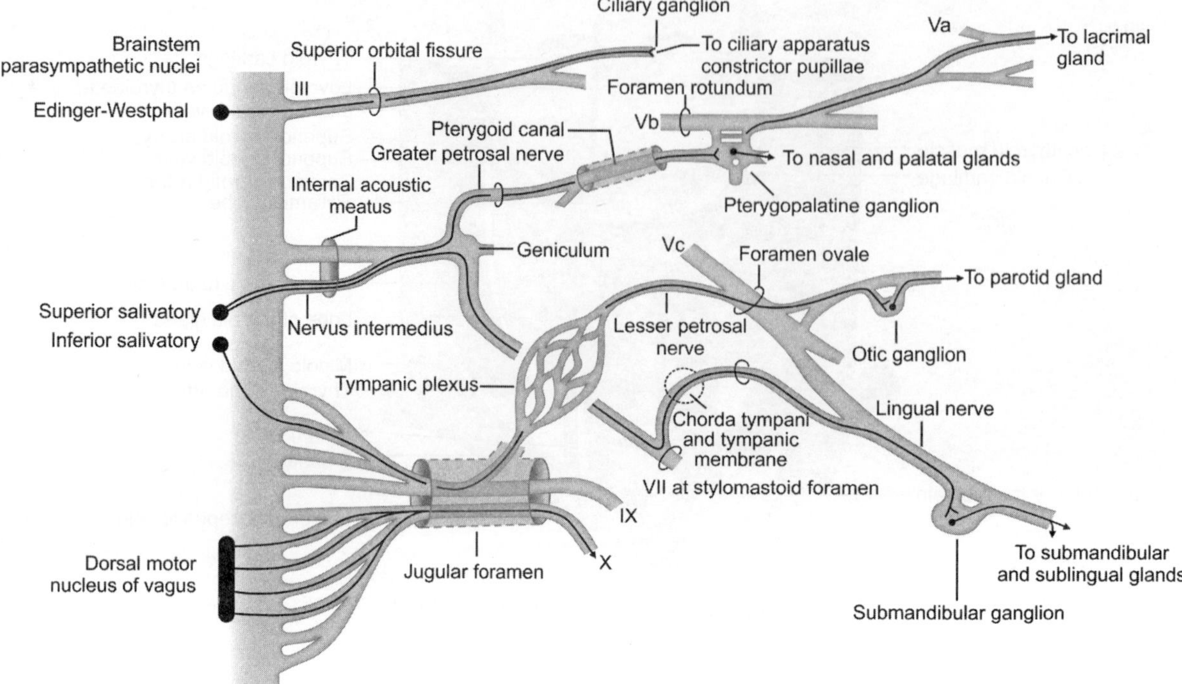

Fig. 213 Head and neck parasympathetics pathways

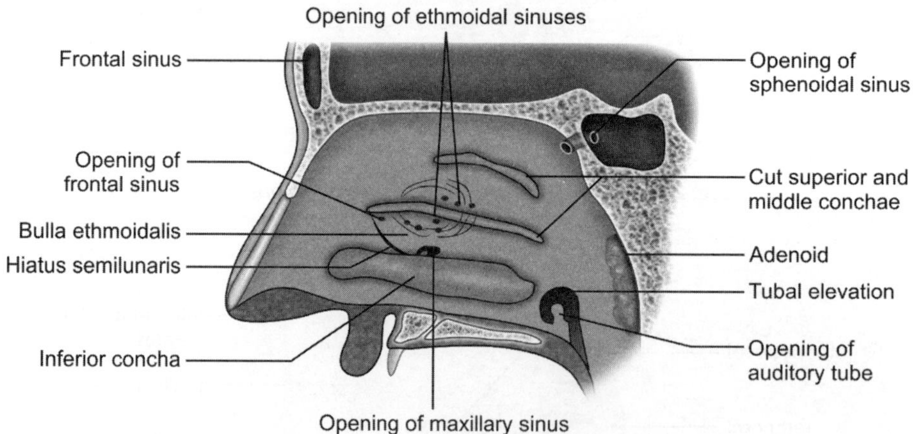

Fig. 214 The lateral wall of the nasal cavity

BRAIN

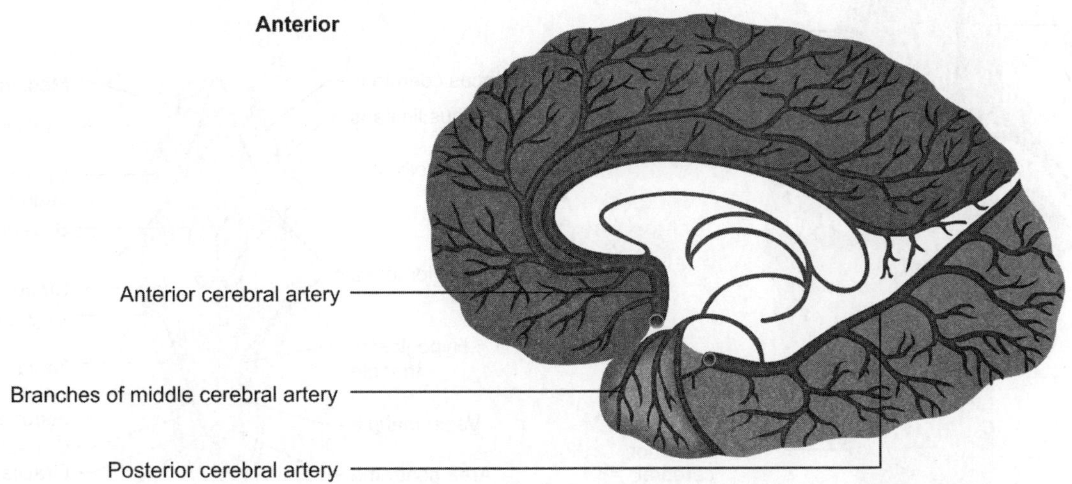

Fig. 215 Blood supply of medical surface of brain

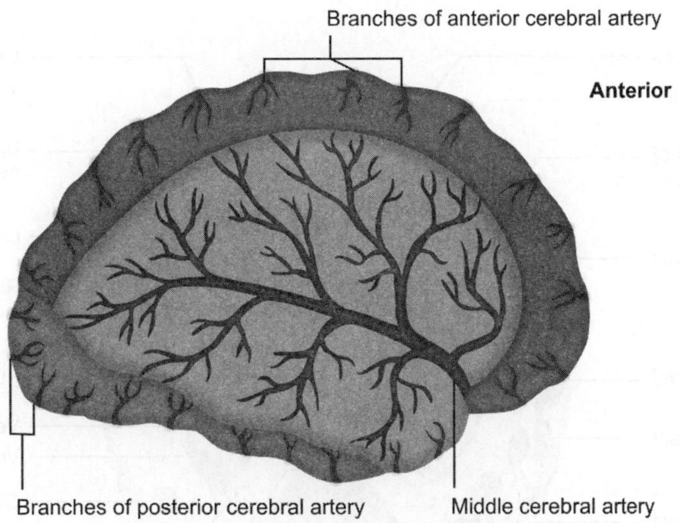

Fig. 216 Blood supply of lateral surface of brain

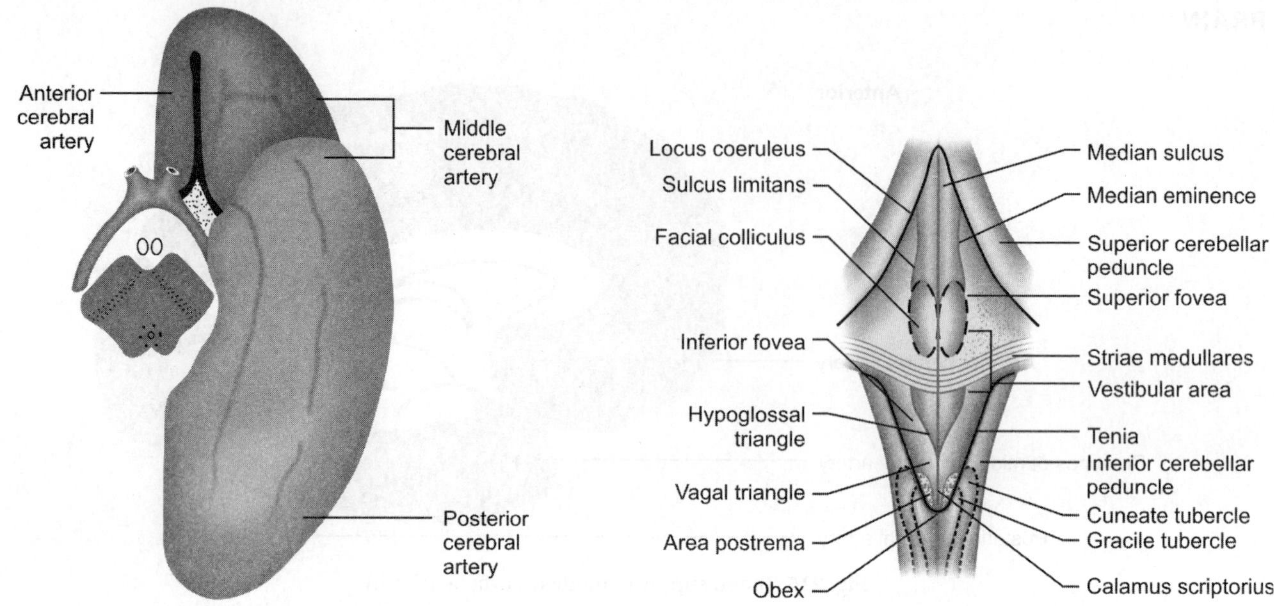

Fig. 217 Blood supply of orbital and tentorial surface of brain

Fig. 218 Floor of fourth ventricle

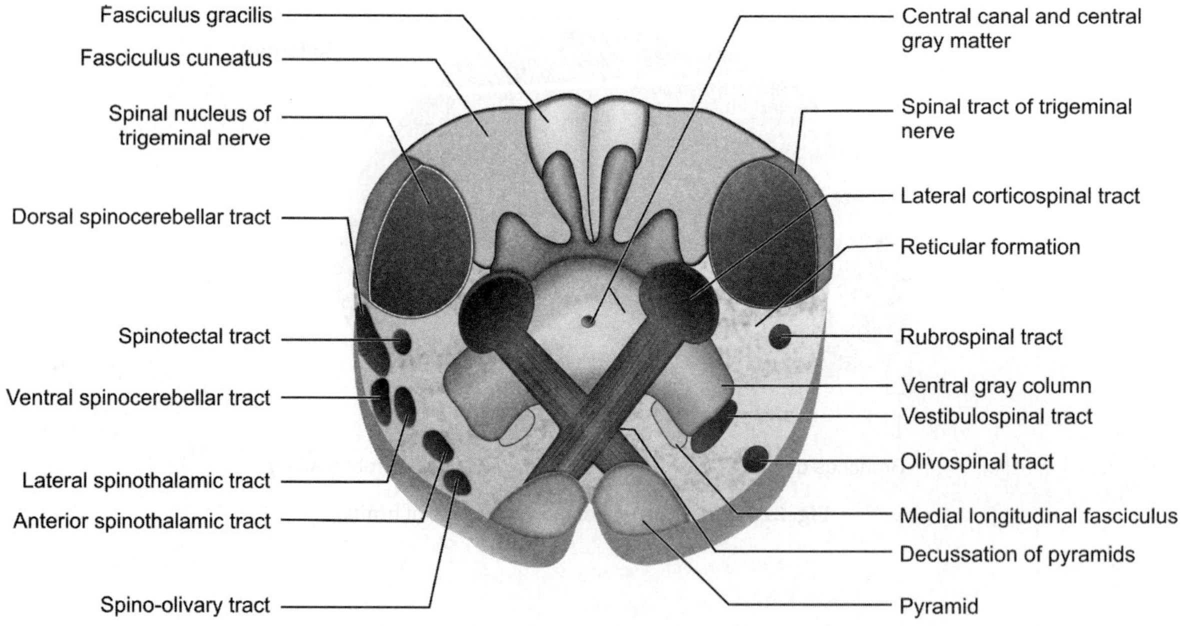

Fig. 219 Transverse section through the medulla at the level of the pyramidal decussation

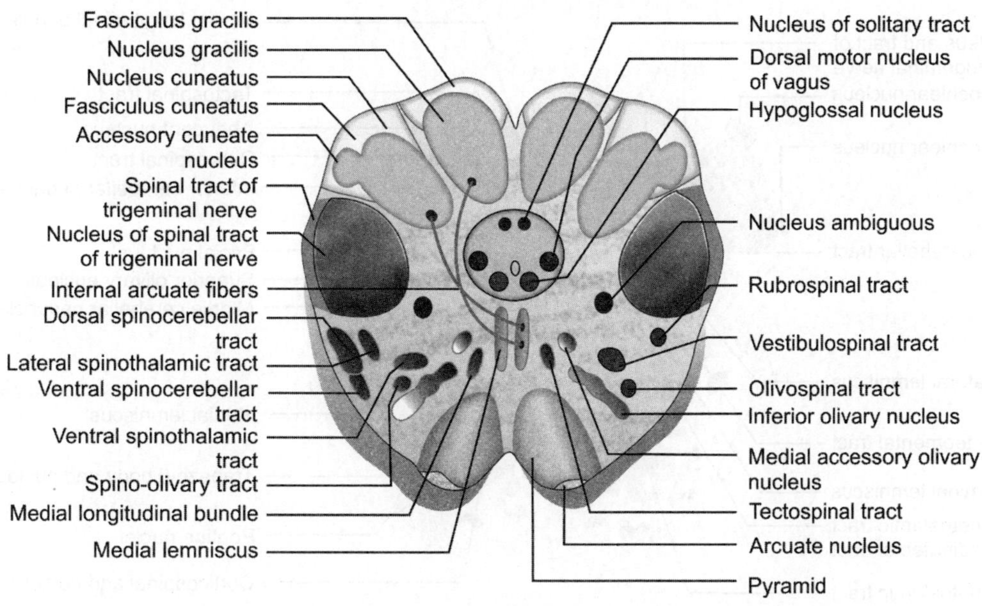

Fig. 220 Transverse section through the medulla a little above the pyramidal decussation

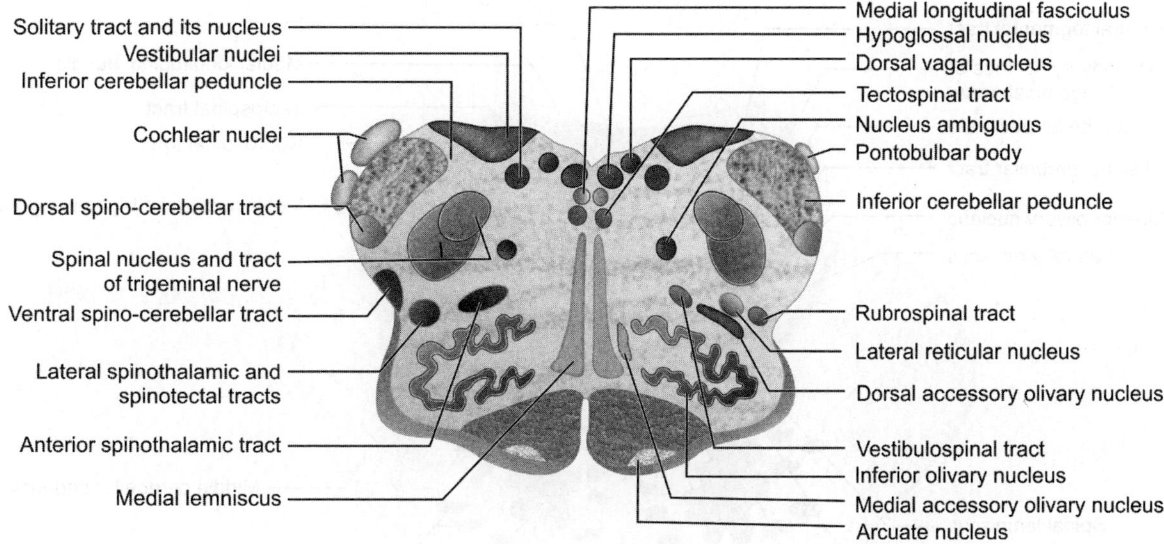

Fig. 221 Transverse section through the medulla at the level or the olive

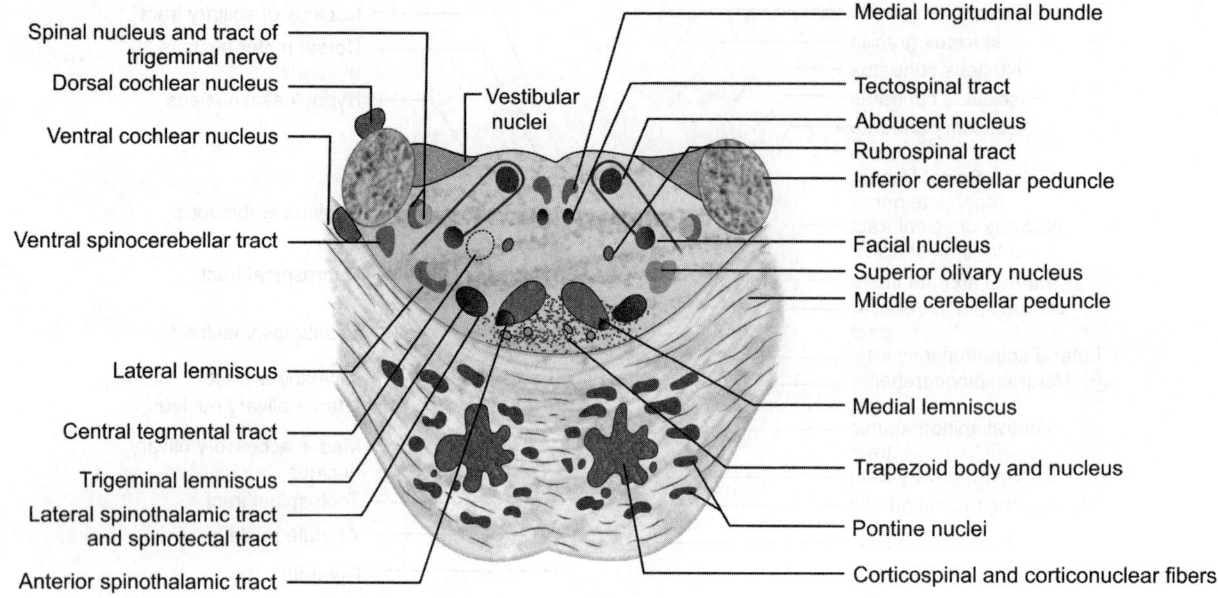

Fig. 222 Transverse section through the lower part of the pons

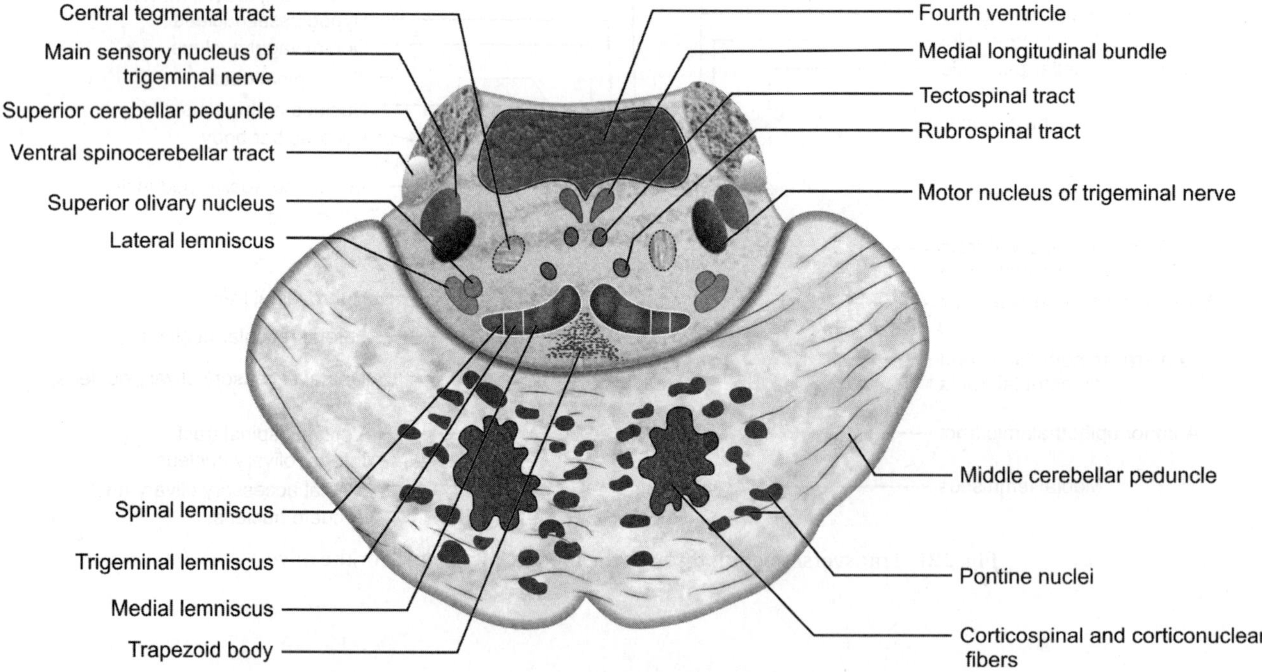

Fig. 223 Transverse section through the upper part of the pons

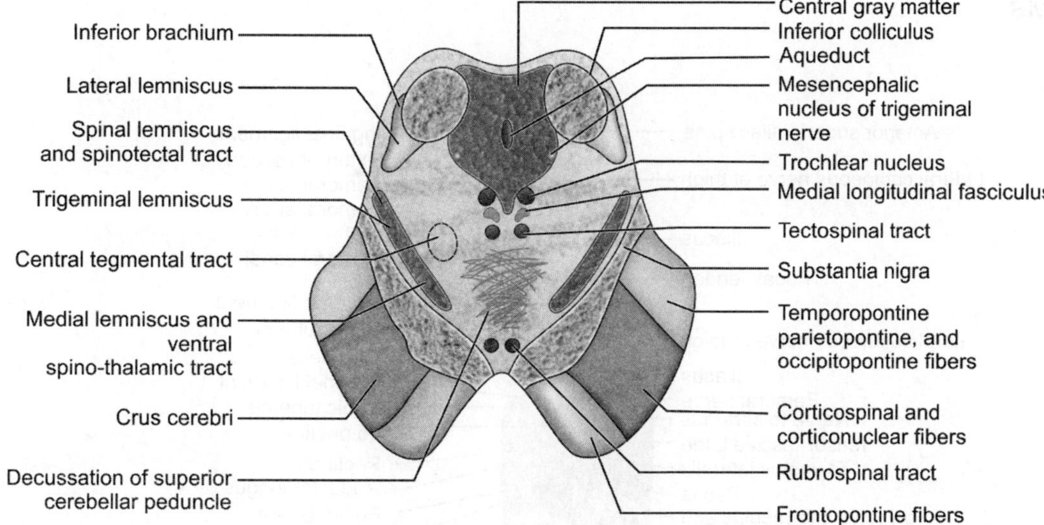

Fig. 224 Transverse section through the lower part of the midbrain

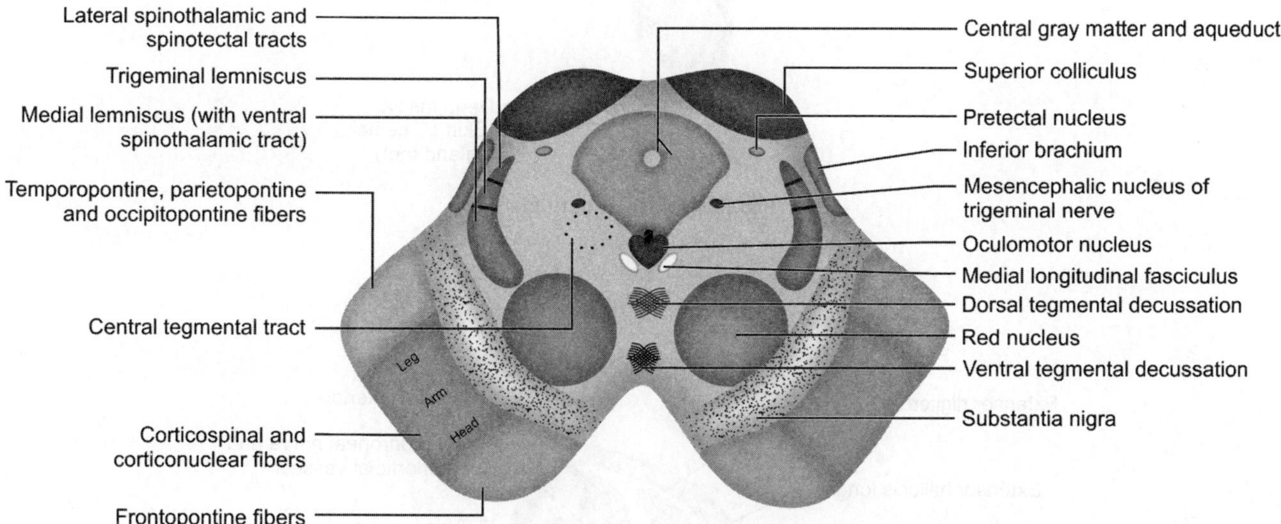

Fig. 225 Transverse section through the upper part of the midbrain

LOWER LIMB

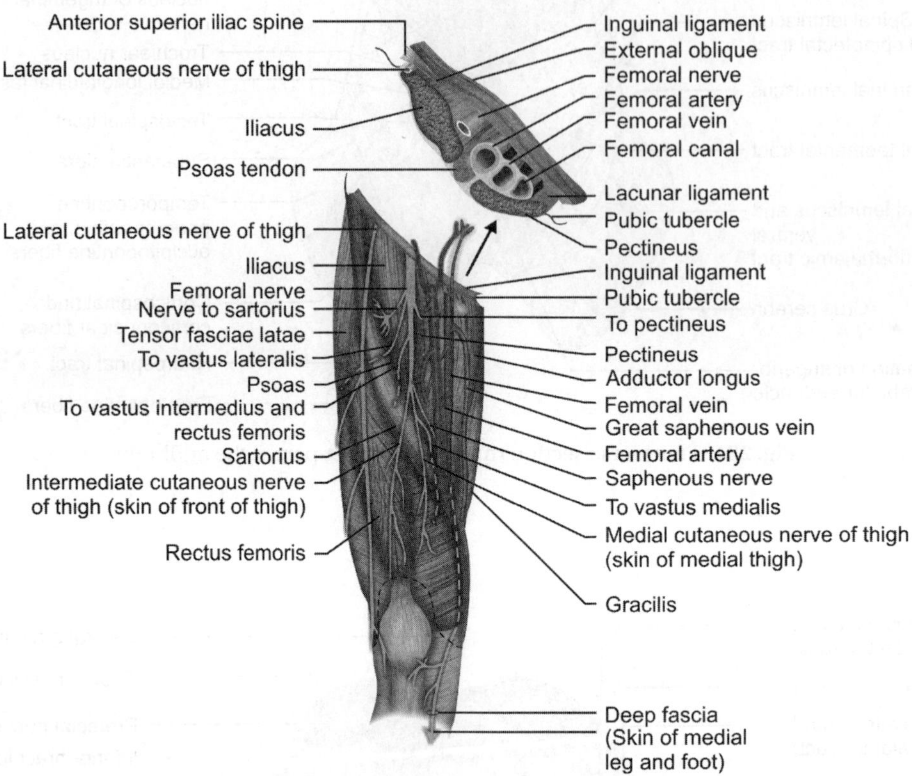

Fig. 226 Muscles in thigh

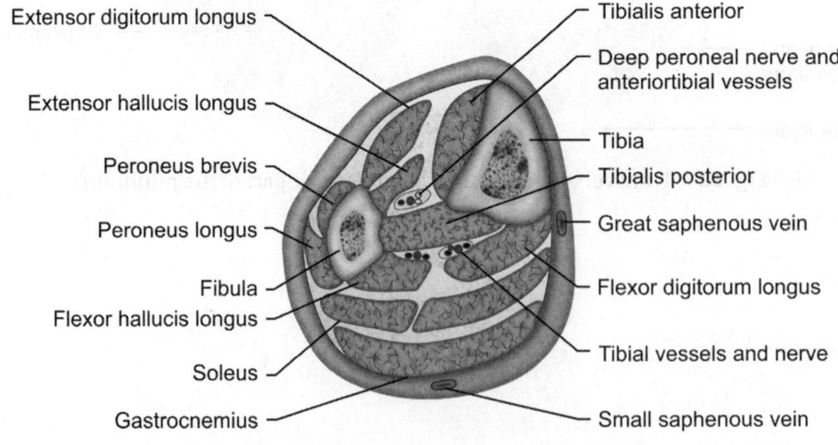

Fig. 227 Cross-section through the leg

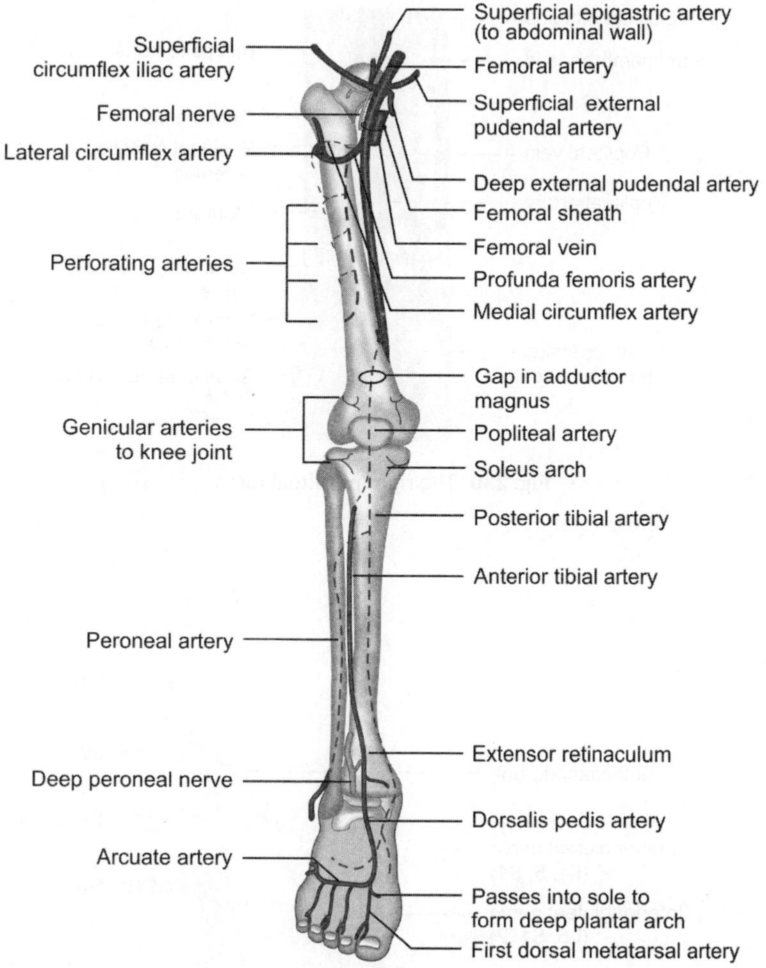

Fig. 228 The course and major branches of the femoral artery and nerve supply to lower limb

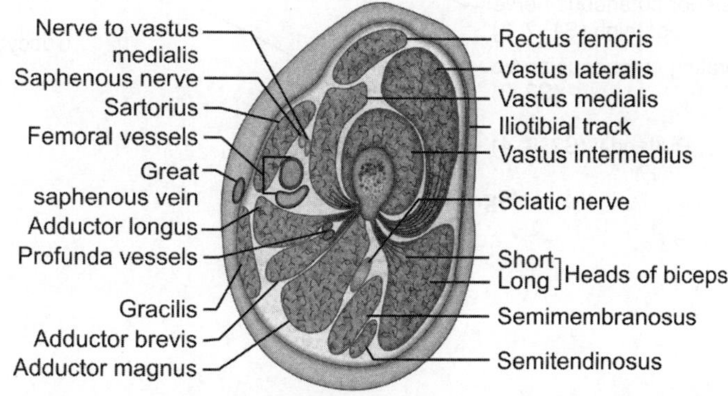

Fig. 229 A section through the thigh to show the adductor (subsartorial) canal

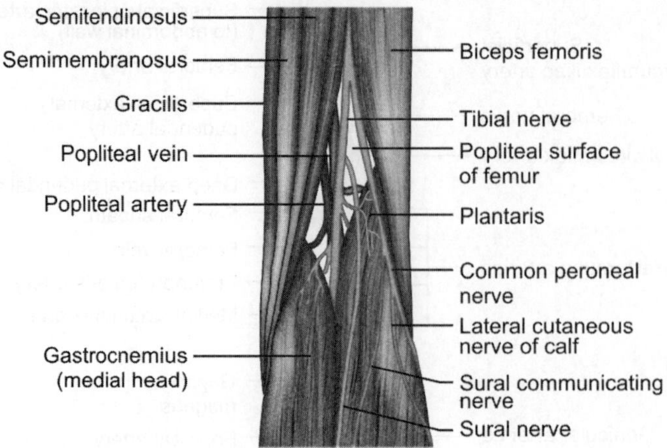

Fig. 230 The right popliteal fossa

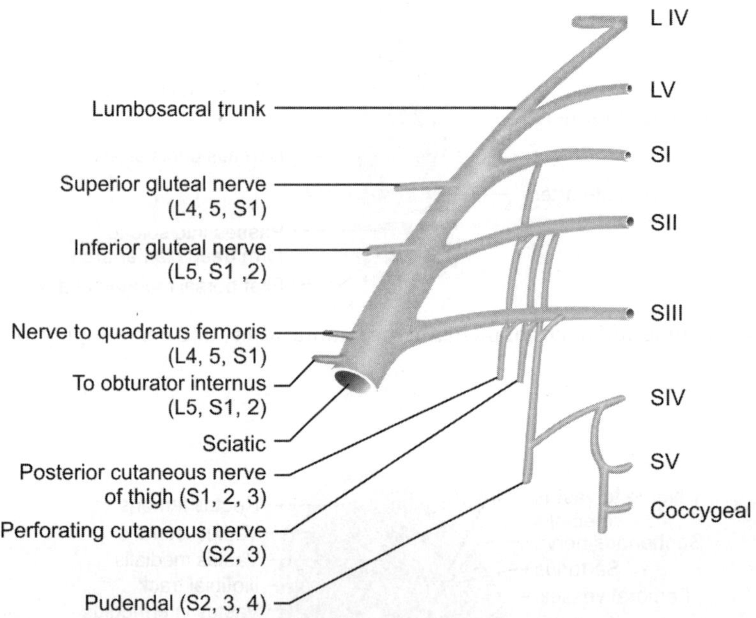

Fig. 231 The sacral plexus

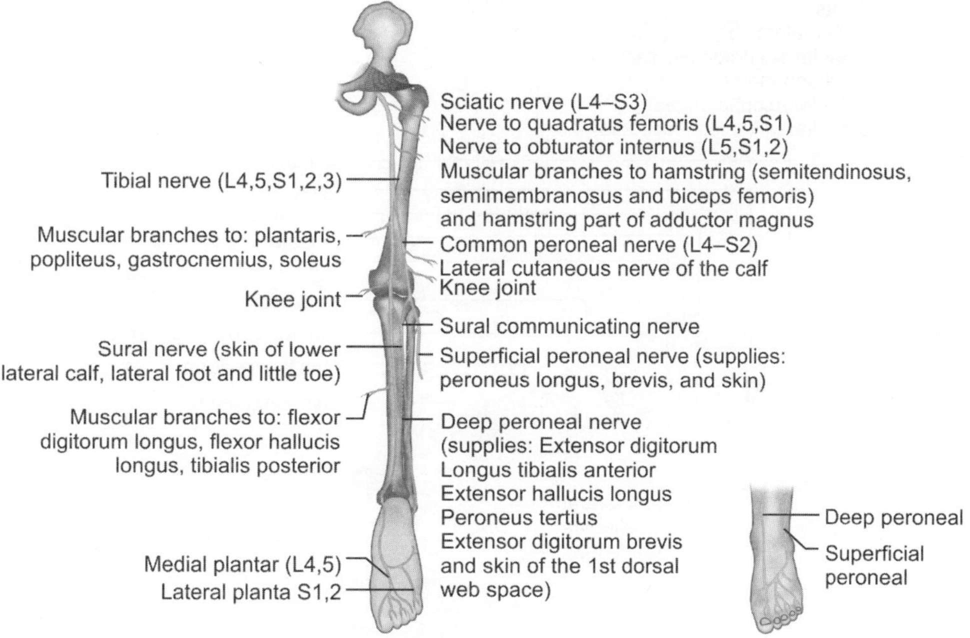

Fig. 232 The sciatic nerve and the major branches

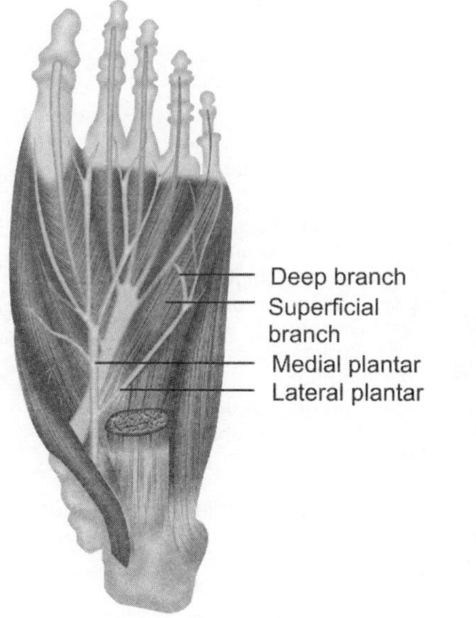

Fig. 233 The medial and lateral plantar nerves

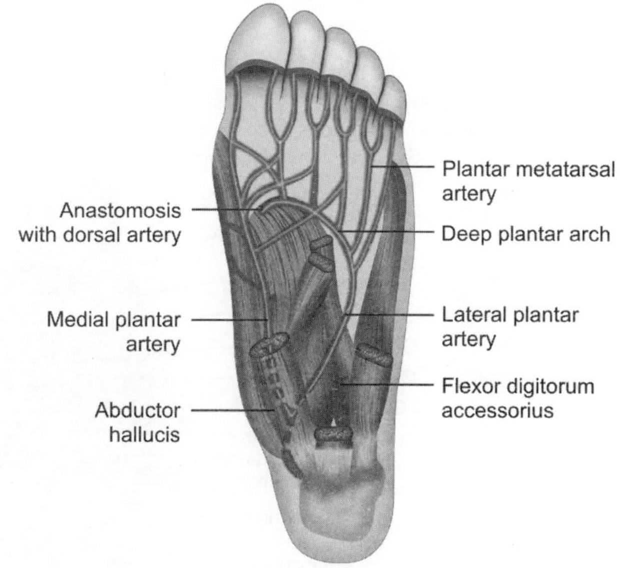

Fig. 234 The medial and lateral plantar arteries

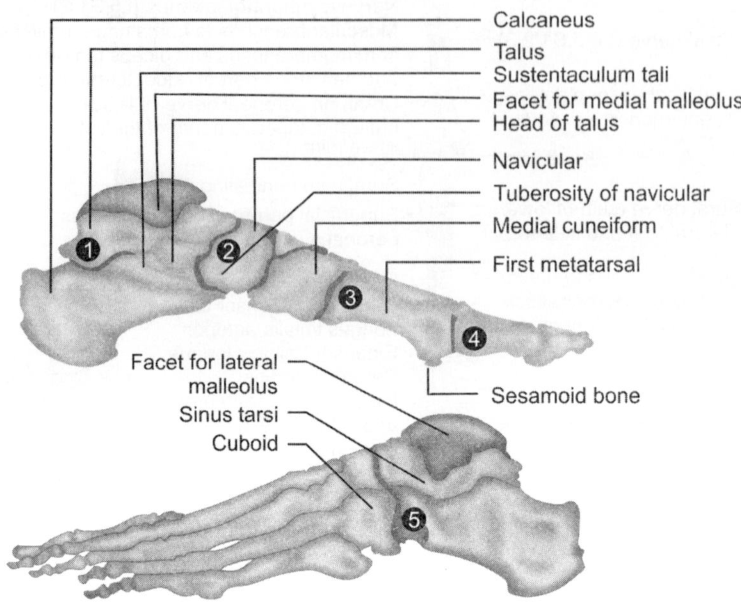

Fig. 235 Bones forming the arch of foot

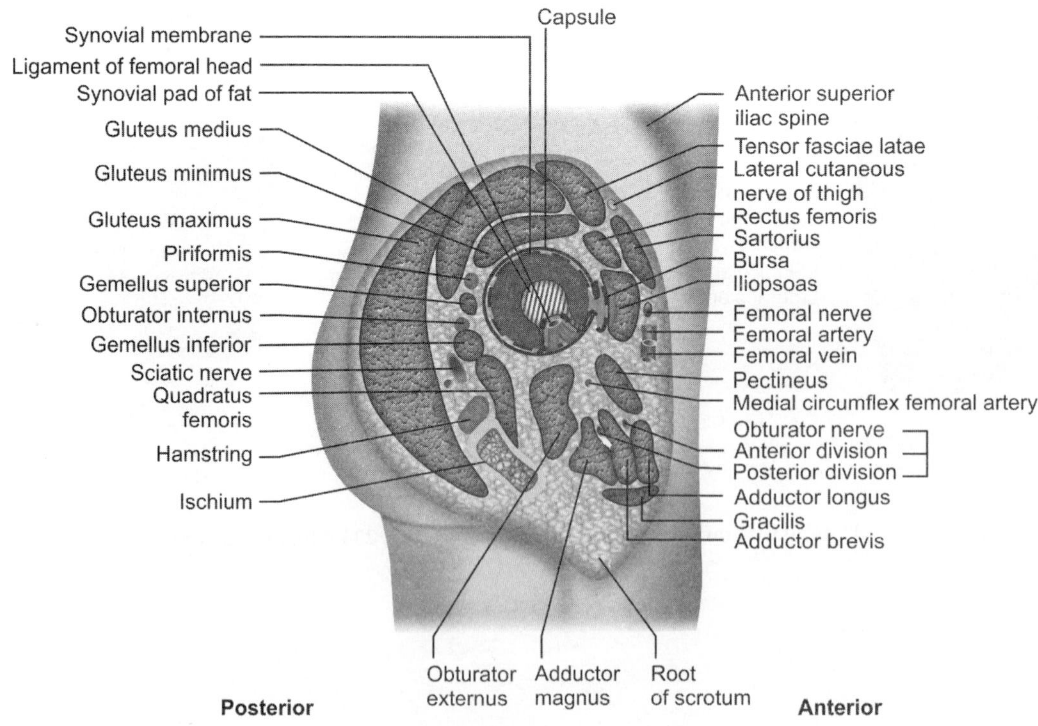

Fig. 236 Structures surrounding the hip joint

NERVES

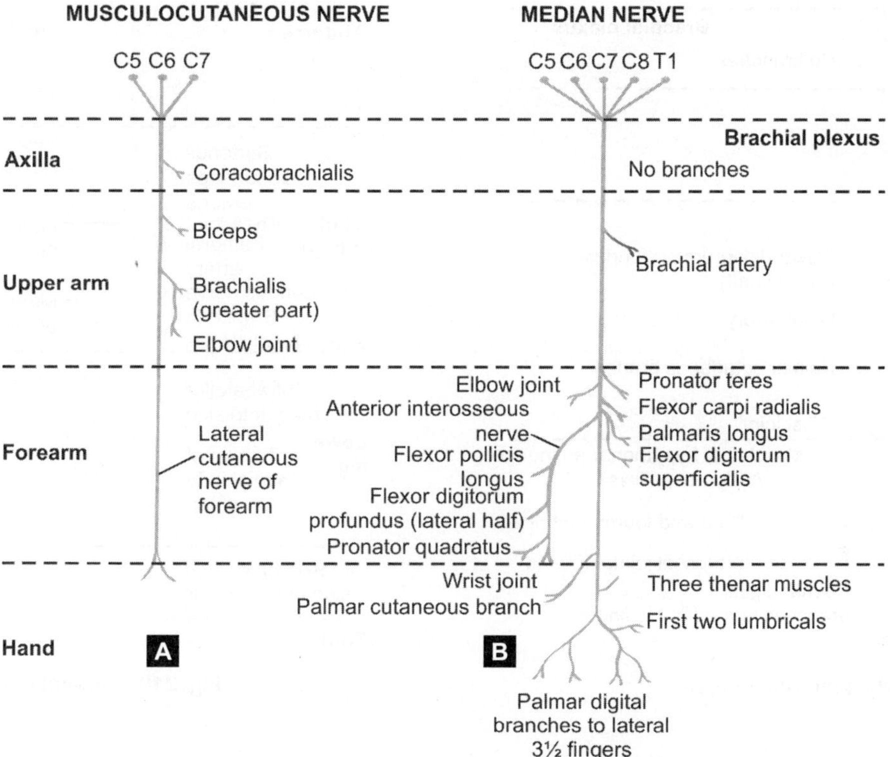

Figs 237A and B (A) Musculocutaneous nerve, (B) Median nerve

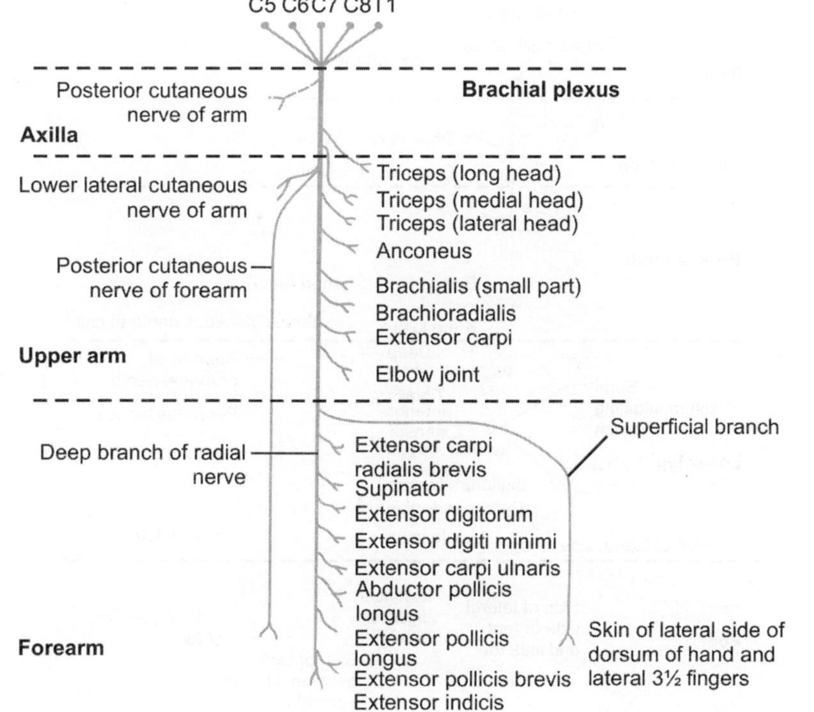

Fig. 238 Radial nerve

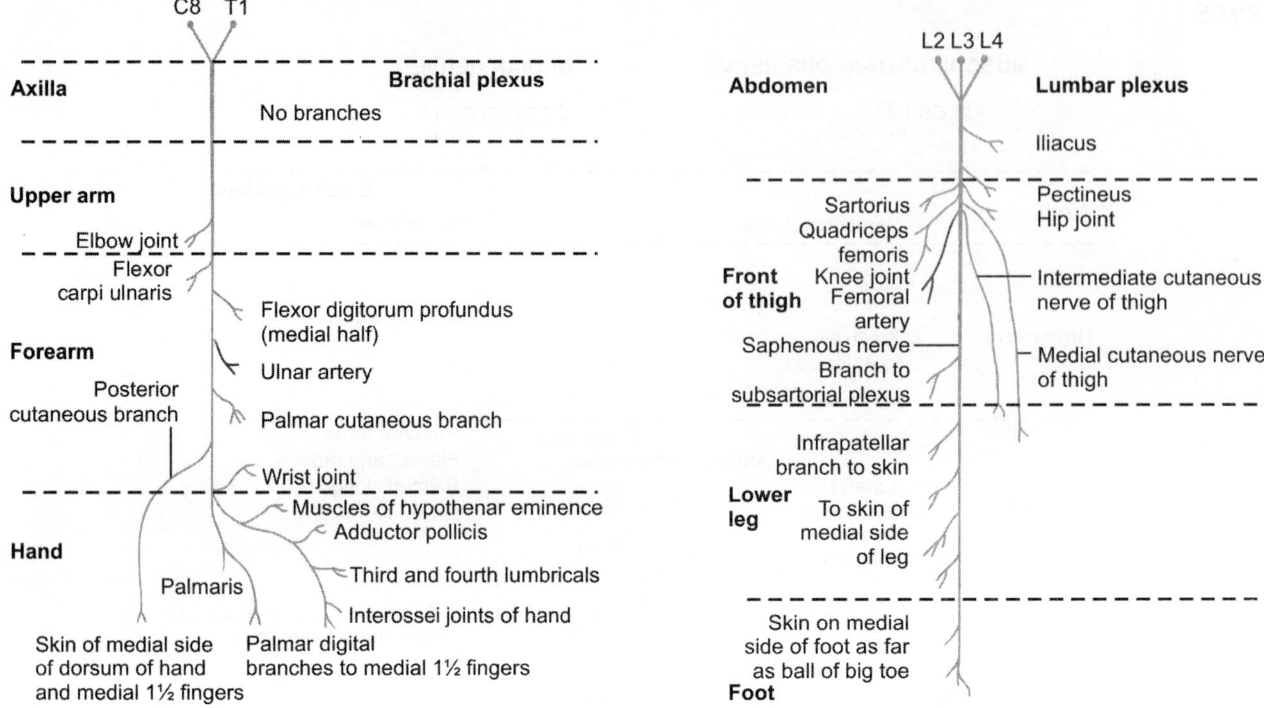

Fig. 239 Ulnar nerve

Fig. 240 Femoral nerve

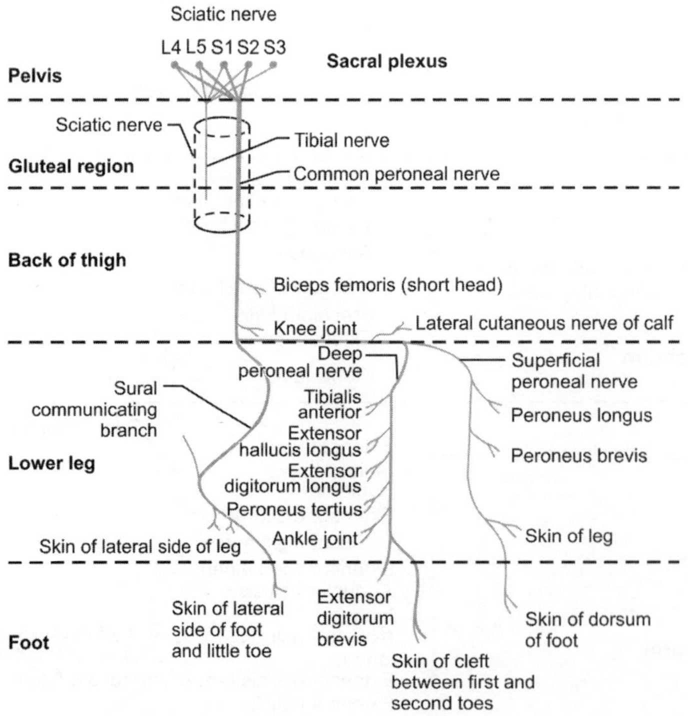

Fig. 241 Sciatic nerve

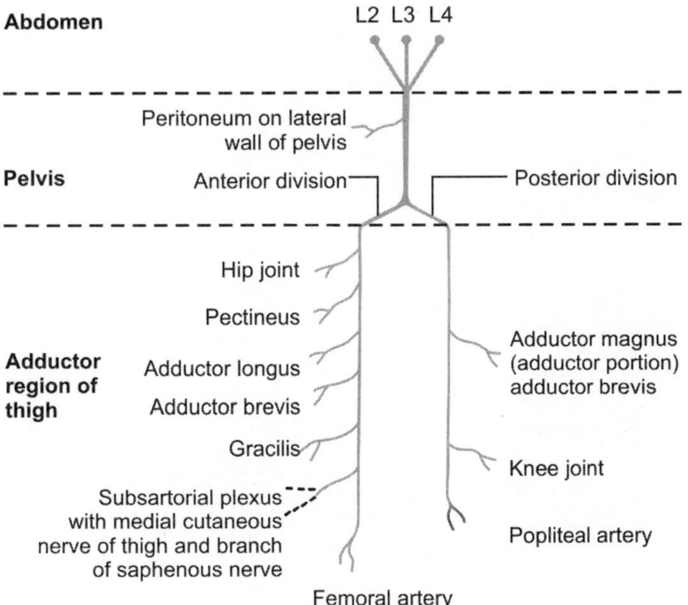

Fig. 242 Obturator nerve

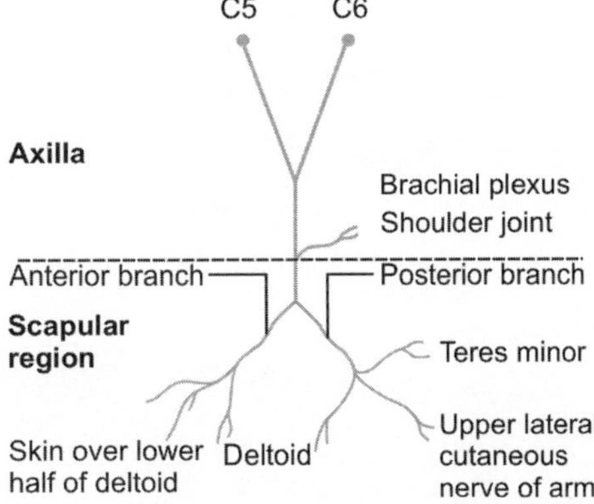

Fig. 243 Axillary nerve

2

Physiology

KERALA UNIVERSITY OF HEALTH SCIENCES (KUHS) SYLLABUS

Theory Paper I	50
Theory Paper II	50
Theory: Internal Assessment	20
Practicals I	20
Practicals II	20
Practicals: Internal Assessment	20
Practical: Viva Voce	20
Total	200

Theory	
Paper I	General Physiology
	Hematology
	Respiratory System
	Cardiovascular System
	Gastrointestinal Tract
	Excretory System
	Temperature Regulation
Paper II	Endocrinology
	Reproductive System
	Central Nervous System
	Special Senses
	Nerve Muscle Physiology

Question Paper Model			
I	Long Essay	10 × 1	10
II	Short Essays	5 × 2	10
III	Write Briefly On	3 × 5	15
IV	Draw and Label	2½ × 2	5
V	Physiological Basis of the Following	2 × 5	10
	Total		50

Practicals		
Viva Voce to be included along with Practicals		
Practical I		
A	Spotting (includes—1 Skill, 2 Graphs, 1 Calculation, 2 Charts, 2 Clinical Application, Peripheral Smear)	10
B	Amphibian Graph Explanation	5
	Hematology: Minor Experiment	5
Practical II		
A	System Examination	10
B	Hematology: Major Experiment (RBC Count, WBC Count, Peripheral Smear)	10
	Total	**40**

THEORY: IMPORTANT QUESTIONS

HEMATOLOGY

IK—Indu Khurana latest edition
NG—N Geetha latest edition
*—Important Questions

Essays

- Erythropoiesis and factors affecting it*(IK-104; NG-78) Fig. 34A in text
- Plasma proteins and its functions (IK-96; NG-67)
- Blood coagulation*(IK-153; NG-103) Fig. 34B in text
- Hemophilia and clotting disorders (IK-109; NG-110)
- Anemia (IK-117; NG-73,83)
- Lymph (IK-230; NG-113)*
- Blood groups and transfusion (IK-165; NG-118,121).

Short Notes

- Composition and functions of blood (IK-95; NG-65)
- Hypoproteinemia (IK-99)
- Reticuloendothelial system (IK-90; NG-90)
- Arneth count (IK-92; NG-92)
- Cellular and humoral immunity (IK-139; NG-93)*
- Helper T cells (IK-144)*
- T lymphocytes (IK-143; NG-88)
- Reticulocytes (IK-104; NG-81)*
- Immunoglobulins (IK-134; NG-96)
- Role of calcium ions in coagulation (IK-156)
- Platelet properties and functions (IK-150; NG-103)
- Anticoagulants (IK-160; NG-108)
- Clotting factors (IK-153; NG-106)*
- Erythroblatosis foetalis (IK-168; NG-122)
- Rh factor (IK-167; NG-120)*
- Cross-matching (IK-165; NG-120)
- Functions of lymph (IK-240; NG-114)
- Tissue macrophages (IK-245; NG-88)
- Fibrinolytic system (IK-159; NG-108)*.

Explain the Physiological Basis

- Reverse anemia occurs after gastrectomy
- Blood does not clot in vivo
- Vitamin B_{12} is given in pernicious anemia, intravenously
- Coagulation of blood in a glass tube
- Aspirin given in MI and stroke
- Streptokinase is used in treatment of MI
- Edema in protein deficiency
- Heparin prevents blood coagulation
- Polycythemia observed in normal individuals residing at high altitude
- Advantages of biconcave shape of RBC.

Diagrams

- Enzyme cascade mechanism of blood coagulation (IK-154; NG-105)
- Stages in erythropoiesis (IK-108; NG-78)
- Acquired immunity (IK-139; NG-97)
- Immunoglobulin (IK-135; NG-96).

CARDIOVASCULAR SYSTEM

Essays

- Blood pressure and regulation (IK-242; NG-174)*
- Conducting system of heart (IK-185; NG-128)
- Cardiac impulse (IK-186)*
- Cardiac output and its regulation (IK-215; NG-167)*
- Cardiac cycle (IK-207; NG-142)*
- Shock (IK-284; NG-182)*
- CVS changes in exercise (IK-369; NG-190)
- ECG diagram (IK-191; NG-132).

Short Notes

- Conduction system of heart (IK-185; NG-128)
- Pacemaker potential (IK-186; NG-52)*
- Stokes-Adams syndrome (IK-257; NG-139)
- Vagal escape (NG-161)
- PR interval and its significance (IK-192; NG-136)
- Jugular venous pressure (IK-210; NG-188)
- End diastolic volume (IK-211; NG-145)
- Arterial pulse (IK-242; NG-187)
- Regulation of Stroke volume (IK-218; NG-168)*
- Fick's principle (IK-216; NG-167)
- Frank-Starlings law (IK-219; 253 ng-166)*
- Bernoulli's principle (IK-232; NG-151)
- Triple response (IK-245; NG-197)
- Laplace law (IK-305; NG-155,220)
- Heart sounds (IK-210; NG-156)*
- Cushing reflex and Benzold Jarish reflex (IK-259)*
- Mary's law (NG-164)*
- Stroke volume and cardiac index (IK-215;NG-168)
- Bainbridge reflex (IK-258,1226)
- Echocardiography (IK-217; NG-169)
- Einthoven's triangle (IK-190; NG-133)
- ECG waves and intervals (IK-192; NG-132)*
- Sinoaortic mechanism (IK-256).

Explain the Physiological Basis

- Hypoxia in circulatory shock
- Bradycardia in raised intracranial tension

- Postural hypotension
- Myocardium is well perfused during diastole
- Fainting during emotions
- BP is first measured by palpatory method
- Increase in heart rate during exercise.

Diagrams

- Graph of pacemaker potential* (IK-187; NG-52)
- ECG (IK-191; NG-132)*
- Left and right pressure changes and aortic changes.

RESPIRATORY SYSTEM

Essays

- Regulation of respiration (IK-335; NG-248)*
- Hypoxia (IK-352; NG-260)
- Respiratory changes in exercise (IK-368, 372; NG-268)*
- Carbon dioxide transport (IK-330; NG-244).

Short Notes

- Respiratory and nonrespiratory functions of lung (IK-295)
- Mechanism of respiration (IK-298; NG-208)
- Surfactant (IK-306; NG-212)*
- Compliance (IK-307; NG-228)*
- Factors that maintain the stability of lung alveoli (IK-321)
- Respiratory centers in brainstem (IK-336)
- Intrapulmonary and intrapleural pressure changes (IK-299; NG-216)*
- Lung volumes and pressure changes (IK-301; NG-222)*
- Timed vital capacity (IK-303; NG-224)
- Dead space (IK-318)
- Ventilation-perfusion ratio (IK-319; NG-233)
- Respiratory membranes (IK-321; NG-237)
- Oxygen transport (IK-325; NG-241)
- Bohr effect (IK-327; NG-243)*
- Chloride shift (IK-331; NG-245)
- Haldane effect (IK-332)
- 2,3 BPG (IK-327)
- Asphyxia (IK-343; NG-260)
- Hypercapnia (IK-355; NG-259)
- O_2 andCO_2 transport (IK-325; NG-244)
- Acclimatization (IK-339; NG-265)
- Cheyne-Stokes breathing (IK-352; NG-258)
- Chemoreceptors (IK-342; NG-181)
- Cyanosis (IK-354; NG-263)
- Dysbarism (IK-263; NG-266)*
- Myoglobin (IK-328; NG-244)
- Oxyhemoglobin (NG-75)
- Oxygen dissociation curve (ODC) (IK-326; NG-242)*

Explain the Physiological Basis

- Acclimatization in high altitude
- Sigmoid shape of oxygen dissociation curve
- Mouth-to-mouth respiration is the best form of artificial respiration
- Change in oxygen carrying capacity in carbon monoxide poisoning.

Diagrams

- Spirogram* (IK-409)
- ODC (IK-439)
- Respiratory center in medulla and pons (IK-336)
- Graphs of intrapulmonary and intrapleural pressure effects (IK-406; NG-216)*
- TCV and FEV (IK-409)
- Respiratory membranes.

GASTROINTESTINAL TRACT

Essays

- Peptic ulcer (IK-477; NG-303)*
- Gastric secretion (phases and regulation) (IK-471; NG-300)*
- Bile (IK-490; NG-309)
- Movements of small intestine (IK-499; NG-329)*
- Pancreatic juice and its regulation (IK-482; NG-306)*
- Jaundice (IK-494; NG-76, 313).

Short Notes

- Functions of saliva (IK-460; NG-287)
- Regulation of salivary secretion (IK-459; NG-288)
- Cephalic phase of gastric secretion (IK-470; NG-300)*
- Mucosal barrier (IK-476; NG-294)
- HCl secretion (IK-486; NG-295)
- Gastric emptying (IK-475; NG-327)
- Hunger contractions (IK-474; NG-326)
- Dumping syndrome (IK-479; NG-305)
- Regulation of pancreatic secretion (NG-482)*
- Gastrin (IK-468; NG-294)*
- Differentiate between gastric and duodenal ulcers (IK-475; NG-303)*
- Bile salts (IK-490; NG-311)
- Secretin and CCK (IK-485; NG-300)
- Enterohepatic circulation (IK-491; NG-76,313)*
- Deglutition (IK-489; NG-323)*
- Gastric movements (IK-473; NG-326)
- Peristalsis (IK-473; NG-330)
- Defecation reflex (IK-507; NG-331)*
- Mechanism of vomiting (IK-477; NG-328).

Explain the Physiological Basis

- Steatorrhea in high altitude
- Gastrocolic reflex
- When food placed in the mouth, salivation increases
- Alkaline urine formed after a heavy meal
- Glucose administration for treatment for diarrhea
- Jaundice in hemolytic anemia
- In obstructive jaundice, presence of clay-colored stool
- After the meals, defecation is a rule in children (gastrocolic reflex)
- Vagotomy for the management of peptic ulcer.

Diagrams

- Layers of gastrointestinal tract (IK-452)
- Mechanism of HCl secretion (IK-466; NG-295)
- Regulation of gastric acid secretion (IK-471; NG-299).

RENAL SYSTEM

Essays

- Glomerular filtration rate (IK-386; NG-352)*
- Renal blood flow (IK-381; NG-350)
- Countercurrent mechanism (IK-403; NG-365)*
- Na^+, glucose and water reabsorption (IK-391)
- Acidification of urine (IK-408; NG-367)*.

Short Notes

- Functions of kidney (IK-307; NG-342)
- Difference between cortical and juxtamedullary nephrones (IK-308; NG-347)*
- Loop of Henle (IK-309; NG-345)
- Autoregulation of renal blood flow (IK-383; NG-496)*
- Juxtaglomerular apparatus (IK-380; NG-347)*
- Renin-angiotensin system (IK-417; NG-354)
- Renal clearance (IK-436)*
- Bartter's syndrome
- Renal threshold and tubular maximum (NG-398)
- Splay (IK-398; NG-360)*
- Innervations of bladder (IK-443; NG-372)
- Micturition reflex (IK-445; NG-374)*
- Atonic bladder, and autonomous bladder (IK-446; NG-374)*
- Cystometrogram (IK-444; NG-374)*
- Diuresis and diuretics (IK-433; NG-375)*
- Nephritic syndrome (IK-433)
- Dialysis (IK-440; NG-370)
- Renal function tests (IK-434; NG-376)*.

Explain the Physiological Basis

- Atonic bladder
- Inulin is used for GFR determination by clearance method
- Cause for polyurea in a individual (NG-369)
- Anemia in chronic renal disease
- Osteomalacia in chronic renal failure (vitamin D deficiency) (NG-376).

Diagram

- Typical nephron (IK-308; NG-344)
- Juxtaglomerular apparatus (IK-380; NG-345)
- Renal corpuscle (IK-309; NG-345)
- Countercurrent system (IK-403; NG-634)
- Cystometrogram (IK-445; NG-379)
- Innervations of bladder (IK-443; NG-373).

CENTRAL NERVOUS SYSTEM (CNS)

Essays

- Properties of synapse and synaptic inhibition (IK-777; NG-502)*
- Touch pathway (IK-693; NG-531)*
- Pain and temperature pathway (IK-699; NG-536)
- Thalamus (thalamic syndrome) (IK-734; NG-541)
- Pyramidal system and lesions (IK-702; NG-548)*
- Transection of spinal cord (IK-708; NG-496)*
- Basal ganglia (IK-726; NG-557)
- Cerebellum (IK-711; NG-563)*
- Hypothalamus—functions (IK-741; NG-586).

Short Notes

- EPSP and IPSP (IK-779; NG-504)*
- Renshaw cell inhibition (IK-782; NG-503)
- Stretch reflex, inverse stretch reflex and withdrawal reflex (IK-825, NG-514)*
- Muscle spindle (IK-821; NG-514)*
- Referred pain and theories (IK-807; NG-539)*
- Muscle tone (IK-822; NG-45,546)
- Hypotonia and hypertonia (IK-822; NG-550)
- Sensory and motor homunculus (IK-753; NG-548)*
- Golgi tendon organ (IK-828; NG-517)
- α-and γ-efferent discharge (IK-820)
- Decorticate and decerebrate rigidity (IK-839; NG-578)
- Extrapyramidal system (IK-703; NG-560)
- Babinski's sign and its clinical significance (IK-708; NG-552)
- Chorea, athetosis and ballism (IK-732; NG-560)
- Brown-Sequard syndrome (IK-709; NG-555)*
- Mass reflex and its significance (IK-831)
- Huntigton's disease (IK-732; NG-562)
- Parkinson's disease (IK-730; NG-10)
- Lead pipe and Cog wheel rigidity (IK-731; NG-561)*
- Cerebellar dysfunction (IK-725; NG-568)
- Functional areas of brain (IK-748; NG-495)
- Functional divisions of cerebellum (IK-715; NG-563)*

- Conditioned reflexes' types (IK-876; NG-289)
- Wernicke's area and Broca's area (IK-747, 875; NG-607, 583)
- Aphasia (IK-845; NG-608)
- Summation and occlusion (IK-784; NG-508)*
- Types of memory (IK-872; NG-595)
- Papez circuit (IK-850; NG-589)
- ECG waves (IK-860; NG-132)
- α-block (IK-861; NG-598)
- REM and NREM sleep (IK-866; NG-599)
- UMN and LMN lesions (IK-711; NG-551)*
- Vestibular apparatus (IK-842; NG-572)*.

Explain the Physiological Basis

- Sensory homunculus
- Spastic paralysis in UMN lesion and flaccid paralysis in LMN lesion (NG-552)
- Reciprocal innervation
- Lesion of basal ganglia causes rigidity
- Intention tremor and hypotonia in cerebellar lesions (NG-569)
- REM sleep is known as paradoxical sleep (NG-599)
- Deep tendon reflexes are very exaggerated in spastic paralysis.

Diagram

- CS of spinal cord (IK-689; NG-497)
- Pre- and postsynaptic inhibition (IK-782)
- Reflex arc (IK-823; NG-492)
- Stretch and inverse stretch reflex (IK-825)
- Sensory pathways (IK-801)
- Pyramidal tract (IK-702; NG-549)
- Brown-Sequard syndrome (IK-710)
- Basal ganglia (IK-728; NG-557).

SPECIAL SENSES

Essays

- Visual pathway and field defects due to lesion at various levels (IK-904; NG-635)*.

Short Notes

- Importance of fovea centralis and macula (IK-899; NG-618, 347)
- Macular sparing (IK-898; NG-634)
- Papillary reflex and accommodation reflex (IK-921)
- Astigmatism (IK-897; NG-623)
- Difference between rods and cones (IK-899; NG-620)*
- Accommodation (IK-894; NG-621)*
- Color vision theories (IK-913; NG-636)*
- Color blindness (IK-914; NG-461)*
- Aqueous humor (IK-920; NG-618)
- Blind spot and fovea centralis (IK-916; NG-618)
- Dark adaptation (IK-920; NG-629)*
- Night blindness (IK-911; NG-628)*
- Presbyopia (IK-897; NG-621)*
- Role of basilar membrane in hearing (IK-932; NG-643)
- Impedance matching (IK-931)
- Travelling wave theory (IK-936)
- Auditory pathway (IK-928; NG-645)*
- Tympanic reflex (IK-925; NG-642)*
- Conduction deafness and nerve deafness (IK-938; NG-647)*
- Olfactory and taste pathway (IK-943; NG-654)*
- Ageusia, hypogeusia, dysgeusia (IK-950; NG-652)
- Anosmia, paraosmia, hyposmia (IK-948).

Explain the Physiological Basis

- Near point of vision recedes rapidly with advancing age (NG-620)
- Bitemporal hemianopia in pituitary tumors
- Reason for macular sparing
- Three primary colors are responsible for the perception of all colors.

Diagram

- Rods and cones (IK-899; NG-627)
- Visual pathway (IK-904; NG-633)
- Dark adaptation curve (IK-210; NG-629)
- Auditory pathway (IK-928; NG-647)
- Taste pathway (IK-947; NG-651).

REPRODUCTIVE SYSTEM

Essays

- Menstrual bleeding (IK-654; NG-384)*
- Hormonal regulation of menstrual cycle (IK-658; NG-489).

Short Notes

- Spermatogenesis (IK-637; NG-458)*
- Factors affecting spermatogenesis (IK-637; NG-459)*
- Regulation of ovulation (IK-654; NG-469)
- Blood testis barrier (IK-637; NG-459)*
- Graafian follicle (IK-649; NG-468)
- Sertoli cells (IK-637; NG-457)*
- Testosterone (IK-640; NG-462)*
- LH surge (IK-658)*
- Fetoplacental unit (IK-666; NG-480)*
- Hormones of pregnancy (IK-665; NG-478)*
- Pregnancy tests (IK-664; NG-481)*
- Placenta (IK-666; NG-879)

- Milk ejection reflex (IK-675; NG-486)*
- Contraception (IK-679; NG-488)
- Neuroendocrine reflex (IK-677; NG-486).

Explain the Physiological Basis

- Sertoli cells are important in spermatogenesis
- LH surge is necessary for ovulation
- Conception not occurs during lactating period.

Diagram

- Hormonal changes in menstrual cycling (IK-656; NG-469)
- Graafian follicle (IK-649; NG-468).

ENDOCRINOLOGY

Essays

- Growth hormones (IK-539; NG-400)
- Thyroid hormone (IK-552; NG-424)*
- Insulin (IK-602; NG-439)
- Regulation of calcium level in body (IK-563; NG-419)
- ADH, regulation of secretion (IK-546; NG-181,362)*
- Mineralo- and glucocorticoids (IK-590; NG-430)*.

Short Notes

- Mechanism of hormonal action (IK-529; NG-389)
- Neuroendocrine reflexes (IK-528; NG-486)*
- Somatomedins (IK-539; NG-396)
- Difference between diabetes mellitus and diabetes insipidus (IK-549, 609; NG-406,441)
- Oxytocine (IK-550; NG-407)*
- Hypoparathyroidism (IK-578; NG-422)
- Acromegaly, gigantism, dwarfism (IK-539; NG-403, 454)*
- Pituitary dwarfism and thyroid dwarfism (IK-539; NG-404)*
- Growth hormones (IK-539; NG-400)*
- Myxedema (IK-559; NG-414)
- Glucagon (IK-606; NG-1714,443)
- Cushing syndrome (IK-593; NG-177,430)*
- Addison's disease (IK-595)*
- Hypocalcemic tetany (IK-578)
- Calcitonin-actions (IK-575; NG-423)*
- Thyroid function tests (IK-559; NG-416)
- Antithyroid drugs (IK-563; NG-417).

Explain the Physiological Basis

- Polyuria and polydypsia in DM
- Exophthalmos is a clinical feature of thyroid dysfunction
- Osteoporosis is common in postmenopausal women
- High level of aldosterone causes diuresis and natriuresis
- Parathyroidectomy leads to signs of neuromuscular excitability
- Carpopedal spasm in tetany (NG-422)
- Exphthalmos in hyperthyroidism and carotenemia in hypothyroidism
- No edema in Conn's syndrome
- Biphasic action of adrenaline
- Exaggerated manifestation of CVS symptoms is seen in pheochromocytoma
- Blood Ca level increases after administration of parathyroid extract.

Diagram

- Regulation of thyroid hormone (IK-554; NG-415)
- Hormonal calcium balance (IK-564)
- Effect of insulin in various metabolic processes (IK-604).

NERVE MUSCLE PHYSIOLOGY

Essays

- Excitation contraction coupling (IK-67; NG-41, 53).

Short Notes

- Action potential (IK-49; NG-48,528)*
- Chronaxie and rheobase (IK-51; NG-30)*
- Neuromuscular junction (IK-63; NG-47)*
- Wallerian degeneration (IK-60; NG-34)*
- Myasthenia gravis (IK-65; NG-49)
- Motor unit (IK-75,1053; NG-44)*
- Rigor mortis (IK-72; NG-43)
- All or none law (IK-181,77; NG-29)*
- Sarcotubular system (NG-38,53)
- Plateau potential*.

Diagram

- Neuromuscular junction (IK-63; NG-47)
- Sarcomere (IK-68,178; NG-39)
- Action potential curve (IK-57; NG-26).

SKIN AND TEMPERATURE REGULATION

- Mechanism of adaptation of body to cold and hot environment (IK-958; NG-350)
- Role of hypothalamus in regulation of temperature (IK-958; NG-586)*
- Pyrexia (IK-960; NG-384)
- Pathophysiology of fever (IK-960; NG-384)*.

HEMATOLOGY EXPERIMENTS

ESTIMATION OF HEMOGLOBIN

Aim

To estimate the hemoglobin content of a person's blood using Sahli's method.

Principle

Hemoglobin contained in a known volume of blood is converted into acid hematin by the action of N/10 HCl. This is then diluted drop by drop till the color matches with the standard brown glass plates provided in the hemoglobinometer.

Normal Values

- *Males:* 14–18 g/100 mL
- *Females:* 12–16 g/100 mL
- *Newborn:* 18–23 g/100 mL.

High value in the newborn is due to the increased RBC count. The value decreases gradually and reaches adult value by 16–18 months (Figs 1A to D).

Objective Structured Practical Examination (OSPE)

Dilute the blood (from the given sample) for estimation of hemoglobin concentration.

Viva Questions

- **Can strong acids (such as nitric, sulphuric acid, concentrated HCl) or alkalies be used in place of decinormal HCl?**
  The strong acids, which are very strong oxidizing agents and alkalies will cause disruption of Hb and thus cannot be used. Only N/10 HCl is used because standardization has been done for acid hematin.
- **Can tap water be used for diluting and color matching?**
  No, it cannot be used because its sail may cause turbidity which will interfere with color matching.
- **Explain the advantages and disadvantages of this method?**
  Advantage: The method is simple and quick.
  Disadvantages:
  - The procedure should be repeated if the sample is over diluted.
  - There is individual variation in color matching.
  - The color in the standard fades with time.
  - Time should be allowed for formation of acid hematin.
  - Interference in color matching by natural substances like plasma proteins and lipids.

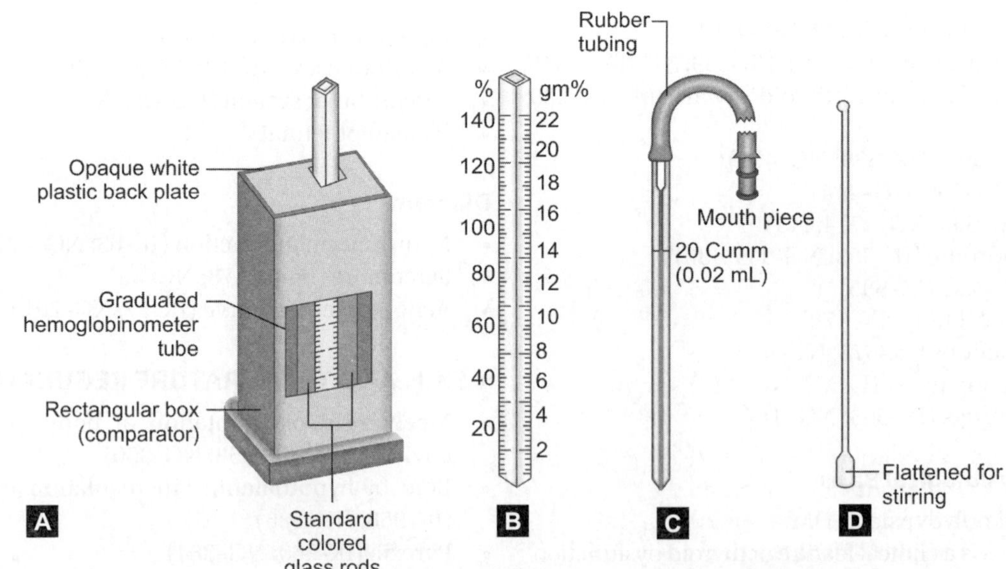

Figs 1A to D (A) Sahli's hemoglobinometer; (B) Graduated hemoglobinometer tube; (C) Hemoglobinometer pipette; (D) Glass rod (stirrer) (*For color version, see Plate 24*)

- **Can N/10 HCl be used instead of distilled water for diluting and color matching?**
Yes, it can be used because it being transparent, it cannot further deepen the color once all the Hb has been converted into acid hematin.
- **What will happen if quantity of N/10 HCl is changed?**
The minimum quantity should be present so as to form complete acid hematin.
- **What are the disadvantages of Sahli's method?**
  - The method estimates only oxyhemoglobin and reduced Hb, other forms such as carboxyhemoglobin and methemoglobin are not estimated.
  - In the long-term use, the standard coloration on the hemoglobinometer may fade and become lighter. This will lead to wrong result.
- **What are the other methods of Hb estimation?**
  - Spectrophotometric methods:
    - Cyanmethemoglobin method
    - Oxyhemoglobin method
    - Haldane's carboxyhemoglobin method
    - Alkaline hematin method.
  - Tallquist's method.
  - Copper sulphate falling drop method.
- **Name some derivatives of hemoglobin.**
  - Oxyhemoglobin
  - Reduced hemoglobin (deoxygenated Hb)
  - Carbaminohemoglobin
  - Carboxyhemoglobin
  - Methemoglobin
  - Cyanomethemoglobin (hemiglobincyanide).
- **Why is it required to allow the solution to stand for 10 minutes before dilution?**
This time is required for complete hemolysis of RBCs and maximum conversion of hemoglobin in blood to form acid hematin.
- **How is heme synthesized from the body?**
Heme portion of Hb is synthesized from glycine and succinyl CoA. Heme is synthesized by cells of erythroid series in red bone marrow.
- **Name the physiological and pathological variations of Hb content in RBC.**
  - *Physiological*
    a. *Age:* Hb% is more in newborn.
    b. *Sex:* Higher in males.
    c. *At high altitudes:* Hb% is increased at high altitudes as hypoxia stimulates eryrhropoiesis, which in turn, increases Hb count.
    d. *Exercise:* Hb content is increased after exercise.
  - *Pathological:* Hb content is increased in polycythemia and decreased in all types of anemias.
- **What would happen if Hb were present freely in the plasma instead of in the red cells?**
Normally, only a very small amount is present in the plasma (about 3 mg/dL), most of it being confined to red cells. If it were present in the plasma, it would increase the viscosity and the osmotic pressure of blood (thus affecting fluid exchanges). It would also be excreted in the urine, besides being taken up and rapidly destroyed by the reticuloendothelial system.

ENUMERATES THE RED BLOOD CELLS (RBC) (FIGS 2A AND B)

Aim

To find out the number of RBCs per cubic mm of blood.

Principle

The number of RBCs in a known volume of diluted blood is counted. From this the number of RBCs in 1 mm^3 of undiluted blood is calculated.

The diluting fluid used in Hayem's fluid

Calculations

Dilution factor – $\frac{\text{Total volume of bulb}}{\text{Volume of blood taken}} = \frac{100}{0.5} = 200$

Side of primary RBC square = 1 mm

Side of secondary RBC square = 1/5 mm

Side of tertiary RBC square = 1/20 mm

Area of one tertiary RBC square = 1/400 mm^2

Depth of the chamber = 1/10 mm

Volume of one tertiary RBC square = 1/4000 mm^3

No. of tertiary squares in which RBC counted = 80

Volume of 80 tertiary RBC squares = 1/4000 × 80 = 1/50 mm^3

Let, N be the number of RBC counted in 1/50 mm^3 of diluted blood

No. of RBC counted in 1 mm^3 of diluted blood = N × 50

No. of RBC counted in 1 mm^3 of undiluted blood

= N × 50 × dilution factor

= N × 50 × 200 = N × 1000

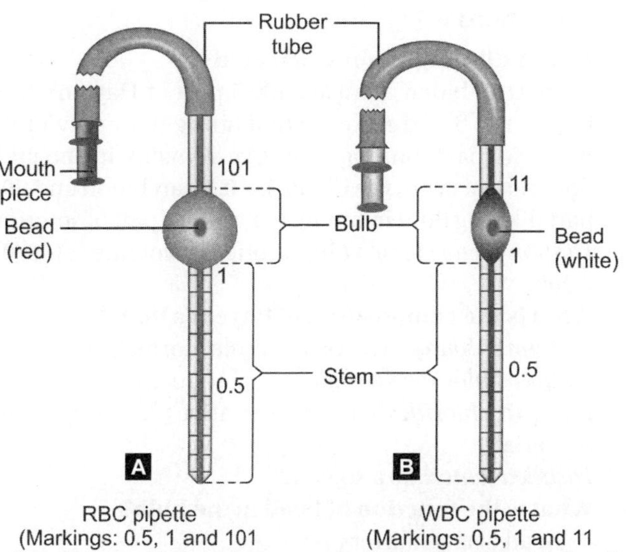

Figs 2A and B RBC and WBC pipettes
(For color version, see Plate 24)

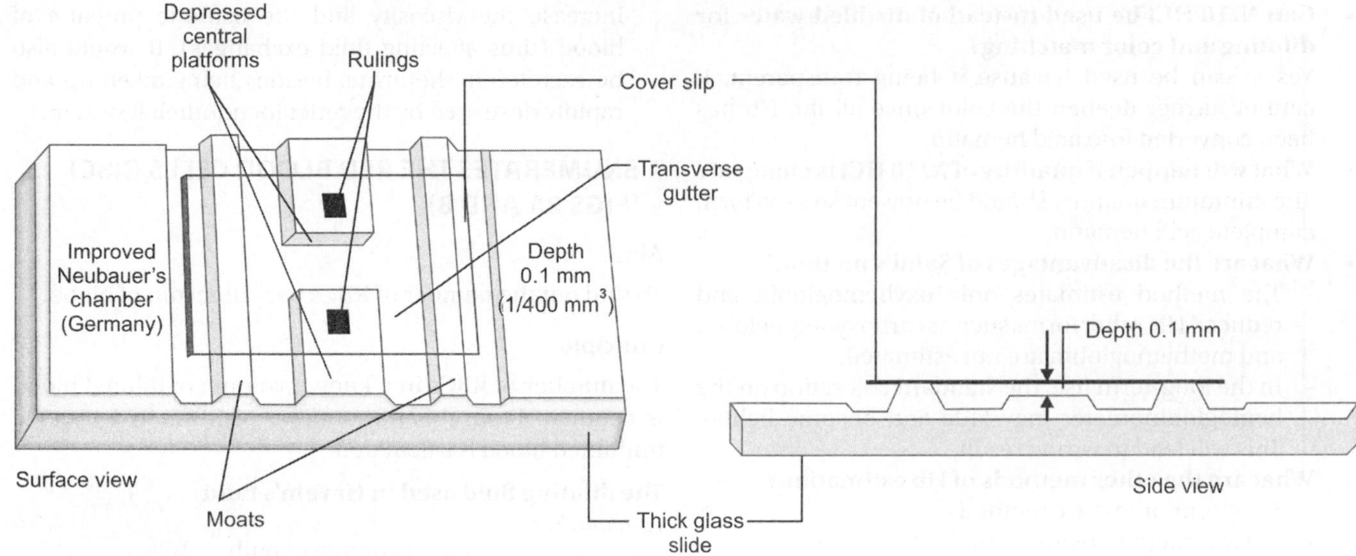

Fig. 3 Hemocytometer

Normal Value

Males: 4.5–6.5 million cells/mm³, average 5.4 million cells/mm³.

Females: 3.9–5.6 million cells/mm³, average 4.8 million cells/mm³.

Newborn: 6–7 million cell/mm³.

Objective Structured Practical Examination (OSPE)

- Dilute the blood for total RBC count.
- Charge the Neubauer's chamber for total RBC count (Fig. 3).

Viva Questions

- **How is diluting factor calculated?**
  0.5 part of blood is mixed 100.5 part of Hayem's fluid in pipette. Blood mixes with diluting fluid only in the bulb. So, part diluting fluid that remains in the stem does not mix with the blood, i.e. 0.5 part blood and 99.5 part diluting fluid in blood, to form 100 paft of solution.
  Diution factor: Final volume/original volume = 100/0.5 = 200.
- **What is the composition of Hayem's fluid?**
  Sodium sulphate: To prevent roulex formation.
  Sodium chloride: To maintain isotonocity of fluid.
  Mercuric chloride: Act as preservative (antifungal/antibacterial).
  Distilled water: As a solvent.
- **What is the function of bead in the bulb?**
  - Bead acts as stirrers.
  - Free rotation of bead in the bulb signifies pipette is dry.
  - Beads are distinguishing feature—red bead for RBC pipette, white bead for WBC pipette.
- **Would not the bead decrease the dilution due to its own volume?**
  The volume of bead is taken into consideration during manufacture of the pipette.
- **Why the fluid in the stem is discarded?**
  The fluid from the stem portion of the pipette is discarded because the actual mixing is taking place only in the bulb and stem contains only the diluting fluid.
- **Since the mature red cells do not contain nuclei, are they dead cells?**
  The RBCs, though without nuclei, are not dead in the usual sense. Since there are no mitochondria (and other organelles), energy is not available from oxidative phosphorylation (Krebs cycle). However, they contain a number of enzymes which control important functions. The cells contain all enzymes nessary for energy supply from anaerobic glucose metabolism via the Embden-Meyerhof pathway (hexose monophosphate shunt). (Glucose enters RBCs by an active process which is insulin-independent).
- **Describe the features of hemocytometer/Neubauer's counting chamber (Fig. 4)?**
  It is solid heavy glass slide. It is divided into three platforms by two deep gutters. The central narrow platform is 1/10 mm lower than those on either side.

  Each counting area has large square of 3 mm side. It is divided into nine primary squares of side 1 mm. Of these the four corner primary squares are used for counting WBCs. The central primary square 1 mm side is divided into 25 secondary squares (of 1/5 mm side) by triple lines or trans lines. Each secondary square is further divided into 16 tertiary squares of 1720 mm side each. For counting the RBCs the central and the four

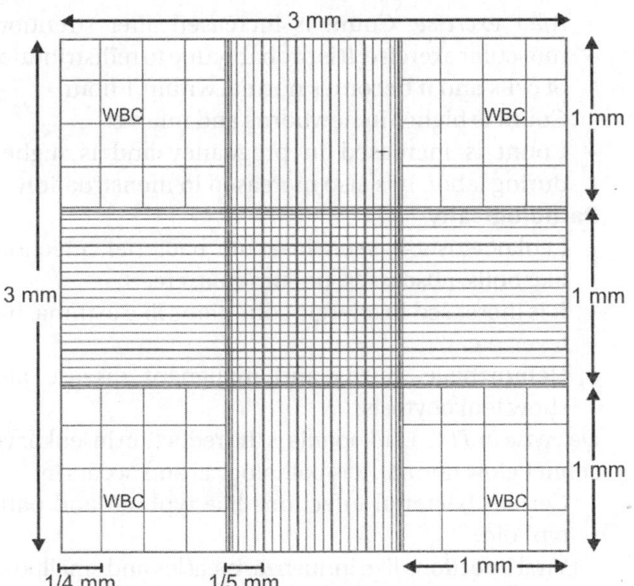

Fig. 4 Counting chamber (Neubauer's chamber) under low power of a compound microscope

corner secondary squares are used, i.e. a total of 16 × 5 = 80 tertiary squares.

For WBC counting the primary squares in the 4 corners are used. Each primary square of 1 mm side is divided into 16 small squares (each of 1/4 mm side). Thus a total of 64 smaller squares are used for counting the WBCs.

- **What are the uses of Neubauer's chamber?**
  It helps in finding out: RBC count, WBC count, sperm count, platelet count and also cells in CSF, peritoneal, pleural fluids, etc.
- **Describe RBC dilution pipette.**
  It has a capillary stem of uniform bore with a conical tip and a bulb above the stem. The capacity of the bulb is 100 times that of the stem. The stem is divided into 10 equal parts and has two markings 0.5 and 1. Just above the bulb there is another mark 101. The bulb contains a red bead which helps in mixing the blood with the diluting fluid, and allows easy identification of the pipette. The other end of the pipette is fitted with a soft and light rubber tubing and a mouth piece.
- **What are the constituents of Hayem's fluid?**
  It contains NaCl—0.5 g, Na_2SO_4—2.5 g, mercuric per chloride—0.25 gm, distilled water up to 100 mL NaCl make the fluid isotonic. Na_2SO_4 prevents Rouleaux formation and also acts as a fixative to preserve the shape of cells. Mercuric per chloride acts as a preservative and prevents growth of any organism.
- **What are the physiological and pathological variations in RBC count?**
  Count is increased:
  A. Physiologically
     In males: High altitude, high temperature, low O_2, tension, after exercise, infants.
  B. Pathologically
     1. Polycythemia vera
     2. Congenital cyanotic heart disease

  Count is decreased
  Decrease in count is seen in anemia.

TOTAL LEUKOCYTE COUNT

Aim

To determine the number of WBCs in one cubic millimeter of blood.

Principle

A known quantity of blood is diluted with a suitable diluting fluid, which destroys the red blood corpuscles and stains the nuclei of white blood cells. The leukocytes are then counted in a hemocytometer and their number in undiluted blood is calculated.
WBC diluting fluid—Turk's fluid.

Normal Values

Adult: 4000–11000/mm^3 of blood.
Newborn: 10000–25000/mm^3 of blood.
Children up to 4 years: 18000 cells/mm^3; count decreases after 4 years.

Calculation

Dilution factor = 10/0.5 = 20
Side of a primary square = 1 mm
Side of one secondary square = 1/4 mm
Area of one secondary square = 1/16 mm^2
Depth of the chamber = 1/10 mm
Volume of one secondary square = 1/16 × 1/10 = 1/160 mm^3
Number of secondary squares in which WBC counted = 64
Volume of 64 sec squares = 1/160 × 64 = 2/5 mm^3
Let N be the number of WBC counted in 2/5 mm^3 of diluted blood
Number of WBC counted in 1 mm^3 of diluted blood = N × 5/2
No. of WBC counted in 1 mm^3 of undiluted blood = N × 5/2 × 20 = N × 50.

Objective Structured Practical Examination (OSPE)

Dilute the blood for total leukocyte count? Charge the Neubauer's chamber?

Viva Questions

- **What is the composition of Turk's fluid?**
  Glacial acetic acid—lyses membrane of RBC, platelets and causes swelling of nucleus of WBC
  Gentian violet—stains nucleus of WBC
  Distilled water—as a solvent.
- **What are the other uses of WBC pipette?**
  The WBC pipette can be used for diluting the blood much less for counting RBCs in cases of severe anemia, or for counting platelets. It can also be used for counting sperms and bacteria.
- **Why are the red cells not seen when counting the leukocytes?**
  The red cells are not seen because they are hemolyzed by glacial acetic acid in the Turk's fluid. The remnants of red cells membranes are faintly visible and they called as ghost cells.
- **How do you differentiate a WBC pipette from a RBC pipette?**

RBC pipette	*WBC pipette*
Calibrations are 0.5 and 1.0 below the bulb and 101 above the bulb	Calibrations are 0.5 and 1.0 below the bulb and 11 above it
The capillary bore is narrow, hence it is a slow speed pipette	The capillary bore is wider, hence it is a fast speed pipette
Bulb is larger and has a red bead	Bulb is smaller and has a white bead
The volume of the bulb is 100 times the volume contained in stem	The volume of the bulb is 10 times the volume of the stem
The dilution can be 1 in 100 or 1 in 200	The dilution can be 1 in 10 or 1 in 20

- **Are WBCs also lyzed while doing WBC count?**
  Yes. WBCs are also lyzed, this is to destroy the plasma membrane to expose the nucleus for staining. So while counting we actually count the nucleus of WBC and not WBC as a whole.
- **What are the physiological and pathological variations in WBC count?**
  Increase in leukocyte count >11000/cumm is called leukocytosis. It generally refers to an increase in neutrophils and hence it is synonymous with neutrophilia.
  Increase in TLC:
  Physiologically
  - *Diurnal variations:* The count is lowest in the morning and rises during midday. It is the highest in the evening. Count is lowest after rest.
  - *After exercise:* Count is increased after strenuous muscular exercise. It is probably due to redistribution of cells and it becomes normal within 1 hour.
  - Count is higher in newborns and infants.
  - Count is increased in pregnancy and is highest during labor. It is also increased in menstruation.

  Pathologically
  - Leukocytosis is seen in acute bacterial infections like boils, abscesses, pneumonia, etc.
  - It is increased in allergic conditions like asthma, hay fever, etc.
  - Hemorrhage, burns and malignant disease also show leukocytosis.

  Decrease in TLC: Leukopenia is the reduction in leukocyte count below normal. It is pathological and occurs in:
  - Certain bacterial infections like typhoid and paratyphoid.
  - Viral infections like influenza, measles and smallpox.
  - Protozoan infections like malaria and kala-azar.
- **What is leukopoiesis? Where does it occur?**
  Leukopoiesis, i.e. production of WBCs occurs both in the bone marrow and lymphatic tissues. The two major lines of WBCs myeloid (for granulocytes and monocyte) and lymphoid (for lymphocyte) arise from pleuripotent hemopoietic stem cells in the bone marrow.
- **What is the lifespan of leukocyte?**
  Normally, the lifespan of granulocytes is about 8–10 hours or a few days. But the lymphocytes recirculate between blood and lymphoid tissue and may survive for months.
- **What is meant by the term agranulocytosis, leukocytosis, leukopenia and leukemia?**
  Agranulocytois: Decrease in the number of granulocytes.
  Leukocytosis: Increase in the number of WBC beyond 1 1,000/mm^3 irrespective of the type of cells (granulocytes, monocytes, leukocytes)
  Leukopenia: Decrease in the number of white cells below 4000/mm^3
  Leukemia: It is a group of malignant neoplasms of WBC (forming organs—bone marrow and lymphoid tissue. The TLC is generally, above 40,000–50,000/mm^3 or even a few lakhs.

DIFFERENTIAL LEUKOCUTE COUNT

Aim

To study the different types of WBCs in a peripheral smear.

Principle

A thin blood smear is prepared, stained with Leishman's stain and examined under the oil immersion objective of microscope. The different types of leukocytes are identified and counted.

Stain used—Leishman's stain.

Characteristic features of different cells

	N	*E*	*B*	*L*	*M*
Diameter	10–14 μm	12–16 μm	10–14 μm	*Small:* 7–10, *Large:* 10–14 μm	14–18 μm
Nucleus	2–7 lobes	Bilobed-2 (spectacle-shaped)	Bilobed Not visible because of granules	Round	Kidney-shaped
Staining by N	Purplish blue	Purplish blue	Purplish blue	Purplish blue	Bluish violet
Cytoplasm	Plenty and pale pink	Bright pink	Plenty	Small—scanty, large—blue	Grayish blue
Granulas	Violet pink	Large, coarse, crimson red granules of uniform size	Large coarse bluish black	Absent	Absent
Function	Phagocytosis, 1st line of defence	Detoxification, role in parasitic infestation, allergic reaction	Anticoagulation by heparin	B-cell and T-cell immunity	Phagocytosis, 2nd line of defence
Increased count	Neutrophilia (PMNL)	Eosinophilia	Basophilia	Lymphocytosis	Monocytosis
Decreased count	Neutropenia	Eosinopenia	Basopenia	Lymphopenia	

Objective Structured Practical Examination (OSPE)

- Prepare a smear from the given sample of blood.
- Stain the supplied smear for DLC.
- Focus a neutrophill/eosinophill, large lymphocyte and monocyte in the given smear, under oil immersion objective.

Viva Questions

- **What are the characteristics of a good smear (Figs 5A and B)?**
  - Should be tongue-shaped with a head, body and tail.
  - It should not touch the edges of the slide and should occupy only the middle 2/3rd of the slide.
  - It should not be serrated or wavy.
  - It should not be too thick or too thin.
  - It should have a thin smooth surface without ridges or holes.
- **What are the criteria for good staining?**
  - There should not be any stain particles.
  - The cell should be uniformly distributed and uniformly stained.
  - The RBCs should be pink in color and just touch each other.
  - The WBCs should take out the appropriate colors.
  - Platelets are seen in groups as small bodies with a central-stained part and pale periphery.
- **What is the composition of Leischman's stain?**
  - *Eosin:* Acidic dye, stains positively charged particles, e.g. nuclei of RBC's, granules of eosinophils.
  - *Methylene blue:* Basic dye, stains negatively charge particles, e.g. nuclei of WBC's, granules of basophils.
  - *Acetone-free methyl alcohol:* Fixative and preserve cells. Blood smear fixed to slide. The methyl alcohol should be acetone free to prevent shrinkage, crenation and lysis of cells.

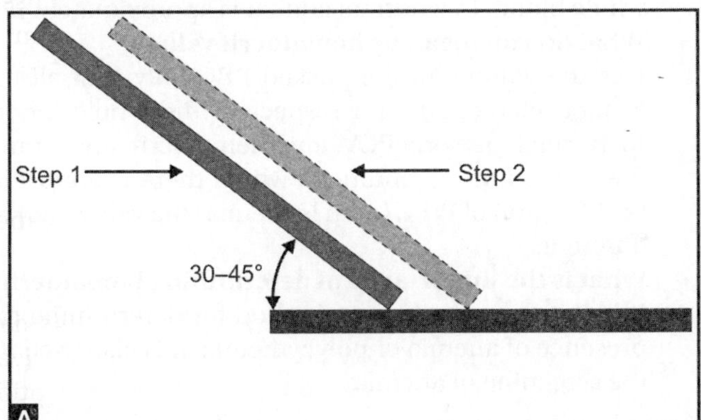

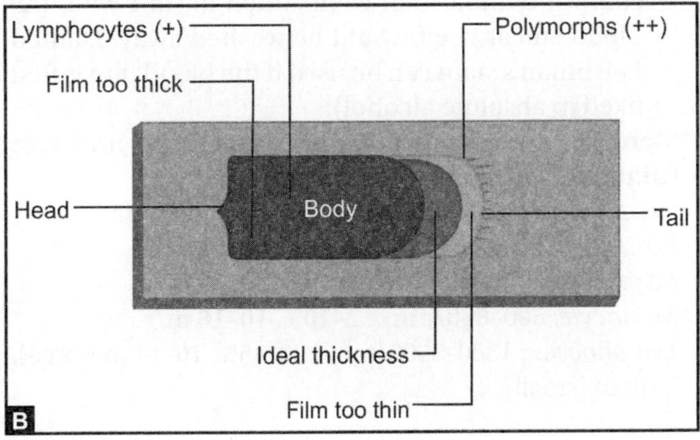

Figs 5A and B Method to prepare a good smear

- **What are the uses of peripheral smear?**
  - To study the alterations in the shape, size and staining characters of red cells or the presence of immature-nucleated red cells in peripheral blood.
  - For differential leukocyte count.
  - Detection of immature and abnormal forms of leukocytes in peripheral blood.
  - To detect the presence of parasites in blood, e.g. malarial parasite.
- **What you meant by differential count?**
  Differential count is the % of different types of WBCs in a smear. Types of WBCs are granulocytes and agranulocytes.
  Granulocytes
  Neutrophils: 50–70%
  Eosinophils: 1–4%
  Basophils: 0–1%
  Agranulocytes
  Lymphocytes: 20–40%
  Monocytes: 2–8%.
- **Discuss the significance of DLC?**
  The differential count is done to find if there is an increase or decrease of a particular type of WBC. Knowing the TLC, the absolute number of each type can be calculated. This information is important in detecting infection or inflammation, allergic and parasitic infections and effects of chemothrerapy and radiation therapy.
- **Why is Leishman's stain diluted after 1–2 minutes? What happens to the blood film during this period?**
  During the fixation period of 1–2 minutes, the pure alcohol serves two purposes:
  - It precipitates the plasma proteins, which act as glue and attach (fix) the blood cells on to the glass slide.
  - It preserves the shape and chemistry of cells to as, near the living state as possible.

    The cells are not stained during this time, because the stain particles cannot enter the cells in their unionized state. Their ionization occurs only when water is added to the salts in the undiluted stain (if diluted stain were added to start with, the blood smear itself would be washed away. Diluted Leishman's stain can be used if the blood film is first fixed in absolute alcohol).
- **Mention the absolute count, percentage and size (diameter) of various leukocytes?**
  Neutrophil: 2000–7500/mm^3, 40–75%, 10–14 m
  Eosinophils: 4–440/mm^3, 1–6%, 10–14 m
  Basophil: 0–100/mm^3, 0–1%, 10–14 m
  Monocyte: 500–800/mm^3, 2–10%, 10–18 m
  Lymphocytes: 1300–3500/mm^3, 20–45%, 10–14 m (large), 7–10 m (small).

PACKED CELL VOLUME/HEMATOCRIT

Aim

To find out the PCV (ratio between volume of red blood cells to the volume of whole blood expressed as percentage.

Principle

The red blood cells are heavier than plasma. When anti-coagulated blood is placed in a tube and centrifuged, the heavier cells settle down and pack themselves because of the centrifugal force.

Observations

The tube shows:

1. An uppermost layer of clear plasma, it is straw colored.
2. A whitish and thin layer of platelets above and leukocytes below just below the plasma layer. This is called buffi coat and is 0.5–1 mm thick.
3. A tall bottom layer of packed red cells. This red cell layer is separated from the buffy coat by the black line. This line is due to the presence of reduced Hb, present in the red cells lying adjacent to the white cells. This line marks the upper limit of red cell layer. Height of the red cell column varies from 4.2–4.7 cm. The packed cell volume percentage is obtained by multiplying the reading obtained by 10.

Normal Value

Adult male: 46 +/– 5%
Adult female: 42 +/– 5%.

Objective Structured Practical Examination (OSPE)

Load the wintrobes tube with the blood supplied for estimation of hematocrit.

Viva Questions

- **What is PCV?**
  It is the volume of cellular elements per unit volume of whole blood. In a normal adult it is approximately 45.
- **What do you mean by hematocrit value?**
  It is the volume of the packed RBC only (not all the formed elements) with respect to the whole blood. In normal person, PCV and hematocrit are almost the same. But in conditions where there is abnormal proliferation of WBC (as in leukemia) the values can be different.
- **What is the importance of determining hematocrit?**
  It is simple and accurate method for determining the presence of anemia or polycythemia. It is also used for the screening of anemia.

- **What cells make up the buffy layer? Mention its clinical significance?**
  The buffy layer consists of packed platelets and leukocyte. A rough estimate of WBC count may be made from the thickness of the buffy coat. A thickness of 1 mm corresponds to 10,000 WBC. The thickness increases in cases of leukemia, severe leukocytosis and primary thrombocytosis. Smears from buffy coat are useful when WBC count is very low and may be of use in detecting blast cells in leukemic leukemia and plasma cells in multiple myeloma.
- **Explain about Wintrobe's hematocrit tube (Figs 6A and B)?**
  It is a heavy cylindrical tube with uniform bore and open at the top. It is 11 cm long and is graduated from 0–10 cm from above downwards on one side and 10–0 cm on the other side. The diameter of the tube is 2.5 mm.
- **What is Pasteur pipette?**
  It is an ordinary glass tube drawn into a long thin nozzle and fitted with a rubber teat.
- **Explain about plasma column obtained in hematocrit?**
  It is normally straw colored. It is red in hemolysis, pale in anemia, yellow in jaundice, milky and opaque in lipemia.
- **What is the effect of a high hematocrit?**
  Increase in Hct, increases the viscosity of blood which leads to an increase in peripheral resistance and thus the blood pressure.
- **Name the conditions where PCV is increased and those where it is decreased?**
  High PCV is seen in:
  Physiological conditions: Newborn, high altitude, after exercise, dehydration resulting from profuse sweating without adequate fluid intake.

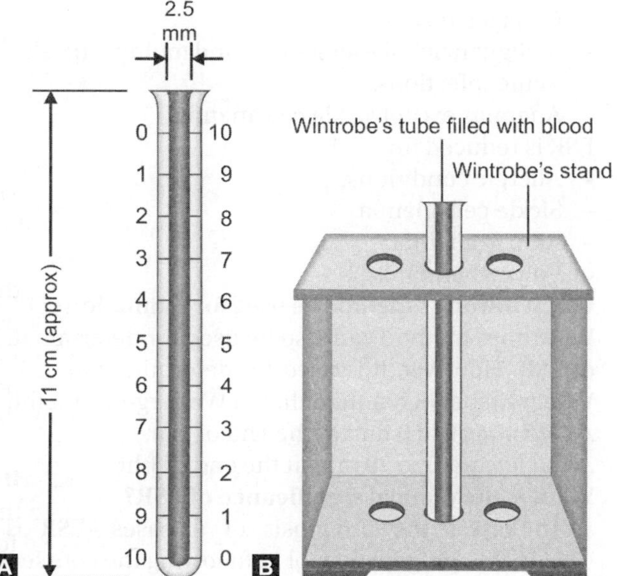

Figs 6A and B (A) Wintrobe's hematocrit tube with its stand (B) (*For color version, see Plate 25*)

  Pathological conditions: Polycythemia, dehydration resulting from severe gastroenteritis, burns leading to hemoconcentration.
  Low PCV is seen in:
  Physiological conditions
  a. During pregnancy due to hemodilution
  b. In females.
  Pathological conditions: In various types of anemias.
- **What are the uses of Wintrobe's method?**
  Estimation of PCV is the primary use. It is also used for the determination of ESR and demonstration of LE cells.
- **What is a true hematocrit?**
  Even under optimum conditions, it is impossible to completely pack the red cells together, and about 2% plasma remains trapped in between the red cells. This percentage is more if the red cells are abnormal in shape (e.g. spherocytosis, sickle cells). To compensate for trapped plasma, the true cell volume (true hematocrit) is obtained by multiplying observed hematocrit value by 0.98.

BLOOD INDICES

Mean Corpuscular Volume (MCV)

It is the volume of a single RBC in cubic microns.
MCV: PCV per 100 mL blood × 10 μm^3/RBC count in million per cu mm.
Normal value: 76–96 cubic microns.

A cell with normal MCV is normocytic. Increased MCV is seen in macrocytic anemia, e.g. pernicious anemia.

Decreased MCV is seen in microcytic anemia, e.g. iron deficiency anemia.

Mean Corpuscular Hemoglobin (MCH)

It is the average amount of Hb in a single RBC in picogram.
MCH: Hb in gm% × 10 pg/RBC count in million/cu mm.
Normal value: 29 +/– 2 pg.

MCH helps in differentiating hypochromic and hyperchromic anemias.

MCH is decreased in hypochromic anemia, e.g. iron deficiency anemia and is increascd in pernicious anemia.

Mean Corpuscular Hemoglobin Concentration (MCHC)

It is the Hb concentration in a single RBC or it is the amount of Hb expressed as % of the volume of a RBC.
MCHC: Hb in gm% × 100/PCV per 100 mL of blood.
Normal value: 34 +/– 2%.

Usually in most types of anemias a decreascd Hb concentration or MCH is associated with a decreased volume of RBC or MCV and vice versa. So that the ratio of MCH to MCV remain normal. But in hypochromic anemias like Fe deficiency anemia the decrease in MCH is greater than the decrease in MCV so that MCHC becomes decreased.

Color Index

It denotes the ratio of Hb to RBC.
Color index: Hb %/RBC%
100% of Hb—14.8 g/100 mL
100% of RBC—5 million/mm
Normal value: 0.85–1.10.

ERYTHROCYTE SEDIMENTATION RATE (ESR)

Aim

To determine the erythrocyte sedimentation rate.

Principle

If blood containing an anticoagulant is allowed to stand in a tube kept vertically and undisturbed, the red cells settle down gradually to the bottom since their specific gravity is higher than that of plasma. Erythrocyte sedimentation rate is the number of millimeters of clear plasma seen above the cell layer, and is expressed in millimeters at the end of the first hour.

Pipette used is—Westergren's pipette.

Normal Values

In males: 1–3 mm/first hour.
In females: 3–7 mm/first hour.
In infants: 0–0.5 mm/first hour.

Objective Structured Practical Examination (OSPE)

- Load the Wintrobe's tube with the supplied blood for determination of ESR.
- Load the Westergren's pipette with the supplied blood for determination of ESR.

Viva Questions

- **Why do the red cells settle down in a sample of anticoagulated blood?**
  Since the blood is not moving, the red cells settle down because they are heavier (specific gravity 1.095) than the plasma specific gravity 1.032) in which they are suspended.
- **What is Rouleaux formation?**
  Rouleaux formation is the piling up of RBC one on top of each other like a stack of coins. Fibrinogen neutralizes the negative charges imparted by sialic acid moieties on the cell membrane and thereby makes the RBCs sticky so that they tend to adhere to each other and form larger Rouleaux.
- **Mention the factors responsible for Rouleaux formation.**
  - Concentration of fibrinogen, albumin and globulin.
  - Bacterial proteins and toxins, products of inflammation and tissue destruction released into the blood neutralize the surface charges of red cells.
  - Concentration of glycoprotein in plasma.
  - Biconcave shape of red cells favors Rouleaux formation.
  - Number of red cells.
- **What are the factors influencing ESR?**
  - Rouleaux formation favors sedimentation.
  - Increase in concentration of fibrinogen in plasma increases the Rouleaux formation and hence increases ESR.
  - Concentration of A and B globulins increases ESR.
  - Albumin decreases ESR.
  - The biconcave disk shape of RBC's help in Rouleaux formation. Variation in size of RBC's or anisocytosis and variations in shape of RBCs or poikilocytosis interferes with Rouleaux formation and hence decreases ESR.
  - *RBC count:* When the RBC count increases ESR decreases.
  - ESR is influenced by viscosity of blood, specific gravity, acid-base balance, temperature, age of the blood since withdrawal and the anticoagulant used. Excess oxalate will slow sedimentation.
  - *Position of the tube:* Slanting position of the tube increases ESR.
- **State the physiological and pathological variations of ESR.**
  Physiological
  - ESR is low in newborn.
  - ESR is high in pregnancy, lactation and old age.
  - ESR is more in females and less in males.

  Pathological
  ESR is increased in:
  - Chronic infections like tuberculosis.
  - Rheumatic fever.
  - Collagen diseases.
  - Malignancies like leukemias and multiple myeloma.
  - Acute infections.
  - Anemias except sickle cell anemia.

  ESR is reduced in:
  - Allergic conditions.
  - Sickle cell anemia.
  - Afibrogenemia.
  - Polycythemia.
- **Can Wintrobe's method be used for estimation of ESR?**
  Wintrobes method can also be used for determination of ESR. However, it is used for determination of PCV. Value will be higher than that in Westergrens method.
  Adult male: 0 to 9 mm at the end of 1 hr.
  Adult female: 0 to 20 mm at the end of 1 hr.
- **What is the clinical significance of ESR?**
  - To assess the prognosis of diseases—ESR is a valuable prognostic tool in following the course of a disease, such as tuberculosis, rheumatoid arthritis, etc; while a patient is on treatment. If a weekly ESR shows a trend towards a decrease, it would indicate

an improvement. But if the ESR shows an increase, it would mean that the disease is deteriorating.

- As an indicator of bodily reaction to tissue injury and inflammation. It is a sensitive indicator of tissue damage. ESR is raised in all organic (pathological) conditions in contrast to functional disorders (anxiety neurosis, hypochondria).

- **Can we use oxalate mixture in Westergren's method and citrate in Wintrobe's method?**
  No. The anticoagulants employed for each method have been standardized and cannot be interchanged. Sodium citrate cannot be used in Wintrobe's method because the blood will be too much diluted as compared to the height of the tube; and this will give high false values for ESR.
- **What are the disadvantages of Wintrobe's method?**
  The disadvantage is that, this method is less sensitive because the column of blood is not as high as is desirable for good results and the chances of errors are high, especially when the ESR is increased, say to over 50 mm.
- **Chart the difference between Wintrobe's and Westergen's tube (Figs 6 and 7).**

Westergen's tube	*Wintrobe's tube*
It is a long tube	It is a short tube
Total length—300 mm	Total length—110 mm
Diameter—2.5 mm	Diameter—3 mm
Both ends are open	Lower end is closed
Marking from top of the tube to the bottom Upper reading—0 mm, Lower reading—200 mm	Marking from top of the tube to the bottom and vice versa Left side—upper reading—0 cm, lower reading—10 cm (right side—vice versa)
For ESR only	For ESR and PCV

BLOOD GROUPING

Aim

To determine the blood group, bleeding time and clotting time of your own blood.

Principle

Surfaces of red cell membrane contain genetically determined antigens—agglutinogens while plasma contains antibodies. Red cells allowed to react with commercially available antisera with agglutinins. Clumping/hemolysis as a result of antigen-antbody reaction.

Blood groups	*RBC antigen*	*Antibody in the plasma*
A	A	Anti-B
B	B	Anti-A
AB (universal receiver)	AB	None
O (universal donor)	None	Anti-A and anti-B

Viva Questions

- **What is agglutination?**
  Clumping and hemolysis of red cells during antigen-antibody interaction.
- **What are the different blood group systems?**
  Different blood group systems include ABO, Rh, M and N, Kell and Duffy, MNS, Lutheran, etc.
- **What is Rh grouping and HDN?**
  Rh factor was discovered in Rhesus monkey and this factor is present in 80–85% of human beings. Rh +ve subjects have Rh antigen on the red cells but their

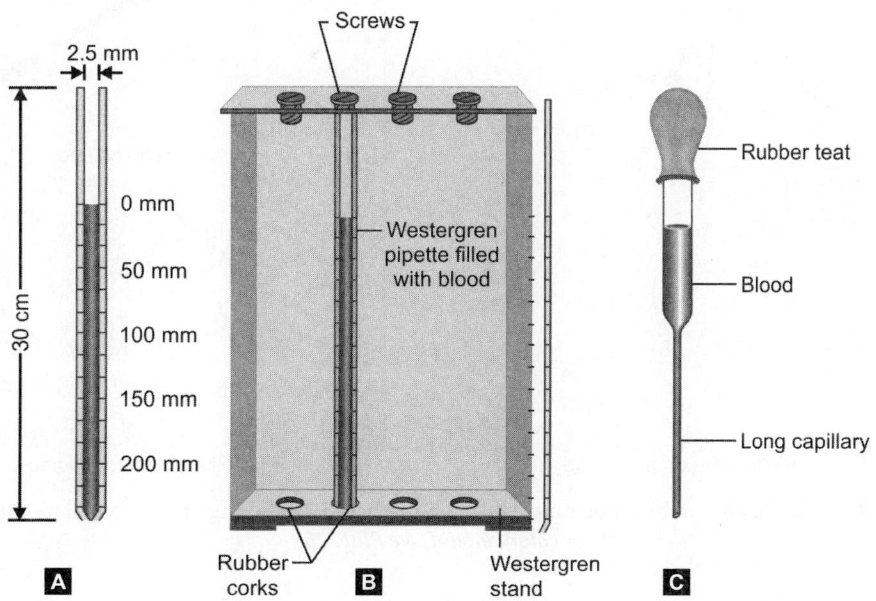

Figs 7A to C (A) Westergren's pipette; (B) with it stand; (C) Pasteur pipette (*For color version, see Plate 25*)

plasma does not contain Rh antibodies. Rh -ve subjects have neither Rh antigen nor Rh antibodies. Antibodies may appear if Rh -ve persons are transfused with Rh +ve blood or during pregnancy.

If Rh -ve mother conceives Rh + fetus. This condition gives rise to erythroblastosis foetails (HDN—hemolytic disease of newborn). The most common Rh antigen is D and its antibody is anti-D.

- **How will you differentiate agglutination from Rouleaux formation?**
  Dilution with saline disperses Rouleaux, but agglutinated cells are not dispersed.
- **What is Bombay blood group?**
  This blood type is a rare phenomenon in which the H antigen is absent. Since there is no H antigen, there is no antigen A or antigen B on the red cells. However, the plasma contains anti-A, anti-B and anti-H antibodies. As a result, such a person can receive blood only from a person having Bombay blood type.
- **What is reverse blood typing?**
  The blood grouping (typing) procedure in which the red cells of a person (whose blood type is to be determined) are tested against anti-A and anti-B sera, is called "blood typing" or "forward blood typing" another but related procedure called "reverse blood typing" (also called "serum wiping" or "backward blood typing"), the serum of the recipient is tested against red cells containing known antigens, i.e. red cells from persons with blood types A, B, AB, and O.
  If agglutination occurs with A and AB red cells, the blood type is B; if agglutination occurs with B and AB red cells, the blood type is A; if agglutination occurs with A, B, and AB red cells, the blood type is 0 and if there is no agglutination in any RBCs the blood type is AB.

BLEEDING TIME AND CLOTTING TIME

Aim

To determine bleeding time and clotting time of your own blood.

Principle

Bleeding time: It is the time taken from the puncture of the blood vessels to the stoppage of bleeding. It can be found by two methods—Duke's method and Ivy's method.

Clotting time: It is the time taken from the puncture of blood vessels to the formation of the fibrin thread. It can be found by two methods—capillary glass tube method and Lee and White method.

BT: Duke's method (Fig. 8A).

Normal time: 2–6 minutes (according to the Duke's method)

CT: Capillary tube method (Fig. 8B).

Normal values: 3–8 minutes at 37°C.

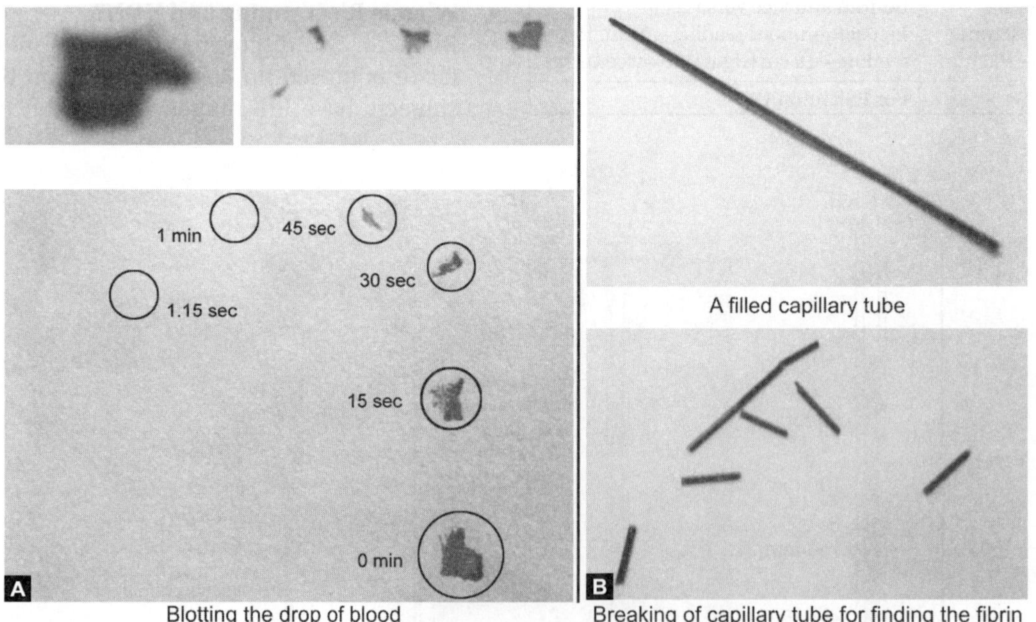

Figs 8A and B (A) Estimation of bleeding time by Duke's method; (B) Clotting time by capillary tube method (*For color version, see Plate 26*)

Viva Questions

- **What is the clinical importance of doing BT and CT?**
  BT and CT are important in the following situations:
  - History of frequent and persistent bleeding from minor injuries, or spontaneous bleeding into tissues.
  - Before every minor and major surgery (tooth extraction, etc.).
  - Before taking biopsy, especially from bone marrow, liver, kidney, etc.
  - Before and during anticoagulant therapy.
  - Family history of bleeding disorders.
- **What are the factors on which BT depends?**
  - Breadth and depth of the wound.
  - Degree of hyperemia of the skin puncture site.
  - Number of platelets and their functional status.
  - Functional status of the blood vessels.
  - Temperature (in cold weather, low temperature promotes vasoconstriction and thus shorten BT).
- **What are the factors on which CT depend?**
  - Increased temperature decreases clotting time.
  - Rough surface decreases clotting time.
  - Vitamin K level in the blood—in deficiency) clotting time is prolonged.
  - Addition of thrombin and thromboplastin—clotting time is reduced.
  - Heparin and other anticoaggulants prolong clotting time.
  - Decreased calcium concentration and decreased temperature also increase clotting time.
- **What are the conditions in which BT is prolonged?**
  Deficiency of vitamin C, thrombocytopenic purpura.
- **What are the conditions in which CT is prolonged?**
  Hemophilia (due to lack of factor VIII), liver disease, lack of Christmas factor (factor IX), vitamin K deficiency.
- **What is hemophilia? Mention the changes of BT and CT in hemophilia.**
  Hemophilia is a disorder in which clotting time is prolonged. In 85% of cases, it is due to deficiency of factor VIII and in about 15% patients it is due to deficiency of factor IX. BT is normal in hemophilic person; only CT is prolonged.
- **How does BT differ from CT? What is the interrelation between them, and which aspects of hemostasis are tested by them?**
  Both BT and CT are done together in all disorders of hemostasis. They are interrelated in the sense that platelets are involved in both tests. The BT tests the platelet plug formation and the condition of the microvessels (arterioles, capillaries, venules), while CT tests the formation of the clot. Increase in BT (e.g. in purpura), or CT (e.g. in hemophilia) usually occur independently of each other.
- **Name the conditions in which only the BT is prolonged while the CT is normal?**
  Low platelet count (thrombocytopenia), functional platelet defects, vessel wall defects.

OSMOTIC FRAGILITY OF ERYTHROCYTES (FIG. 9)

Aim

To determine the osmotic fragility of RBCs of one's own blood.

Principle

Normal red cells can remain suspended in isotonic saline solutions for many hours without rupturing and releasing the hemoglobin into the saline. When red cells are placed in a medium of hypotonic saline they swell up due to endosmosis. This is because the osmotic pressure is higher inside the cells and fluid passes into them. When they cannot swell any further, they burst liberating the hemoglobin content.

Viva Questions

- **What is osmotic fragility?**
  Osmotic fragility of red cells is the ease with which red blood cells undergo hemolysis when suspended in hypotonic solutions.
- **What is the principle behind osmotic fragility of erythrocytes?**
- **Normally, at what strength of saline solution, hemolysis starts and get completed?**
  Hemolysis starts normally at 0.45% saline and it is completed at 0.55% saline.
- **What are the physiological and pathological variations of osmotic fragility?**
  Physiological: Fragility is increased:
  - In the cells of the venous blood
  - In the cells of the newbom
  - At low temperature.

  Pathological:
  Fragility is increased in:
  - Hereditary spherocytosis
  - Acquired hemolytic anemia
  - Drug induced hemolysis.

  Fragility is decreased in:
  - Sickle cell anemia
  - Thalassemia
  - Iron deficiency anemia.

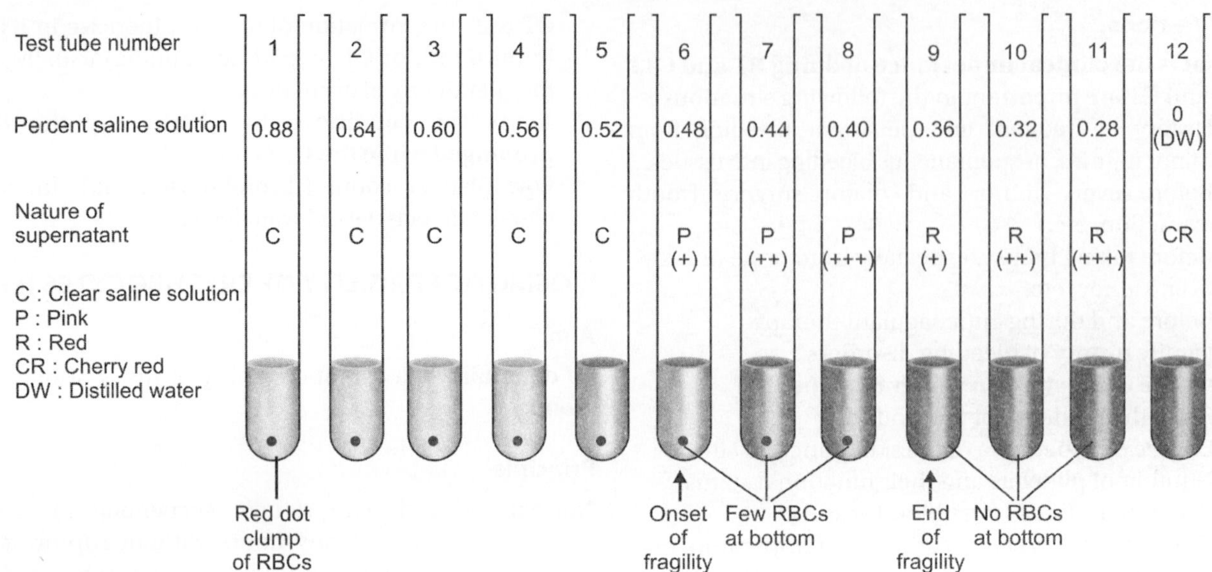

Fig. 9 Osmotic fragility of erythrocytes (*For color version, see Plate 26*)

- **What happens in hereditary spherocytosis? How can you induce hemolysis? Mention different ways?**
  Osmotic fragility may increase during hereditary spherocytosis.
  Hemolysis can be induced by:
  - Mechanically by shaking with glass beads
  - By fat dissolving chemicals like ether, chloroform and alcohol
  - Bile salts
  - Chemicals like acid and alkali and saponin, a fat solvent
  - Snake poisons.

CLINICAL EXAMINATION

HUMAN ARTERIAL BLOOD PRESSURE

Aim

To record the blood pressure of a normal individual in sitting, standing, recumbent position and after exercise. Measurement is done by two methods.

1. Palpatory method
2. Auscultatory method.

For which the instrument commonly used is a sphygmomanometer (Fig. 10).

Normal Values

Systolic BP: 100–140 mm Hg
Diastolic BP: 60–90 mm Hg
Average: 120/80 mm Hg.

Viva Questions

- **Describe the parts of sphygmomanometer?**
  Sphygmomanometer has three important parts:
  1. *Mercury manometer*
     - It has a long limb graduated from 0–300 and each division corresponds to 2 mm Hg.
     - A short broad limb of manometer acts as a reservoir from which mercury can be pushed into the long limb.
     - A rubber tube is attached to the opening at the top of reservoir and it leads to an inflatable rubber bag with linen cuff (compression armlet) or **Riva Rocci cuff**.

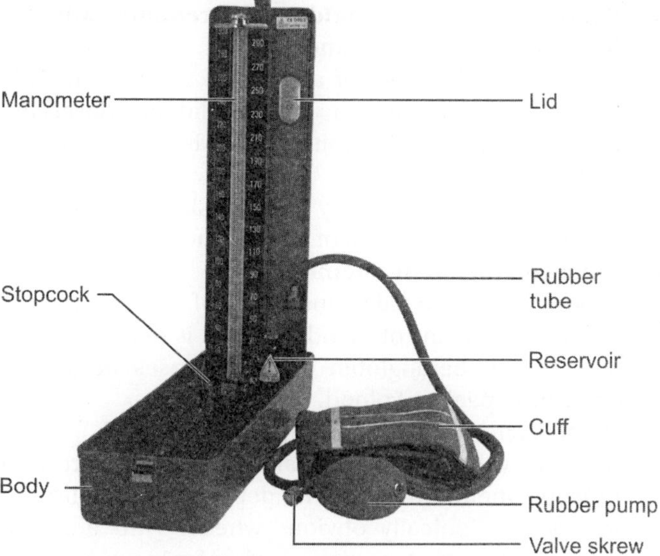

Fig. 10 Sphygmomanometer

  2. *Rubber bag with linen cuff*
     - This is a soft elastic rubber bag and has got two pressure rubber tubings attached to it.
     - One of the rubber tubings is attached to the air pump and the other to the Hg reservoir through an air-tight metal adapter, width of the cuff varies for adults and children.
  3. *Air pump*
     - A thick but flexible rubber balloon.
     - It has two openings guarded by valves and allows air flow only in one direction.
- **What is the width of Riva Rocci cuff?**
  Adult: 12.5 cm
  Children: 8 cm.
- **What is Korotkoff sound?**
  Series of sounds heard during deflation are called sounds of Korotkoff.
  It is divided into five phases:
  - *Phase I:* Sudden appearance of a clear-tapping sound. It becomes louder during 10–15 mm Hg fall of pressure.
  - *Phase II:* Sound becomes soft and murmuring in the next 10–15 mm Hg fall of pressure.
  - *Phase III:* Murmuring character continues but becomes louder and clear in the next 5–7 mm Hg fall of pressure.
  - *Phase IV:* Sound becomes soft and muffled.
  - *Phase V:* Sound completely disappears.
- **What is the basis of Korotkoff's sound?**
  Normal blood flow is laminar and stream lined and is always silent. Flow through a partially-occluded vessels produces turbulence, hence a sound is produced. There is no sound in a completely-occluded vessel. When the vessel is partially occluded by the pressure cuff, there is turbulence. These sounds of vibration are transmitted and heard by auscultation. Appearance and disappearance of sounds are observed which corresponds to systolic and diastolic BP respectively.
- **What is auscultatory gap and what is its significance?**
  In some patients of hypertension, there may be a gap in the Korotkoff sound. As the Hg is lowered, a few faint sounds are heard which soon disappear only to reappear once again at a lower pressure. This brief interruption, which may range from 40–60 mm Hg is called the 'auscultatory' or 'silent gap'.

  If the Hg column is raised to this gap and then the pressure lowered, one may miss the first appearance of sounds, which indicate systolic pressure and thus record a false low systolic pressure. To avoid this mistake, the BP should always be recorded by the palpatory method first. Then during auscultatory method, the Hg column must be raised 30-40 mm Hg above the level found by palpatory method. If we record BP only by auscultatory method, systolic BP may be underestimated due to the presence of auscultatory gap (particularly in HT individuals). But, during palpatory method this gap is not seen so there will be an idea of actual BP. So, palpatory method is done before auscultatory method to get an approx value of systolic BP.

- **What are the variations in the blood pressure?**
  Physiological:
  - *Diurnal:* Lowest in the morning and highest in the afternoon.
  - *Age:* Minimum at birth. As age increases, BP increases. Atherosclerosis and old age add to this.
  - *Sex:* Females in the reproductive age group. It increases after menopause.
  - *Body build:* BP is high in obese people.
  - *Meals:* Systolic BP show changes with meal.
  - *Sleep:* Systolic BP falls in undisturbed sleep. If sleep is disturbed by dreams, systolic BP shoots up.
  - *Emotion:* Anxiety, worries, etc. increases BP.
  - *Gravity:* Pressure is high in vessels below heart level.
  - *Posture:* Systolic BP is maximum in the supine position. In the supine position venous return increases which leads to increase in cardiac output and increase in systolic BP.

    Diastolic pressure is maximum in standing position. On standing up there is a fall in arterial pressure in the upper part of body. This cause less stimulation of baroreceptors, which in turn, causes strong sympathetic discharge and elevates the diastolic BP.
  - *Exercise:* Systolic BP moderately rises. Diastolic BP remains unchanged or it may fall in severe exercise. Increased systolic BP is due to sympathetic stimulation. Fall in diastolic BP is due to peripheral vasodilation.

  Pathological
  - *Increased BP:* Hypertension
    a. Primary or idiopathic—essential hypertension
    b. Secondary—due to many causes.
  - *Decreased BP:* Hypotension.

GENERAL EXAMINATION (FIGS 11A TO J)

Biodata

Name: Age: Sex:
Occupation: Addresss:

General examination

- Appearance:
- Conscious and cooperation:
- Build and nourishment:
- Height:
- Weight:
- Pallor:
- Jaundice/icterus:
- Cyanosis:
- Clubbing:
- Lymphadenopathy:
- Edema:
- Skin, hair and nail:
- Other features
  Gait:
  Thyroid swelling or any other swelling:
  Varicose vein:

Vital signs

- Temperature: febrile/afebrile
- Pulse
  Rate: Normal range—60-120/mt
  Rhythm: Regular/irregular/reg irregular
  Volume: Low/normal/high
  Character: Pattern of pulse
  Condition of vessel wall: Normal/thickened
  Radiofemoral delay:
  Peripheral pulsations:
- Blood pressure:
- Jugular venous pressure:
- Respiratory:
  Rate:
  Rhythm:
  Type: Male—abdominothoracic
  Female—thoracoabdominal

"Examiner should be taken permission from the patient before the test procedure performed on him."

Viva Questions

- **What is pallor? How could we differentiate pallor?**
  It suggests pale appearance of skin. It gives a rough assessment of degree of anemia of the patient. It is looked for by retracting the lower eyelids and observing the color of palpebral conjunctiva. It is normally red in color.

  Pallor is also noted by color of skin, especially of palms, nail bed, mucosa of tongue and oral cavity.
- **What you meant by anemia?**
  Pallor suggest the pale appearance of skin but anemia suggests the color of blood. Anemia is defined as the decrease in hemoglobin level decreases in oxygen carrying capacity of blood.
- **What is icterus? How could you examine it?**
  It is the yellowish discoloration of skin, sclera and mucous membrane due to deposition of bilirubin in tissues. Clinically obvious when serum bilirubin exceeds 2 mg/dL. Jaundice is looked for in upper sclera by asking the patient to lower his eyeballs.

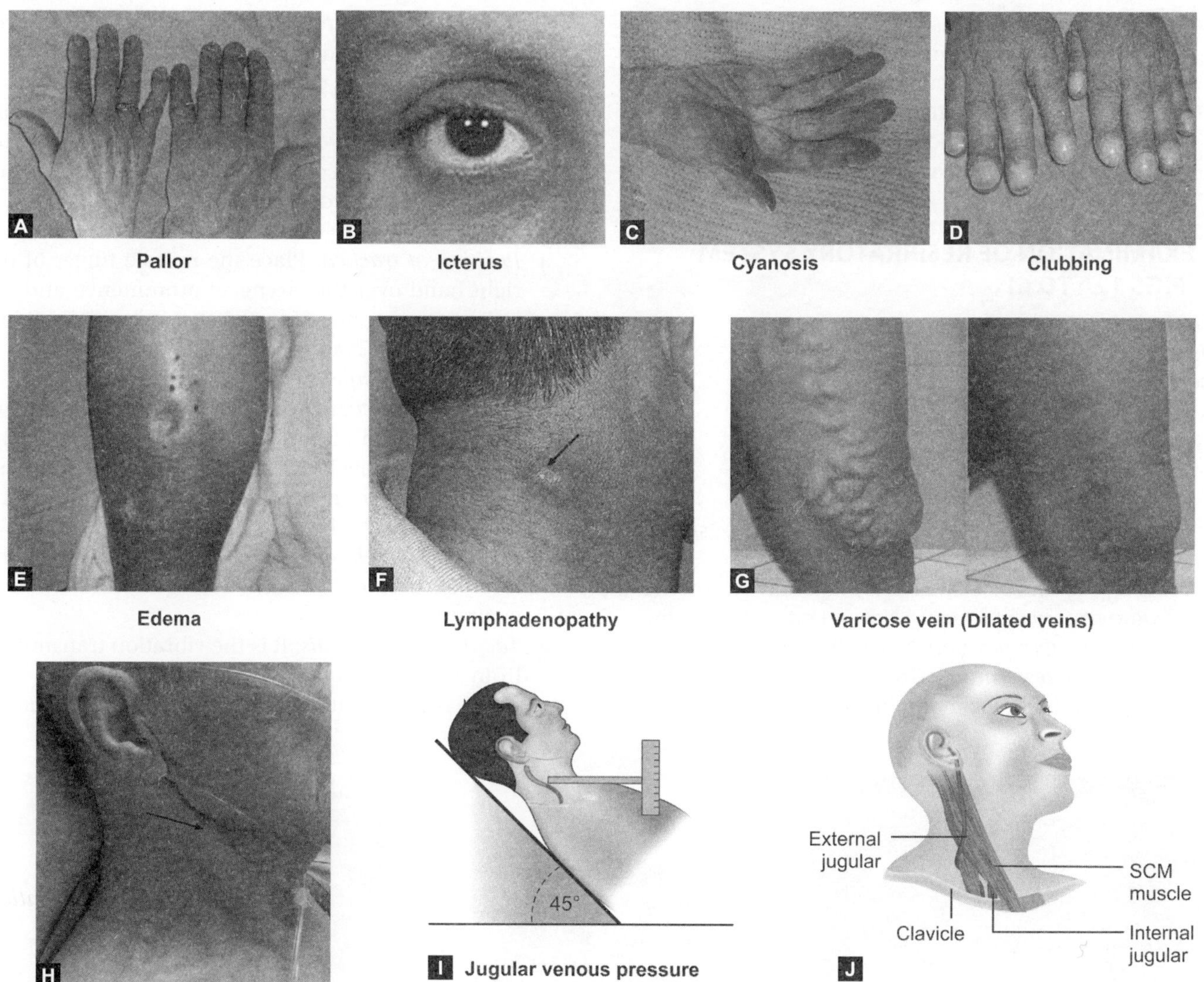

Figs 11A to J General examination (*For color version, see Plate 27*)

- **Explain cyanosis?**
  It is the bluish discoloration of the skin and mucous membrane due to an increase in amount of reduced Hb in blood above 5 gm%. Peripheral cyanosis is looked for at fingertips, ear lobes, tip of nose, etc. and central cyanosis at tongue and lips. Central cyanosis results from imperfect oxygenation of blood or from mixing of arterial and venous blood. It is more generalized. In central cyanosis extremities are warm whereas in peripheral cyanosis extremities are cold due to defective peripheral circulation.
- **What is clubbing?**
  It is the thickening of tissues at base of nail associated with obliteration of angle between nail base and adjacent skin of the finger and increase in convexity of the nail.
- **What you meant by lymphadenopathy?**
  Different groups of lymph nodes are palpated, e.g. cervical, axillary, inguinal, etc.
- **Explain edema?**
  Accumulation of fluid in subcutaneous tissue. Presence of dependent edema in ambulant person is usually detected by applying sustained firm pressure with the thumb against medial malleolus or shaft of tibia (for about 30 sec) and see for pitting or depression at pressure point.
- **What is the peculiarity in case of examining skin, hair and nail?**
  The texture of skin, abnormal pigmentation, texture and distribution of body and scalp hair are also noted. Nails are examined for pitting, ridges, spooning, hemorrhagic spots, nodules, etc.

- **Explain jugular venous pressure?**
The internal jugular veins are in direct continuity with right atrium. So observations of jugular venous pulsations give direct information about pressure changes and is an important guide to cardiovascular functions.
To look for neck veins, patient should be reclining at a angle of about 45°.

EXAMINATION OF RESPIRATORY SYSTEM (FIGS 12A TO C)

Biodata

Name: Age: Sex:
Occupation: Addresss:
General examination:

Systemic examination

1. *Inspection:*
   a. *Nasal alae:* It do not move usually.
   b. *Position of trachea:* Usually central in position. A slight shift towards right is normal.
   c. *Shape of chest:* Normally it is bilaterally symmetrical.
   d. *Respiratory movements:* Normal rate—14-16/min.
   e. *Rhythm of respiration:* Normally regular.
   f. *Types of respiration:* Usually abdominothoracic in male and thoracoabdominal in female.
   g. *Movements of chest wall:* Normally chest moves equally on both sides.
   i. *Apex beat:* It is defined as the lowermost and outermost point on precordium where definite cardiac impulse can be seen or felt. In adult normally it is seen or felt in 5th left intercostal space 1 cm medial to midclavicular line.
2. *Palpation:*
   a. *Position of trachea:* Place the middle finger of the right hand over the laryngeal prominence and the index and ring finger on the sternoclavicular joints on either side. Trace the trachea downwards.
   b. *Position of the apex beat:* Palpate the apex beat.
   c. *Movement of chest wall:* Placing the finger tips of both hands on either side, so that the tips of the thumbs just meet in the midline in front of the chest. The distance of movement of the thumb from the midline indicate the extent of expansion.
   d. *Expansion of chest:* Using a measuring tape at the level of nipple measure during inspiration and expiration.
   e. *Tactile vocal fremitus:* It is the vibration transmitted from the trachea and bronchus to the chest wall which is appreciated with the ulnar border of hand.

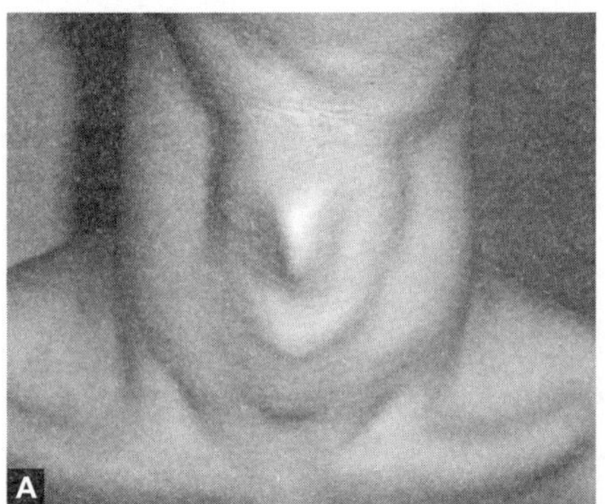

A Position of trachea—central

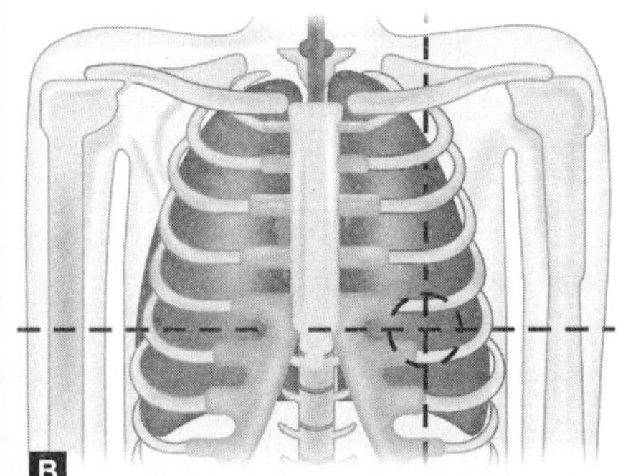

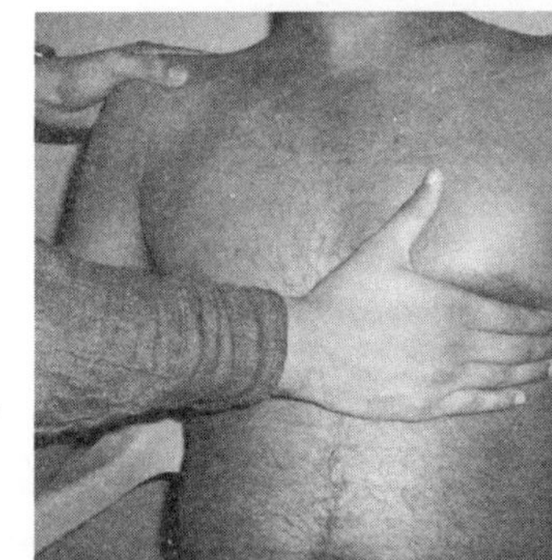

B Apex beat

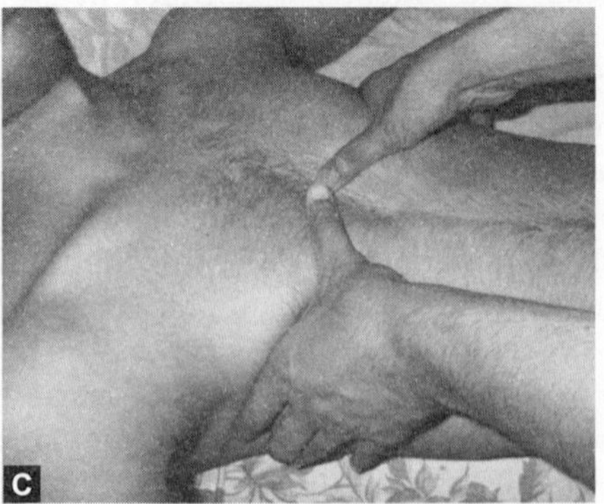

C Movement of chest

Figs 12A to C Examination of respiratory system

Here, ask the patient to say "one", or '99' repeatedly while placing the ulnar border of the paim over the chest wall on corresponding areas on either side of chest.

3. *Percussion:* Normally the lower border of right lung lies over the liver.
   Chest area: Normal lung resonance in either side with equal intensity.
   Liver dullness: Upper border of liver dullness is on the right 5th intercostals space in the midclavicular line.
   Cardiac dullness: Left border corresponds to apex beat. Right border corresponds to right margin of sternum. Normally, right 2nd intercostals space is resonant.
4. *Auscultation:* Breath sounds
   a. *Over chest:* Normal vesicular breath sound
   b. *Over trachea:* Normal bronchial breath sound
   Vocal resonance: Ask the subject to say 'one, one' repeatedly and auscultate different areas in corresponding areas of both sides
   Report: On examination the respiratory sytem of given subject is in normal limits.

Viva Questions

- **What are the abnormal shape of chest (Figs 13A to D)?**
  Abnormalities:
  - *Pigson chest (Pectus carinatum)* is a common sequel to chrome respiratory disease in childhood. It consists of a localized prominence of the stemum and adjacent costal cartilages, often accompanied by in drawing of the ribs to form symmetrical horizontal grooves (Harison's sulci) above the coase margins. Rickets also produce this type of deformity.
  - *Barrel chest:* Seen in chronic bronchitis and emphysema. Here the anteroposterior diameter is equal to transverse diameter. Chest assumes barrel shape.
  - *Kyphosis:* Forward bending of the vertebral column.
  - *Scoliosis:* Lateral bending of vertebral column. Combination of these two—kyphoscoliosis produced by either disease of spine or lung tissue.
  - *Funnel-chest deformity (Pectus excavatum)* is a developmental defect in which there is either a localized depression of the lower end of the sternum or depression of the whole length of the body of the sternum and of the costal cartilage attached to it.

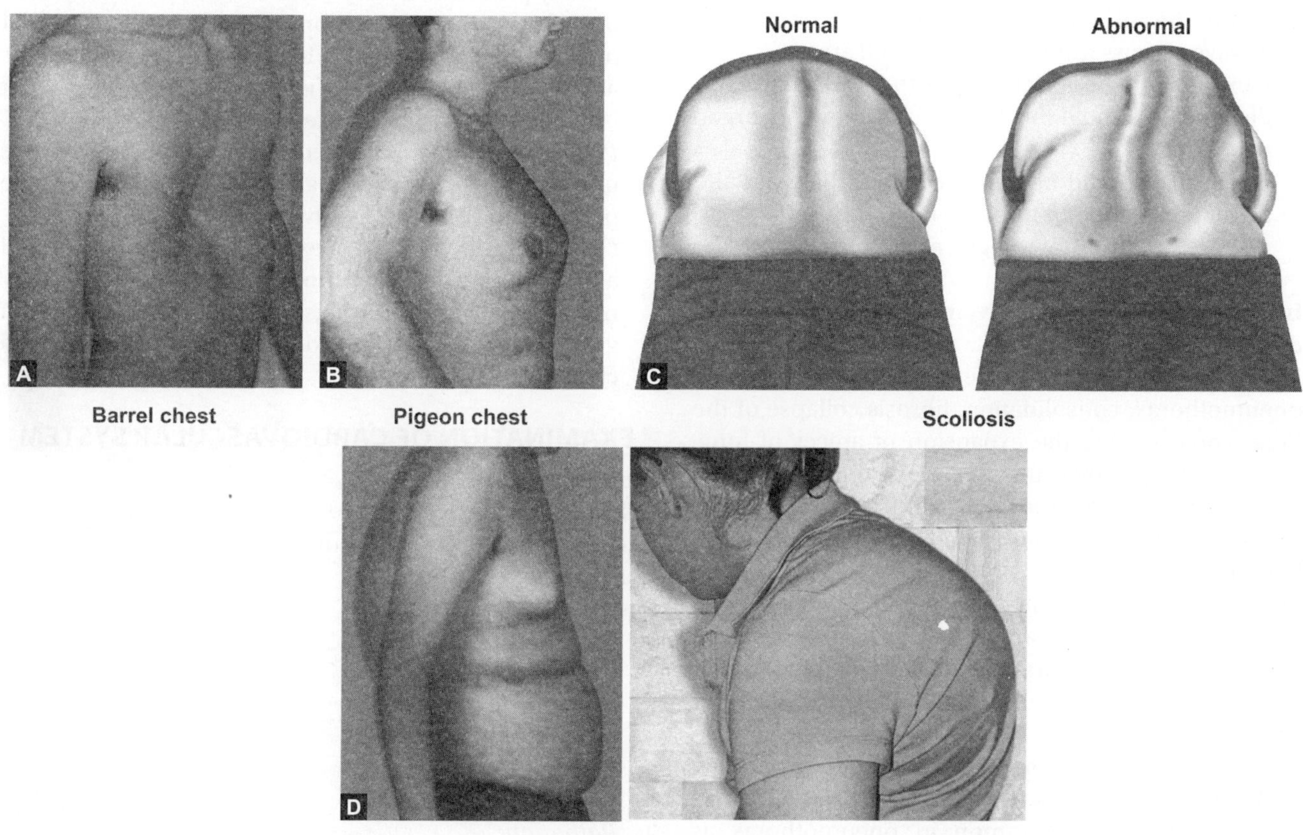

Figs 13A to D Abnormal shapes of chest

- **What are the variations in respiratory rate?**
  Increased rate—tachypnea. Seen in exertion, fever, thyrotoxicosis, nervous excitement, hypoxia. Decreased rate—bradypnea. Seen in narcotic poisoning.
- **In what all conditions, respiratory rhythm varies?**
  In tracheal and laryngeal diseases inspiration is prolonged. In bronchial and pulmonary disease the expiratory phase is prolonged. The rhythm of respiration is varied in Biot's and Cheyne-Stokes breathing.
- **What are the conditions in which position of trachea varies?**
  In fibrosis and collapse of lung, trachea is polled towards the affected side. In pleural effusion and pneumothorax, trachea is pushed towards the opposite side.
- **How does percussion performed?**
  Middle finger of the left hand is pleximeter. Middle finger of the right hand is plexor. Pleximeter finger is placed firmly over the part to be percussed. With the tip of the plexor finger strike the middle phalanx of the left middle finger. The movement should come from the wrist joint.
- **What are the rules of percussion?**
  - Always percuss from resonant to dull area.
  - Plexor should be at right angles to the pleximeter.
  - Pleximeter should be kept parallel to the organ percussed.
  - The stroke should be delivered from the wrist and finger joints and not from the elbow or shoulders
  - As soon as the blow is given the plexor must be raised.
- **In what condition, the movement of chest wall will decline?**
  Diminished movement is seen in pleural effusion, pneumothorax, consolidation, fibrosis collapse of the lung. For assessing the expansion of apices of lung, place the fingers over the shoulder from behind, the thumbs meeting over the lower cervical vertebrae.
- **What are the areas to be examined for 'tactile vocal fremitus'?**
  The areas to be examined are: Supraclavicular area, infraclavicular area, mammary area, inframammary area, axillary area, infra-axillary area, suprascapular area, interscapular area, infrascapular area, scapular area.
- **What are the conditions in which hyper-resonance and dullness is percused over chest area?**
  Hyper-resonance is common in pneumothorax as well as in emphysema. Dullnesss is seen in fibrosis, consolidation, collapse of lung and effusion. In pleural effusion, we get stony dullness.
- **What are different breath sounds?**

Breath sounds heard over chest	*Breath sounds heard over trachea*
Expiratory sound is less intense, audible only in early part	Expiratory sound is more intense than inspiration audible in all phases high pitched and harsh
Inspiratory phase which is continuous with a short expiratory phase	Equal inspiratory and expiratory phase
The vesicular breath sounds are produced when air passes in and out of lung tissue	The bronchial breath sounds are produced when air passes in and out of trachea and bronchi
There is no gap between the inspiratory and expiratory phase	A definite gap between inspiratory and expiratory phase

- **What are the adventitious sounds heard during auscultation?**
  Rhonchi or wheeze: It is prolonged uninterrupted sounds arising in bronchi due to partial obstruction of lumen. Partial obstruction can be produced by mucosal swelling, viscid secretions or bronchial smooth muscle spasm resulting in turbulent outflow. Rhonchi are usually heard in bronchial asthma. Rhonchi are musical in character.
  Crepitations: They are discontinuous crackling sounds usually produced by secretion collected within alveoli or in bronchi or in pulmonary cavities. There can be fine or coarse crepitations. In certain cases crepitations are precipitated or intensified following cough. Then it is known as post-tussive crepitations.
  Pleural rub: Seen in pleurisy. This pleural rub is unchanged following cough. They occur during late part of inspiration and early part of expiration.
  Crackles: They are short explosive sounds described as bubbling or clicking noises. They are not usually need by moistness in lungs but by sudden changes in gas pressure related to sudden opening of previously closed airways.

EXAMINATION OF CARDIOVASCULAR SYSTEM

Biodata

Name: Age: Sex:

Occupation: Addresss:

General examination:

Systemic examination

1. *Inspection:*
   a. Shape of chest:
   b. Shape of precordium:
   c. Site of apex beat:
   d. Enlarged vein:
   e. Other pulsation:
2. *Palpation:*
   a. Position of apex beat:
   b. *Character of apex beat:* Whether normal tapping/forceful or heaving.

c. *Palpability of heart sounds,* e.g. 2nd heart sound is palpable in pulmonary area in pulmonary hypertension.
d. *Left parasternal heave:* Medial aspect (ulnar surface) of palm is kept over the left sternal margin to feel for an impulse.
e. *Thrills:* A thrill is a palpable murmur.
f. Other pulsations:

Percussion:

Left border: It corresponds with apex beat.

Right border: Pleximeter finger is placed on the right side of the chest in the 2nd ICS 4–5 cm away from sternum and note the resonance.

Upper border: Resonant note is obtained over clavicle. Normally 2nd ICS shows resonance.

Lower border: It is in relation with diaphragm and left lobe of liver below it. Hence it cannot be defined by percussion.

Auscultation:

Mitral area: S1 and S2 sounds are heard—normal intensity (S1 louder).

No additional sounds and no murmer/click/pericardial rub.

Tricuspid area: S1 and S2 sounds are heard—normal intensity (S1 louder).

No additional sounds and no murmer.

Pulmonary area: S1 and S2 sounds are heard—normal intensity (S2 louder).

No additional sounds and no murmer.

Aortic area: S1 and S2 sounds are heard—normal intensity (S2 louder).

No additional sounds and no murmer.

Report: On examination, the cardiovascular system of the given is within normal limit.

Viva Questions

- **In which case, left parasternal heave is seen?**
  This is obtained in right ventricular hypertrophy.
- **How does the precordium is divided for the sake of auscultation?**
  Mitral area: 5th intercostals space 1 cm medial to the midclavicular line.
  Tricuspid area: Lower end of sternum to the left side.
  Aortic area: 2nd right intercostals space close to the sternum.
  Pulmonary area: 2nd left intercostals space close to the sternum.

EXAMINATION OF SENSORY SYSTEM

Biodata

General examination:

Examination of nervous system—higher function

General appearance and behavior: Normal

Level of consciousness: Conscious

Mental and emotional state: Cooperative

Delusion and hallucinations: No delusions and hallucinations

Orientation of time, place and person: Well oriented in time place and person

Memory

- *Short-term:* Normal
- *Long-term:* Normal

General intelligence: Normal

Speech: Normal

Sleep: Normal

Gait: Normal.

Sensory System

"Examiner should be taken permission from the patient before the test procedure performed on him."

Sensation				*Trunk*				*Limbs*							
		Face		*Front*		*Back*		*Upper limb*				*Lower limb*			
		Rt	*Lt*	*Rt*	*Lt*	*Rt*	*Lt*	*RF*	*RB*	*LF*	*LB*	*RF*	*RB*	*LF*	*LB*
Touch	Fine touch	N	N	N	N	N	N	N	N	N	N	N	N	N	N
	Crude touch	N	N	N	N	N	N	N	N	N	N	N	N	N	N
	Tactile localization	N	N	N	N	N	N	N	N	N	N	N	N	N	N
	Tactile descrimination	N	N	N	N	N	N	N	N	N	N	N	N	N	N
Pain	Superficial pain	N	N	N	N	N	N	N	N	N	N	N	N	N	N
	Deep pain	N	N	N	N	N	N	N	N	N	N	N	N	N	N
Temp	Warmth	N	N	N	N	N	N	N	N	N	N	N	N	N	N
	Cold	N	N	N	N	N	N	N	N	N	N	N	N	N	N

Sense of position: It implies the ability to imitate on the opposite side of the body with eyes closed.

Passive movements:

Stereognosis: It is the ability to recognize common objects like pen, pencil, key, etc. with eyes closed.

Vibration sense: It is a tingling sensation felt when the foot of a vibrating tuning fork is applied on the skin over an underlying bone.

Abnormal sensations: Not present.

Report: On examination the sensory system of the given subject is within normal limits.

Viva Questions

- **Demonstrate 'tactile sensibility'?**
  Light touch or fine touch: A wisp of cotton wool is used to test fine touch. Ask the subject to say 'yes' each time he feels the touch sensation. Test all over the body on both sides starting from face downwards.
  Pressure touch or crude touch: It is tested with a blunt object like a pencil or finger tip carefully, without applying too much pressure to avoid pain or any discomfort. Ask whether he can appreciate it or not.
  Tactile localization: It is tested in the same way as above. But ask the subject to localize the point of application of the stimulus either by describing or pointing out the spot.
  Tactile discrimination or two point discrimination: Ability to discriminate between two points touched simultaneously is called tactile discrimination. This can be tested using dividers. A minimum separation of 2 mm is needed between the 2 points to be appreciated in highly-sensitive areas like fingertips where touch receptors are more in number. A wider separation is needed in less sensitive areas like back, pulp of toes, etc.
- **How is superficial and deep pains are tested?**
  Superficial pain: Tested by using the point of a pin. Don't confuse the subject for pain sensation and sharpness of the object. Even in the absence of pain sensation subject can recognize the sharpness of the object.
  Pressure pain or deep pain: Tested by squeezing the muscle or pinching the Achilles tendon.
- **How do we test thermal stability?**
  Tested by using test tubes containing hot and cold water touched in turn on the part to be tested. The subject is asked to say whether he feels hot or cold.
- **How is position sense tested?**
  Ask the subject to close his eyes. One of his limbs is held in examiners hand and moved passively in different directions. Finally keep it in any definite position. Ask him to imitate the position on the opposite side. While the sense of position is being tested, the part being tested should not touch any other part of the body.
- **How is stereognosis tested?**
  To test this, take some familiar objects like pen, pencil, books, etc. in the palm and ask to identify them with eyes closed. Two objects differing only in size are placed on the palm and ask the subject to say which is smaller or larger. Absence of this sensation is called astereognosis. This occur in parietal lobe and posterior column lesions.
- **How is vibration sense tested (Fig. 14)?**
  Ask the subject to say at once when vibrations stop. Immediately place the foot of the fork over the examiners body over the same bony prominence and see whether the examiner can perceive the vibration. If vibration sense is lost the subject cannot feel the vibration. If the vibration sense is decreased, the examiner can perceive the vibration after taking the tuning fork from the subject.

EXAMINATION OF MOTOR SYSTEM

Biodata

General examination:

Exmination of nervous system—higher function

Examination of motor system

Bulk of muscle: Circumference of different parts of the limb is measured

Tone: It is a state of tension or contraction found in healthy muscles.

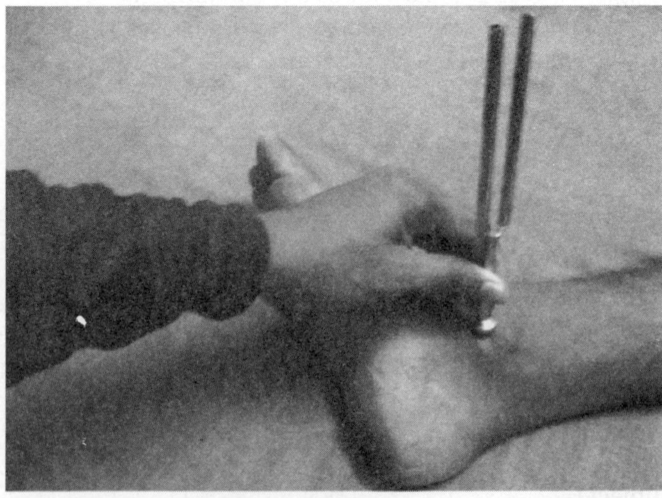

Fig. 14 Sense of vibration

Strength of Muscle (Figs 15 and 16)

	Right	*Left*
Muscles of upper limb		
Abductor pollicis brevis	Grade?	Grade?
Opponens pollicis	Grade?	Grade?
First dorsal interosseous	Grade?	Grade?
The interossei and lumbricals	Grade?	Grade?
Flexors of finger	Grade?	Grade?
Flexors of wrist	Grade?	Grade?
Extensors of wrist	Grade?	Grade?
Brachioradialis	Grade?	Grade?
Biceps	Grade?	Grade?
Triceps	Grade?	Grade?
Supraspinatous	Grade?	Grade?
Deltoid	Grade?	Grade?
Infraspinatous	Grade?	Grade?
Pectorals	Grade?	Grade?
Serratous anterior	Grade?	Grade?
Latissimus dorsi	Grade?	Grade?
Trunk	Grade?	Grade?
Lower Limb		
Dorsiflexion and plantar flexion	Grade?	Grade?
Extensors of knee	Grade?	Grade?
Flexors of knee	Grade?	Grade?
Extensors of hip	Grade?	Grade?
Flexors of thigh	Grade?	Grade?
Rotators of the thigh	Grade?	Grade?

Coordination of Movements

Upper Limbs

Finger nose test: Normal on both sides
Dysdiadochokinesia: Normal.

Lower Limbs

Heel knee test: Normal on both sides
Romberg's sign: Normal (negative)
Gait: Normal
Involuntary movements: Not present
Report: On examination the motor system of the given subject is found to be within normal limits.

Viva Questions

- **What are the characteristics of muscle wasting?**
  If there is wasting or atrophy, the muscles are smaller, softer and more flabby than normal. When wasting is accompanied by fibrosis, the muscle feels hard and inelastic and difficulty to stretch passively. This is called contracture. Generalized wasting may be due to chronic debilitating diseases.
  Localized atrophy may be due to injury or disease at a joint. In such cases, strength is preserved. The main neurological cause of muscle wasting is lower motor neuron lesion. In upper motor neuron, lesion wasting may occur due to prolonged disuse (Disuse atrophy).
- **What you meant by 'hypotonia and hypertonia'?**
  Hypotonia: There is little or no resistance to passive movements of the limbs and when the limb is lifted and let go, limb falls down inertly. They are also abnormally soft and flabby to palpation. Hypotonia is seen physiologically in sleep and on treatment with certain drugs. Pathologically, it is seen in LMN lesions, lesions of afferent pathways and cerebellar lesions.
  Hypertonia is of different types:
  - *Spasticity:* Hypertonia is seen following UMN. Lesions, e.g. lesions of corticospinal tract. This type of spasticity is referred to as clasp knife spasticity. This is characterized by increased resistance to passive movement, which is maximal at the beginning of movement and suddenly decreases as the passive movement is continued. It occurs predominantly in flexor muscles of upper limb and extensor muscle of lower limb.
  - *Rigidity:* Increase in resistance to passive movement is uniformly present throughout the range of movement and is known as " lead pipe" rigidity. This is seen in Parkinsonism. Sometimes, there is a series of "catches" during passive motion, due to tremor being superimposed on rigidity. This is known as "Cog Wheel Rigidity".
- **Describe the 'grading' of muscle strength?**
  Grade 0: Complete paralysis
  Grade I: A flicker of contraction only
  Grade II: Power detectable only when gravity is excluded by appropriate postural adjustments
  Grade III: Limbs can be held against the force of gravity but not against the examiner's resistance.
  Grade IV: There is movement against resistance but not to normal extent. There is some degree of weakness.
  Grade V: Normal power is present.

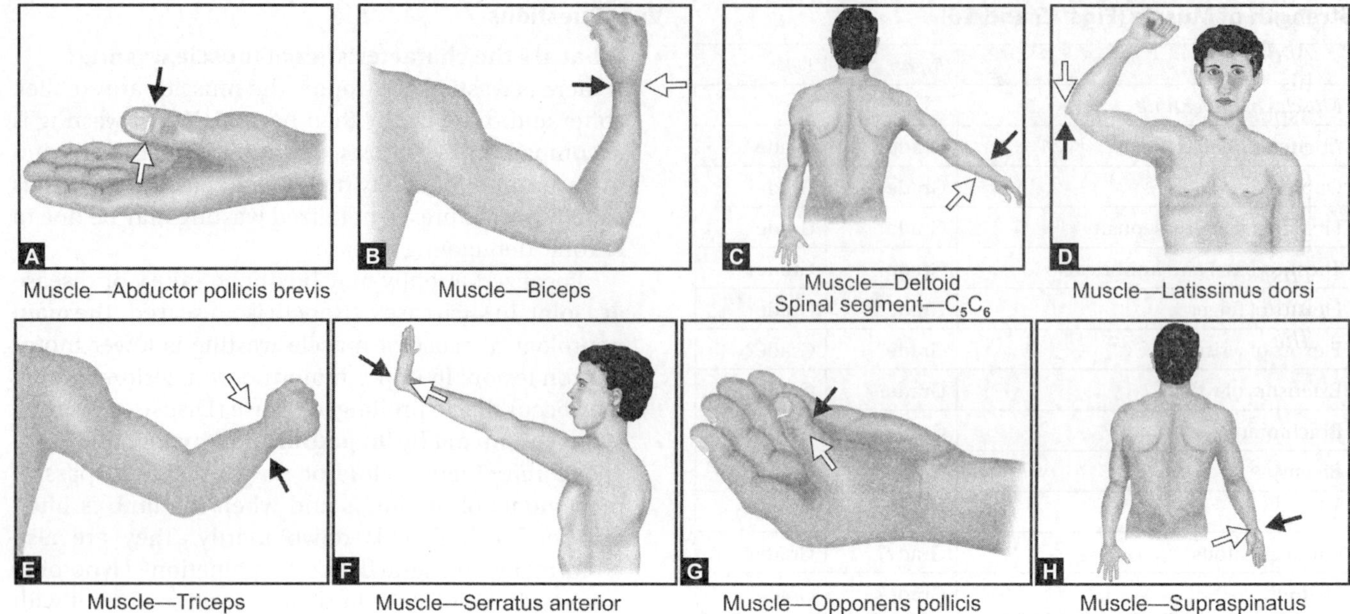

Figs 15A to H Examination of power of muscles

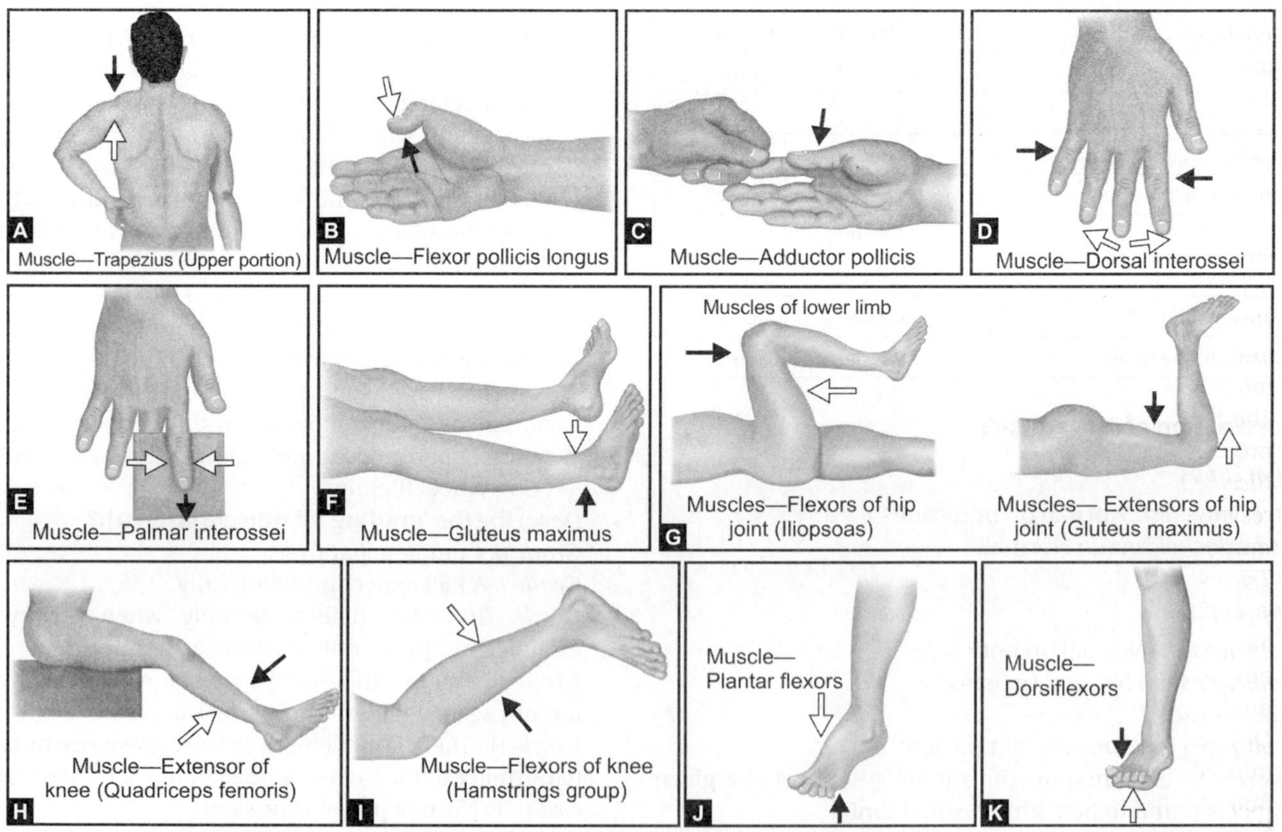

Figs 16A to K Examination of power of muscles

- **Describe the testing of muscles of upper limb?**

Abductor pollicis brevis: The subject is asked to abduct his thumb in a plane at right angles to the palmar aspect of index finger against resistance of examiner's own thumb. The muscles can be seen and felt.

Opponens pollicis: Ask the subject to touch the tip of his little finger with the point of his thumb. Oppose the movement with your thumb or index finger.

First dorsal interosseus: Ask the subject to abduct his index finger against your resistance

The interossei and lumbricals:

- Ask the subject to flex the metacarpophalangeal joints and extend the interphalangeal joints.
- Ask him to adduct and abduct his fingers.
- Give the subject a piece of paper or a card and ask him to grip it between the fingers—card test. When the muscles are weak the subject will either be unable to grip it or will offer poor resistance to its withdrawal. When these muscles are paralyzed, a claw-hand deformity is produced. The first phalanges are over-extended and the distal ones are flexed.

Flexors of fingers: Ask the subject to squeeze your fingers and assess the strength of the grip.

Flexors of wrist: Ask him to bring the tips of his finger towards the front of the forearm.

Extensors of wrist: Ask the subject to make a fist, which results in contraction of both extensor and flexors of the wrist. Then forcibly try to flex the wrist against resistance. It is almost impossible to overcome the wrist extensors. The wrist flexors can also be tested similarly. Radial nerve palsy leads to weakness of the extensors, resulting in a condition called wrist drop.

Brachioradialis: Place the arm midway between prone and supine positions. Ask the subject to bend up the forearm while the examiner opposes the movement. The healthy muscle will be seen and felt to stand out prominently.

Biceps: Ask the subject to bend up the forearm against resistance with the forearm in full supination. The muscle will stand out prominently.

Triceps: Ask the subject to extend the forearm against your resistance.

Supraspinatus: Ask the subject to lift his arm straight out at right angles to his side. The first 30° of this movement is brought out by supraspinatus.

Deltoid: The next 60° of shoulder abduction is by the middle fibers of deltoid. The anterior and posterior fibers help to draw the abducted arm forwards and backwards.

Infraspinatus: Ask the subject to tuck his elbow into his side with forearm flexed to a right angle. Then ask him to rotate the limb outwards against the examiner's resistance, the elbow being held against the side throughout. The muscle can be seen and felt to contract.

Pectorals: Ask the subject to sketch his arm out in front of him and then to clasp his hands together while the examiner tries to hold them apart.

Serratus anterior: Elevating the arm above right angles or pushing forwards with the hands against resistance result in winging of scapula, if the muscle is paralyzed.

Latissimus dorsi: Subject is asked to clasp his hands behind his back while the examiner standing behind him offers passive resistance to the downward and backward movement.

Testing the muscles of the trunk:

- Make the subject to lie on his back with legs extended. Ask him to rise up without using hands. If there is weakness of abdominal muscles, the subject is unable to do it. In spastic paralysis of the leg, the affected limb will rise first. This is Babinski's rising up sign.
- Ask the subject to lift up his head from the pillow against resistance. With paralysis of lower region of anterior abdominal wall the umbilicus moves upwards. When the upper segment is affected the umbilicus is pulled downwards—Beevor's sign.
- To test erector spinae and muscles of the back, make the subject to lie on his face and try to raise his head from the bed by extending the neck and back. The muscles, if healthy, will stand out prominently during this effort. The trapezius is tested by asking the subject to shrug his shoulders while the examiner tries to press them down from behind.

Lower limbs:

Dorsiflexion and plantar flexions of feet and toes are tested by asking the subiect to elevate or depress the part against resistance.

Extensors of knee: Bend up the subject's knee. Ask him to try to staighten it out again.

Flexors of knee: Raise the leg up from the bed supporting the thigh with examiner's left hand and holding the ankle with your right. Ask the subject to bend his knee against resistance.

Extensors of hip: Lift the subject's foot off the bed with his knee extended. Ask him push it down against resistance.

Flexors of the thigh: Ask the subject to raise his leg from the bed with the leg extended against resistance.

- *Adductors of thigh:* Abduct the limb and ask the subject to bring it tack to the midline against resistance.
- *Abductors of thigh:* Place the subject's legs together and ask him to separate the against resistance.

Rotators of the thigh: With the lower limb extended on the bed ask the subject to roll outwards or inwards against resistance.

- **How does coordination tests are performed?**
  Upper limb
  Finger nose test: Ask the subject to touch first his nose and then your finger with his index finger. Repeat with the other hand also. If he performs the movement naturally and without making errors coordination is normal. In persons with cerebellar ataxia, this is not possible (Figs 17A and B).
  Dysdiadochokinesia: Impaired ability to execute rapidly repeated movements. The subject is asked to flex his elbow to a right angle and then altemately supinate and pronate his forearm as rapidly as possible. When dysdiadochokinesia is present the movements are slow, awkward, incomplete, irregular and impossible after a few attempts. This is seen characteristically in cerebellar ataxia (Fig. 17D).
  Lower limbs
  - Ask the subject to walk along a straight line. If in coordination is present he will soon deviate to one side or the other.
  - *Heel-knee test:* If the person cannot walk, ask him as he lies on the bed to lift one leg high in the air to place the heel of his leg on the opposite knee and then slide the heel down his shin towards the ankle with his eyes open. In cerebellar ataxia, irregular side to side errors in the direction of movements occurs (Fig. 17C).
  - *Romberg' s sign:* The subject is asked to stand with his feet close together. If he can do this he is asked to close his eyes. If Romberg's sign is positive, he begins to sway about or may even fall as soon as his eyes are closed that is, the patient is more unsteady standing with eyes closed than open. This sign is positive in posterior column disorders (Sensory ataxia).
- **Explain gait? Explain how the gait is tested? Give examples for various types of gaits?**
  The legs should be adequately exposed for examining the gait. The feet should be bare. The subject is asked to walk away from the observer, to turn around at a point and come towards him again.
  If there is any abnormality exclude local causes like old injury of a joint or local pain. Certain well-recognized abnormal types of gait are:
  - Spastic gait, e.g. hemiplegia
  - Stamping gait, e.g. sensory ataxia
  - Reeling gait (or drunken gait), e.g. cerebellar lesion
  - Festinant gait, e.g. parkinsonism
  - Waddling gait, e.g. myopathies, muscular dystophies
  - High stepping gait, e.g. common peroneal nerve palsy.
- **What are the different types of involuntary movements?**
  In certain diseases of the nervous system, involuntary unintended movements occur either at rest or during voluntary movement. Most of them are due to diseased basal ganglia and extrapyramidal system. Epilepsy, myoclonus, tremor, athetosis, chorea, dystonia, tics.

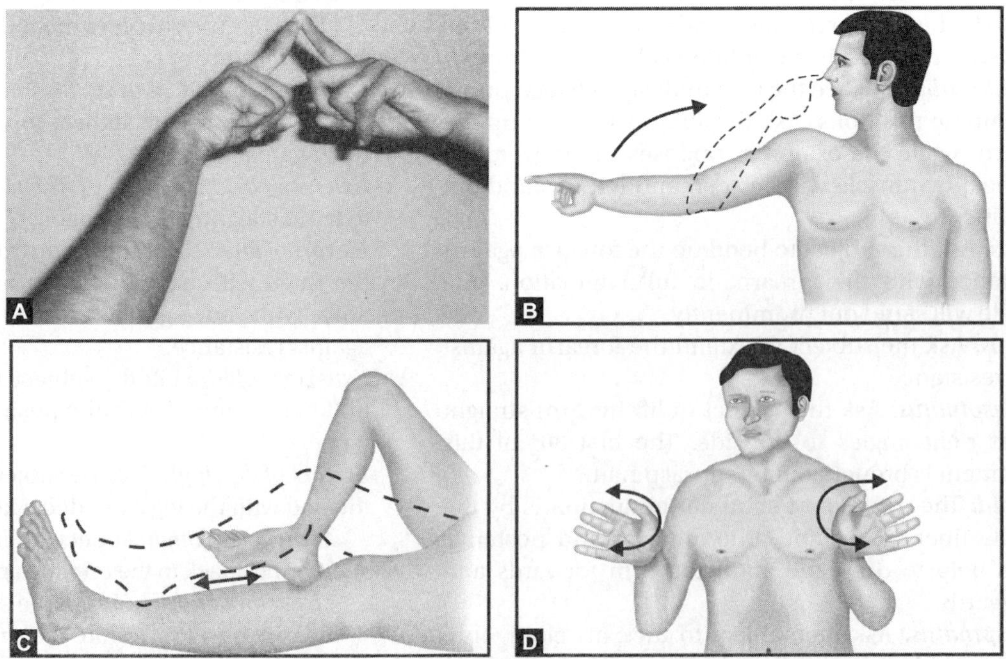

Figs 17A to D (A and B) Finger-nose test; (C) Hell-knees test; (D) Dysdiadochokinesia

EXAMINATION OF REFLEXES (FIGS 18A TO H)

Biodata

General examination:

Examination of nervous system—higher function

Examination of reflexes:

Reflexes are classified into three types: Superficial, deep and visceral/sphincteric reflexes.

Superficial reflex

a. *Conjunctival reflex:* Blinking of eyes on both sides
b. *Corneal reflex:* Blinking of eyes on both sides
c. *Pupillary reflex*
   Direct light reflex:
   Indirect light reflex:
   Accommodation reflex:
d. *Superficial abdominal reflexes:* Contraction of underlying abdominal muscles
e. *Plantar reflex:* Flexor plantar reflex on both sides
f. *Anal reflex:* Not tested
g. *Cremasteric reflex:* Not tested
h. *Bulbocavernosus reflex:* Not tested

Deep reflex

a. *Knee jerk:* Brief extension of knee, caused by contraction of quadriceps
b. *Ankle jerk:* Contraction of calf muscles
c. *Triceps jerk:* Contracts causing etension
d. *Biceps jerk:* Contracts causing flexion of elbow and supination of forearm
e. *Supinator jerk:* Sudden flexion and supination of forearm
f. *Jaw jerk:* Absent

Sphincteric reflexes:

Deglutition reflex: Normal
Micturition reflex: Normal
Defaecation reflex: Normal

Clonus

Patellar clonus: Not present
Ankle clonus: Not present

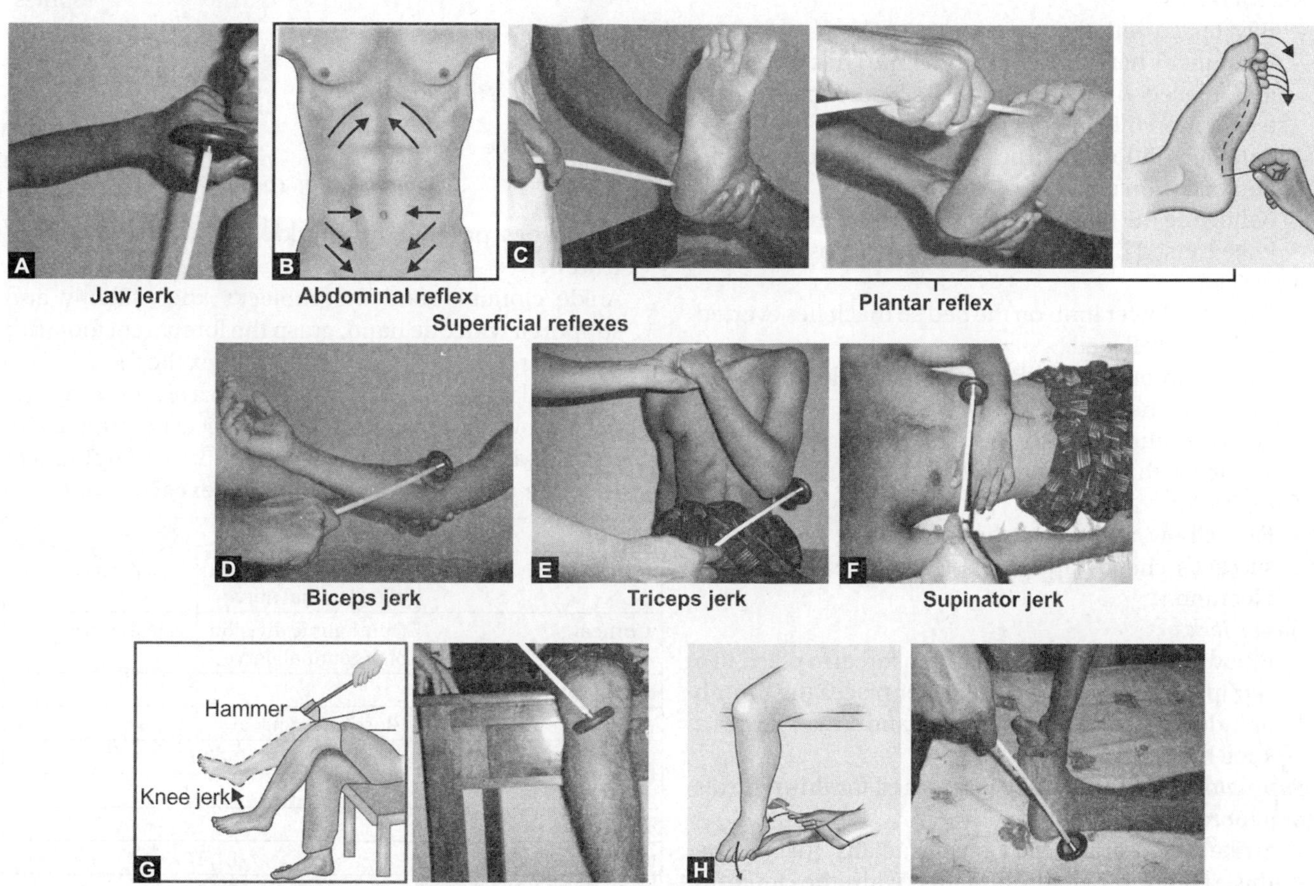

Figs 18A to H Examination of reflexes

Viva Questions

- **How does the following reflexes are demonstrated?**
  - *Superficial abdominal reflexes:* Ask the subject to lie relaxed in the supine position with abdomen uncovered. A light stimulus like a key is passed over the abdominal skin from outer aspect towards the midline. Contraction of underlying musculature is seen.
  - *Plantar reflex:* Muscles of the lower limb are relaxed, Outer segment of the sole of foot is stimulated by gently scratching with a key or stick from the heel towards the little toe and medially across the metatarsals up to the base of the big toe. In healthy adults even a slight stimulus produce contraction.
  - *Anal rellex:* Stroking or scratching of skin near anus produces contraction of anal sphincter.
  - *Cremasteric reflex:* Movements of testicle upwards when skin on the medial side of thigh is stroked.
  - *Bulbocavernosus reflex:* Pinching of glans penis produces contraction of the muscle.

  Knee jerk:
  - Best tested with the subject supine.
  - Examiner's hand is passed under the knee of subject and placed upon the opposite knee, knee to be tested is on the dorsum of examiner's wrist.
  - Patellar tendon is struck midway between origin and insertion with knee hammer.
  - Following the blow, there will be a brief extension of knee caused by contraction of quadriceps.

  Ankle jerk:
  - Place the lower limb on the bed so that it lies everted and slightly flexed.
  - Then with one band slightly dorsiflex the foot so as to stretch the Archilles tendon.
  - With the other hand strike the tendon on its posterior surface with a knee hammer.

  Triceps jerk:
  - Flex elbow and allow the forearm to rest on the subject's chest. Tap triceps tendon just above the olecranon.

  Biceps Jerk:
  - Elbow is flexed to right angle with forearm placd in a semipronated position. Examiner places the thumb or index finger on biceps tendon and strikes it with a knee hammer.

  Supinator jerk: The muscle concerned for this reflex is brachioradialis.
  - Strike the tendon of brachioradialis just above the styloid process of radius with the forearm semipronated and semiflexed at the elbow. There is sudden flexion and supination of forearm

  Jaw jerk: Ask the subject to open the mouth a little. Place one finger firmly on his chin. Then tap it with the other hand as in percussion. Contraction of the muscles that close the jaw occurs.

- **Explain the grading of tendon reflexes?**
  Tendon reflexes are graded as:
  0—Absent
  1—Present (as in normal ankle jerk)
  2—Brisk (as in normal knee jerk)
  3—Very brisk
  4—Clonus
- **What you meant by clonus (Figs 19A and B)?**
  When a muscle is subjected to a sudden continued stretch, a regular oscillation of contraction and relaxation occur, which is called clonus. Sustained clonus is abnormal and is an evidence of UMN lesion. Phenomenon is elicitable especially at the ankle.

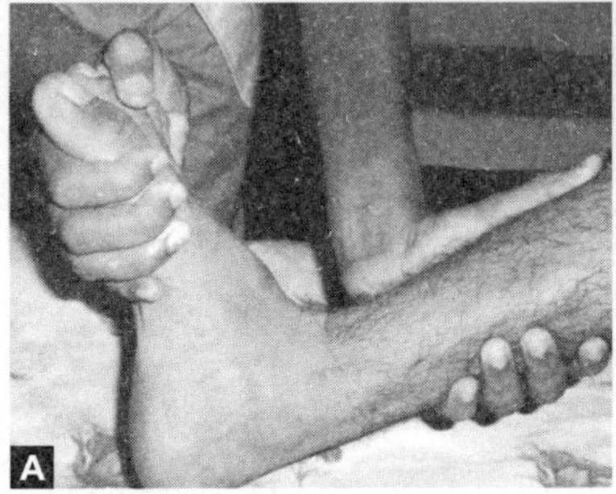

Ankle clonus

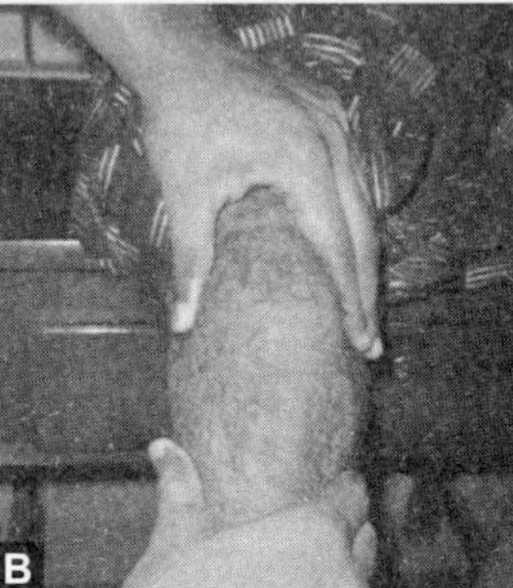

Patellar clonus

Figs 19A and B Clonus

- **How does patellar and ankle clonus are demonstrated?**
  Ankle clonus—bend the subject's knee slightly and support it with one hand, grasp the forepart of foot with the other hand and suddenly dorsiflex the foot.
  Patellar clonus is elicited by sharply pushing the patella towards the foot while the subject lies supine and relaxed with his knee extended and supported by the bed.
- **Give the neuronal pathways of reflexes?**

Reflex	*Afferent*	*Efferent*
Conjunctival reflex	Ophthalmic division of trigeminal nerve	Facial nerve
Corneal	Ophthalmic division of trigeminal nerve	Facial nerve
Pupillary		
Palatal	Glossopharyngeal	Vagus
Superficial abdominal	T7-T12	
Plantar reflex	L5, S1	
Anal reflex	S3, S4	
Cremasteric	L1, L2	
Bulbourethral	S3, S4	
Knee jerk	L2-L4	
Ankle jerk	S1, S2	
Triceps jerk	C6, C7	
Biceps jerk	C5, C6	
Supinator jerk	C5, C6	

EXAMINATION OF CRANIAL NERVES

Biodata

General examination:

Examination of nervous system—higher function:

Examination of cranial nerves:

Cranial nerve	*Cranial nerve testing*	*Right*	*Left*
Olfactory nerve	Test for sense of smell		
Optic nerve	Visual acuity		
	Distant vision		
	Near vision		
	Field of vision		
	Color vision (ishihara chart)		
	Presence of squint, nystagmus, and ptosis		
Occulomotor	Size and shape of pupil		
Trochlear	Ocular movements		
Abducent	Light reflex		
	Direct		
	Indirect		
	Accomodation reflex		
Trigeminal	*Test for sensory functions*		
	Sensation over face		
	Corneal reflex		
	Conjunctival reflex		
	Jaw jerk		
	Test for motor functions		
	Ask the patient to clench his teeth		
	Ask the patient to open his mouth		
Facial nerve	*Test for sensory function*		
	Taste sensation over anterior 2/3rd		
	Test for motor functions		
	Look for wrinkle over forehead		
	Ask the subject to close his eyes tightly and then tell him to open it against resistance		
	Look for nasolabial folds		
	Ask the subject to smile		
	Ask the subject to inflate both cheeks		
	Ask the subject to inflate both cheeks		
	Ask the subject to whistle		
Vestibulocochlear nerve	Watch test		
	Rinne's test		
	Weber's test		
	Schwabach's test		

Contd...

Contd...

Cranial nerve	*Cranial nerve testing*	*Right*	*Left*
Glossopharyngeal nerve	*Test for sensory functions*		
	Taste sensation over posterior 1/3rd		
	Sensation of mucous membrane of soft palate and palate		
	Test for motor functions		
	Pharyngeal reflex (gag reflex)		
Vagus nerve	Nasal regurgitation		
	Nasal tone to voice		
	Position of uvula		
	Dysphagia		
	Palatal reflex		
Spinal accessory nerve	Ask the subject to shrug his shoulders against resistance		
	Ask the subject to turn his head against resistance with a hand on side of face		
	Look for any deviation on protrusion of tongue		
Hypoglossal nerve	Movement of tongue		
	Look for any fasciculations, wasting and tremors of tongue		
	Look for protrusion of cheek on pushing with cheek		

Viva Questions

- **Demonstrate the tests done for examination of cranial nerves.**

  Olfactory nerve (Fig. 20)

  To test sensation of smell: Take three bottles containing oil of clove, oil of peppermint and tincture of asafoetida.

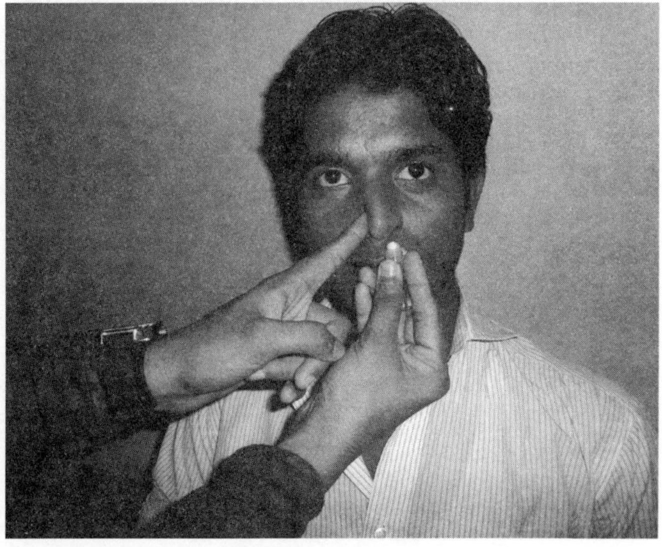

Fig. 20 Olfactory nerve

Ask the subject to close his eyes and present these to each nostril of the subject separately. Ask him to recognize them. Avoid using irritant substances as these may partially stimulate the trigeminal nerve.

Optic nerve (Fig. 21)

a. *Visual acuity:* Far vision is measured with Snellen's chart, in this a series of letters of varying size are constructed so that the top letter is visible to the normal eye at 60 m and subsequent lines at 36 m, 24 m, 18 m, 12 m, 9 m, 6 m, and 5 m respectively. Visual acuity (V) is recorded according to the formula.

   V = d/D Where, d = distance at which letters are read
   D = distance at which they should be read.

   The subject is placed at a distance of 6 m from the chart (d = 6).

   Test for near vrsion: Visual acuity at reading distance is assessed by using reading text types of varying sizes. Near vision is recorded as the smallest type which the person can read comfortably.

b. *Visual fields*

   Confrontation test: The subject is seated opposite the exarniner at a distance of about 1 m from him. If the subjects right eye is to be tested his left eye is covered and he is asked to look steadily at the examiner's left eye. The examiner should cover his right eye with the hand and gaze steadily at the subject's right eye. Then the examiners left hand is held up in a plane midway between the patient's face and his own at almost a full arm's length to the side. The hand is brought nearer while moving the fingers until the examiner can just see the movements of the fingers with the tail of his eye. Ask the subject whether he can see the movements while fixing his gaze on examiners eye. If he fails to see the fingers, keep bringing the hand nearer until he can see them. Test the field in this manner in each direction, upwards, downwards to the right and to the left. Test the other eye in the same way.

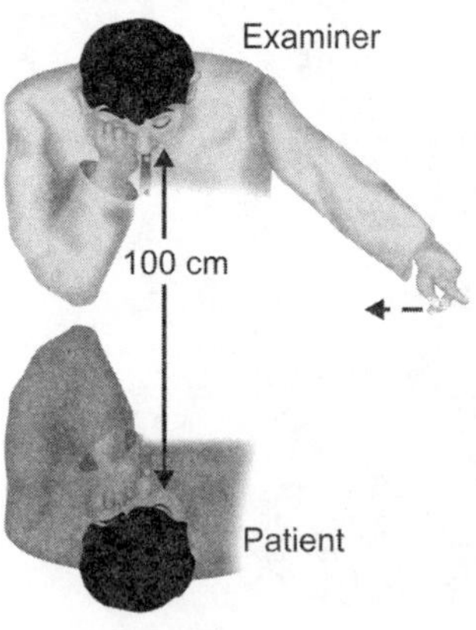

Figs 21 Optic nerve

   Perimetry: Instrument used to measure the monocular field of vision and can be used to assess the visual fields.

c. *Color vision:* Most easily tested (using Ishihara's charts). People with defective color vision confuse certain colors. Ishihara's charts are so constructed that a person with abnormal color vision will read a different number from a normal person on the same color plate.

Oculomotor, trochlear and abducent nerves

These three nerves are tested together because they function as a physiological unit in the control of ocular movements. The trochlear nerve innervates the superior oblique muscle and abducent nerve innervates the lateral rectus. All the other extraocular muscles, sphincter pupillae and levator palpebrae superioris are supplied by the oculomotor nerve.

Ocular movements: Look for horizontal movements adduction and abduction and vertical movements elevation and depression. Intorsion and extorsion are involuntary and so cannot be tested. Recti act as depressors and elevators when the eye is in abduction and the oblique act as elevators and depressors when the eye is in adduction. Medial and lateral recti act directly in single plane.

Look for the presence of squint or ptosis (Figs 22A and B). In abducent nerve lesion the person is unable to move the eye outwards and diplopia will be present on looking in that direction. In trochlear nerve lesion downward movements of eye in adducted position is lost. In complete oculomotor palsy there is ptosis and eye is displaced downwards and outwards.

Pupil: Size, shape and mobility of pupils are studied.

Size: Compare the size of the pupils first in bright light and then in dim light.

Shape: Note whether the pupil is circular or whether its contour is irregular.

Direct light reflex: The subject is seated in an indirectly illuminated place. Ask him to look into the distance. Each eye is examined separately. Shine a bright light into the eye to be tested. The pupil should constrict almost immediately. When the light is switched off, the pupıl will rapidly dilate to its previous diameter.

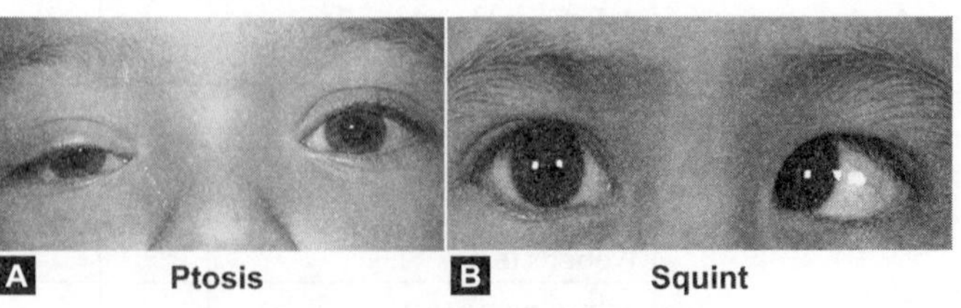

Figs 22A and B 3, 4, 6th nerves

Indirect light reflex (Consensual light reflex): Keep one eye shaded. Shine a bright light into the other eye. The pupil of the shaded eye is also seen to contract.

Reaction to accommodation: Hold up one finger close to the subject's nose. Ask him to look away at a distant object and then to look quickly at your finger. As the eyes converge to accomplish this, the pupils become smaller.

Trigeminal nerves

Test for sensory functions

1. Test for touch pain and temperature sensations on both sides of the face.
2. *Corneal reflex:* Tested using a bit of cotton twisted into a fine hair. Ask the subject to gaze into a distance and lightly touch the lateral end of the cornea at its conjunctival margin with the cotton wisp. If the reflex is present, the subject blinks. The cornea should not be wiped with cotton and central part of cornea should never be touched.
3. *Conjunctival reflex:* A bit of cotton is used to touch the conjunctiva. This results in closure of the eye.

Test for motor functions

1. Ask the subject to clench his teeth. Feel for the contraction of the masseter and temporalis on both sides. They stand out with equal prominence on both sides. If there is paralysis on one side, the muscles on that side will fail to become prominent.
2. Ask the subject to open his mouth. If there is paralysis on one side, on opening the mouth, the jaw will deviate towards the paralyzed side. This is because the paralyzed side is being pushed over by the healthy lateral pterygoid muscle.

Facial nerve (Figs 23A and B)

1. Ask the subject to shut his eyes as tightly as he can. Then examiner tries to open the eyes while the subject attempts to keep them closed. If the orbicularis oculi is acting normally, it is impossible to make the eyes open with normal effort. In paralysis of orbicularis the closure of eye is not normal.
2. Ask the subject to look upward without moving his head. Look for wrinkling of the forehead.
3. Ask the subject to smile or show his upper teeth. In facial nerve lesion, there is deviation of angle of mouth to normal side.
4. Ask the subject to whistle.
5. Ask the subject to inflate his mouth and blow-out his cheeks. The examiner tries to press on the cheeks. Air escapes easily on the weak or paralyzed side.
6. Test the sense of taste on the anterior 2/3rd of tongue by placing strong solution of sugar or salt using a rod on the surface of the tongue. Ask the person whether he can appreciate its taste before withdrawing the tongue to his mouth.

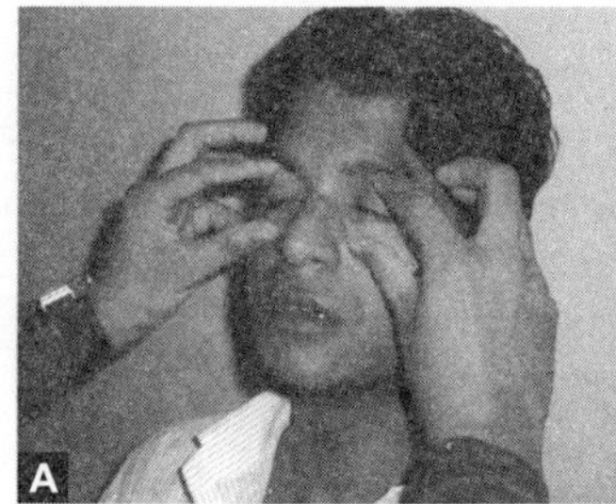

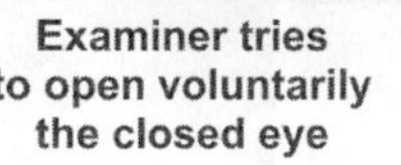
Examiner tries to open voluntarily the closed eye

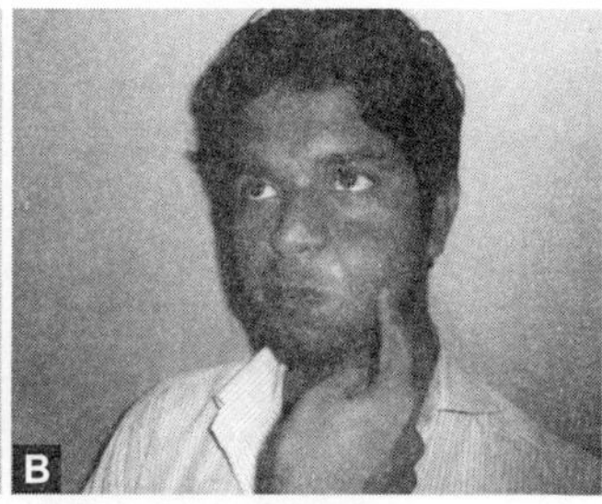

Examiner pressing over the blowed cheek

Figs 23A and B Facial nerve

Vestibulocochlear nerve (Figs 24A to C)

1. *Watch test:* Ask the subject to shut his eyes. Close the opposite ear. Place a sound source such as wrist watch at the probable range of hearing. Bring it gradually nearer to the ear. Ask the subject to tell whether he can hear it or not.
2. *Tuning fork test (frequency of tuning fork - 256):* The hearing impairment can be either due to defect of the nerve or of middle ear. Differentiation can be made by tuning fork test.
   a. *Rinne's test:* Place the charged tuning fork over the mastoid process. When it becomes inaudible, bring it close to the ear and ask the subject whether he can hear the sound. Normally, it can be heard, i.e. air conduction is better than bone conduction. In middle ear diseases bone conduction is greater than air conduction. In neurological damage, both bone and air conduction are impaired.
   b. *Weber's test:* Place the base of a sounding tuning fork at the middle of the forehead. The conducted sound through the bone is heard in both ears with equal intensity in normal persons. If there is middle ear disease, the sound through the bone is better heard on the side of lesion.
   c. *Absolute bone conduction test (Schwabach test):* Place the base of the sounding tuning fork on the mastoid process of the subject. Ask him to tell when the sound dies off. Immediately place the base of the tuning fork on the examiner's mastoid process. If the examiner can still hear the sound, absolute bone conduction is reduced in the subject, there is some sensorineural loss. If the patient's hearing is better, there is some conduction defect.

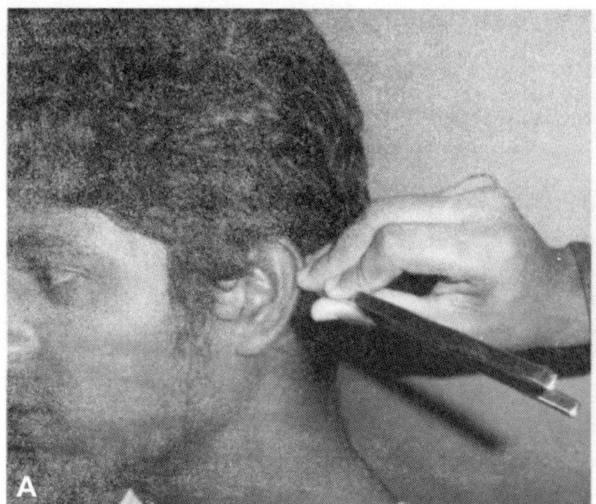
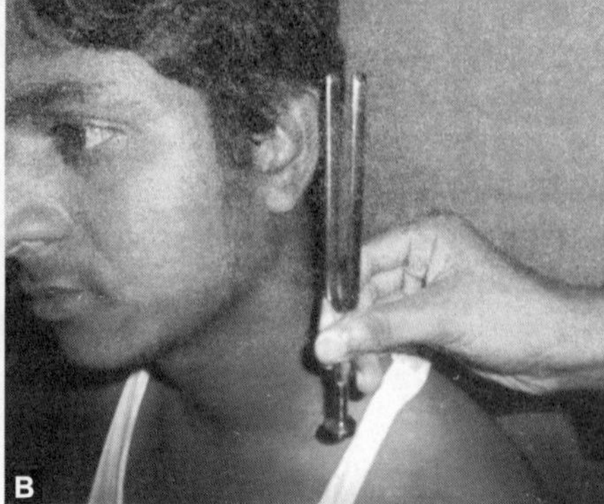
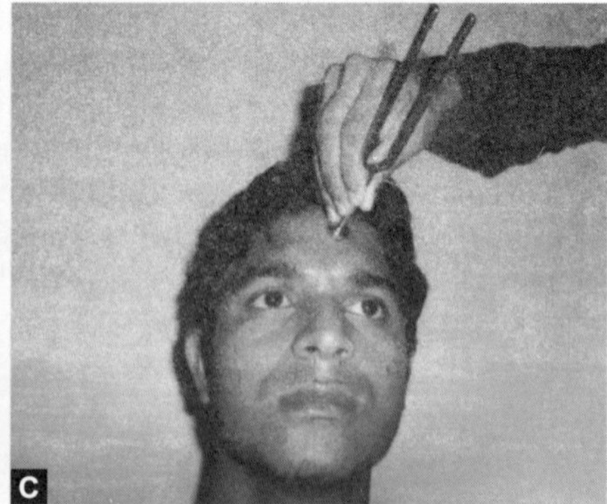

Figs 24A to C Vestibulocochlear nerve. (A and B) Rinne's test; (C) Weber's test

Glossopharyngeal nerve

Test for sensory function

Test the taste sensation on the posterior 1/3rd of tongue.

Test for motor functions

Test the gag reflex or pharyngeal reflex by touching the posterior part of the pharynx with a swab.

Vagus nerve

1. Ask the patient whether there is nasal regurgitation or history of dysphagia.
2. Observe whether there is any nasal tone to the voice. Check the ability to say words like 'egg' and 'rub' which require complete closure of nasopharynx.
3. Ask the subject to open his mouth. See the position of uvula. Normally it is in the midline.
4. Ask the subject to say 'ah' and see if the palate arches upwards. If the vagus on one side is affected the palate on that side and the median raphe is pulled towards the healthy side.
5. Test for palatal reflex. Touch the palate with the tip of a twisted cotton wool.

Spinal accessory nerve (Figs 25A and B)

1. Stand behind the subject and ask him to shrug his shoulders against resistance. Then trapezius becomes prominent.
2. Ask the subject to tum his face towards the opposite side, while resistance is offered to the chin. The sternomastoids become prominent.

Hypoglossal nerve (Figs 26A and B)

1. Ask the subject to put out his tongue as far as possible. In XII nerve palsy, tongue will deviate to the paralyzed side.
2. Ask the subject to move his tongue from side to side and push each cheek with it. Also do it against resistance.
3. See whether there is any wasting of tongue.
4. Look for fibrillation and fasciculations of the tongue. The fasciculations should be noted with the tongue relaxed in the mouth.

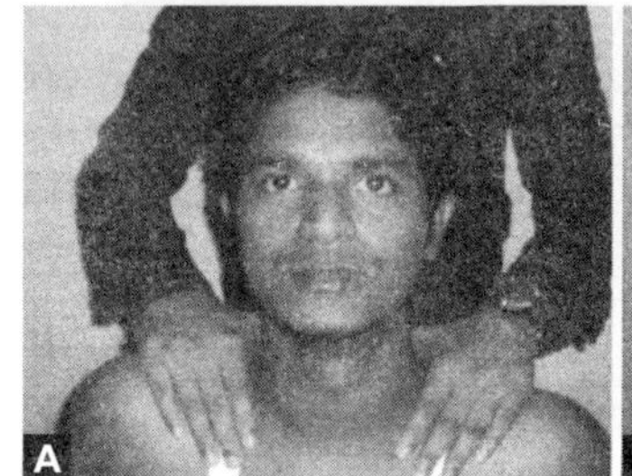
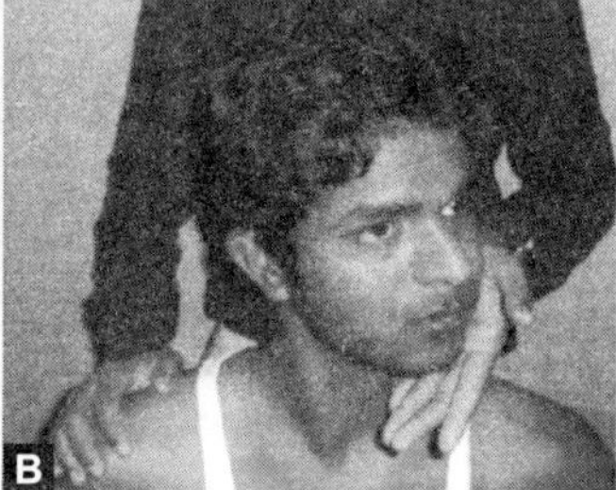

Figs 25A and B Spinal accessory nerve

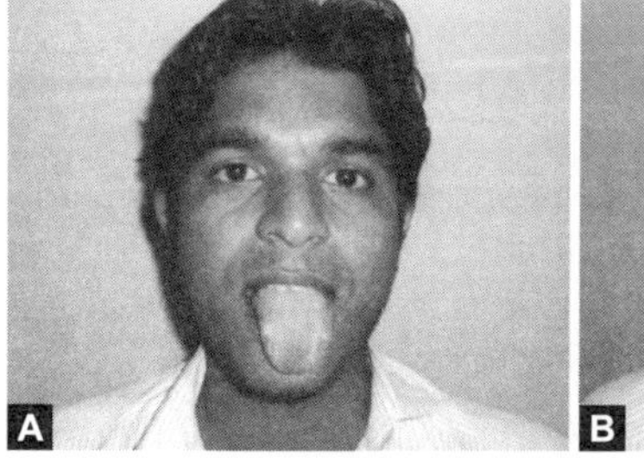
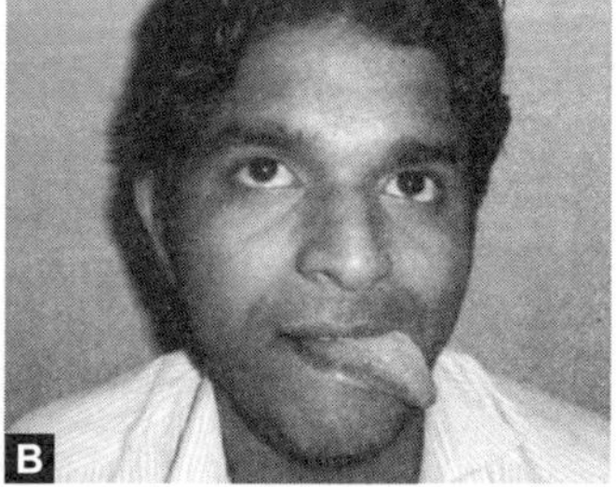

Examination of tongue

Figs 26A and B Hypoglossal nerve

Objective Structured Practical Examination (OSPE)

Planning for OSPE incudes making the valid, appropriate and important questions, and preparing an accurate checklist suitable for evaluating the students performance.

1. **Human arterial blood pressure**
   Record the effect of standing,on blood pressure of the given subject and report your findings.
2. **Respiratory system**
   - Clinically assess the expansion of the lower part of the chest.
   - Elicit vocal fremitus from the infraclavicular region of the chest of the given subject and report your findings.
   - Elicit vocal resonance from the infraclavicular region of the chest of the given subject.
   - Percuss the infraclavicular region of the chest of the given subject and report your findings.

3. **Cardiovascular system**
   - Locate the apex beat of the subject and report your findings
   - Examine the neck veins of the subject and report your findings
   - Auscultated the apex beat of the subject and report your findings.
4. **Examination of sensory motor system**
   - Elicit touch sensation of anterior aspect of the forearms of the subject and report your findings
   - Elicit crude touch sensations of the anterior aspect of the forearms of the subject and report your findings
   - Elicit two point discrimination of anterior aspect of the right forearm of the subject and report your findings.
5. **Examination of motor system**
   - Measure the bulk of the muscle of the right arm of the subject.
   - Assess the tone of the flexors and extensors of the right elbow of the subject.
   - Assess the strength of the biceps muscles of the right side of the subject.
   - Elicit biceps jerk of the right side of the subject.
   - Elicit triceps jerk of the right side of the subject.
   - Elicit triceps jerk of the right side of the subject.
   - Elicit right side supinator jerk of the jerk.
   - Elicit knee jerk of the right side in supine position of the subject.
   - Elicit ankle jerk of the right side in supine position of the subject.
   - Elicit plntar reflex of the subject.
   - Elicit abdominal reflex of the subject in the supine position.
   - Perform finger nose test of the subject.
   - Perform heel-knee test of the subject in supine position.
6. **Examination of cranial nerves**
   - Check the acuity of vision of the subject by confrontation test.
   - Examine III, IV and VI cranial nerves of the subject and report your findings.
   - Examine VII cranial nerves of the subject and report your findings.
   - Examine IX cranial nerves of the subject and report your findings.
   - Examine XII cranial nerves of the subject and report your findings.

AMPHIBIAN EXPERIMENTS

SIMPLE MUSCLE TWITCH (FIG. 27)

Aim

To record a simple muscle twitch.

Principle

A single induction shock passed into the nerve results in a momentary twitch like contraction of muscle followed by relaxation. The graphic record of contraction and relaxation of a voluntary muscle is known as a simple muscle twitch. A standard simple muscle twitch is 7–9 cm in amplitude. It has got a point of stimulation (PS), point of contraction (PC), point of maximum contraction (PMC), and point of relaxation (PR). Total duration is 0.1 sec. There is a latent period, contraction period and a relaxation period and a few shatter curves in each twitch.

Observation

Application of a single adequate stimulus causes a single brief contraction of the muscle followed by relaxation. The contaction does not begin immediately after application of stimulus, but after a brief interval, i.e. the latent period.

Viva Questions

- **What is latent period? Causes for LP?**
  It is the period between the point of stimulation and the point of contraction.
  Normal value: 0.01–0.012 sec.
  Causes:
  1. The time taken for the generation of the impulse
  2. The time taken for the impulse to travel along the nerve fiber
  3. Neuromuscular delay
  4. The time taken for the impulse to spread along the muscle fibers
  5. Mechanical inertia of the lever.

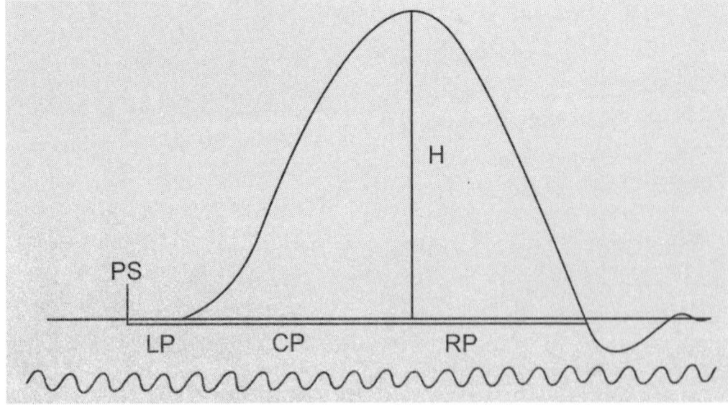

Fig. 27 Graph for simple muscle twitch

- **What are the factors influencing LP?**
  1. The point where the electrode is placed
  2. Increase in temperature shortens the latent period
  3. Increase in pH increase the latent period
  4. Increases latent period.
- **What is contraction period?**
  It is the period between the point of contraction and the point of maximum contraction.
  Normal value: 0.04 sec.
- **What are the factors influencing CP?**
  1. Fatigue increases the contraction period
  2. Increase in temperature shortens contraction period.
- **What is relaxation period?**
  It is the period between the point of maximum contraction and the point of relaxation.
  Normal value: 0.05–0.06 sec.
- **What are the facors affecting contraction period?**
  1. Fatigue increase the relaxation period
  2. Increase in temperature shortens relaxation period.
- **What you meant by amplitude?**
  It is the height of the curve and it depends on:
  1. Initial length of the muscle fiber.
  2. Intensity of stimulus.
  3. Distance of fulcrum from the point of tying the thread.
  4. Fatigue of the muscle decreases the amplitude.
- **Chart the differences between isometric and isotonic muscle contraction?**

Isometric	*Isotonic*
The muscle is not allowed to shorten, i.e. contraction of muscle without shortening	The muscle shortens in length depending on the load
The recording of simple muscle twitch shows no change in latent period. But there is much longer contraction and relaxation period	There is no change in latent period. Contraction and relaxation periods are shortened
The tension developed is greater and depends on strength of stimulus	The tension developed is comparatively less and depends on load applied
The muscle does no work	The muscle does the work
Heat produced is more	Heat produced is less
For example, contraction of the postural muscles against gravity	For example, lifting up a weight with the hand, there is shortening of biceps

EFFECT OF TWO SUCCESSIVE STIMULI ON MUSCLE CONTRACTION (FIGS 28A AND B)

Aim

To study the efect of successive stimuli on muscle contraction.

Observation

When the second stimulus is applied after the relaxation period of the first one, the second curve obtained is of higher amplitude. This is called beneficial effect.

Inference

In skeletal muscle, the second stimulus is effective during relaxation period and contraction period, but ineffective during latent period.

Viva Questions

- **What are the different causes of beneficial effect?**
  1. Rise in temperatue due to metabolic reactions. The temperature increases and the chemical reactions are speeded up. These changes occur readily in the second contraction and so the amplitude increases.
  2. *Viscoelastic changes:* These occur during the first contraction. It will not come to the original state before the second contraction. Elasticity is increased and viscosity is decreased. These also help the second contraction.
  3. During the first contraction glycogen is converted to lactic acid. So the pH decreases and the muscle contracts more rapidly.

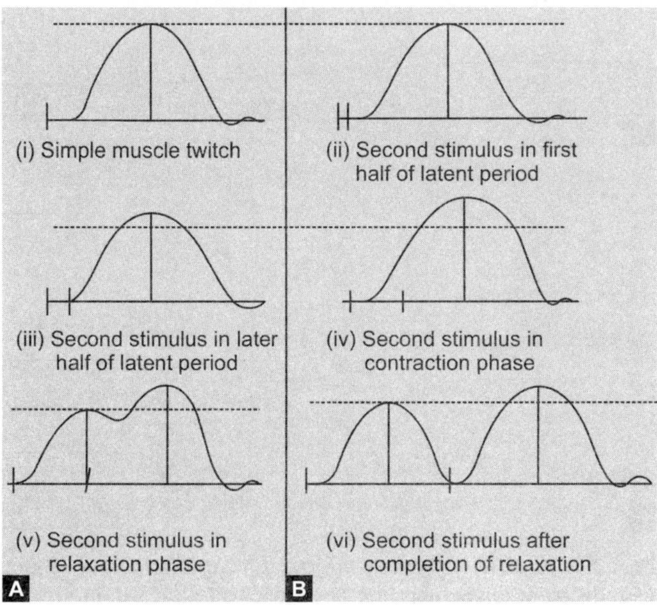

Figs 28A and B Effect of two successive stimulation

- **What you meant by superposition (Fig. 28A)?**
  When the second stimulus falls during the relaxation period, the second curve obtained is superimposed on the first. The second contraction will be of higher amplitude.
- **What is summation?**
  This results when the second stimulus falls during the contaction period of the first. The effects of the two stimuli are fused together and leads to a forceful contraction. The curve has a higher amplitude and a broader base than the normal curve and also it has 2 points of stimulation.
  There are two types of summation.
  1. Wave/temporal summation
  2. Multifiber/quantal summation.

  Wave summation: The stimuli are of same strength but the frequency of stimuli are increased and the contractions are fused.
  Quantal summation: The strength is increased, so that the number of motor units contracting is increased.
- **What you meant by refractory period?**
  Refractory period is the period after the application of the first stimulus during which a second stimulus of adequate strength fails to produce a response. In skeletal muscle the refractory period is less than .005 sec and is represented by the early part of latent period in the simple muscle twitch.
- **What are different types of refractory periods?**
  1. Absolute refractory period is the period during which a second stimulus will not produce response, whatever be the intensity of the stimulus.
  2. *Relative rcfractory period:* It is the period during which a second stimulus of stronger intensity can produce a response.
- **What is the effect, when 2nd stimulus applied on the contraction phase of cardiac muscle (Fig. 28B)?**
  In cardiac muscle no effect is seen when the second stimulus is applied during contraction poiod. This is because in cardiac muscle, the whole of systole and early part of diastole is in absolute refractory period and the later part of diastole is in relative refractory period.

FATIGUE AND RECOVERY (FIG. 29)

Aim

To study the effect of repeated stimuli on muscle nerve preparation and to demonstrate the phenomenon of fatigue and recovery.

Observation

Amplitude of first few contractions increases due to beneficial effect. After that gradually the amplitude decreases

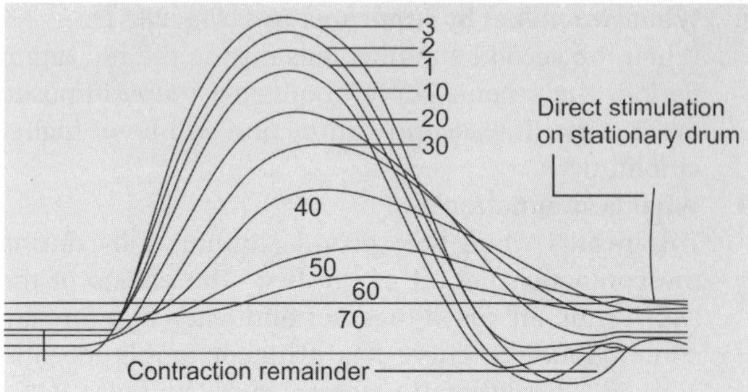

Fig. 29 Fatigue and recovery

and there is increase in latent period, contraction period and relaxation period. The last few curves fail to touch the baseline during relaxation period, this is contraction remainder. This is because of incomplete relaxation of muscle due to depletion of ATP.

Inference

Repeated stimulation causes fatigue of muscle. Site of fatigue is the neuromuscular junction in an isolated gastrocnemius—sciatic preparation. Fatigue is a reversible process.

Viva Questions

- **What you meant by the term 'fatigue'?**
  Fatigue is defined as the inability of muscle to respond to a stimulus following repeated stimulation. At this stage if the muscle is stimulated, it contracts showing that the muscle is not fatigued. By CRO it can be shown that the nerve is not fatigued. Thus nerve and muscle are not the sites of fatigue but the neuromuscular junction is the site of fatigue in muscle nerve preparation. By allowing the muscle nerve preparation to rest and by washing it with saline, recovery curve is obtained.
- **What are the different causes of fatigue?**
  1. Anoxia
  2. Accumulation of metabolic waste products like lactic acid. Small amounts of lactic acid increases excitability, but high concentrations decreases it.
  3. Depletion of acetylcholine
  4. Shortage of energy producing substances like glycogen, creatine phosphate, etc.
  5. Failure to re-establish the electrical potential due to repeated stimulation.
- **What are the different factors affecting fatigue?**
  Fatigue is enhanced by:
  1. Increasing the frequency of stimulation
  2. By application of load
  3. Increase in temperature
  4. Lack of O_2

  Factors favoring recovery:
  1. Giving rest
  2. Giving O_2
  3. Removal of waste products of metabolism.

EFFECTS OF AFTERLOAD AND FREELOAD ON MUSCLE CONTRACTION (FIGS 30A AND B)

Aim

To prove Starling's law (to understand the effect of freeload and afterload in muscle contraction).

Observation

With increase in load, the amplitude decreases. When work done is calculated, it is seen to increase with increase in weight up to a certain limit, then it decrcases. In freeload the contraction obtained for a given weight is of higher amplitude than that obtained for the same weight in afterload. This is because in freeload, the initial length of muscle is increased. So there is increase in force of contraction. This proves Starling's law. For example:

- *For freeload:* Throwing the ball in shot put.
- *For afterload:* Lifting a weight from the ground.

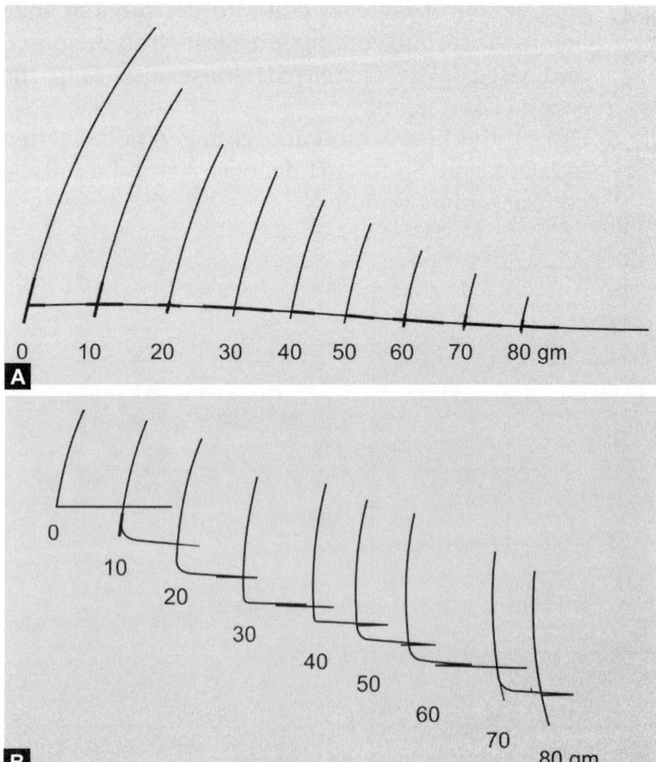

Figs 30A and B (A) Muscle contraction in afterload condition with different loads in grams; (B) Muscle contraction in preload (freeload) condition with different loads in grams

Inference

Starling's law is proved.

Viva Questions

- **Explain 'Starling's law'?**
  It states that the force of contraction is directly proportional to the initial length of muscle fiber within physiological limits.
- **Explain afterload?**
  It is load acting on the muscle after it starts contracting. It has no effect on the muscle before it contracts and so there is no initial stretching of the muscle fiber.
- **Explain freeload?**
  It is the load acting on the muscle even before it starts contracting. It will stretch the muscle fiber before it contracts.
- **How does Starling's law is proved in cardiac muscle?**
  This law is also applicable to cardiac muscle. When venous retum to the heart is increased, the end diastolic volume is increased. So there is an increase in the initial length of the muscle fiber and force of contraction is increased.

GENESIS OF TETANUS (FIG. 31)

Aim

To study the effect of repeated stimuli of various frequencies on muscle contraction.

Observation

- At a frequency of 5 vib/sec the individual contractions are recorded separately. Here the individual contractions fall only after the complete relaxation of the previous one. The subsequent ones will show beneficial effect.

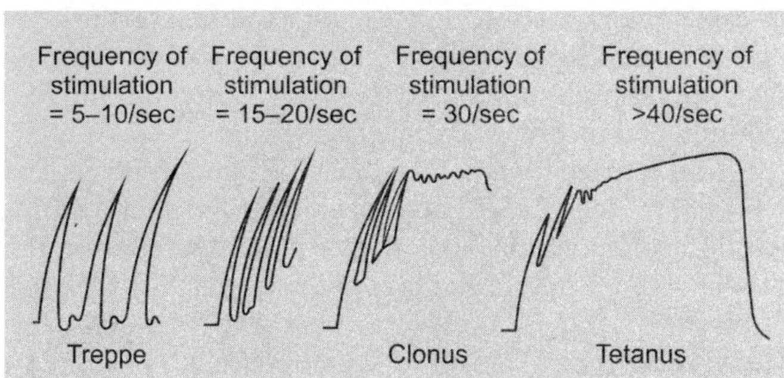

Fig. 31 Genesis of tetanus

- With a frequency of 7 vib/sec contractions are seen much closer but still separate.
- With a frequency of l0 vib/sec, the curves move still closer. The duration of one simple muscle twitch is 0.1 sec. So we do not get fusion of contractions up to a frequency of 10 vib/sec.
- At a frequency of 15 vib/sec, the curves do not touch baseline.
- At a frequency of 20 vib/sec, there is partial fusion of individual contractions. This is because of incomplete relaxation and curves do not touch the baseline. This is called clonus. Here the subsequent stimuli fall during the relaxation period of the previous one.
- At a frequency of 30 vib/sec, complete fusion of contractions takes place, thus producing a smooth sustained contraction called tetanus. Here the subsequent stimuli fall during the contraction period of previous one. Hence, there is mechanical fusion of the contractions.

Viva Questions

- **What you meant by the term 'clonus'?**
  It is incomplete tetanus where subsequent stimuli fall during relaxation period of the previous one. So the curves obtained will have a wavy appearance.
- **What is 'tetanus'?**
  It is a smooth sustained contraction due to mechanical fusion of curves. Here subsequent stimuli fall during contraction period of previous one, but electrical potentials are separate. Tetanus is not possible in cardiac muscle because the confection period is refractory and hence subsequent stimuli will have no effect.

  Minimum frequency at which tetanus occurs is called critical fusion frequency.
- **What is 'tetany'?**
  It is a clinical condition where there is a spasm of muscle due to hypocalcemia, alkalosis, etc.
- **What is the relation between critical fusion frequency (CFF) and contraction period?**
  The critical fusion frequency depends on duration of contraction period. It is inversely proportional to the contraction period of the muscle.

  In small muscles like thigh, calf muscles, etc. contraction period is long. So tetanus is produced by low frequency stimuli. Conditions which increase the contraction period such as cold, fatigue, etc, will decrease the CFF.

EFFECT OF TEMPERATURE ON MUSCLE CONTRACTION (FIG. 32)

Aim

To study the effect of variations of temperature on muscle contraction.

Observation

	With warm saline	*With cold saline*
Latent period	Decreased	Increase
Slope of contraction	Steeper	Not
Amplitude	Increase	Decrease
Contraction period	Decrease	Increase
Relaxation period	Decrease	Increase
	This is because at higher temperature the muscle's enzymatic and chemical changes are increased, conduction velocity is increased, elasticity is increased and viscosity is decreased	Decrease in the metabolic rate, decrease in conduction velocity, increase in viscosity and decrease in elasticity

Inference

With warm saline, latent period is decreased contraction period is dectease, relaxation period is decreased and amplitude is increased. With cold saline, latent period is increased, contraction period is increased, relaxation period is increased and amplitude is decreased.

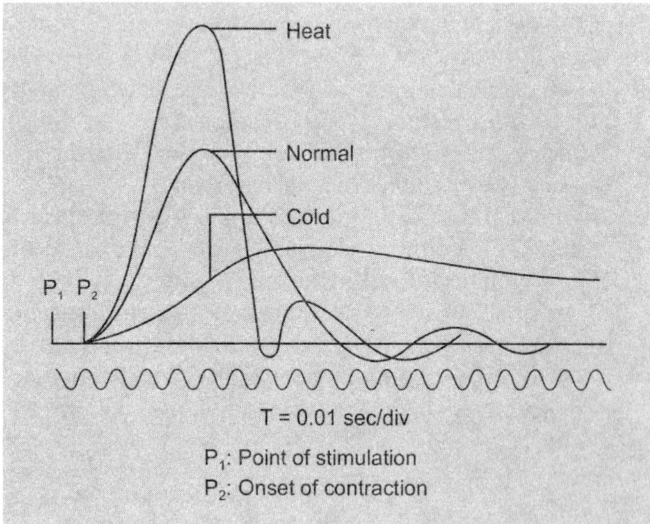

Fig. 32 Effect of temperature on muscle contraction

Viva Questions

- **What you meant by 'cold stiffening'?**
  With very low temperature the muscle fails to contract. This is known as cold stiffening, which is a reversible process.
- **What is 'heat rigor'?**
  At temperature above 42°C, the muscle proteins coagulate causing a condition known as heat rigor, which is an irreversible process.
- **What is 'rigor mortis'?**
  It is the postmortem stiffening. In the muscle which appears 1-2 hours after death. Rigor mortis first appear in the involuntary muscles and then in the voluntary muscles.

  In the voluntary muscles rigor mortis occurs in a definite course. It first occurs in the eyelids, next in the muscles of the back of the neck and lower jaw, then those of front of neck, face, chest, upper extremities, muscles of abdomen and lower extremities in that order. It appears last in the small muscles of the fingers and toes. It passes off in the same sequence.

NORMAL CARDIOGRAM OF FROG AND EFFECT OF TEMPERATURE ON FROG'S HEART (FIGS 33 AND 34)

Aim

To record normal cardiogram of frog's heart and to study the effect of heat and cold on sinus venosus and the ventricle.

Effect of Heat and Cold on Sinus Venosus and Ventricle

Record a normal cardiogram. Then heat the glass tube over the flame of the spirit lamp. Test the intensity of the heat by blowing over the back of your hand. Blow moderately warm air over the sinus venosus for about half a minute. Record the contraction, pour Ringer's solution on the heart and then record a normal cardiogram. Now blow warm air over the ventricle and record its effect. Again pour Ringer's solution and record a normal cardiogram.

Hold a small piece of ice near the sinus venosus and record the effect. Record normal cardiogram after washing with Ringer's solution. Hold the ice piece near the anterior aspect of the ventricle and record the effect.

Observation

Cardiogram is the recording of the mechanical activity of the heart. The heart rate is between 50-60/mt. The upstroke is due to systole with a small auricular component and a large ventricular component. The downstroke is due to diastole. Each beat is followed by a distinct pause.

	Effect of heat		*Effect of cold*	
	Sinus venosus	Ventricle	Sinus venosus	Ventricle
Heart rate	Increases	Remains same	Decreased	Remains same
Amplitude	Decreases	Increased	Increased	Decreased
Reason for change in HR	The rate is increased because the metabolism of sinus venosus is increased	The rate remains the same as the ventricle is not the pacemaker	Rate is decreased as the metabolism of sinus venosus is decreased	The rate remains the same as the ventricle is not the pacemaker
Reason for change in amplitude	As the rate increases filling time decreases and end diastolic volume decreases, so the initial length of the muscle fiber is decreased and hence the force of contraction is decreased (Starling's law)	The amplitude is increased as the metabolism of the ventricle is increased	When rate is decreased filling time is increased and end-diastolic volume is increased. Initial length of muscle fiber is increased and force of contraction is increased	Amplitude is decreased as the metabolism of the ventricle is decreased and force of contraction decreased

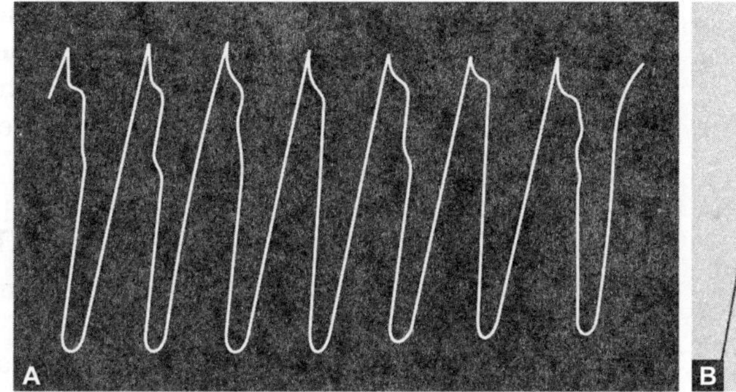

Record showing only atrial and ventricular events

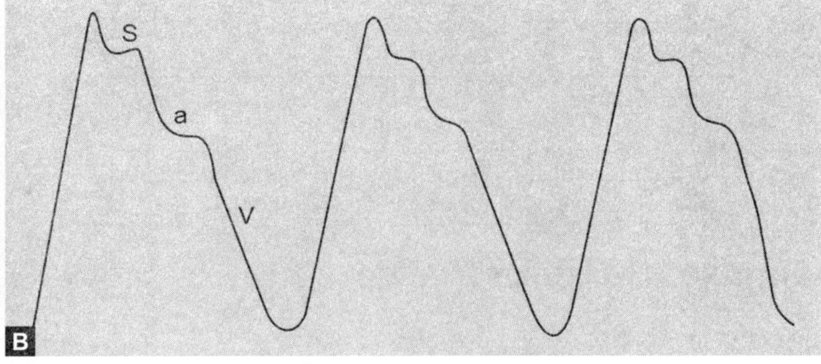

Record showing contractions of sinus (S), atria (a) and ventricle (V)

Figs 33A and B Normal cardiogram on frogs

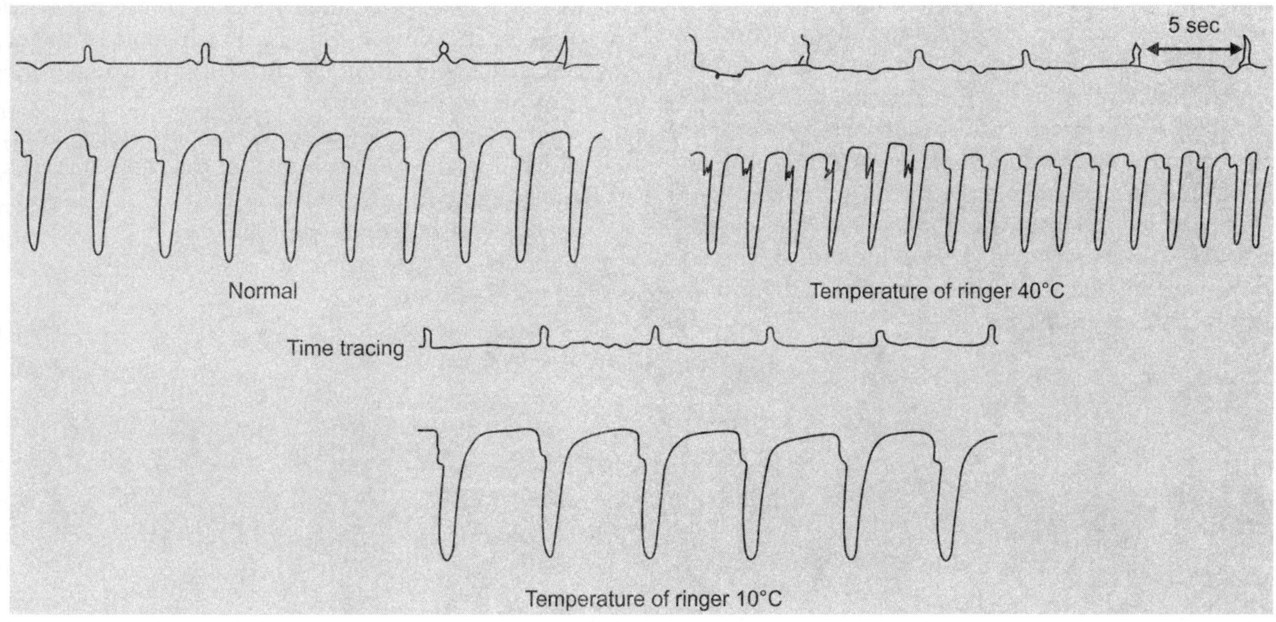

Fig. 34 Effect of temperature on normal cardiogram

Inference

Sinus venosus is the pacemaker of the heart and it controls the rate of the heart. The ventricles determine the force of contraction.

Viva Questions

- **What is the difference between mammalian heart and frog's heart?**

Frog's heart	*Mammalian heart*
Three chambered	Four chambered
Sinus venosus is the pacemaker of heart	SA node is pacemaker
Nutrition of the heart is from the surrounding tissue fluid	Nutrition is from the coronary blood vessels which supply the heart
Chamber perfusion	Coronary perfusion
Specialized conducting system is absent	Specialized conducting system is present
Ringer's solution is used in the experiment	Ringer-Locke solution is used in the experiment
Oxygen, pressure and temperature need not be maintained	Oxygen, pressure and temperature have to be maintained

STANNIUS LIGATURES (FIG. 35)

Aim

To study the mode of origin and transmission of cardiac impulses by applying ligatures.

Discussion

Application of ligature is an attempt to block the transmission of cardiac impulse from sinus venosus to auricles in the first ligature and from atria to venticles in the second ligature. After the first ligature, the heart stops except at the sinus venosus, due to the blockage of impulses coming from the sinus venosus. After some time, the atria and ventricle start contacting. This is the auricular rhythm.

When the second ligature is applied, the ventricle stops contracting whereas the auricles continue to contract. Later the ventricle starts to contract at its own rhythm. This is the idioventricular rhythm.

Inference

Sinus venosus is the pacemaker of frog's heart and ventricle can contact at its own rhythm.

Viva Questions

- **Why ligature experiments are not performed in mammals?**
  In mammals, SA node is situated in the posterior wall of the right atrium near the opening of superior vena cava. So the first ligature is not possible in mammalian heart. Similarly in the mammalian heart, coronary vessels are seen in the atrioventricular groove. So the blood supply to the heart will be stopped if the second ligature is applied. So the second ligature also cannot be applied to mammalian heart.
- **What are the important theories regarding impulse production?**
  - Myogenic theory is the most widely accepted theory. According to this impulses are produced within the cardiac muscle and it travels through the heart.
  - *Neurogenic theory:* According to this theory specialized nervous tissue is present in the cardiac muscle and is concerned with impulse production:
    a. Remak's ganglion situated in the white crescenteric line is mainly inhibitory in nature.
    b. Ludwig's ganglion is situated in the interatrial septum and inhibitory in nature.
    c. Bidder's ganglion in the atrioventricular groove which is also inhibitory.
- **What about the pacemaker of frog's heart and in mammals?**
  In frog's heart the sinus venosus is the pacermaker because the rate of impulse production in the sinus venosus is more than the atrial and ventricular rate. It controls the heart rate.

  In mammals, SA node is the pacemaker and it is situated in the posterior wall of the right atrium near the opening of superior vena cava.
  Average rate of impulse production:
  SA node—72/mt
  AV node—50/mt
  Venticle—30/mt.

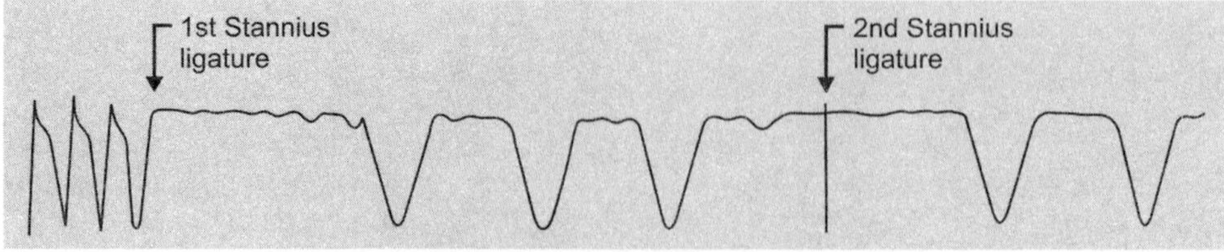

Fig. 35 Effects of Stannius ligature on frog's heart

EFFECT OF STIMULATION OF VAGUS NERVE ON FROG'S HEART (FIGS 36A AND B)

Aim

To demonstrate the effect of continuous stimulation of vagus nerve on ftrog's heart and the phenomenon of vagal escape.

Observation

With weak stimuli the heart may beat faster and more forcefully due to the excitation of sympathetic fibers present in the vagal trunk. With increase in the strength of stimuli, the heart beat becomes slower and weaker. Finally the heart stops in diastole. This is called vagal inhibition.

With continued stimulation of vagus, the heart starts beating at a slower rate in spite of the stimulation, which is the idioventricular rhythm. This phenomenon is called the vagal escape. Then stop the stimulation. The heart beats normally.

The parasympathetic supply to the heart is through the vagus. It has an inhibitory action on heart. In mammalian heart the right vagus supplies the SA node and the left vagus supplies the AV node and the rest of the conducting system. The ventricle gets the least supply.

Inference

Vagus has inhibitory effect on heart. But continuous stimulation can cause vagal escape.

Viva Questions

- **What is 'vagal escape'? What are the common causes of vagal escape?**
  It is the escape of the heart from the inhibitory effect of vagus.

  Causes:
  1. Depletion of acetylcholine due to continuous stimulation.
  2. *Idioventricular rhythm:* The lower 1/3rd of the venticle is not supplied by the vagus. So it starts contracting on its own even while the vagus is being stimulated.
  3. Stimulation of sympathetic fibers present in the vagal nerve.
- **What are the additional causes of vagal escape in an unpithed frog?**
  1. *Marey's law:* It states the heart rate is inversely proportional to blood pressure. When BP is low, the baroreceptors of the great vessels are stimulated, which cause an increase in heart rate.
  2. *Bainbridge reflex (cardioaccelerator reflex):* Whenever BP falls there will be pooling of blood in the right side of the heart, which results in the congestion of the right auricle. Receptors in the right atrium will respond to increase in pressure inside the atrium and send impulses though the vagus nerve to the cardioinhibitory center. The center responds by inhibiting the vagal tone. Thus heart rate increases and prevents pooling of blood in the veins, atrium and pulmonary circulation.
- **What you meant by 'vagal tone'?**
  The continuous inhibitory effect of vagus on heart in normal state is called vagal tone. In infants the tone is reduced. So the heart rate is increased. In the adults vagal tone is increased. So heart rate is less. The tone can be increased by training and experience as in athletes. Vagal tone can be abolished by the administration of atropine, which causes paralysis of vagus nerve. Vagal tone is maintained by the cardioinhibitory centers.

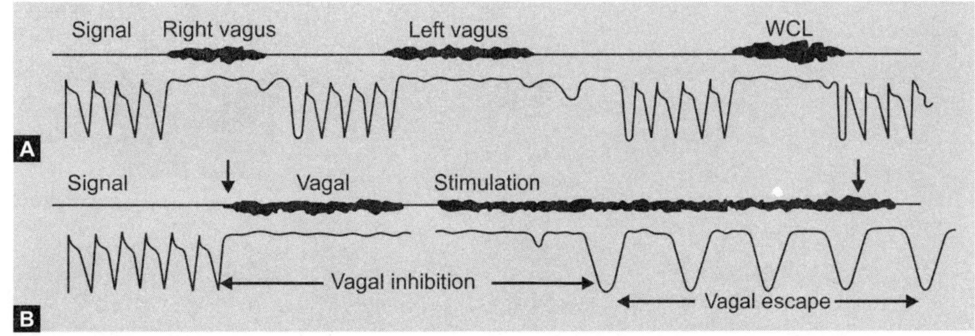

Figs 36A and B (A) Effect of electrical stimulation of vagosympathetic trunk and WCL; (B) Phenomenon of vagal escape

SPOTTERS

1. A young adult male has the following white cell count?
   Total WBC count: 12000/cu mm^3
   Differential count: Neutrophills: 82 percent
   Eosinophill: 2 percent
   Basophill: 0 percent
   Lymphocytes: 12 percent
   Monocytes: 4 percent
   a. Comment on these values?
   b. What can be the probable cause of the change from the normal pattern?
   c. What are the normal values?

Ans. Neutrophilia count increased in infection.

2. An 8-year-old boy presented to the outpatient department with profuse bleeding after dental extraction. On investigation, Hb—8 gm percent; BT—2 min; CT—15 min; platelet count—2 lakhs
   a. What is the probable diagnosis?
   b. Write its mode of inheritance?

Ans. Hemophilia (coagulation disorder).

3. In a test, the urine-creatinine concentration is 196 mg/mL. Plasma-creatinine concentration is 1.4 mg/mL and urine flow is 1 mL/min. What would be the creatinine clearance value?

Ans. Creatinine clearance—uv/p
$196 \times 1/1.4 = 140$

4. In a test the subjects inspiratory capacity is 3.3 Lt, FRC is 2.2 Lt, and the residual volume is 1.2 Lt. His body surface area is 1.5 m^2. Calculate the vital capacity and vital index?

Ans. Vital capacity—IRC + FRC – RV
$3.3 + 2.2 - 1.2 = 4.3$ Ltr
Vital index = VC × surface area
$4.3 \times 1.5 = 6.45$

5. Identify the given chart? What is the point indicated by 'A', 'B' and 'C'?

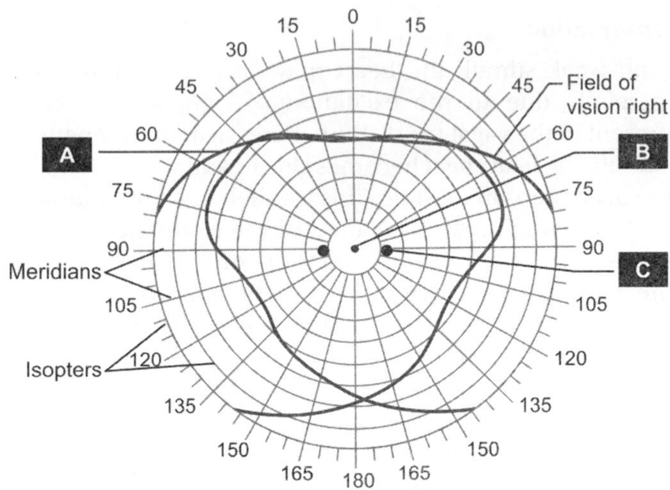

Ans. (A) Field of vision of eye; (B) Visual axis; (C) Blind spot.

6. A. What is the name of this endocrine disorder?
   B. What are the causes of this disorder?

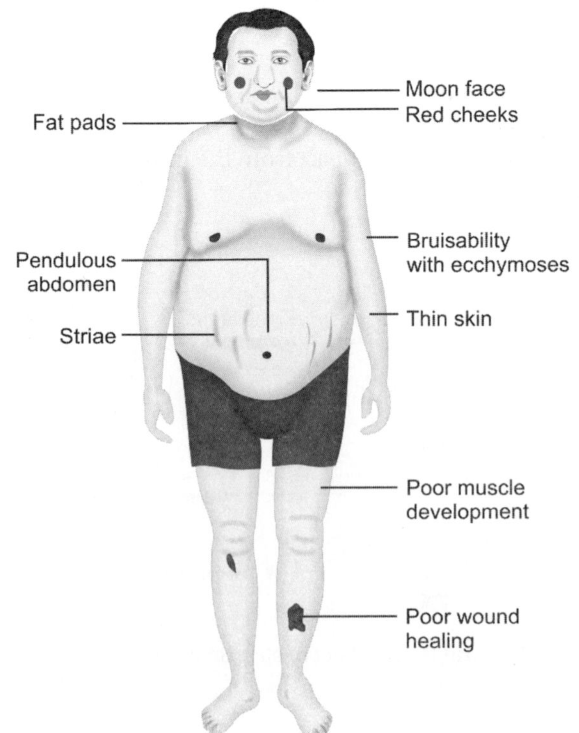

Ans. Cushing syndrome.

7. A. What is the duration of 'QRS' complex?
   B. What is meant by QT interval and its duration?

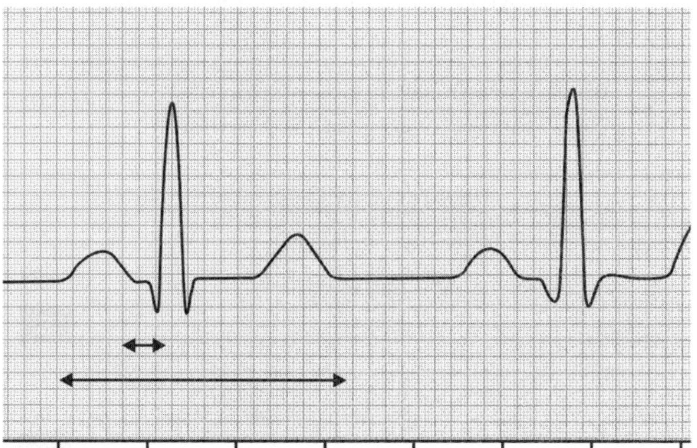

Ans. QRS complex—0.8 sec.
QT-time from the start of QRS complex to the end of T wave = 0.4 sec.

8. A. Name the volumes/capacities represented by A, B, C and D?
   B. Give the normal values of each?

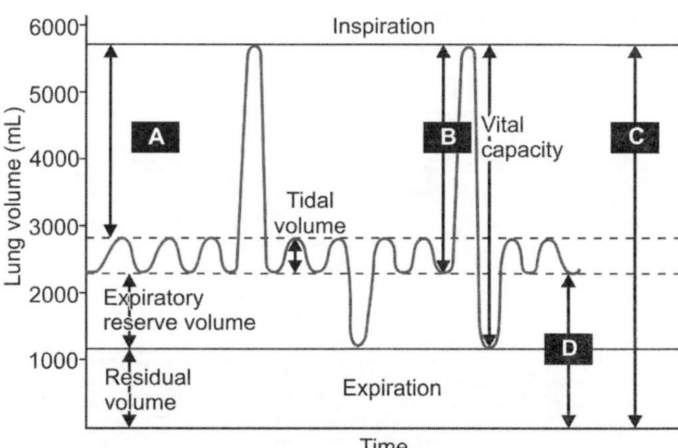

Ans. A—inspiratory reserve volume
B—inspiratory capacity
C—total lung capacity
D—functional residual capacity.

9. A. What is indicated by A and B?
   B. Their functions?

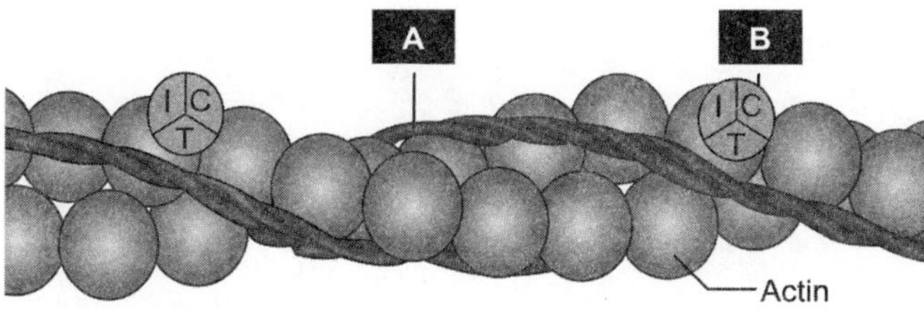

Ans. A—tropomyosin
B—troponin.

10. GFR rate of a patient is 125 mL/min and renal plasma flow is 625 mL/min then calculate the filtration fraction?

Ans. FF = GFR/RPF
125/625 = 0.2

11. A doctor can diagnose a patient by hearing the sound of the patient. What is the clinical condition? How does he diagnose?

Ans. Thyrotoxicosis

12. Calculate the heart rate of the patient from the given data?
R-R interval—20 mm
Speed of the paper—1500 mL/min.

Ans. 1500/20 = 75/min.

13. Calculate the MCH and MCHC of the patient from the given data:
Hb—12 gm percent
PCV—37 percent
RBC count—5 million cells/cu mm.

Ans. MCH = Hb g/L divided by RBC count/liter
MCHC=HB g% divided by PCV/100 mL.

14. A. Which pathway?
    B. What is the effect, when lesion occurs at 'A', 'B', 'C', and 'D'?

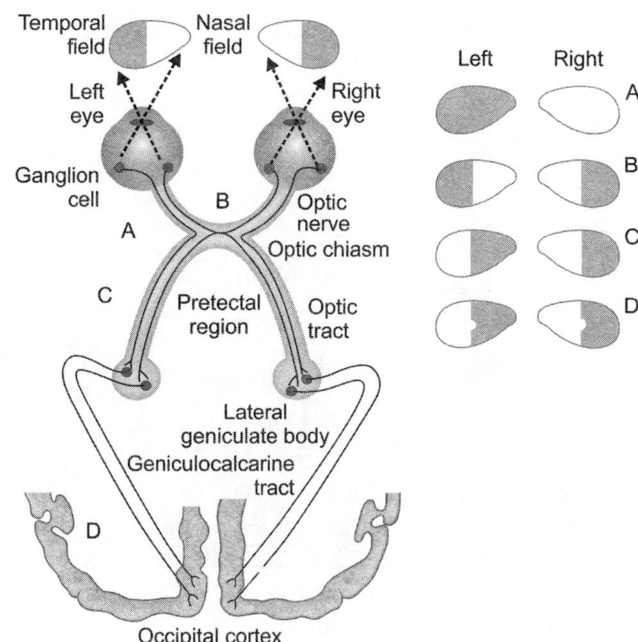

Ans. A—anopia at left side
B—bitemporal hemianopia
C—homonymous hemianopia
D—homonymous hemianopia sparing macula.

15. A. What is the diagram representing?
    B. Name the layers marked as A, B, C and D?

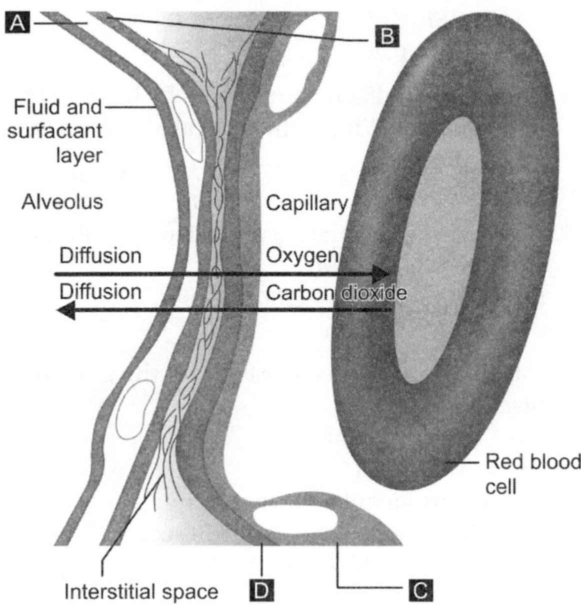

Ans. (A) Alveolar epithelium; (B) Epithelial basement membrane; (C) Capillary endothelium; (D) Capillary basement membrane.

16. (i). What is the structure shown in the given diagram?
    (ii). Identify the points A, B and C?

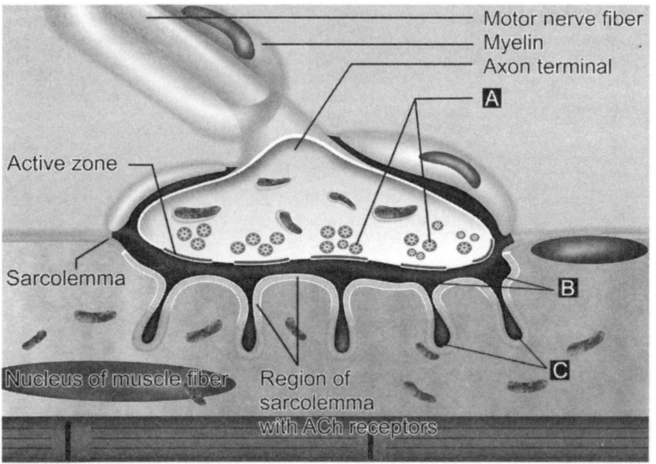

Ans. (i) Neuromuscular junction
(ii) A—synaptic vessicle
B—synaptic cleft
C—junctional folds.

17. Refer the graphs of amphibian experiments (questions can be asked by showing the amphibian charts).

Ans. Refer to page no. 206 (Amphibian Experiments).

18. A. This is a graphical representation of ________?
    B. Time at which each graph is produced?

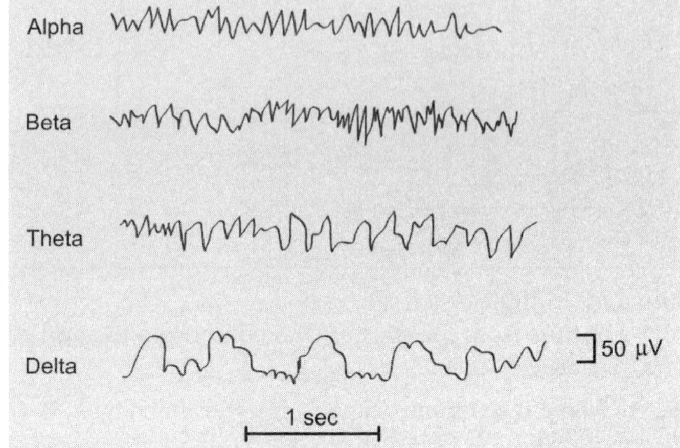

Ans. Electroencephalogram.

19. A. What is the diagram representing?
    B. Explain the theory?

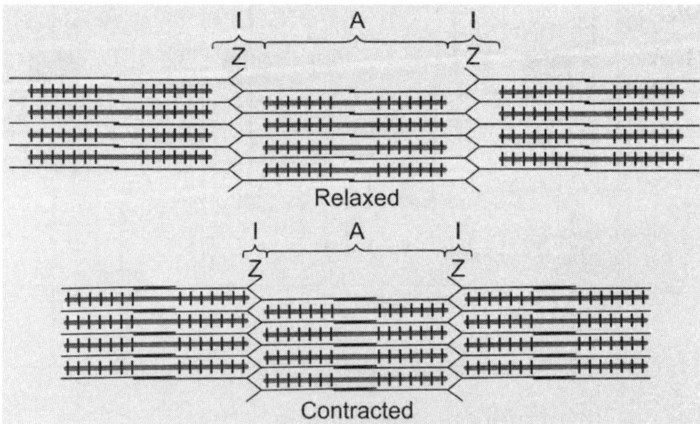

Ans. A—sarcomere.
B—sliding theory.

20. What is the diagram representing?

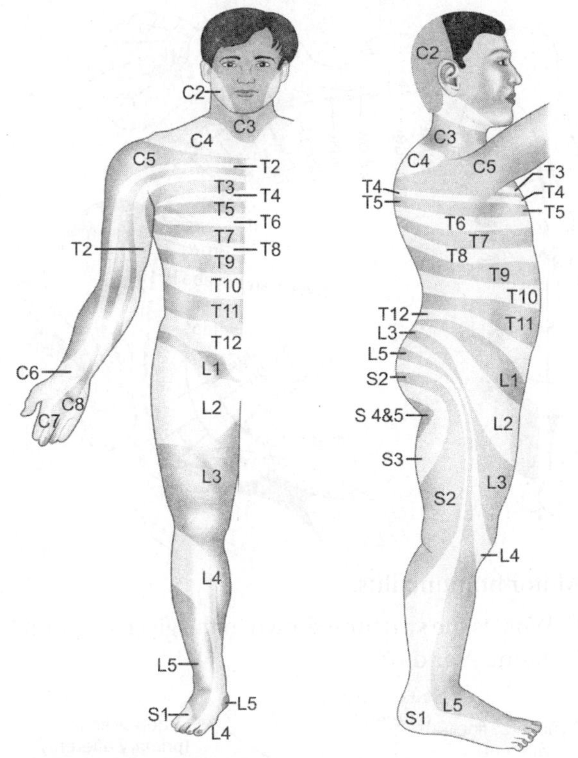

Ans. Dermatomes.

21. A. Which is the tract?
B. Importance of this tract?

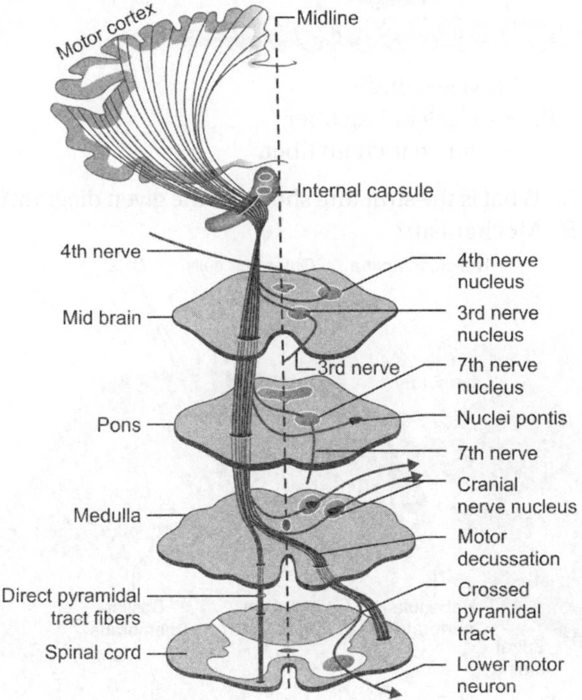

Ans. A. Pyramidal/corticospinal tract.
B. Main motor pathway.

22. What is the structure shown in the given diagram?

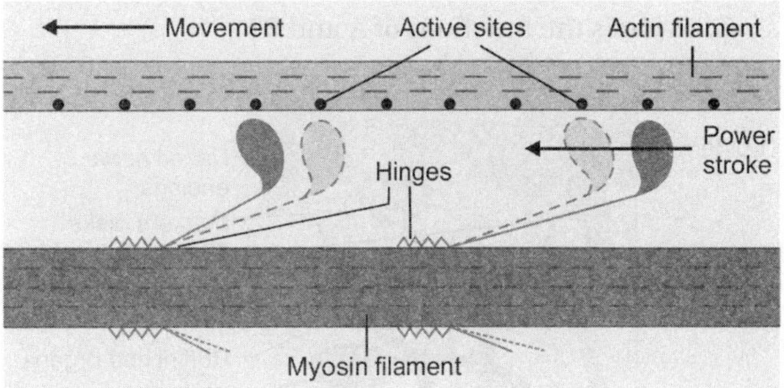

Ans. Walk along theory.

23. What is the structure shown in the given diagram?

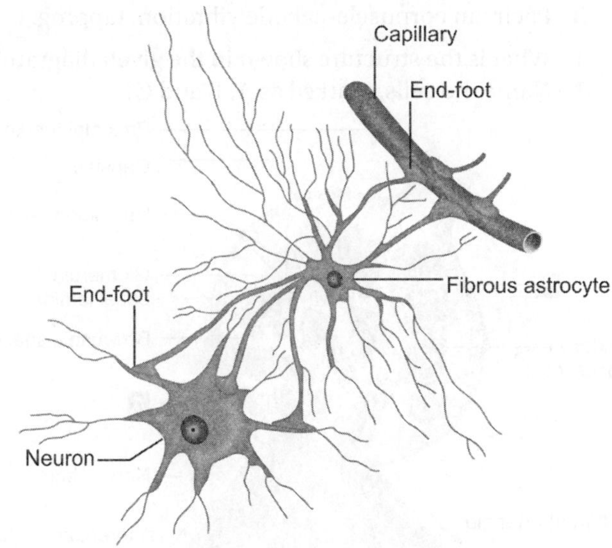

Ans. Astrocyte.

24. What is the structure shown in the given diagram?

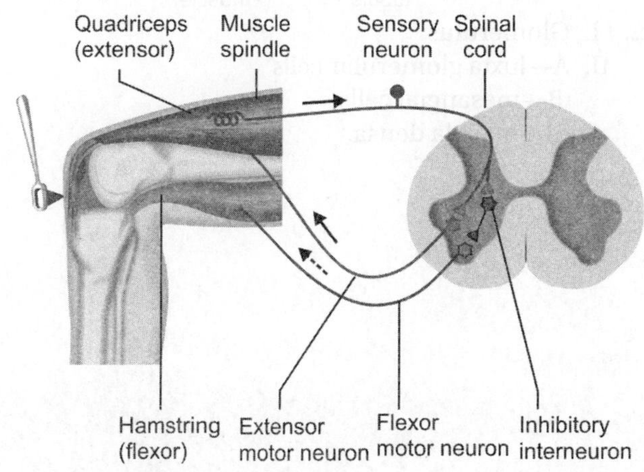

Ans. Reflex arc.

25. A. What is the structure shown in the given diagram?
    B. What is A and B?
    C. What is the functions of A and B?

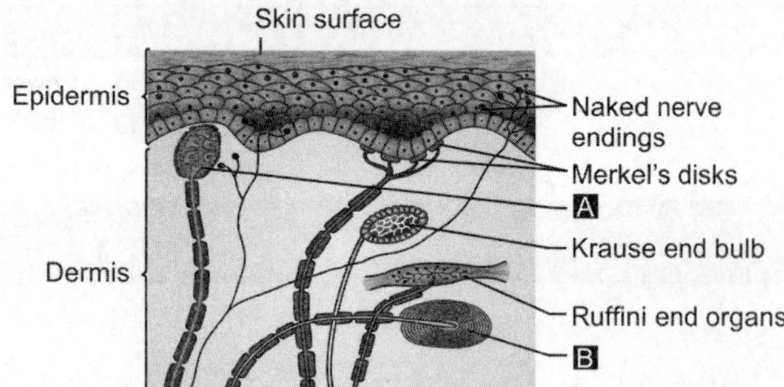

Ans. A. Meissner's corpuscle-encode speed of stimulus application.
B. Pacinian corpuscle-encode vibration, tapping.

26. I. What is the structure shown in the given diagram?
    II. Name the cells, marked as A, B and C?

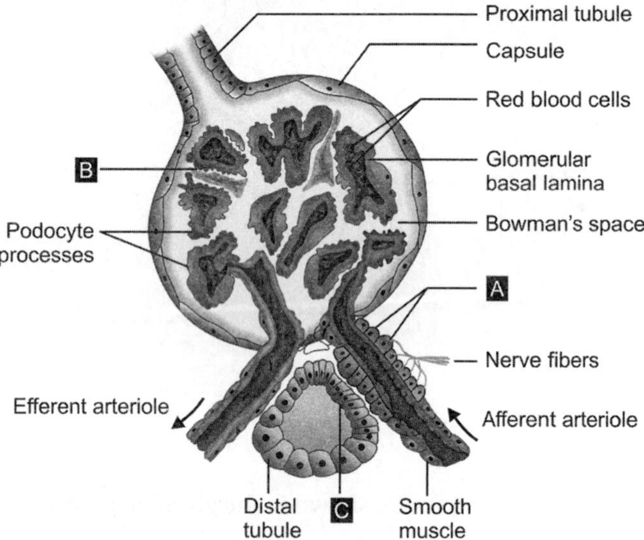

Ans. I. Glomerulus
II. A—juxta glomerular cells
B—mesangial cells
C—macula densa.

27. What is the structure shown in the given diagram?

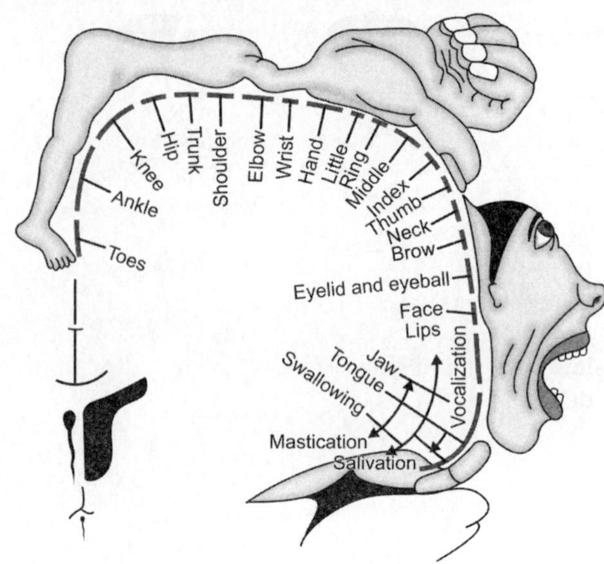

Ans. Motor homunculus.

28. I. What is the structure shown in the given diagram?
    II. Name A and B?

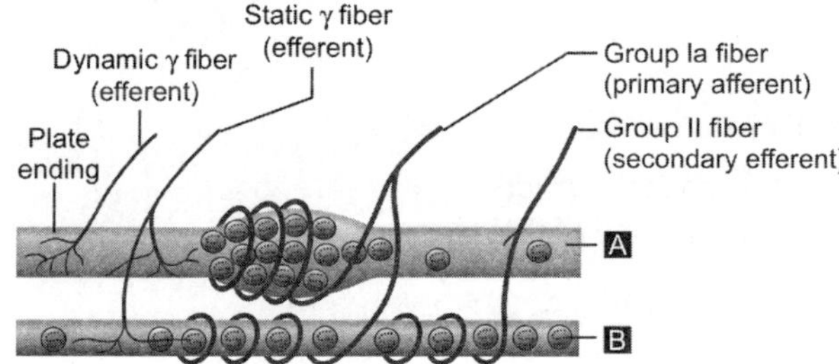

Ans. I. Muscle spindle
II. A—nuclear bag fiber
B—nuclear chain fiber.

29. A. What is the structure shown in the given diagram?
    B. Mechanism?

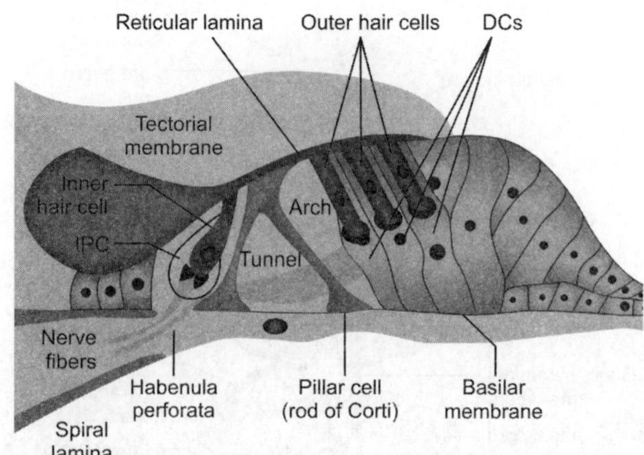

Ans. Organ of Corti.

SKILLS

- Demonstration of pallor
- Demonstration of cyanosis, clubbing, etc.
- Demonstration of edema
- Examination of pulse
- Palpating apex beat
- Demonstration of power of muscle
- Examination of individual muscles of upper limb, lower limb and trunk (biceps, triceps, supraspinatus, deltoid, serratus anterior, etc.)
- Demonstrate—biceps jerk, knee jerk, ankle jerk, etc.
- Demonstrate coordination tests—finger nose, heel-knee test
- Test cranial nerve 3, 4, 6
- Test cranial nerve 7
- Rinne's test
- Weber's test
- Schwabach's test
- Test cranial nerve—9, 10, 11.

THEORY: VIVA VOCE

HEMATOLOGY

- Name the formed elements.
- List the plasma proteins.
- What are the functions of plasma proteins?
- Name the anucleated cells.
- What is the shape of RBC?
- What is the normal red cell count?
- What are the functions of blood?
- What is the normal Hb count?
- What are the types of Hb?
- What are the functions of Hb?
- What is sickle cell Hb?
- Define erythropoiesis.
- What are the stages of erythropoiesis?
- What is the life span of RBC?
- Define anemia.
- How will you classify anemia?
- What is polycythemia?
- What is the normal RBC count?
- List the physiological conditions where there is increase in red cell.
- What are the functions of RBC?
- What is phagocytosis?
- What are the stages of phagocytosis?
- Name the blood group antigens.
- What is HDN?
- What are the types of blood groups?
- What are the indicators of blood transfusion?
- What is autologous transfusion?
- Enumerate the functions of platelets.
- Hemostasis.
- What are the steps of hemostasis?
- Define bleeding and clotting time.
- Name few conditions where BT and CT are prolonged.
- What is the normal prothrombin time?
- What are the mechanisms that prevent intravascular clots?
- What is Bombay blood group?
- Define Landsteiner's law.
- What is hemophilia?
- What is purpura?
- What is von Willebrand's disease?
- Define immunity. How do you classify immunity?
- What are the difference between passive and active immunity?
- What is the peripheral smear picture of iron deficiency?
- What is the function of intrinsic factor?
- What is PCV?
- What is the normal ESR?
- What are red cell indices?

CARDIOVASCULAR SYSTEM

- Define cardiac output with its values.
- Define stroke volume and cardiac index.
- Define arterial pressure, pulse pressure and mean arterial pressure with its normal values.
- What is Bezold-Jarisch reflex, baroreceptor reflex, bainbridge reflex?
- What is hypertension and types of hytertension?
- Define shock and types of shock with examples.
- Causes and features of heart sounds.
- ECG waves with amplitude and definition.
- What is Stokes-Adams syndrome?
- Definition, functions and composition of lymph.
- Types of cardiac failure.
- Why is SA node called the pacemaker?
- What is vagal tone and vagal escape?
- What is idioventricular rhythm?

RESPIRATORY SYSTEM

- Layers of respiratory membrane.
- Definition and values of lung volume and capacities.
- Definition of surfactants—source, composition and function.
- Factors shifting ODC to right and left.
- Modes of oxygen and carbon dioxide transport.
- Name the respiratory center.
- Normal respiratory rate.
- Hering-Breuer reflex.
- Stages of dysphasia.
- Types of periodic breathing with examples.
- Definition and types of cyanosis.
- Mechanism of inspiration.
- Definition and types of dead space.
- Name the pulmonary pressures and their normal values.
- Types of artificial respiration.
- What is oxygen doubt?

GASTROINTESTINAL TRACT (GIT)

- Name the GI hormones.
- Functions of GI hormones.
- Functions of salivary juice.

- Functions of liver.
- Functions of bile.
- Functions of gallbladder.
- Functions of large intestine.
- Source of HCl.
- Source, functions of intrinsic factors.
- Functions of pancreatic juice.
- What is succus entericus?
- Functions of succus entericus.
- Types of intestinal motility.
- Steps of deglutition.
- Types of jaundice.
- Name the bile pigment.
- What is Hirschsprung's disease?
- What is dumping syndrome?
- What is mucosal barrier?
- Define jaundice and its types.

EXCRETORY SYSTEM

- Define GFR.
- What is the normal GFR?
- What are aquaporins?
- Name the cells of juxtaglomerular apparatus.
- Where does maximum reabsorption take place?
- Name the hormones acting on the tubules.
- What are the types of water reabsorption?
- What are the types of counter-current mechanism?
- What are the functions of kidney?
- What is the normal urine output?
- What is atonic bladder?
- What is automatic bladder?
- What is neurogenic bladder?

CENTRAL NERVOUS SYSTEM (CNS)

- List the properties of neuron.
- What is reflex action?
- What is reflex arc?
- Classify reflexes.
- What is stretch reflex?
- Give examples of monosynaptic and polysynaptic reflexes.
- What is synapse and what are the types of synapse?
- List the functions of basal ganglia.
- List the functions of thalamus.
- List the functions of hypothalamus.
- List the functions of cerebellum.
- List the receptors for pain, heat, cold and pressure.
- Parkinsonism.
- State chorea, athetosis and ballism.
- State astereognosis.
- List the functional lobes of cortex.
- What is aplasia? Types?
- Types of sleep and difference?
- Types of memory?
- What is amnesia?
- Source and functions of CSF.
- Difference between UMNL and LMNL.
- What is upper and lower motor neuron?
- Difference between spasticity and rigidity.
- What is decerebrate rigidity?
- What is decorticate rigidity?
- Define muscle tone.
- Examples of hypotonia and hypertonia.

SPECIAL SENSES

- Name the refractive errors.
- Name the pupillary reflexes.
- What are the changes taking place during accommodation?
- What is the visual cortex?
- What are the functions of aqueous humor?
- What is the normal intraocular pressure?
- What is glaucoma? How is it checked?
- Name the visual receptors with their pigments.
- Which is blind spot?
- Where is fovea centralis?
- List the theories of color vision.
- What is color blindness?
- What is visual acuity? How is it determined?
- What is field of vision?
- What are the primary colors?
- What is scotopic and photopic vision?
- What is nystagmus?
- What is binocular vision?
- List the functions of middle ear.
- What is organ of Corti?
- List the theories of hearing.
- Which is the receptor for hearing?
- What is endocochlear potential?
- What is the audible range of hearing?
- Name the ear ossicles.
- Functions of cochlea.
- What is deafness? Types?
- Name the gustatory receptors.
- Name the gustatory cortex.
- What are the primary tastes?
- What is the olfactory receptors?
- What is anosmia, name few causes?

ENDOCRINOLOGY

- What are second messengers and examples?
- Define hormone.

- Hormone classification.
- Name the amino acid present in thyroid hormone.
- Name the substance/element required for the thyroxine synthesis.
- List the steps involved in thyroxine synthesis.
- List the functions of thyroxine.
- What is cretinism and its features?
- What is myxedema and its features?
- Graves disesase.
- Goiter, types.
- Name the calcitrophic elements and their functions?
- What is tetany and its features?
- Name the posterior pituitary hormone.
- What are the functions of ADH?
- Name the neuroendocrine hormones.
- What is neuroendocrine reflex?
- What are the functions of oxytocin?
- What is milk ejection reflex?
- What is diabetes insipidus and types?
- Name the anterior pituitary hormone.
- List the functions of growth hormone.
- List the difference between cretinism and dwarfism.
- What is gigantism and what are its features?
- What is acromegaly and its features?
- List the functions of melatonin.
- List the functions of aldosterone, cortisol, etc.
- What is permissive action?
- What is Cushing syndrome and its features?
- What is Addisons disease?
- What is Addisonian crisis?
- What is the normal calcium level?
- Name the hormones of pancreas.
- What is diabetes mellitus and what are its types?
- Enumerate the difference between type I and type II of DM.
- How many amino acid are present in α and β chains of insulin?
- What are poitrogens?

REPRODUCTION

- Define ovulation.
- When does ovulation take place?
- What is corpus luteum?
- Functions of corpus luteum.
- Name the ovarian hormones, and their functions.
- What are the steps of ovarian cycle?
- Define spermatogenesis.
- What are the stages of spermatogenesis.
- Functions of testosterone.
- What is endometrial cycle?
- What is the duration of endometrial cycle?
- What are the stages of endometrial cycle?
- Enumerate the functions of placenta.
- List the pregnancy tests.
- What is lactation?
- What are the stages of lactation?
- Where does fertilization take place?
- Where does implantation take place?
- What is contraception?
- What are the types of contraception?
- What is Graafian follicle?
- What is zona pellucida?
- What are the test for ovulation?

NERVE-MUSCLE PHYSIOLOGY

- Name the neuroglial cells.
- What are the functions of neuroglia?
- Name the contractile proteins.
- What is myasthenia gravis?
- What is rigor mortis?
- Types of muscle fibers.
- Types of muscle contractions.
- What is motor unit?
- List the properties of skeletal muscle.
- What is rheobase and chronaxie?
- What is tetanus and clonus?
- What is salutatory conduction?

CLINICAL QUESTIONS

1. A person who have been living at sea level, migrates to a region at an altitude of about 18,000 ft and stays there for 10 years.—**Physiological polycythemia**
   a. Give the physiological adjustments that make it possible for him to live at this high altitude?
   b. Give the normal arterial pCO_2 and pO_2 at sea level?
   c. What is mountain sickness?
2. A 50-year-old man came to the OPD with complaints of passing large volume of urine, general weakness and weight loss.
   Investigations: Blood sugar—250 mg percent
   Urine sugar: ++
   a. Identify the probable condition.—**Diabetes mellitus**
   b. Give the physiological basis of polyuria.
   c. Comment on the investigation values giving reason.
   d. How can you account for weight loss?
3. A 50-year-old obese lady was admitted to the hospital at MES with complaints of lethargy, hoarseness of voice and dryness of skin. On questioning the patient admits that she had sensitivity to cold and constipation. Her resting pulse rate was 60/min.
   a. What is the probable diagnosis?—**Hypothyroidism**
   b. What will be the cause of lethargy and sensitivity to cold?
   c. What is the cause of dryness of skin?
4. A 25-year-old man complaints of severe headache and enlargement of his hands and feet. Wide spaces could be observed between his teeth and his lower jaw was abnormally prominent.
   a. Mention the probable nature of the abnormality and state how it gives rise to the symptoms mentioned. —**Acromegaly**
   b. Explain any probable change in his glucose tolerance
   c. How would the symptoms be different if the disorder has started during childhood?
5. Routine investigations in a man aged 40 years who presented himself for general health check up revealed the following:
   Cardiac index: 3.21/min; resting pulse—70/min; ejection fraction—65 percent; blood pressure—130/80 mm Hg; no murmur; no cyanosis; ECG—normal; but he complaints of pain in the chest (retrosternal) when he exerted himself and the pain was proportional to the amount of exertion.
   a. Comment on the values obtained on investigation give their normal range also.
   b. Define murmur and mention two causes for it.
   c. Define cyanosis and give two examples when it can be seen.
   d. Explain the physiological basis for pain experienced by this subject and how does this pain differ from reffered pain?
6. A 35-year-old man came to the doctor and complained that he had headache and that his driving was dangerous as if it was difficulty to see the vehicles on the right and left. The doctor examined him and noticed that his palms were rather large.—**Suprasellar pituitary tumors**
   a. What can be the probable diagnosis?
   b. Which organ is at fault?
   c. Explain the reason for difficulty to see the vehicles on the right and left while driving.
7. A middle-aged female complaints of palpitation, diarrhea, weight loss and menorrhagia. On examination, swelling on the neck and exophthalmos were noticed.
   a. What is the probable endocrine abnormality? —**Hyperthyroidism**
   b. List the functions of the hormone.
   c. Explain the causes of signs and symptoms in that patient.
   d. Name three salient investigations to come to a diagnosis.
8. When a vibrating tuning fork was applied on the forehead of a person he heard the sound better on the left side.—**Weber's test**
   a. Name the probable cause of it.—**Conductive deafness on left side**
   b. Name another test whih may help in this case.
9. An obese diabetic patient decided to start on exercise program to lose weight. He got up in the morning, ate a light breakfast, took his regular daily dose of insulin and started running. He was found unconscious some time later.—**Hypoglycemia**
   a. What is the blood sugar value of this patient likely to be at time of loss of consciousness? **<63 mg/dL**
   b. What would you do immediately to save the patient? —**Give sweets**
   c. What is the cause for loss of consciousness?
10. A school teacher with an RBC count of 7 million/mm^3 has normal activities except for the erythematous skin.
    a. What may be the probable condition?—**Polycythemia vera.**
    b. Mention one abnormal physical property of her blood which can cause high blood pressure?

11. A young man, during his driving test said he was unable to clearly distinguish the red (stop) light.
    a. What is the condition?—**Color blindness**
    b. Name the theory on which your diagnosis based on?
12. A 35-year-old business executive complained of burning pain in his upper abdomen. Pain is relieved by taking food.
    a. What is the likely diagnosis?—**Duodenal ulcer**
    b. Mention 2 substances which provoke gastric secretion?
13. A 55-year-old business man was brought to casualty with a history of acute chest pain radiating to left shoulder. On examination the patient was sweating; and systolic BP 100 mm Hg.
    a. What is the probable diagnosis?—**Myocardial infarction (MI)**
    b. What immediate bed side investigation can help to confirm the diagnosis?
14. A 30-year-old man was admitted to the hospital with complaints of tendency to fall right side while walking and inability to stand straight. On examination there was marked hypotonia of the muscles of right limb, nystagmus and intention tremor of right hand.
    a. Identify the clinical condition?—**Cerebellar lesion**
    b. Give reason for the hypotonia of muscle?
    c. Mention type of knee jerk in this case (pendular knee jerk).
15. A young healthy soldier was found on the ground in the war front unable to move both lower limbs. On examination, muscles of lower limb showed flaccid paralysis. Cremasteric and abdominal reflex were absent and loss of sensation below T8.
    a. What can be the probable diagnosis?—**Paraplegia**
16. A 50-year-old man entered the doctor's room with short quick steps. The doctor smiled at him but his face showed no expression. The doctor noticed a mild tremor of his hands.
    a. What is the diagnosis?—**Parkinsonism**
    b. Where is the lesion?
    c. Mention two causes of the disease?
17. A 14-year-old girl was brought to the OPD with complaints of irregular menstrual cycles and profuse bleeding during menstrual period. After routine investigations, it was concluded to be due to anovulatory cycles.
    a. Give the basis of profuse bleeding in the girl during menstruation?—**Dysfunctional uterine bleeding**
    b. Mention the hormones involved in ovulation.
    c. Explain the uterine, ovarian and cervical changes during different phases of normal menstrual cycle.
18. A 40-year-old man was admitted to the casuality after a car accident with paralysis and absence of all sensations in both lower limbs.
    a. Identify the probable site of lesion.—**L_1**
    b. Mention the tracts involved.
    c. Outline the immediate and delayed effects with the physiological basis of each.
19. A 10-year-old girl prescribed to ENT with bleeding from nose since 3 days. History of bleeding from gums are also present since brushing.

    Laboratory investigations:

    i. RBC count—3.8 million
    ii. WBC count—25000
    iii. BT and CT—normal
    iv. Peripheral smear—presence of immature cells in WBC series.

    a. Identify the condition.—**Leukemia**
    b. What other interpretations would you suggest to establish the diagnosis?
20. A 30-year-old man was brought to the causuality with history of road traffic accident. BP—90/70 mm Hg, respiratory rate—10/minute.

    Examination of CVS: S1, S2 are prolonged

    Urinary intolerance—increased

    Examination of CNS: Pupils reacting to light, sensation absent below cervical region, Motor system—all reflexes are absent, power 0 in both upper and lower limbs.

    a. Identify the condition.—**Quadriplegia**
    b. Discuss the condition in detail.
21. A 40-year-old man came to the OPD with a gait characterized by raising his feet unnecessarily high and bringing it down in a stamping manner (stamping gait). He also stood with his feet wide apart and tended to fall to the right with the eyes closed.
    a. Where is the lesion?—**Dorsal column**
    b. Describe the neural tract with diagram.
    c. What are the sensations carried by this tract?

NORMAL VALUES

Hematology		
RBC count	Male	5.4 milion cells/μL
	Female	4.8 million cells/μL
	Infants	6.8 million cells/μL
WBC count	Adult	4000–11000 cells/μL
	Infants	18000–20000 cells/μL
Granulocyte		
Neutrophils		3000–6000 cells/μL (50–70%)
Eosinophils		150–300 cells/μL (1–4%)
Basophils		0–100 cells/μL (0–1%)
Agranulocyte		
Lymphocyte		1500–4000 cells/μL (20–40%)
Monocyte		300–600 cells/μL (2–8%)
Platelets		1.5–4 lacs/μL
Hematocrit (Hct)	Male	46 +/–5%
	Female	42 +/–5%
Hemoglobin count	Male	14–18 gm%
	Female	12–16 gm%
	Infant	18–22 gm%
Mean corpuscular volume (MCV)	Male	76–96 cubic microns
	Female	76–96 cubic microns
Mean corpuscular hemoglobin (MCH)	Male	29 +/–2 pg
	Female	29 +/–2 pg
Mean corpuscular hemoglobin concentration (MCHC)	Male	34 +/–2%
	Female	34 +/–2%
Protein—total		6-8 g/dL
Albumin		3.5–5 g/dL
Globulin		1.5–3 g/dL
Fibrinogen		0.3 g/dL
Bilirubin—total		0.2–0.8 mg/dL
Bilirubin—conjugated		0–0.2 mg/dL
Bilirubin—unconjugated		0.2–0.6 mg/dL
Erythrocyte sedimentation rate (ESR)	Male	1–3 mm/one hour
	Female	3–7 mm/one hour
Bleeding time		2–6 minutes
Clotting time		3–8 minutes

Contd...

Contd...

Respiratory System		
Arterial blood		
pO_2		90–100 mm Hg
pCO_2		35–45 mm Hg
Hb saturation		97%
O_2 content		19.8 mL O_2/dL
Venous blood		
pO_2		40 mm Hg
pCO_2		45 m Hg
Hb saturation		75%
O_2 content		15.2 mL O_2/dL
Tidal volume	Male	500 mL
	Female	500 mL
Inspiratory reserve volume (IRV)	Male	3300 mL
	Female	1900 mL
Expiratory reserve volume (ERV)	Male	1000 mL
	Female	700 mL
Residual volume (RV)	Male	1200 mL
	Female	1100 mL
Vital capacity (VC)	Male	4800 mL
	Female	3100 mL
Inspiratory capacity (IC) (TV+ IRV)	Male	3800 mL
	Female	2400 mL
Expiratory capacity (EC)	Male	1500 mL
	Female	1200 mL
Functional residual capacity (FRC)	Male	2200 mL
	Female	1800 mL
Total lung capacity (TLC)	Male	6000 mL
	Female	4200 mL
Respiratory rate		14–16/min
Intrapleural pressure		754–757 mm Hg
Intra-alveolar pressure		759–761 mm Hg
Cardiovascular System		
Normal cardiac output		5L/min (4.5–6)
Cardiac index		2.5–3.6 L/min.m^2
Stroke volume		70–90 mL
Heart rate		60–100/min
ECG waves duration		
PR interval		0.18 sec

Contd...

Contd...

QRS duration	0.08 sec
QT interval	0.40 sec
ST interval	0.32 sec
Conduction speed	
SA node	0.05 m/s
Atrial pathways	1 m/s
AV node	0.05 m/s
Bundle of His	1 m/s
Purkinje system	4 m/s
Average rate of impulse production	
SA node	72/min
AV node	50/min
Ventricle	30/min
Cardiac cycle	
Atrial systole	0.1 sec
Ventricle systole	0.3 sec
Ventricular diastole	0.5 sec
Atrial diastole	0.7 sec
Normal blood pressure	
Systolic pressure	100–140 mm Hg
Diastolic pressure	60–90 mm Hg
Pulse pressure	50 mm Hg
Mean arterial blood pressure	90 mm Hg

Contd...

Contd...

Gastrointestinal Tract		
Gastric emptying time		3–4 hours
pH of saliva		7–8
pH of gastric juice		1–2
Excretory System		
Glomerular filtration rate (GFR)		125 mL/min or 180 L/day
Filtration fraction		0.16–0.2
Transport maximum for glucose	Male	375 mg/min
	Female	300 mg/min
Renal threshold value		300 mg/dL
Renal blood flow (RBF)		1273 mL/min
Actual renal plasma flow		700 mL/min
Effective renal plasma flow		625 mL/min
Inulin clearance value		125 mL
Endocrinology		
Growth hormone		3 ng/mL
Thyroid binding globulin (TBG)		7–17 mg/L
Thyroxine (T4)		70–140 nmol/L
Tri-iodothyronine (T3)		1.2–3 nmol/L
Parathyroid hormone (PTH)		10–55 pg/mL
Insulin		0.3–2 ng/mL
Reproductive System		
Sperm count		80–120 million/mL
AV volume of semen per ejaculate		2.5–3.5 mL
Blood loss during menustration		30–80 mL

DIAGRAMS

BLOOD

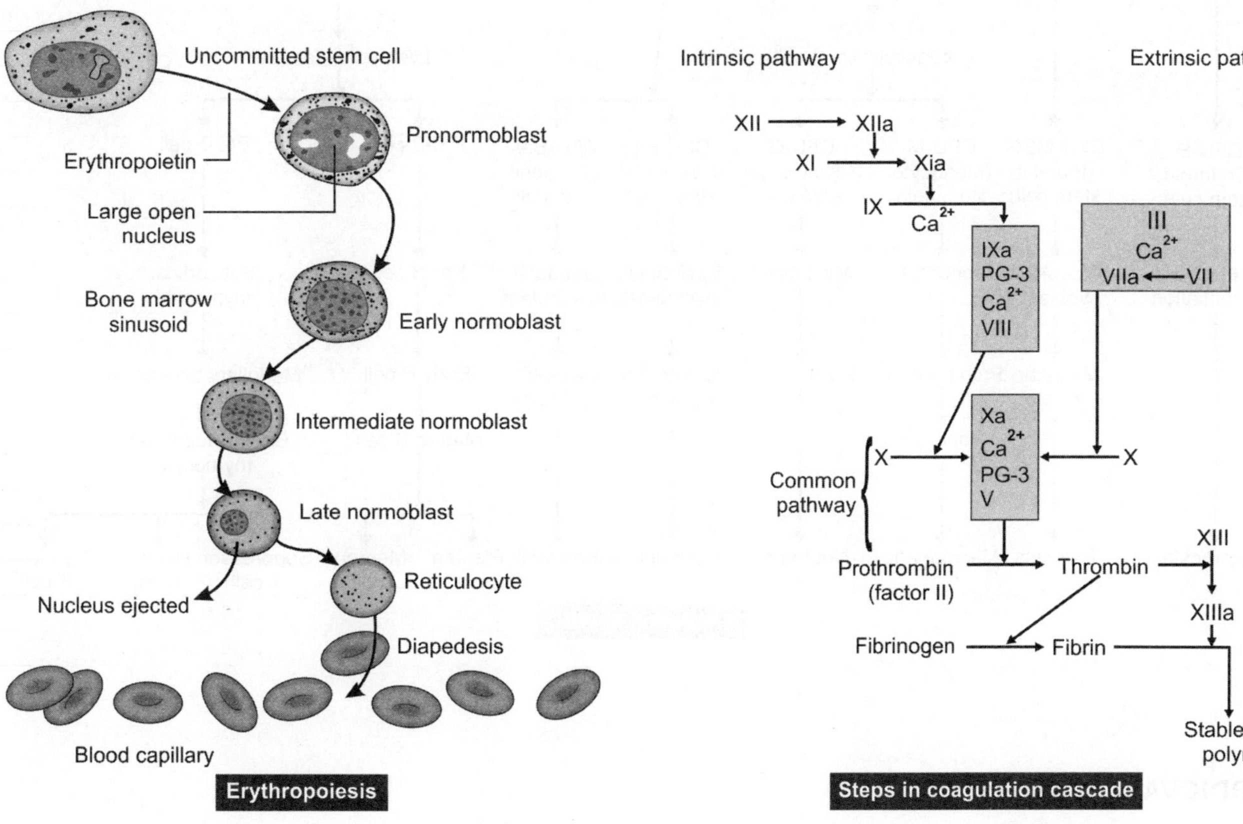

Erythropoiesis

Steps in coagulation cascade

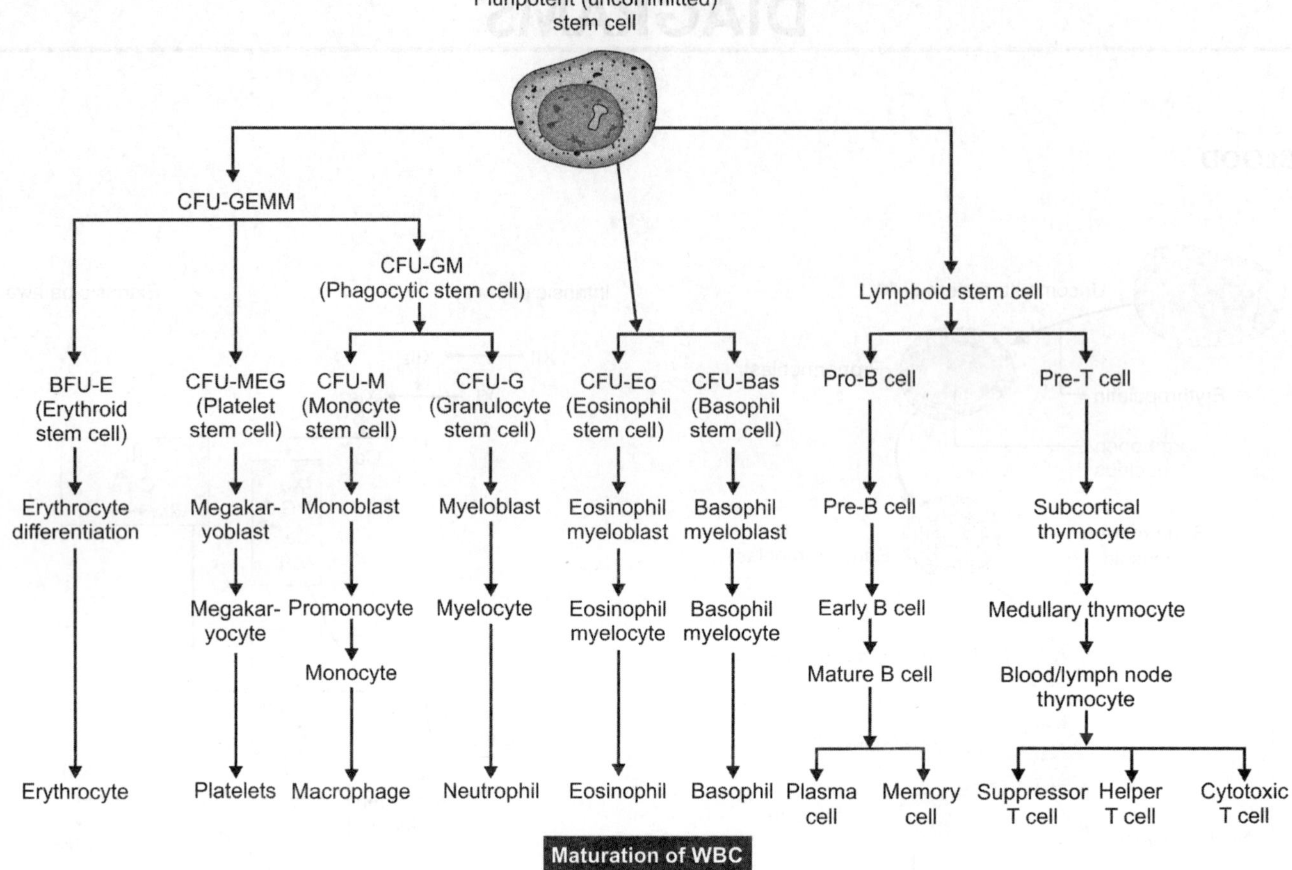

Maturation of WBC

CARDIOVASCULAR SYSTEM

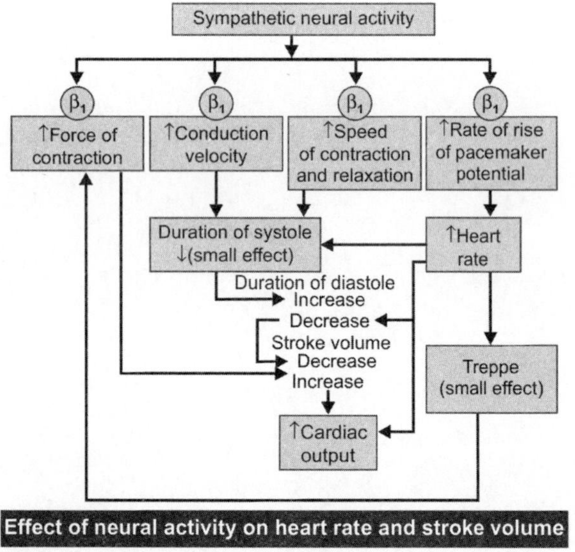

Effect of neural activity on heart rate and stroke volume

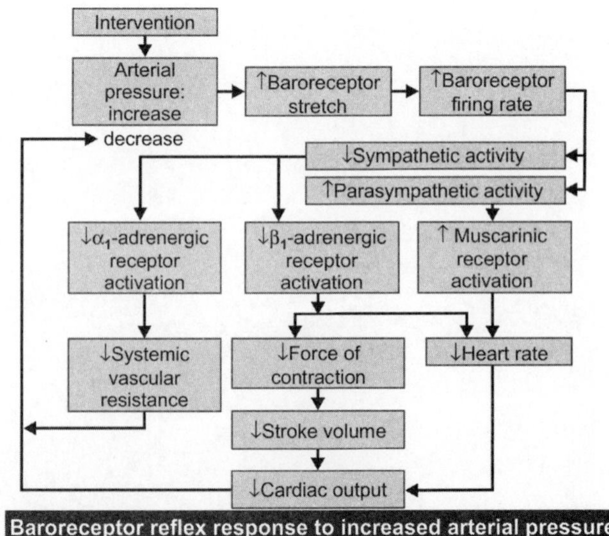

Baroreceptor reflex response to increased arterial pressure

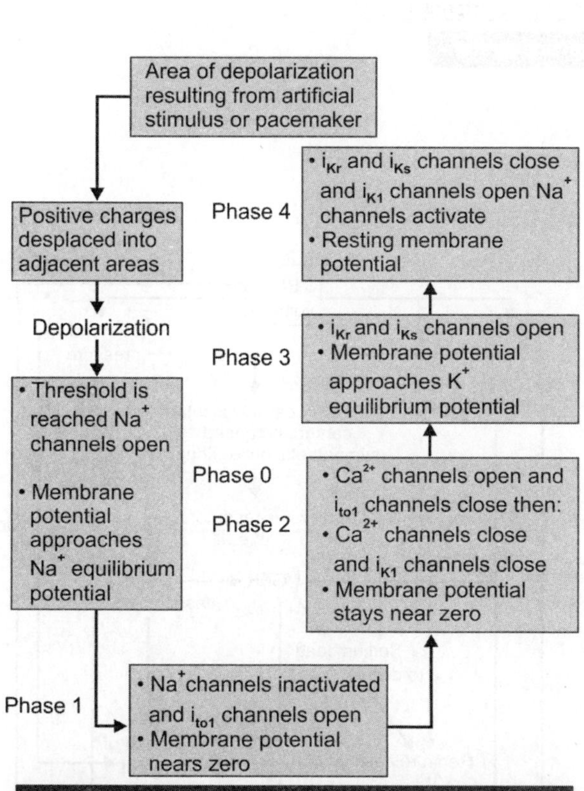

Events associated with ventricualar action potential

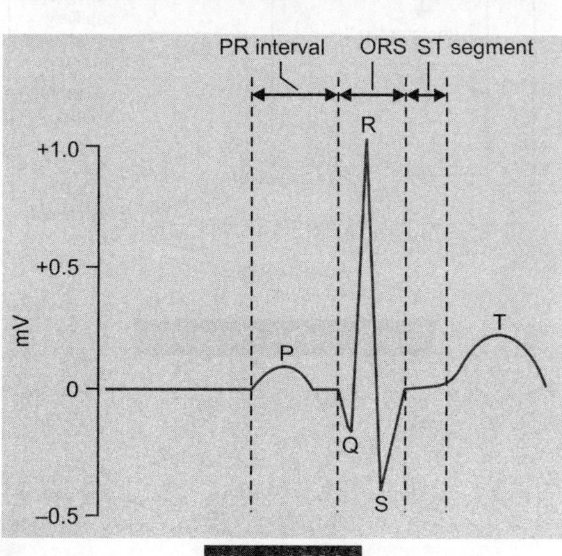

Normal ECG

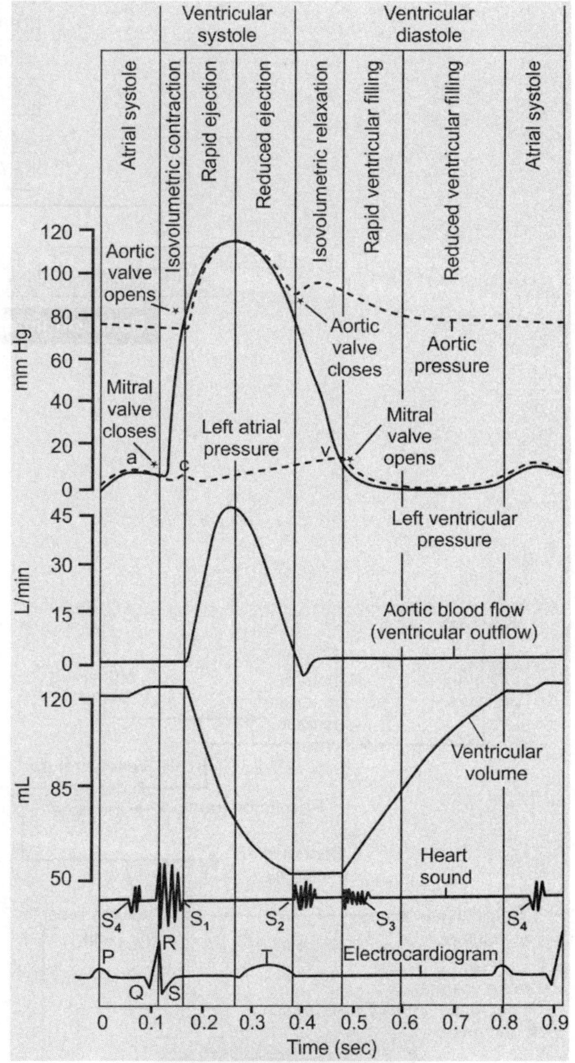

Events in cardiac cycle

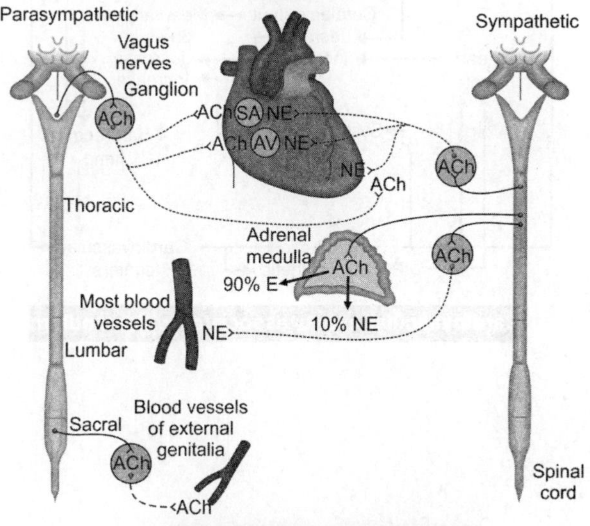

Autonomic innervation of CVS

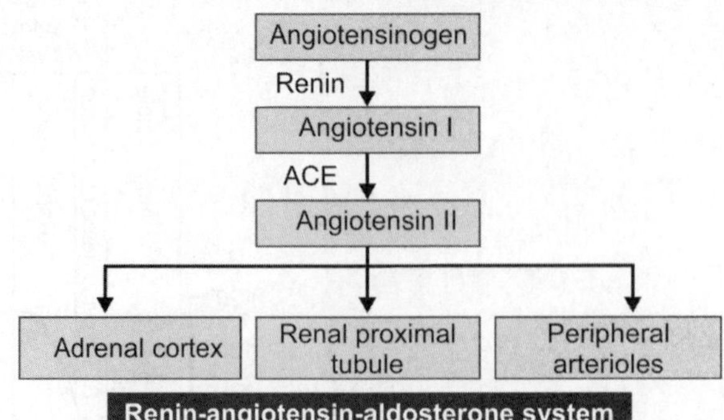

Renin-angiotensin-aldosterone system

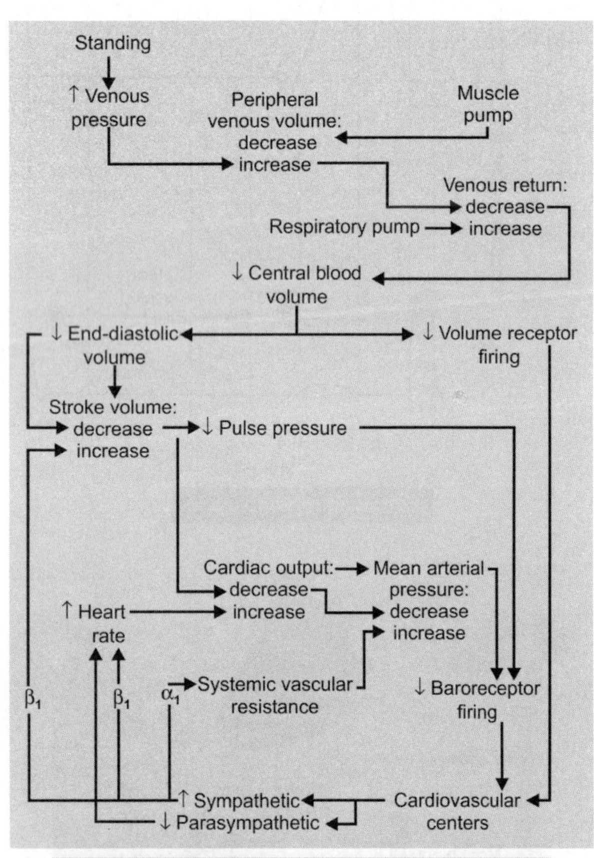

Cardiovascular events associated with standing

↓ Blood volume
+
↓ Atrial volume
↓ Arterial pressure
↑ AVP ↓ ANP
Medullary cardiovascular center: increased sympathetic nerve firing
β-receptors
α-receptors
↓ GFR
Renal vasoconstriction
↓ Sodium load to distal tubules
↑ Renin release
↓ Stretch of afferent arterioles
↑ Angiotensin I
↓ Peritubular capillary hydrostatic pressure
↑ Angiotensin II
↑ Aldosterone
↑ Plasma volume
↓ Sodium excretion
↓ Water excretion
↑ Extracellular fluid volume
↑ Intake of sodium and water

Regulation of blood volume

RESPIRATORY SYSTEM

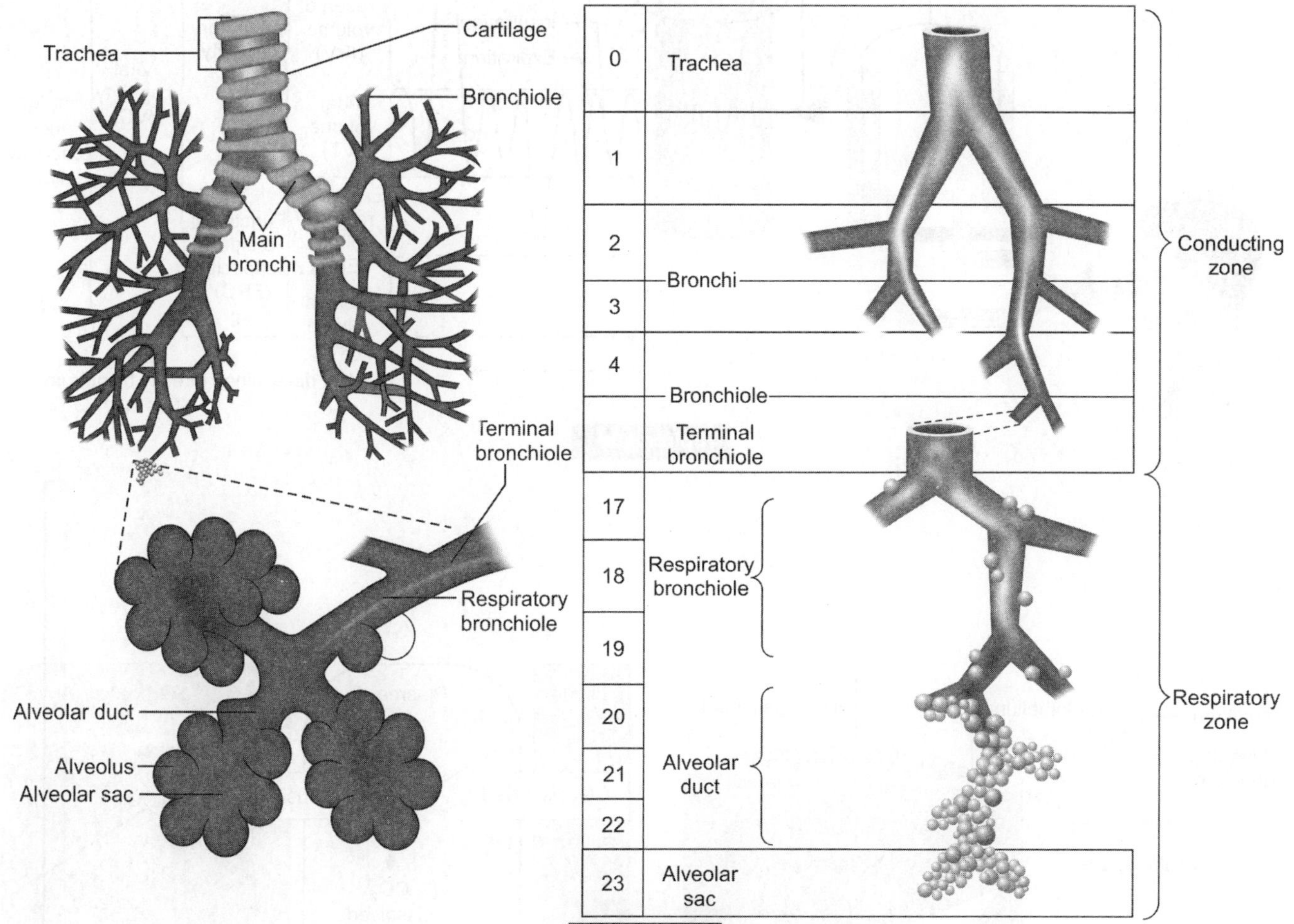

Trachea
Cartilage
Bronchiole
Main bronchi
Terminal bronchiole
Respiratory bronchiole
Alveolar duct
Alveolus
Alveolar sac

Generation	Airway	Zone
0	Trachea	Conducting zone
1		Conducting zone
2	Bronchi	Conducting zone
3	Bronchi	Conducting zone
4	Bronchiole	Conducting zone
	Terminal bronchiole	Conducting zone
17	Respiratory bronchiole	Respiratory zone
18	Respiratory bronchiole	Respiratory zone
19	Respiratory bronchiole	Respiratory zone
20	Alveolar duct	Respiratory zone
21	Alveolar duct	Respiratory zone
22	Alveolar duct	Respiratory zone
23	Alveolar sac	Respiratory zone

Airway tree

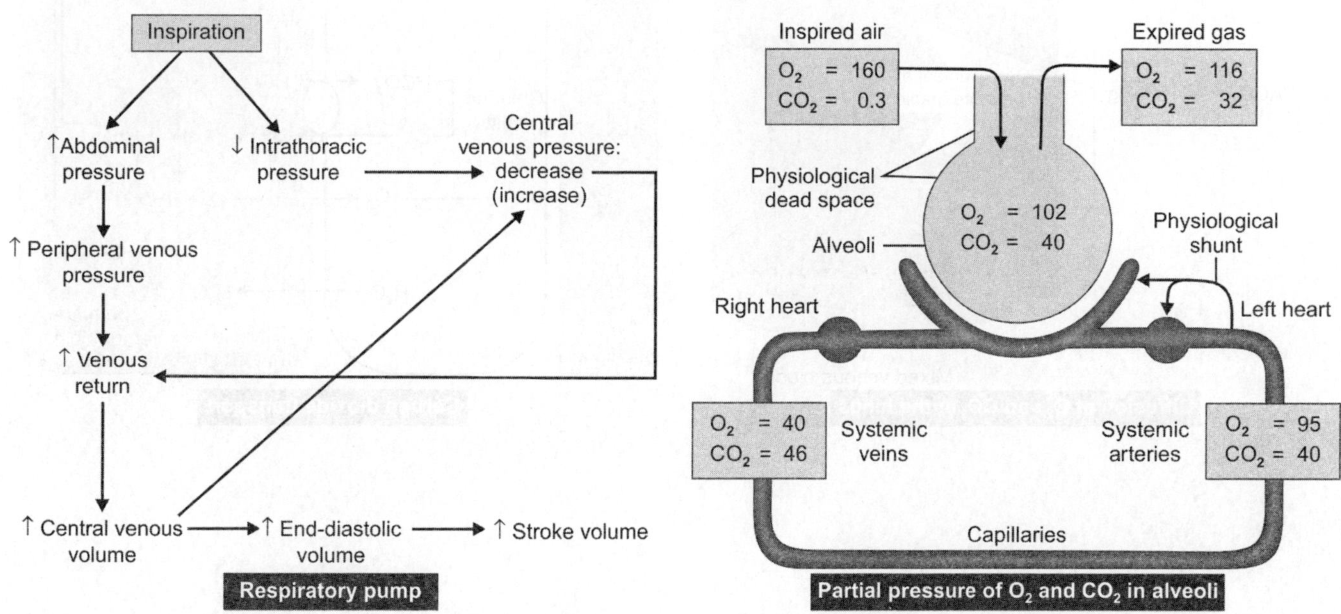

Respiratory pump

Partial pressure of O_2 and CO_2 in alveoli

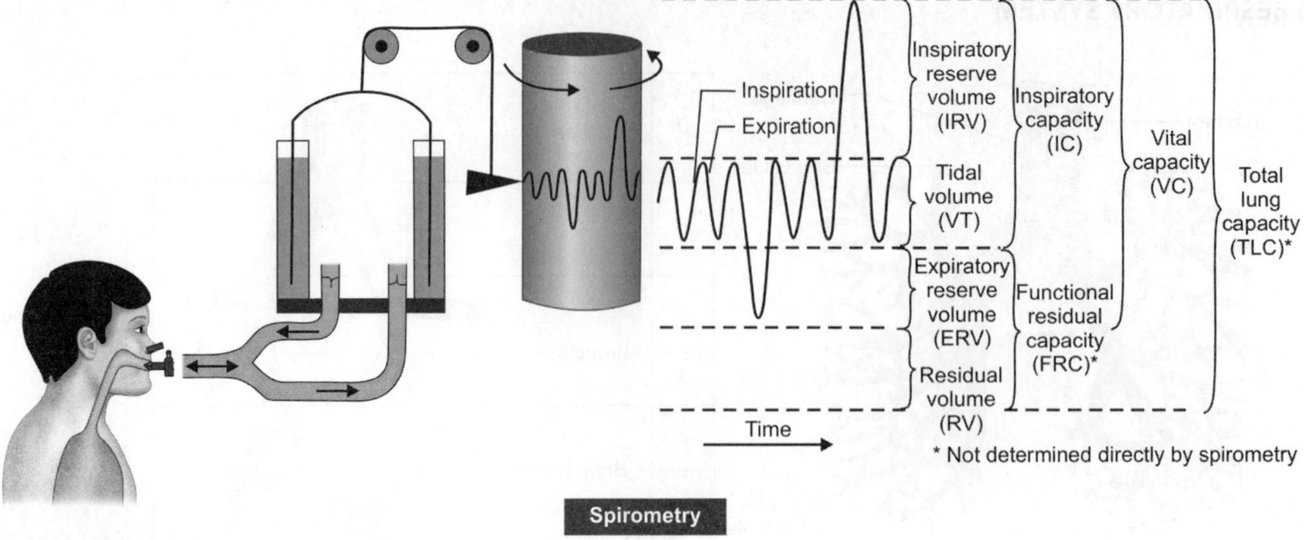

Spirometry

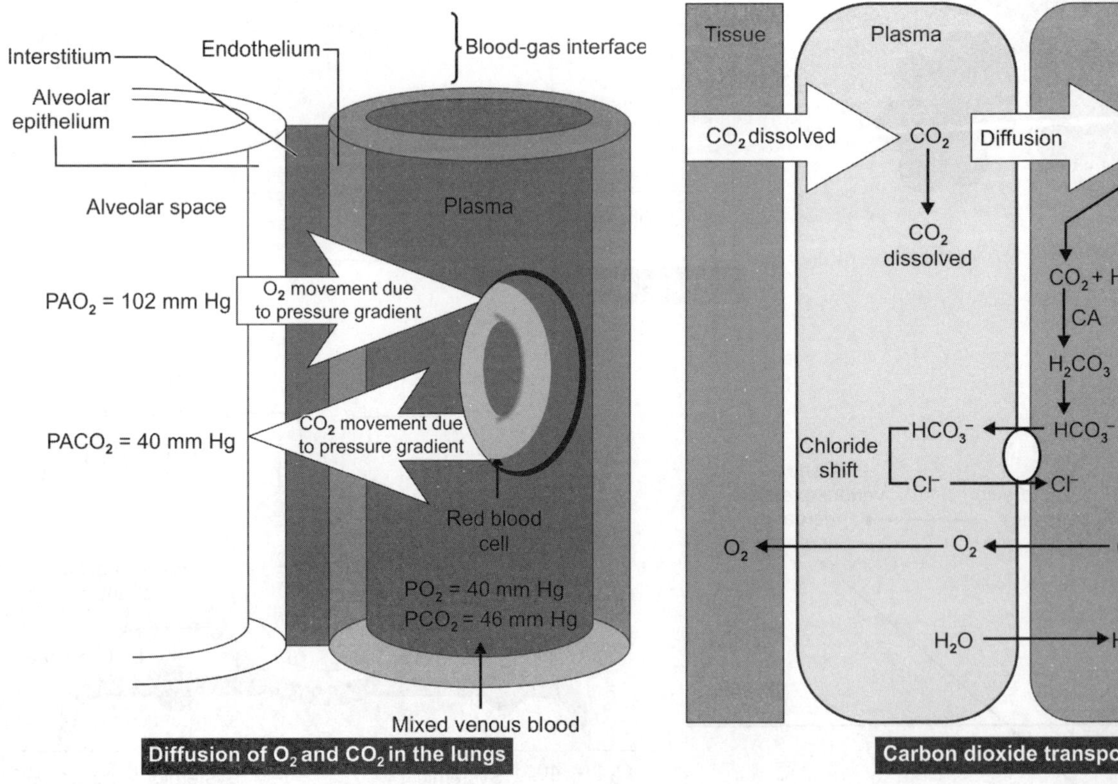

Diffusion of O_2 and CO_2 in the lungs

Carbon dioxide transport

RENAL SYSTEM

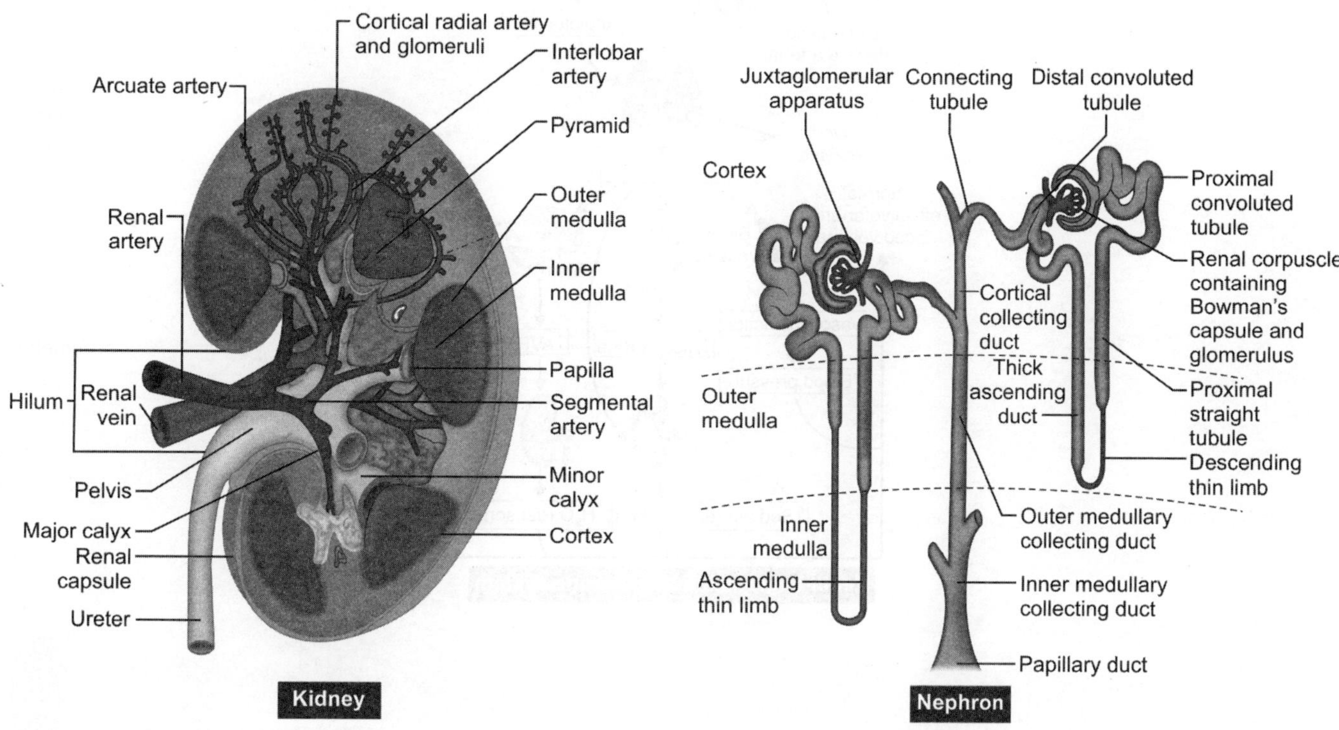

Kidney

Nephron

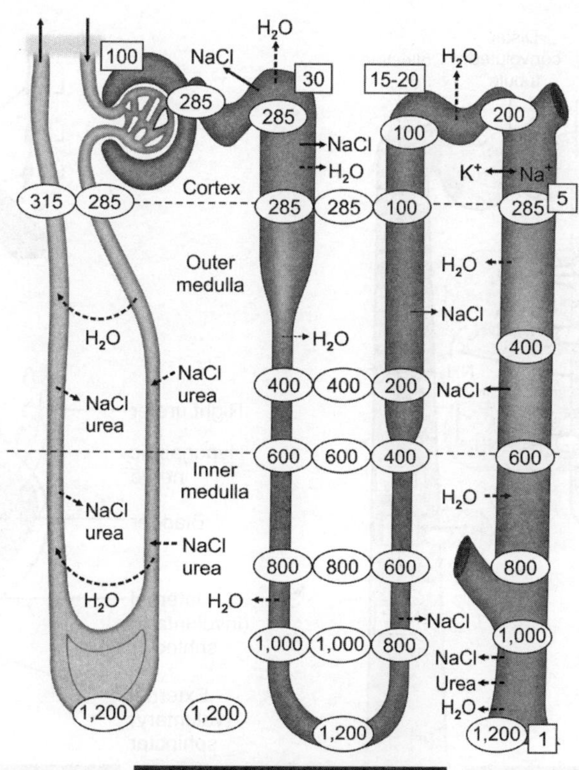

Counter-current mechanism

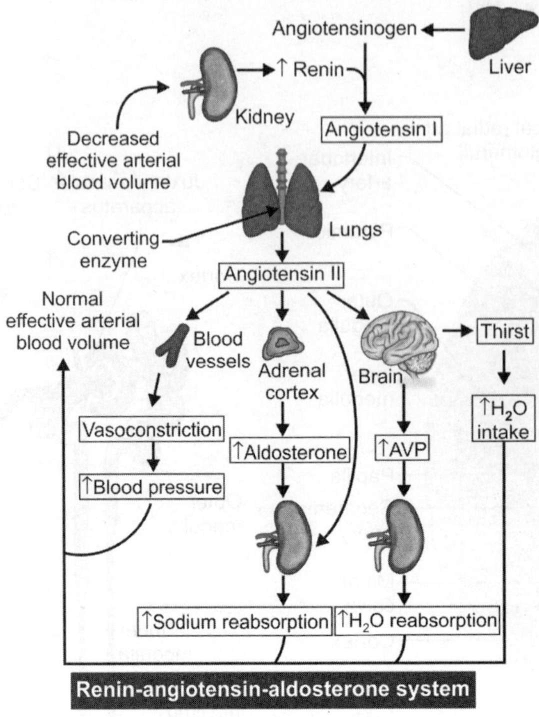

Renin-angiotensin-aldosterone system

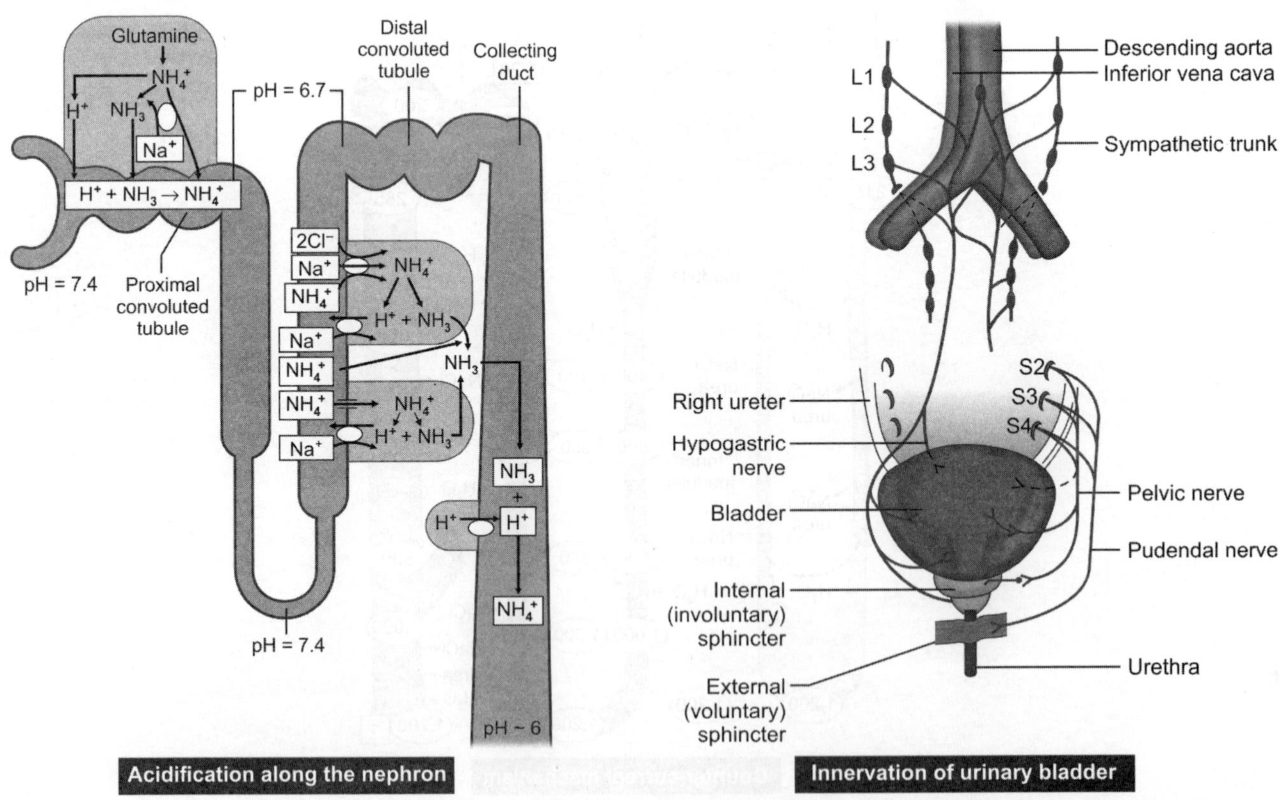

Acidification along the nephron

Innervation of urinary bladder

GASTROINTESTINAL TRACT

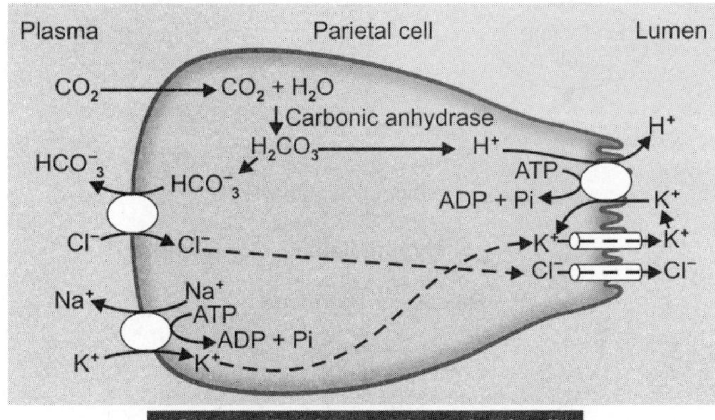

HCl secretion by gastric parietal cells

TEMPERATURE REGULATION

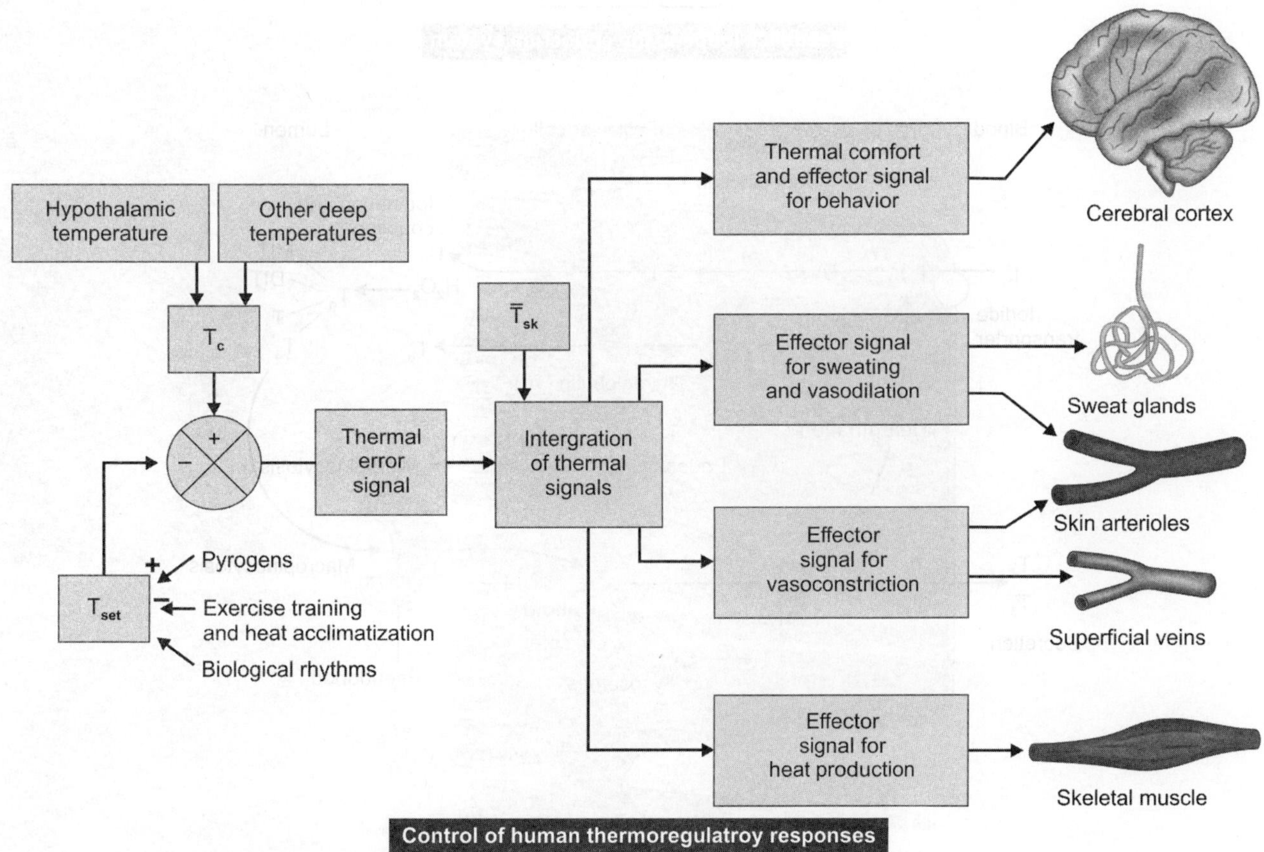

Control of human thermoregulatroy responses

ENDOCRINOLOGY

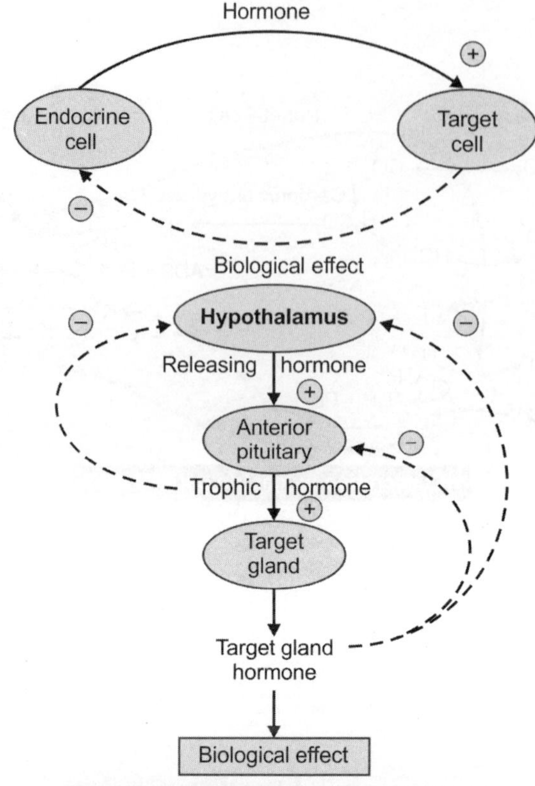

Feedback loops in the endocrine system

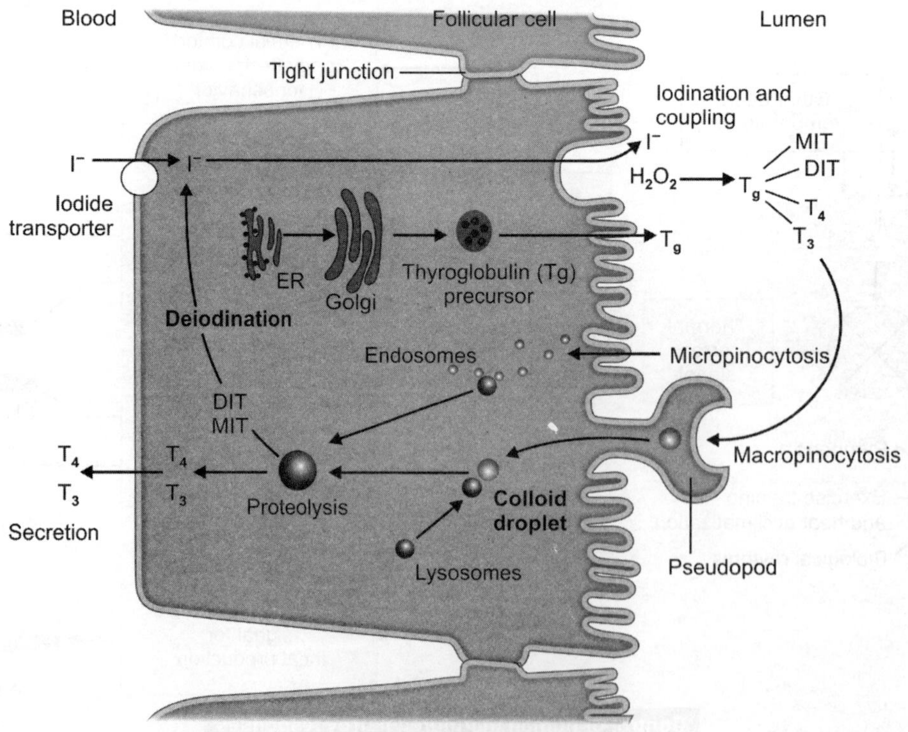

Thyroid hormone synthesis and secretion

CENTRAL NERVOUS SYSTEM

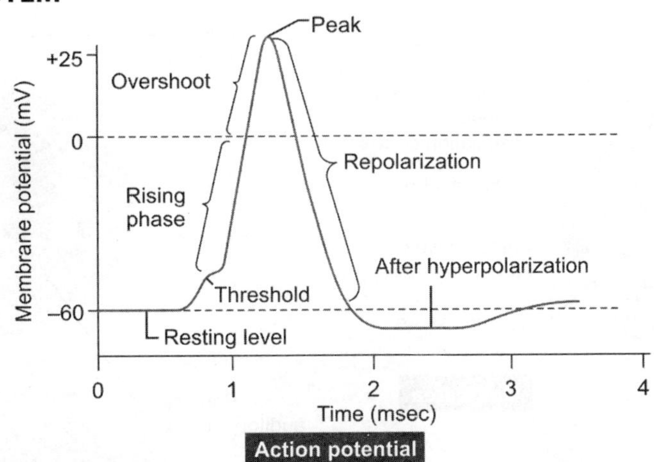

Action potential

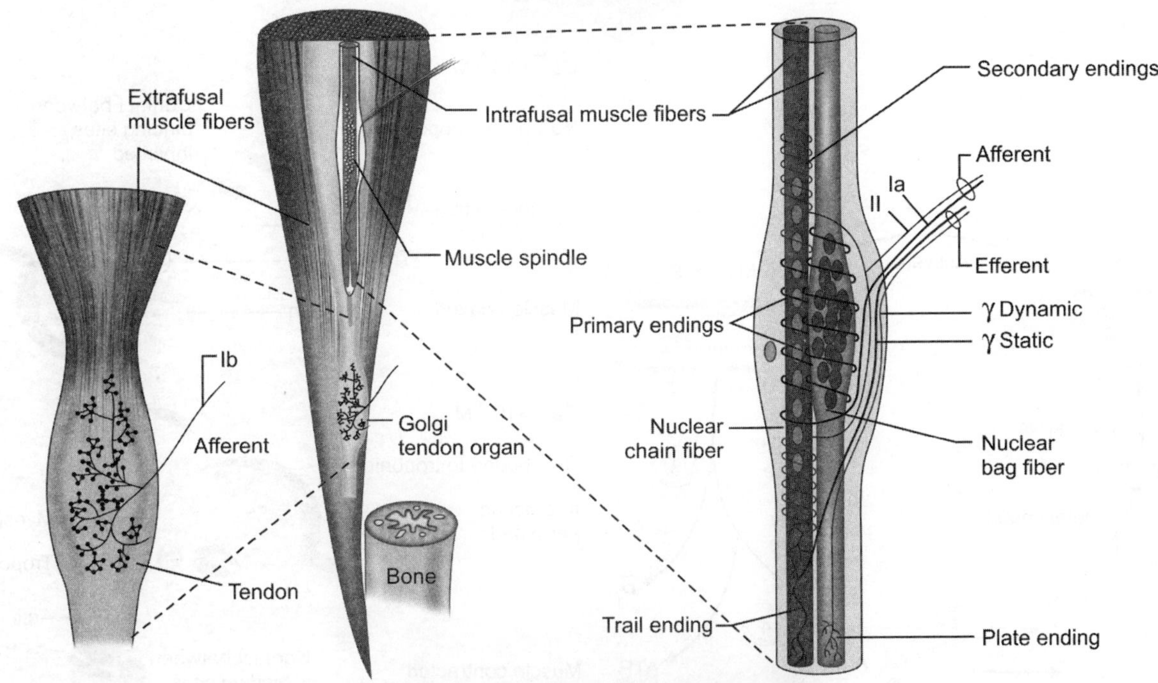

Muscle spindle and Golgi tendon organ

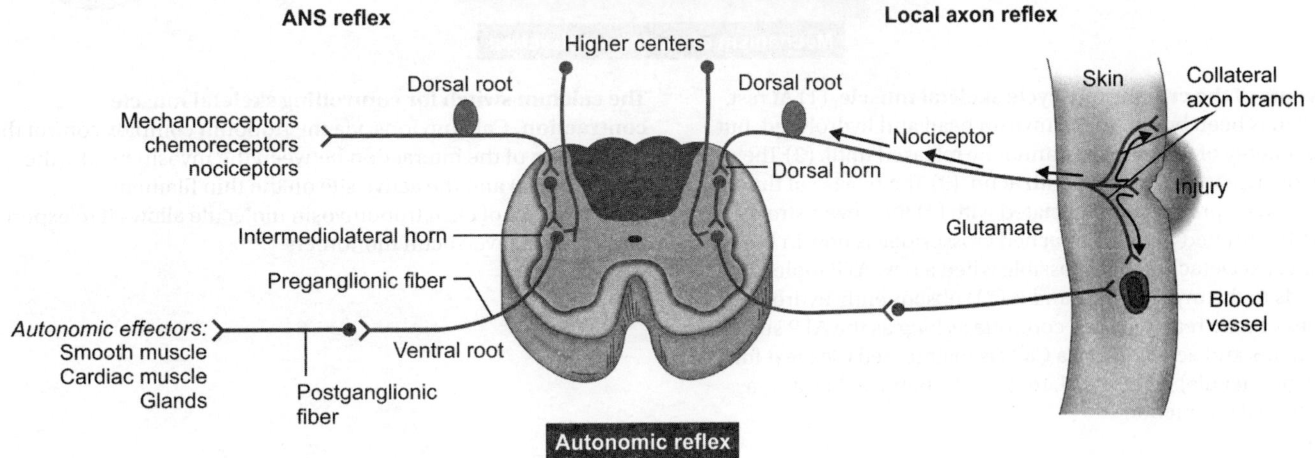

Autonomic reflex

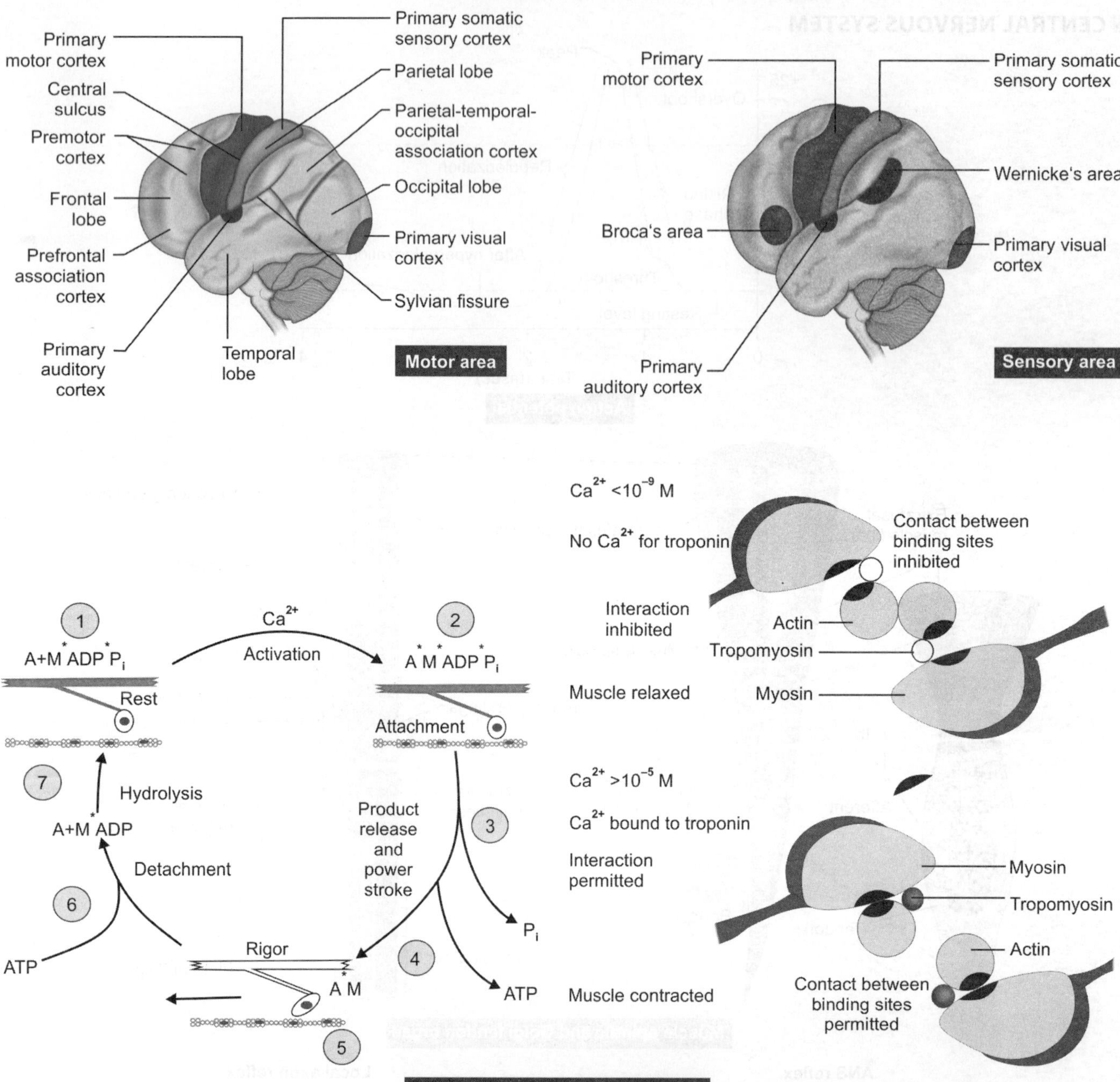

Events of the crossbridge cycle skeletal muscle. (1) At rest, ATP has been bound to the myosin head and hydrolyzed, but the energy of the reaction cannot be released until. (2) The myosin head can interact with actin. (3) The release of the hydrolysis products is associated with (4) the power stroke. (5) The rotated and still-attached crossbridge is now in the rigor state. (6) Detachment is possible when a new ATP molecule binds to the myosin head and is (7) subsequently hydrolyzed. These cyclic reactions can continue as long as the ATP supply remains and activation (via Ca^{2+}) is maintained (See text for further details). A, actin, M, myosin; *, chemical bond; +, a potential interaction

The calcium switch for controlling skeletal muscle contraction. Calcium ions, via the troponin complex control the unblocking of the interaction between the myosin heads (the crossbridges) and the active site on the thin filaments. The geometry of each tropomyosin molecule allows it to expert control over seven actin monomers

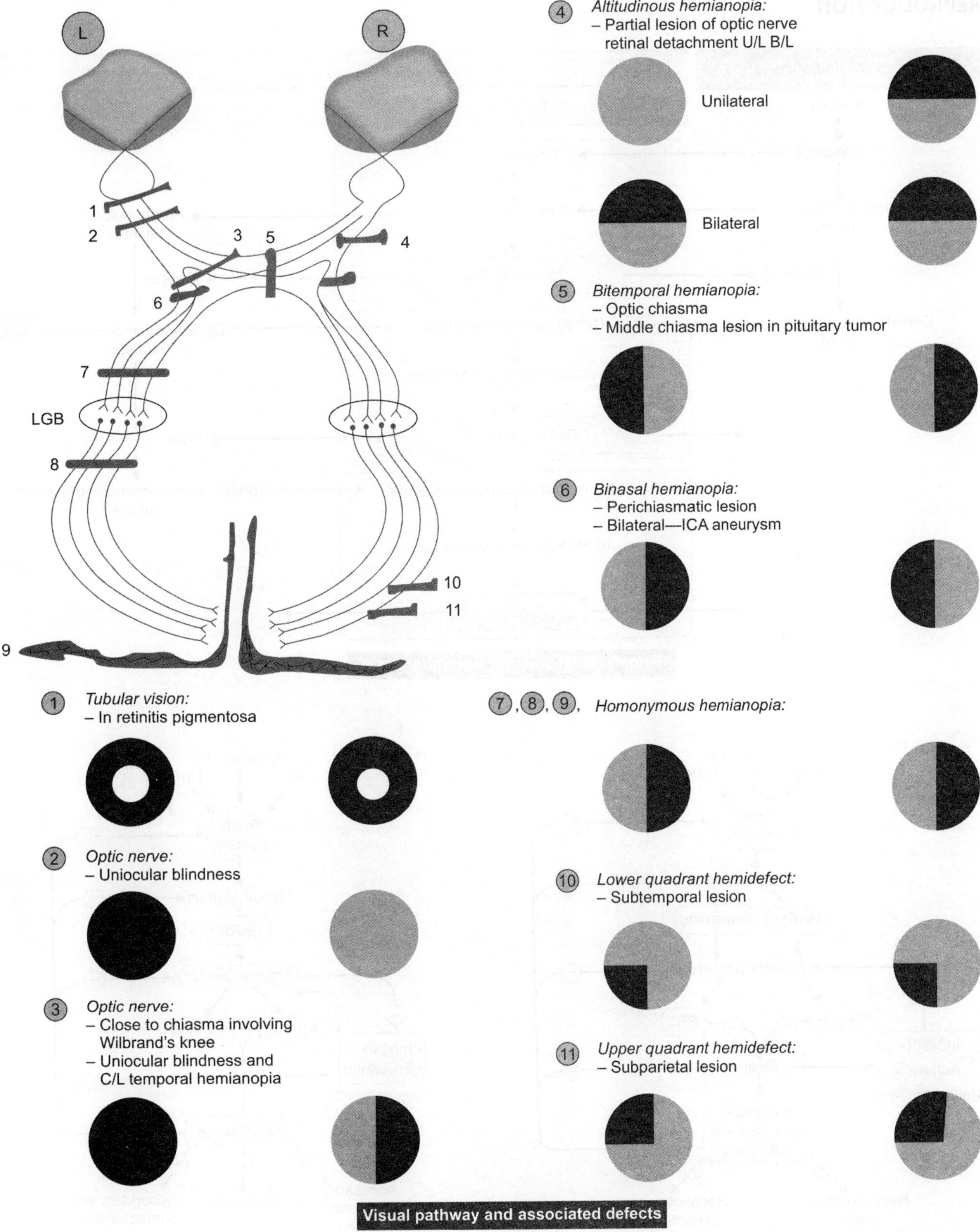

Visual pathway and associated defects

REPRODUCTION

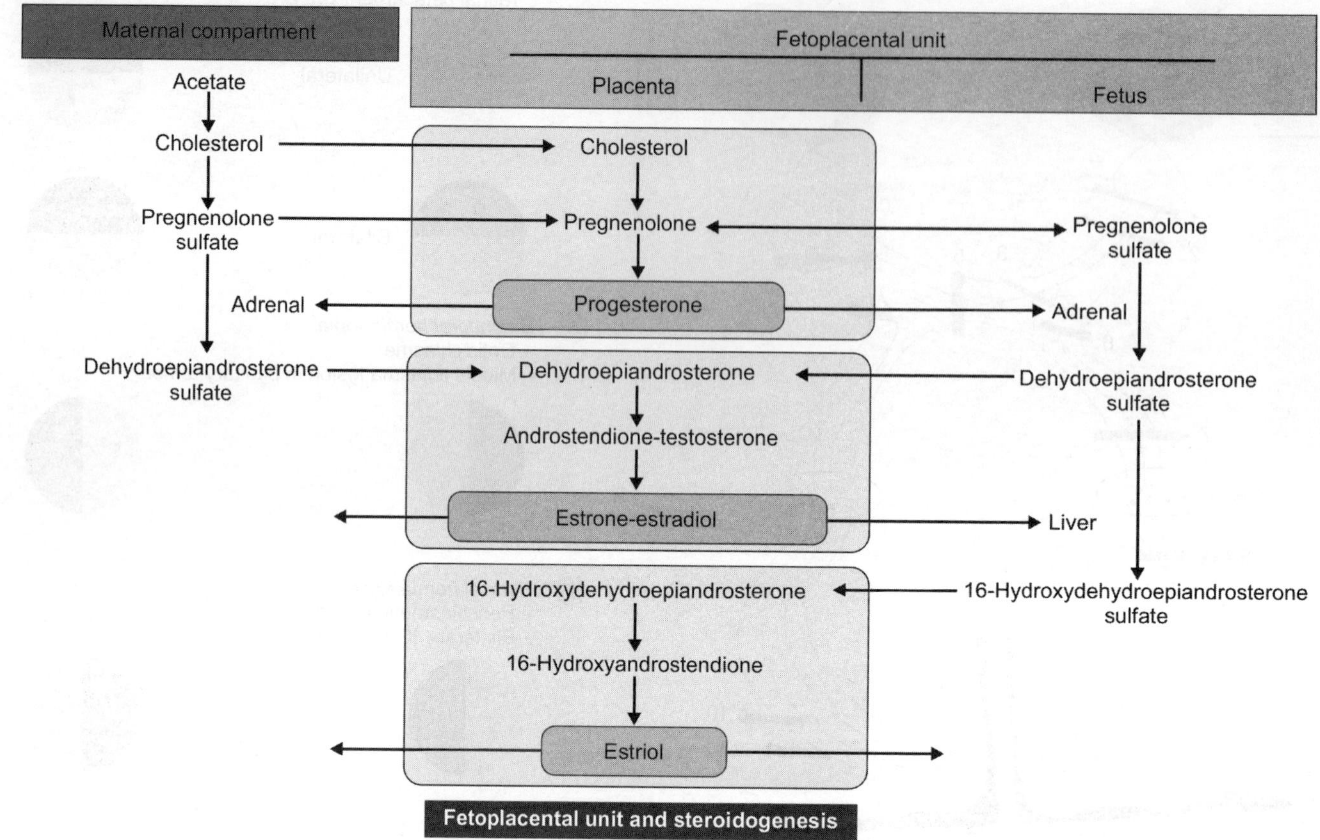

Fetoplacental unit and steroidogenesis

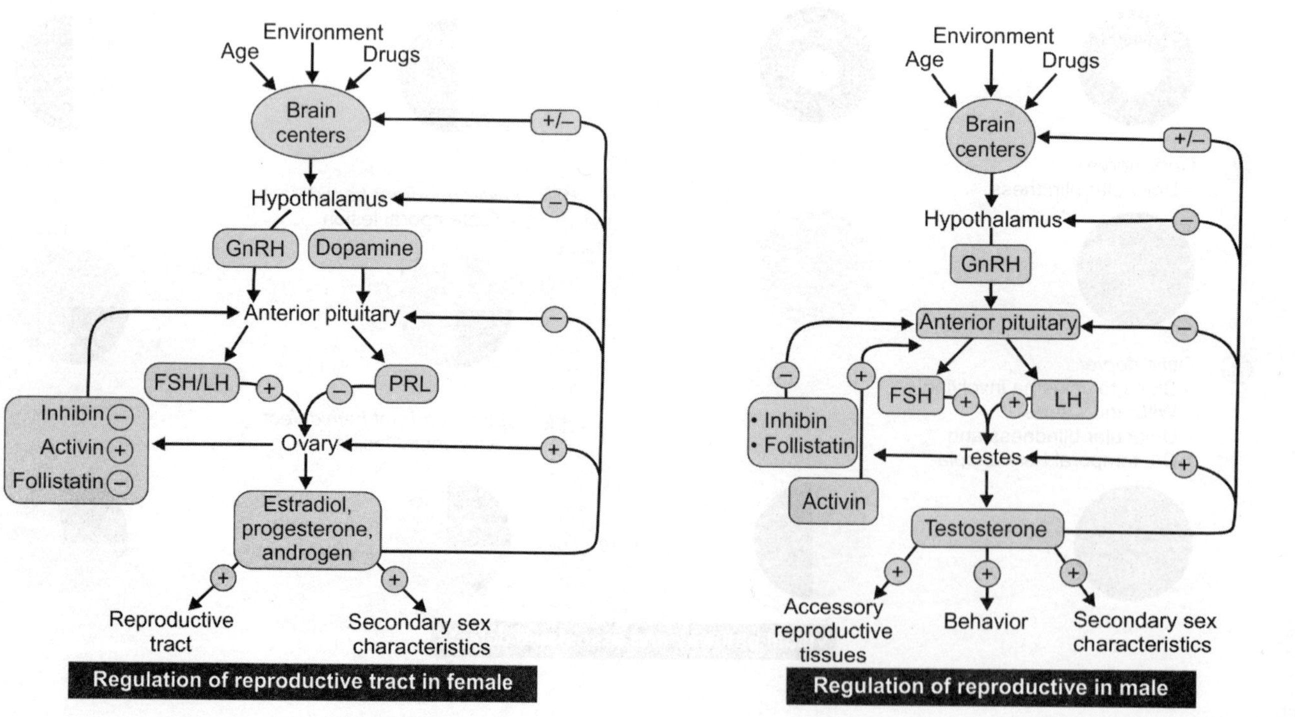

Regulation of reproductive tract in female

Regulation of reproductive in male

3

Biochemistry

KERALA UNIVERSITY OF HEALTH SCIENCES (KUHS) SYLLABUS

Theory Paper I	50
Theory Paper II	50
Theory: Internal Assessment	20
Practical I	20
Practical II	20
Practical: Internal Assessment	20
Practical: Viva Voce	20
TOTAL	200

Theory	
Paper I	Introduction to Biochemistry, Enzymology, Metabolism of Carbohydrates, Metabolism of Lipids, Metabolism of Proteins, Biological Oxidation, Clinical Enzymology and Clinical Markers, Regulation of Blood Glucose, Insulin and Diabetes Mellitus
Paper II	Vitamins, Mineral Metabolism, Heme Synthesis Breakdown and Hemoglobin, Free Radical and Antioxidant, Detoxification and Biotransformation of Xenobiotics, Nucleotides, DNA—Structure and Replication, Transcription and Translation, Molecular Genetics and Control of Gene Expression, Recombinant Technology and Gene Therapy, Immune Chemistry, Clinical Biochemistry

Question Paper Model			
I	Long Essay	10 × 1	10
II	Discuss the Following	5 × 2	10
III	Write Short Notes on	3 × 5	15
IV	Write Briefly	2 × 5	10
V	Give Precise Answers	1 × 5	5
	TOTAL		50

Practicals		
Viva Voce to be included along with Practicals		
Practical I		
A	Quantitative Experiment—Estimation of Blood Urea, Glucose, Total Protein, Albumin, Creatinine, etc.	10
B	Charts for Discussion, Interpretation of Data/Problem-solving Exercise	10
Practical II		
A	Spotting (Graph, Test, Reagent, Microscopy, Instrument, Molecule, etc.)	5
B	Evaluation of Records	5
C	Qualitative Experiments	10
	TOTAL	40

THEORY: IMPORTANT QUESTIONS

GENERAL BIOCHEMISTRY

VSK—Textbook of DM Vasudevan, Sreekumari S and Kannan Vaidyanathan, 7th edition
*—Important Questions

Short Notes

- Marker enzymes (VSK-8)
- Donnan membrane (VSK-8)
- Lysosomes (VSK-12,14,199)
- Peroxisomes (VSK-13)
- Fluid mosaic model* (VSK-14)
- Ionophores (VSK-19)
- Transport mechanism* (VSK-20).

CARBOHYDRATES

Essay

- Glycolysis—regulation, energy yield, rate limiting steps* (VSK-108)
- Gluconeogenesis* (VSK-117)
- Glycogenolysis* (VSK-124)
- Glycogen synthesis* (VSK-125)
- Regulation of blood glucose (VSK-311)
- Hexose monophosphate (HMP) shunt pathway—significance* (VSK-129)
- Krebs cycle—significance, functions, energy yield, rate limiting step* (VSK-253).

Short Notes

- Epimerism (VSK-71)
- Anomerism (VSK-71)
- Mucopolysaccharides* (VSK-80)
- Glycosides (VSK-75)
- Absorption of carbohydrates (VSK-106)
- Glycosaminoglycans* (VSK-80)
- Glucose transporters* (VSK-107)
- Glycogen storage diseases* (VSK-128)
- G6PDH deficiency (VSK-113)
- Rapoport-Luebering cycle (VSK-115)
- Metabolic fate of pyruvate* (VSK-117,118)
- Glucuronic acid (VSK-547)
- Essential pentosuria* (VSK-135)
- Fructose metabolism (VSK-137)
- Hereditary fructose intolerance* (VSK-144)
- Galactosemia* (VSK-139).

LIPIDS

Essays

- Digestion (VSK-147,148)
- Beta oxidation of fatty acid* (VSK-151)
- De Novo synthesis of fatty acid* (VSK-156)
- Ketone body metabolism* (VSK-163)
- Cholesterol synthesis, regulation, fats* (VSK-170)
- Lipoproteins—classification, composition and function (VSK-176)

Short Notes

- Polyunsaturated fatty acids* (VSK-186)
- Phopholipids (VSK-89,495)
- Liposomes* (VSK-90)
- Lecithin (VSK-90)
- Cardiolipin (VSK-91)
- Omega-3-fatty acids (VSK-163)
- Absorption of lipids (VSK-147,148)
- Chylomicrons* (VSK-149,175)
- Oxidation of odd chain fatty acids* (VSK-154)
- Advantage of multienzyme complex (VSK-66, 210)
- Metabolism of adipose tissue (VSK-161)
- Fatty liver and lipotropic factors* (VSK-162)
- Micelle formation (VSK-89)
- Ketosis (VSK-164)
- Apolipoproteins (VSK-174)
- Very-low-density lipoprotein (VLDL) (VSK-177)
- Low-density lipoprotein (LDL) and high-density lipoprotein (HDL) (VSK-179)
- Formation of bile salts (VSK-182)
- Polyunsaturated fatty acid (PUFA)—significance* (VSK-186)
- Essential fatty acids (VSK-187)
- Prostaglandins* (VSK-188)
- Lipid storage diseases* (VSK-193).

PROTEINS

Essays

- Structure of amino acids* (VSK-25)
- Urea cycle** (VSK-203)
- One carbon metabolism* (VSK-207)
- Glycine metabolism and function (VSK-211)
- Sulfur containing amino acids (VSK-216, 217)
- Phenylalanine* (VSK-233)
- Tryptophan* (VSK-239).

Short Notes

- Transamination* (VSK-201)
- Peptide bond (VSK-31)
- Structure of proteins* (primary, secondary and tertiary) (VSK-34)
- Denaturation (VSK-42)

- Classification of proteins* (VSK-42)
- Formation of ammonia (VSK-200)
- Detoxification of ammonia* (VSK-203)
- Disorders of urea cycle (VSK-205)
- Homocystinuria* (VSK-220)
- Cystinuria* (VSK-219)
- Cystathioninuria (VSK-221)
- GABA metabolism (VSK-224)
- Polyamines (VSK-229)
- Maple syrup urine disease* (VSK-230)
- Phenylketonuria* (VSK-236)
- Alkaptonuria* (VSK-237)
- Albinism (VSK-238)
- Catecholamines (VSK-234)
- Hartnup disease* (VSK-242)
- Serotonin (VSK-239).

ENZYMES

Essays

- Enzyme inhibition* (VSK-59)
- Classification of enzymes* (VSK-48).

Short Notes

- Mode of action of enzymes (VSK-51)
- Active center (VSK-54)
- Michaelis constant* (VSK-57)
- Competitive inhibition* (VSK-59)
- Noncompetitive inhibition (VSK-60)
- Allosteric inhibition (VSK-62)
- Isoenzymes* (VSK-66)
- Suicide inhibition (VSK-62)
- Factors affecting enzyme action* (VSK-56).

BIOLOGICAL OXIDATION

Essays

- Tricarboxylic acid (TCA) cycle* (VSK-247)
- Organization of ETC with diagram (VSK-260).

Short Notes

- High energy compounds* (VSK-258)
- Cytochrome oxidase* (VSK-257)
- ATP synthase (complex V)* (VSK-264)
- Chemiosmotic theory* (VSK-263)
- Inhibitors of ATP synthesis* (VSK-265)
- Substrate level phosphorylation* (VSK-256)
- Uncouplers* (VSK-265)
- TCA cycle inhibitors* (VSK-254).

HEME SYNTHESIS AND BREAKDOWN AND HEMOGLOBIN

Essays

- Heme synthesis and regulation* (VSK-272)
- Porphyrias* (VSK-274)
- Heme catabolism (VSK-276)
- Jaundice (VSK-280).

Short Notes

- Structure of heme (VSK-270)
- Van den Bergh test* (VSK-279)
- Microsomal heme oxygenase system (VSK-279)
- Crigler-Najjar syndrome* (VSK-279)
- O_2 and CO_2 transport (VSK-285, 287)
- Heme-heme interactions (VSK-287)
- Oxygen dissociation curve (ODC)—Bohr effect* (VSK-285, 286)
- Hb derivatives (VSK-289)
- Hb variants (VSK-290)
- Thalasssemia* (VSK-293)
- Myoglobin (VSK-294).

CLINICAL ENZYMOLOGY AND BIOMARKERS

Short Notes

- Cardiac biomarkers* (VSK-302)
- Creatinine kinase* (VSK-302)
- Lactate dehydrogenase* (VSK-303)
- Alkaline phosphatase (VSK-305)
- Acid phosphatase (VSK-306)
- Glucose-6-phosphate dehydrogenase (VSK-307)
- Enzymes as therapeutic agents* (VSK-308; tab-23.4)
- Amylase* (VSK-307)
- Immobilized enzymes (VSK-309)
- CRP (VSK-383)
- Alpha 1 antitrypsin (VSK-384).

REGULATION OF BLOOD GLUCOSE, INSULIN AND DIABETES MELLITUS

Essays

- Regulation in glucose in fasting state* (VSK-311)
- Diabetes mellitus* (VSK-323).

Short Notes

- Oral glucose tolerance test (OGTT) (VSK-314)
- Impaired glucose tolerance (VSK-315)

- Impaired fasting glycemia (VSK-315)
- Alimentary glycosuria* (VSK-316)
- Renal glucosuria (VSK-316)
- Reducing substances in urine* (VSK-316)
- Action of insulin and glucagon (VSK-318)
- Metabolic syndrome (VSK-325)
- Metabolic derangements in diabetes (VSK-326)
- Diabetic ketoacidosis* (VSK-326)
- Splay*
- Ketosis (VSK-327)
- Lactic acidosis (VSK-328)
- Glycated hemoglobin* (VSK-329)
- DM—management (VSK-330).

VITAMINS

Fat-soluble Vitamins

Essays

- Vitamin A* (VSK-464)
- Vitamin D (VSK-469).

Short Notes

- Wald's visual cycle* (VSK-465)
- Night blindness and keratomalacia* (VSK-467)
- Rickets and osteomalacia (VSK-472)
- Antioxidant role of vitamin E (VSK-473).

Water-soluble Vitamins

Essays

- Vitamin C* (VSK-495).

Short Notes

- Physiological role of thymine (VSK-478)
- Beriberi (VSK-478)
- Coenzyme role of niacin (VSK-480)
- Pellagra (VSK-481)
- Functions of vitamin-B_6 (VSK-483)
- Enzyme activity of biotin* (VSK-484)
- Biotin antagonists (VSK-486)
- Folate trap* (VSK-490)
- Folate antagonist (VSK-491)
- Functional role of vitamin B_{12} (VSK-493)
- Deficiency manifestations of vit-C* (VSK-497).

MINERAL METABOLISM

Essays

- Ca metabolism* (VSK-503)
- Fe metabolism* (VSK-514).

Short Notes

- Action of calcitonin, calcitriol and PTH (VSK-505)
- Hypo- and hypercalcemia (VSK-507)
- Iron toxicity (VSK-520)
- Wilson disease* (VSK-521)
- Ceruloplasmin (VSK-520)
- Aceruloplasminemia (VSK-520)
- Metabolism of zinc* (VSK-522)
- Se-containing enzymes (VSK-523)
- Se-biochemical role (VSK-523)
- Fluorosis (VSK-522).

ENERGY METABOLISM AND NUTRITION

Short Notes

- Calorific value (VSK-527)
- Respiratory quotient (VSK-527)
- Resting metabolic rate (VSK-528)
- Protein energy malnutrition* (VSK-534)
- Glycemic index (VSK-540).

ACID-BASE BALANCE

Essays

- Maintenance of normal blood pH (buffers of body fluid, renal and respiratory mechanisms)* (VSK-395).

Short Notes

- Henderson-Hasselbalch equation (VSK-392)
- Anion gap* (VSK-399)
- Metabolic acidosis* (VSK-399)
- Metabolic alkalosis* (VSK-402)
- Respiratory acidosis* (VSK-403)
- Respiratory alkalosis* (VSK-403)
- Metabolic alterations in diabetes mellitus and diabetes insipidus.

FREE RADICALS AND ANTIOXIDANTS

Short Notes

- Free radical scavenging enzymes* (VSK-435)
- Polyphenols (VSK-435)
- Lipid peroxidation (3 phase) (VSK-437)
- Role of antioxidants (VSK-439).

DETOXIFICATION AND BIOTRANSFORMATION OF XENOBIOTICS

Short Notes

- Phases of detoxification* (VSK-545, 546)
- Cytochrome P450 (VSK-545)

- Conjugations (VSK-547)
- Examples for each reactions* (VSK-545-547)
- Detoxification of ammonia* (VSK-203).

NUCLEOTIDES

Essays

- De Novo synthesis, salvage pathway* (VSK-564)
- Degradation and disorders of purine and pyrimidine metabolism* (VSK-566-67)
- Gout* (VSK-566).

Short Notes

- Structure and source of purine and pyrimidine ring* (VSK-560)
- Purine synthesis inhibitors (VSK-565)
- PRPP synthesis (VSK-563)
- Disorders of purine metabolism (VSK-566)
- Lesch-Nyhan syndrome* (VSK-568)
- Regulation of pyrimidine synthesis (VSK-570)
- Orotic aciduria (VSK-570)
- CPS 1 and CPS 2* (VSK-570).

DNA: STRUCTURE AND REPLICATION

Essays

- DNA replication* (VSK-579).

Short Notes

- Watson-Crick model of DNA structure* (VSK-576)
- Base pairing rule (VSK-576)
- Wobble hypothesis (VSK-599)
- Histones* (VSK-576)
- Nucleosomes* (VSK-576)
- Introns, EXONS, cistrons (VSK-578)
- DNA polymerase and inhibitors (VSK-580)
- DNA repair mechanisms and disorders* (VSK-583)
- Telomere and telomerase* (VSK-585)
- Inhibitors of DNA replication* (VSK-586).

TRANSCRIPTION AND TRANSLATION

Essays

- Transcription* (VSK-589)
- Translation* (VSK-599).

Short Notes

- Types of RNA (VSK-587)
- t-RNA* (VSK-596)
- RNA polymerase (VSK-589)
- TATA box (VSK-590)
- Post-transcriptional processing* (VSK-591)
- Spliceosomes (VSK-592)
- Ribozymes (VSK-592)
- Reverse transcriptase (VSK-592)
- Inhibitors of RNA synthesis* (VSK-593)
- Genetic codon-features* (VSK-598)
- Polysomes (VSK-602)
- Chaperons* (VSK-604)
- Heat-shock proteins (VSK-604)
- Post-translational processing* (VSK-603)
- Inhibitors of protein synthesis (VSK-605)
- Mitochondrial DNA and RNA (VSK-605)
- Antisense therapy (VSK-595)
- OXPHOS disease (VSK-606).

MOLECULAR GENETICS AND CONTROL OF GENE EXPRESSION

Essays

- Mutations (VSK-612)
- Cell cycle regulation of gene expression (VSK-614).

Short Notes

- Mutagens* and mutagenesis (VSK-614)
- Apoptosis* (VSK-616)
- Prions* (VSK-616)
- Retinoblastoma (VSK-615)
- Oncosuppressor proteins* (VSK-615)
- Hormone responsive elements (VSK-619)
- Lac operon* (VSK-617)
- Oncogenes (VSK-709, 710).

RECOMBINANT TECHNOLOGY AND GENE THERAPY

Essays

- Recombinant DNA technology* (VSK-626–629).

Short Notes

- Application of recombinant DNA technology* (VSK-624)
- Vectors (VSK-626,629)
- Restriction endonucleases (VSK-625)
- Gene therapy (VSK-629)
- Retroviruses (VSK-629).

CANCER AND AIDS

Short Notes

- Antimutagens (VSK-707)
- Oncogenic viruses (VSK-707)
- Oncogenes* (VSK-709)
- Protooncogene (VSK-709)
- Tumor markers* (VSK-713).

IMMUNE CHEMISTRY

Short Notes

- Structure and function of immunoglobulins (VSK-687)
- Multiple myeloma (VSK-690)
- Bence-Jones proteins* (VSK-690)
- Acute phase proteins* (VSK-383)
- Immune electrophoresis (VSK-448).

CLINICAL BIOCHEMISTRY

Short Notes

- Therapeutic application of radioisotopes in biochemistry (VSK-733,736)
- Liver function test* (VSK-346)
- Kidney function test (VSK-361)
- Electrophoresis* (VSK-448)
- Chromatography (VSK-448)
- Rf value (VSK-449)
- Radioimmunoassay* (VSK-731)
- ELISA* (VSK-453)
- Creatinine clearance* (VSK-367)
- Urea clearance* (VSK-369)
- Southern blot* (VSK-634)
- Restriction fragment length polymorphism (RFLP)* (VSK-637)
- Polymerase chain reaction (PCR)* (VSK-638, 645)
- Monoclonal antibodies (VSK-717)
- Western blot* (VSK-700).

QUALITATIVE EXPERIMENTS

IDENTIFICATION OF BIOLOGICALLY IMPORTANT SUBSTANCES

Physical Tests

- Color
- Odor
- Appearance
- Reactions to litmus

Chemical Tests

Flow chart 1 Biologically important substances

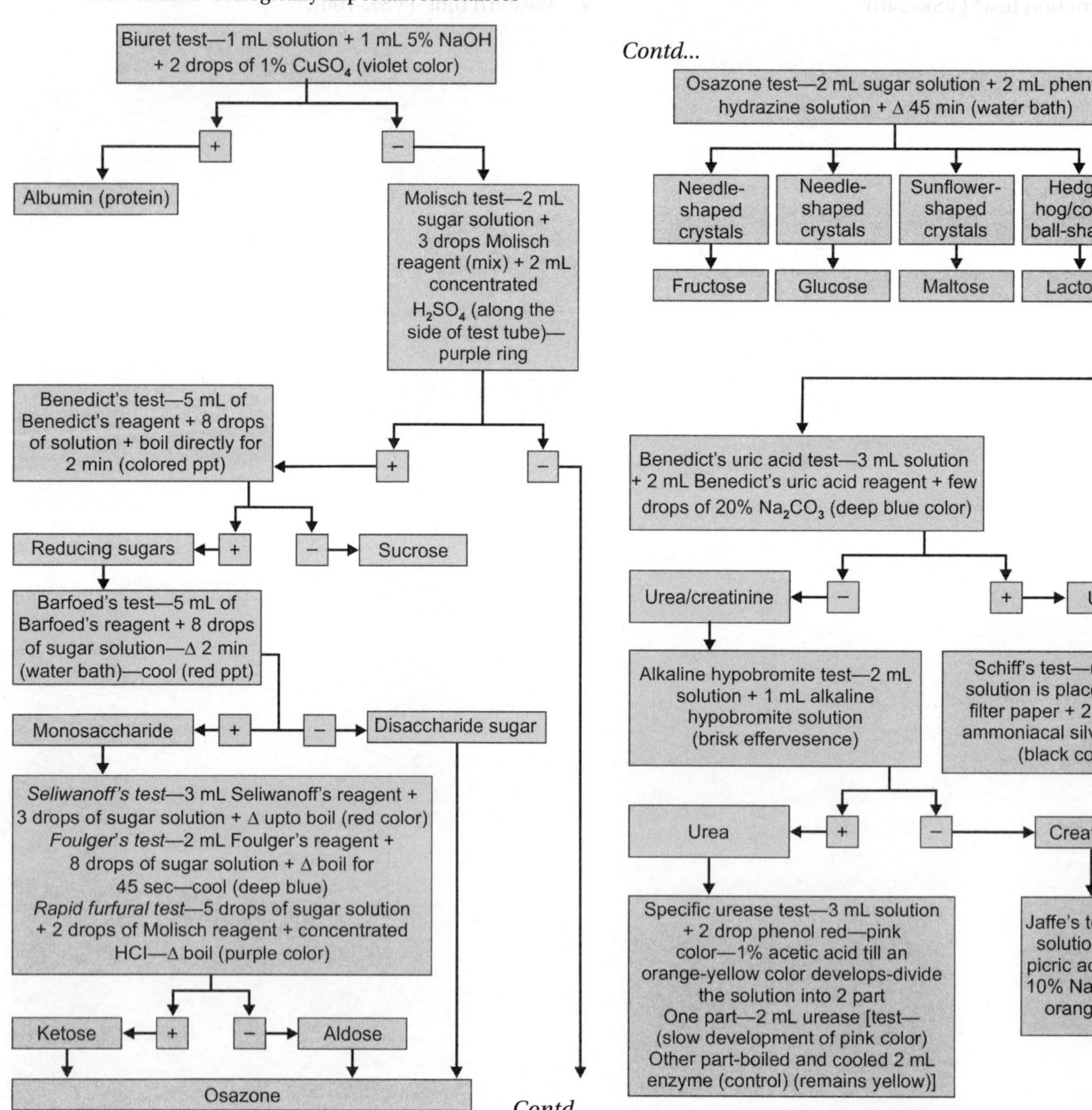

Reactions of Glucose (Flow chart 1)

Procedure	*Observation*	*Inference*
i. Molisch test	Purple ring is formed at the junction of two liquids	Glucose is a carbohydrate
ii. Benedict's test	Colored precipitate—green/yellow/orange/red	Glucose is a red sugar
iii. Barfoed's test	Red precipitate is formed at the bottom of the test tube.	Glucose is a reducing monosaccharide
iv. Osazone test	Yellow crystals of osazone seperate out. The crystals are needle-shaped/'sheaves of corn'	Glucosazone is formed

- **Define carbohydrates.**
  These are aldehyde or keto derivatives of polyhydric alcohol or compounds that yield these compounds on hydrolysis.
- **Classify carbohydrates.**
  Monosaccharides—Glucose, fructose
  Disaccharides—Lactose, maltose, sucrose
  Oligosaccharides—Maltotriose
  Polysaccharides—Starch, glycogen, dextrin.
- **What are the ingredients of Molisch reagent?**
  It is α(alpha)-naphthol in alcohol. The furfural derivatives condense with α-naphthol in alcohol to form the purple colored product.
- **What is the principle of Molisch test?**
  Carbohydrates get dehydrated and form-furfural/hydroxyl methyl furfural derivatives by the action of concentrated sulfuric acid on sugar. The furfural derivatives condense with phenols to give characteristic colored products.
- **What are the ingredients of Benedict's reagent?**
  It is constituted by copper sulfate (provides cupric ions), sodium carbonate (makes medium alkaline) and sodium citrate (improves shelf-life).
- **What is the principle of Benedict's test?**
  Sugar solution in the presence of dilute alkali, undergoes molecular rearrangement (tautomerization) to form enediols, which are powerful reducing agents). Cupric ions take electrons from enediols and get reduced to cuprous ions (Molisch reagent gets oxidized to sugar acids). Cuprous ions combine with hydroxyl ions to form cuprous hydroxide, which is highly unstable on heating it is converted to cuprous oxide, which is precipitated. Cupric hydroxide is insoluble in water but is made soluble with the help of citrate, tartrate, etc.
- **Why is Benedict's test called the semiquantitative test?**
  Benedict's solution changes through a range of colors (blue, green, yellow, orange, red) according to how much reducing sugar is present in the sample. Because of that it is called semiquantitative test.
- **Name the non-carbohydrate reducing substances.**
  Non-sugar reducing substances such as ascorbic acid, homogentisic acid, salicylic acid, uric acid and creatinine, when present in excess, also give a positive test.
- **What are the ingredients of Barfoed's reagent?**
  Barfoed's reagent is copper acetate in acetic acid.
- **What is the principle of Barfoed's test?**
  Reduction within 2 minutes in a boiling water bath indicates the presence of monosaccharides. Here reduction is carried out in acidic medium. Acidic medium is unfavorable for reduction, but usually strongly reducing carbohydrates, i.e. monosaccharides give a positive test.
- **What is the principle of osazone test?**
  Phenyl hydrazine reacts with sugars to form hydrazone and having characteristic crystalline shape osazones in presence of acetate buffer.
- **Why does lactose show the Barfoed's test negetive?**
  Lactose is a disaccharide. Monosaccharides reduce the cupric ions even in acidic medium and the precipitate formed is of cuprous oxide.
- **What is the difference between Benedict's and Barfoed's test even though both are based on the reducing property of sugars?**
  Reducing monosaccharides is more reducing than reducing disaccharides, only strong reducing sugars can reduce cupric ions at acidic pH (Barfoed's reagent is acidic).
- **Why does glucose, fructose and mannose give the same shape for osazone crystals?**
  Glucose, fructose and mannose give same type of osazone because they differ only at first two carbon atoms, which are masked by attachment of two molecules of phenylhydrazine.
- **Name some reducing sugars.**
  Glucose, fructose, mannose, lactose, maltose and galactose, etc.
- **Name some non-reducing sugars.**
  Sucrose, trehalose.
- **Name some non-sugar reducing sugars.**
  Non-sugar reducing substances such as ascorbic acid, homogentisic acid, salicylic acid, uric acid and creatinine.
- **What is the shape of maltosazone?**
  Sunflower shaped/petal-shaped crystals.

Reactions of Fructose (Flow chart 1)

Procedure	*Observation*	*Inference*
Molisch test	Purple ring	Fructose is a carbohydrate
Benedict's test	Green/yellow/orange/red precipitate	Fructose is a reducing sugar
Barfoed's test	Red ppt	Fructose is a red monosaccharide
Osazone test	Needle/'sheaves of corn' shaped crystals	Fructosazone is formed
Rapid furfural test	Purple color—indicate the presence of ketoses	Fructose is a ketohexose
Seliwanoff's test	Cherry red color—indicate the presence of ketoses	Fructose is a ketohexose
Foulger's test	Deep blue color—indicate the presence of ketoses	Fructose is a ketohexose

- **What is the principle of rapid furfural test?**
  Ketoses are dehydrated rapidly than aldoses to form furfural derivatives. The color is due to the complex formed by furfural derivative with alpha naphthol. This test helps to differentiate between glucose and fructose.
- **What are the ingredients of Seliwanoff's and Foulger's reagent?**
  Seliwanoff's reagent is resorcinol in con. HCl
  Foulger's reagent is urea, stannous chloride (40% in H_2SO_4).
- **What is the principle of Seliwanoff's test and Foulger's test?**
  When sugar solution is boiled with Seliwanoff's reagent, ketoses are dehydrated to form furfural, which condenses with resorcinol to form red color.
- **Why aldoses give Seliwanoff's, Foulger's and rapid furfural tests negative?**
  Ketoses are dehydrated more rapidly than aldoses to form furfural compounds and they further condens with alcohol to form colored precipitate.
- **What are the monosaccharide units in lactose, maltose and sucrose?**
  Lactose—glucose + galactose
  Mannose—glucose + glucose
  Sucrose—glucose + fructose

Reactions of Lactose (Flow chart 1)

Procedure	*Observation*	*Inference*
Molisch test	Purple ring	Lactose is a carbohydrate
Benedicts test	Green/yellow/orange/red precipitate	Lactose is a reducing sugar
Barfoeds test	No characteristic precipitate	Lactose is a reducing disaccharide
Osazone test	Puff-shaped/cotton ball-shaped osozon crystals are seen. It is also described as pin cushion or flower of "touch me not" plant	Lactosazone is formed

- **What is the linkage in lactose?**
  Lactose is formed by β 1-4 glycosidic linkage b/w the anomeric carbon of β galactose and 4th -OH group of glucose.
- **What is the shape of maltosazone?**
  It has petal shaped or sun-flower like crystals.

Reactions of Sucrose (Flow chart 1)

Procedure	*Observation*	*Inference*
Molisch test	Purple ring is formed	Sucrose is a carbohydrate
Benedict's test	No characteristic precipitate	Sucrose is a non-reducing sugar
Specific sucrose test	Green/yellow/orange ppt is formed	Prescence of sucrose is confirmed
Rapid furfural test	Purple color formed	Presence of ketohexose in sucrose
Seliwanoff's test	Cherry red color formed	Presence of ketohexose in sucrose
Foulger's test	Deep blue color develops	Presence of ketohexose in sucrose

- **Why sucrose hydrolysis is known as inversion?**
  Sucrose is optically active and rotates the polarized light plane to the right (dextrorotatory). When hydrolyzed, sucrose yields equimolar amounts of glucose and fructose, a mixture that turns the polarized light to the left (levorotatory) due to predominant levorotation of fructose. So, hydrolysis of sucrose "inverts" the polarized light plane from right to left and the reaction is called inversion.
- **What is the principle of specific sucrose test?**
  The color is formed because sucrose is hydrolyzed to glucose and fructose by heating with acid. Thymol blue is added as indicator. Its pH range is 1.2–2.8. The color change is pink to yellow. The monosaccharides can reduce Cu^{3+} to Cu^{2+} and forms Cu_2O giving a red precipitate.

Reactions of Albumin (Flow chart 1)

Procedure	*Observation*	*Inference*
Biuret test	Violet color	Presence of protein
Precipitation by organic solvents 2 mL soln + 2 mL acetone	White precipitate is formed	Presence of proteins
Precipitation by heat and acid 10 mL soln-hold the tube in a slanting position and over the flame – Δ upper part + few drops of 1% acetic acid	White cloudy precipitate formed in the upper part	Coagulation takes place and albumin gets denatured
Heller's test 2 mL con HNO_3 + soln along the sides of the test tube	White ring formed at the jn of two liquids	Presence of albumin (ring due to formation of metaprotein)

Contd...

Contd...

Procedure	*Observation*	*Inference*
Heat coagulation test 5-10 mL soln + 2 drops of chlorophenol red + 1% acetic acid drop by drop—till pink color disappears—Δ till coagulum comes to top—divide it into 2 parts: One part—2% Na_2CO_3 Other part—1% acetic acid	A coagulum appears which is insoluble in both alkali and acid	Presence of albumin
Half saturation with $(NH_4)_2 SO_4$ 3 mL soln + 3 mL $(NH_4)_2 SO_4$ + stand for 5 min + perform biuret test by using 40% NaOH	Violet color develops	Albumin is not completely precipitated by half saturation
Full saturation with $(NH_4)_2 SO_4$ 3 mL soln + add $(NH_4)_2 SO_4$—till it becomes saturated—stand for 5 min—perform biuret test by using 40% NaOH	No violet color develops	Albumin is completely precipitated by half-saturation
Color reaction		
Ninhydrin test 1 mL soln + 4 drops ninhydrin soln—Δ2 min—cool	Blue/purple color develops	Presence of protein
Xanthoproteic test 2 mL soln + 1 mL con HNO_3—Δ till the soln turns yellow—cool—divide into 2 parts To one part—+ 1 mL, 40% NaOH (compare the color with the other part)	Yellow color deepens to orange	Presence of amino acids containing benzene ring (aromatic amino acids)
Millon's test 2 mL soln + 1 mL mercuric sulfate + Δ30 sec—cool—8 drops of 1% sodium nitrite	White ppt formed, which turns red	Presence of tyrosine
Aldehyde tests (Hopkin-Cole Reaction) 1 mL soln + few drops of formalin + 1 drop of mercuric sulfate in H_2SO_4 + 2 mL con. H_2SO_4 along the side	Purple/violet colored ring is formed at the junction of the two liquids	Presence of tryptophan
Folin-ciocalteau test 1 mL soln + 1 mL 10% NaOH + few drops of folin ciocalteau reagent	Deep blue color	Presence of tyrosine
Sakaguchi's test 1 mL soln + 8 drops of 40% NaOH + 2 drops of molisch reagnt + 2 mL bromine water	Bright red color	Presence of arginine

Contd...

Contd...

Procedure	*Observation*	*Inference*
Pauly's test (diazo reaction) 2 mL soln + 0.5 mL sulfanillic acid + 0.5 mL 0.5% sodium nitrite—allow 2 min—+ 1 mL 10% sodium carbonate	Deep cherry red color	Presence of histidine
Sulfur test 2 mL soln + 1 mL 40% NaOH—Δ2 min—+ 0.5 mL lead acetate	Brownish black color	Presence of sulfur containing amino-acids

- **Name plasma proteins.**
  Albumin, globulin, fibrinogen.
- **What are the functions of albumin?**
  - It contributes to colloidal osmotic pressure
  - It acts as a carrier protein and helps in transport of various hydrophobic substances such as bilirubin, non esterified free fatty acids, drugs like sulpha drugs, aspirin, salicylates, dicumarol, phenytoin, steroid hormone, thyroxine, Ca, Cu, and heavy metals.
  - It has maximum buffering capacity.
  - It also acts as the transport form of essential amino-acids from liver to extra hepatic cells.
- **What is isoelectric pH?**
  The pH at which the molecule carries no charge. They exist as zwitterion.
  Isoelectric pH of albumin is 4.8.
- **What is the principle of 'precipitation by organic solvents'?**
  Addition of organic solvents such as acetone and alcohol decreases dielectric constants of solvents and displaces some water molecules associated with proteins and decreases the concentration of water in solution. This effect tends to decrease solubility of proteins.
- **What is the principle of 'precipitation by heat and acid' method?**
  Proteins are easily denatured when subjected to heat, as heating of proteins causes disorganization of peptide chain, as a result breaking of cross-linkage with resultant unfolding of chain and marked changes in properties occur. This is called denaturation.
- **What is the principle of biuret test?**
  - In alkaline medium, cupric ions form a violet colored complex with peptide bond nitrogen of peptides and proteins.
  - This test is also answered by other compounds having NH-CO bond and also metaproteins, proteoses, peptones and polypeptides with 2 or more peptide bonds.
  - Dipeptides and individual amino acids will not answer the test.

- **What is the importance of biuret test?**
It is a general test for all proteins. This test is also answered by other compounds having NH-CO bonds and also metaproteins, proteoses, peptons and polypeptides with 2 or more peptide bonds. Dipeptides and individual amino acids will not answer the test.
This reaction is used for quantitative estimation also. Excess of $CuSO_4$ may mask the development of color. Magnesium and ammonium sulfates interfere with the reaction.
- **Which all amino acids will answer the 'sulfur test'?**
Sulfur containing amino acids such as cysteine and cystine will answer the test. But methionine will not answer the test.
- **What is the normal serum level of albumin?**
Normal serum level is 3.5–5 g/dL.
- **What are complete proteins?**
These are proteins containing all essential amino acids.
- **What are limiting amino acids?**
Certain proteins are deficient in one or more essential amino acids. These amino acids which are deficient in the particular proteins are called limiting amino acids.
- **What is hypoalbuminemia?**
Decreased serum albumin level is termed as hypoalbuminemia. Decreased levels of serum albumin is seen in cirrhosis of liver, chronic liver failure, malnutrition, malabsorptin syndrome and nephrotic syndrome.
- **What is albuminuria? And what are the causes?**
Presence of albumin in urine is called albuminuria. Large quantities of proteins are lost in nephritic syndrome.
Causes
Prerenal—pregnancy, severe dehydration, heart disease, impaired renal circulation, inflammatory conditions.
Renal—glomerulonephritis, nephrotic syndrome
Postrenal—urinary tract infections.
- **What is Bence-Jones proteinuria?**
This is a disorder seen in patients with multiple myeloma. Light chain immunoglobulins are excreted in urine. Multiple myeloma is characterized by proteinuria. This is due to increased production of H and L chains or due to deletion of portions of L chains so that they can not combine with H chains.
The Bence-Jones proteins are get precipitated when heated b/w 45–60°C. but redissolved at 80–90°C. They precipitate and dissolve on cooling. These proteins may block kidney tubules, leading to renal failure.
- **What are essential amino acids? Give examples.**
These amino acids are compulsory for growth. Their carbon skeleton cannot be synthesized by human beings and so performed amino acids are to be taken in food for normal growth.
Essential amino acids—Isoleucine, Leucine, Threonine, Lysine, Methionine, Phenylalanine, Tryptophan, Valine.
- **What is the principle of Heller's test?**
White rings are formed due to formation of metaproteins which are hydrolytic products formed by action of acids or alkalies on proteins. They are generally soluble in dilute acids and alkalies but insoluble in neutral solvents.
- **What is the principle of 'heat coagulation test'?**
When heated at isoelectric pH, some proteins denature irreversibly producing the floating precipitate called coagulum. Albumin is easily coagulated.

Reactions of Uric Acid (Flow chart 1)

Procedure	*Observation*	*Inference*
Benedict's uric acid test	Deep blue color	Indicates presence of uric acid
Schiff's test	Black color	Presence of uric acid

- **What is Benedict's uric acid (BUA) reagent?**
It is arsenophosphotungstate.
- **What is the principle of Benedict's uric acid test and Schiff's test?**
BUA reagent is reduced by uric acid to tungsten blue in alkaline medium.
In case of Schiff's test, uric acid reduces silver nitrate to metallic silver in alkaline medium, which appears black.
- **What is its biological importance and its normal serum level?**
Uric acid is sparingly soluble in water, but dissolves in alkali. It is a powerful reducing agent and reduces metals such as silver, copper, and compounds such as phosphotungstate, phosphomolybdate, etc.
Normal serum uric acid level in male: 2–5 mg/dL
In females: 3–7 mg/dL
Normal daily excretion is 500–700 mg.
- **Explain hyperuricemia.**
Hyperuricemia causes gout and gouty arthritis. Hyperuricemia may or may not be associated with increased uric acid excretion in urine, called uricosria. Hyperuricemia can be primary with increased purine synthesis due to enzyme defects.
It can be secondary to malignancies, following radiotherapy and chemotherapy, starvation, renal failure.

Reactions of Urea (Flow chart 1)

Procedure	*Observation*	*Inference*
Alkaline hypobromite test	Brisk effervescence	Presence of urea
Specific urease test	Test—slow development of pink color—confirms presence of urea Controls—remains yellow	Presence of urea

- **How is urea formed?**
Urea is the diamide of carbonic acid (NH_2CONH_2). It is the endproduct of protein metabolism. Ammonia

released as a result of protein catabolism is highly toxic to brain cells. Ammonia is converted into non-toxic urea in liver cells by urea cycle/ornithine cycle/Krebs-Hansleit cycle. Urea is water-soluble and excreted through kidney.

- **What is its biological importance and normal serum level?**
  Urea is the diamide of carbonic acid (NH_2CONH_2). It is the end-product of protein metabolism.
  Normal blood urea level—20–40 mg/dL
  Average excretion of urea is 15–30 g/day.
- **Give the clinical significance.**
  Uremia is the term used for raised blood urea level, which is seen in renal failure and acute glomerulonephritis. Decreased levels of urea is seen in liver diseases.
- **What is the principle of hypobromite test?**
  Effervescence is due to release of nitrogen.
  $$(CO(NH_2)_2 + 3NaBrO + 2NaOH \rightarrow N_2 + Na_2CO_3 + 3NaBr + 3H_2O$$
  Carbon dioxide formed is absorbed by alkaline medium.
- **What is the principle of specific urease test?**
  Urease converts urea to NH_3 and CO_2 which combine to form ammonium carbonate
  $$NH_2CONH_2 + 2H_2O \rightarrow (NH_4)_2CO_3$$
  Phenol red is pink in alkaline medium. So the test is pink. In control, the enzyme is inactivated by heating to give test –ve.
- **What is urea clearance? How is it calculated?**
  It is the volume of plasma/blood which is completely cleared of urea by kidneys per minute. The urea clearance is less than GFR, because urea is partially reabsorbed.
  Urea clearance = U × V/P
  U-mg of urea per mL of urine
  P-mg of urea per mL of plasma
  V-mL of urine excreted per minute
  The normal value is 75 mL/min.

Reactions of Creatinine

Procedure	*Observation*	*Inference*
Jaffe's test	Deep orange color	Presence of creatinine

- **How is creatinine formed?**
  Creatinine is the end-product of creatine metabolism.
- **What is its biological importance and normal serum level?**
  Creatinine is present as creatine phosphate in muscles and brain. It is synthesized from 3 amino acids—arginine, glysine and methoinine. Creatinine is phosphorylated into creatine phosphate by creatine phospho kinase. Creatine phosphate is converted into its anhydride creatinine. Creatinine is excreted in urine. Levels of creatinine in blood and urine remains more or less constant as long as the muscle mass is not affected. Noramal serum level is 0.7–1.4 mg/dL.
- **Its clinical significance.**
  It is increased in renal failure, myopathies, fever and muscle injuries. Normal excretion is 1–2 g/day.
- **What is the principle of Jaffes' test?**
  Orange color is due to the formation of alkaline creatinine picrate.
- **What is creatinine clearance? How is it calculated?**
  It is the volume of blood or plasma which is cleared of creatinine by the kidney per minute. Creatinine excreted in a minute by kidneys.
  C = U × V/P
  U-mg of creatinine per mL of urine
  P-mg of creatinine per mL of plasma
  V-mL of urine excreted per minute
  The normal value is 80–110 mL/min.

URINE EXAMINATION

Examination of urine can be studied under 3 headings—physical, inorganic and organic constituents.

Physical Characteristics

Volume

Normal daily urine output—1.5 L/day. Minimum volume of urine needed to remove daily waste product is 500 mL.

Color

Normal urine is straw-colored or amber-yellow in color. Normal urine color is due to urochrome.

Appearance

Normal urine is clear and transparent when freshly voided. But on keeping it may become turbid. This is due to the action of bacteria which convert urea to ammonia. Ammonia makes urine alkaline and causes precipitation of phosphates of calcium and magnesium.

Odor

Urine is faintly aromatic when freshly voided, due to the presence of minute amounts of volatile organic compounds. Bacterial action converts urea in urine to ammonia which gives an unpleasant ammoniacal odor.

Specific Gravity

It is a measure of dissolved substances in urine. Normal specific gravity is 1.015–1.025.

pH of urine: Normaly pH value is 5.5–7.5. pH of urine is dependent on the relative proportions of monobasic phosphates of sodium and potassium which are acidic and dibasic phosphates of sodium and potassium which are basic.

Viva Questions

- **What are the conditions in which normal urine volume is altered?**
  Polyuria is the condition in which urine volume is increased to more than 2500 mL/day. It is seen in increased water intake, salt intake, high protein diet, diabetes insipidus, diabetes mellitus, etc.
  Oliguria is the condition in which urine output is less than 500 mL/day. It is seen in low blood pressure, dehydration, acute nephritis, ADH over-activity, etc.
  Anuria is the condition in which urine output is less than 100 mL/day. It is seen in acute glomerulonephritis, acute renal failure and shock.
- **What are the abnormal states in which different colors of urine is produced?**
  Yellow in color in cases of jaundice. Reddish color of urine indicates hematuria, while brown color is seen in hemoglobinuria. Urine becomes black on standing in cases of alkaptouria. Yellow color of urine becomes intense on standing if there is excess of urobilinogen in urine.
- **What are the various odors produced by different conditions?**
  In diabetic ketoacidosis there is a fruity odors due to the presence of acetone. Excretion of certain drugs in urine may produce characteristic odors.
- **How is specific gravity determined?**
  Specific gravity is determined using an instrument called urinometer. This consists of a bulbous portion and a narrow stem. The narrow stem above has graduations from above downwards starting from 1.000.
  Procedure: Early morning sample is taken in the cylindrical container upto 3/4th level. Remove all the froth from the surface. Immerse the urinometer in urine so that it floats without touching the sides of the cylinder. Read off the specific gravity from the graduation, corresponding to the meniscus, keeping it at eye-level. Specific gravity decreases in excessive water in-take, chronic nephritis, diabetes insipidus, etc. Specific gravity increases in diabetes mellitus.
- **What is the effect on pH after meal?**
  A few hours after a heavy meal, urine becomes alkaline due to secretion of HCl in stomach, which makes blood more alkaline. To counteract this, kidney eliminates more alkaline urine by secretion of more bicarbonate. This is called post-prandial alkaline tide.
  Diets rich in protein make urine acidic due to the production of excess phosphates and sulfates which are excreted in urine. Pathologically acidic urine is found in diabetic ketoacidosis and chronic respiratory acidosis and fever. Diet rich in vegetables makes urine alkaline.

Inorganic Constituents

Chloride

It is the chief inorganic constituent of urine, mainly sodium chloride is present. Chloride content is usually 10–15 g/24 hours.

Inorganic Sulfate

Urinary sulfur occurs as 2 types, inorganic and organic. Inorganic sulfur is in the form of sulfate. Inorganic sulfates are derived from sulfur containing amino acids. Normal excretion of inorganic sulfate is 0.8 g/day.

Phosphates

It is derived from phosphates of nucleic acids, phospo proteins and phospholipids. Normal excretion of phosphates is 1 gm/day.

Calcium

Daily calcium excretion is 0.22 g.

Ammonia

About 0.59 of ammonium salt is excreted per day.

Tests		
Test for chloride 3 mL urine + con. HNO_3 + few drops of silver nitrate	White ppt	Presence of chloride (Con. HNO_3 prevents the precipitation of phosphates)—Silver chloride
Test for sulfates 5 mL soln + con. HCl + 1.5 mL $BaCl_2$	White ppt	Presence of sulfate-Barium sulfate
Test for phosphates and calcium 10 mL soln + liq NH_3 + - Δ - white ppt—wash and filter it + 2 mL of hot 20% acetic acid—divide it into 2 parts:	Canary yellow ppt of ammonium phosphomolybdate.	Presence of phosphates in urine—Ammonium phosphomolybdate
One part—few drops con. HNO_3 + few drops ammonium molybdate—Δ Other part—+ potassium oxalate	White ppt of calcium oxalate	Presence of calcium—Calcium oxalate
Test for ammonia 3 mL soln + Δ + few drops of phenolphthalein + add dil NaOH till pink color appears + Δ + place the red litmus paper at the mouth of the test tube	Red litmus changed to blue in color	Presence of ammonia

Organic Constituents

The important organic constituents of urine are urea, uric acid, creatinine. Small amounts of ethereal sulfate and urinary pigments may also be present.

Test for urea		
Alkaline hypobromite test	Brisk effervescence	Presence of urea
Specific urease test	Slow development of pink color	Presence of urea
Test for uric acid		
Benedict's uric acid test	Deep blue color	Indicates presence of uric acid
Schiff's test	Black color	Presence of uric acid
Test for creatinine		
Jaffe's test	Deep orange color	Presence of creatinine
Test for indican 3 mL urine + 3 drops of Molisch reagent + 3 drops of H_2O_2 + 3 mL con HCl	Blue color	Presence of indican (ethereal sulfate)
Ehrlich's test 10 mL urine + 1 mL of Ehrlich's reagent —10 min	Observe the color through the top/mouth of the test tube	A pink color indicates presence of urobilinogen

Viva Questions

- **What is indican? What is the principle of 'test for indican'?**
  It is the potassium salt of indoxyl sulfuric acid. Indoxyl arises from bacterial decomposition of tryptophan in the intestine. Normal excretion is 20–40 mg/day.
  A blue color gradually develops which intensifies on standing. Indican is hydrolyzed to indoxyl which reacts alpha naphthol to give a colored ring.
- **What are urinary pigments?**
  The chief pigments of normal urine is urochrome. Small amount of urobilinogen may also be present. The oxidation of urobilinogen to urobilin is supposed to be the reason of deepening in color of urine on standing. Urobilinogen excretion is increased in fever and hemolytic conditions.
- **What is Ehrlich's reagent?**
  Ehrlich's reagent is para dimethyl amino benzaldehyde in hydrochloric acid. Normal urine contains only traces of urobilinogen. So this test may not be positive but in hemolytic jaundice and in liver diseases when there is increased urobilinogen, this test is positive.

Abnormal Constituents of Urine

Substances that are not present in easily detectable quantities in urine of healthy people but are known to occur in certain pathological or abnormal conditions are called abnormal constituents of urine. Abnormal constituents usually detected in urine are:

1. Protein
2. Blood
3. Reducing sugar
4. Ketone bodies
5. Bile salts
6. Bile pigments.

Protein

The amount of protein excreted in normal urine is insignificant and constitutes 20–80 mg/24 hrs. presence of protein in urine is described as proteinuria. Protein usually excreted in urine is albumin (albuminuria).

Proteinuria is of two types—functional and pathological.

Blood

Hematuria is presence of blood in urine. It is seen in renal stones, malignancy of kidney, a/c glomerulonephritis, trauma to kidney, malignant hypertension, TB, schistomiasis, etc. In hamaturia RBCs are seen in urine. Red colored urine without RBCs are seen in incompatible blood transfusion, burns, snake bites, black water fever, etc.

Reducing Sugars

The most common reducing sugar seen in urine is glucose. The condition is known, glucosuria. Other reducing sugars which appear in urine are fructose, lactose, galactose, pentose, etc. Glucosuria can be benign or pathological.

1. *Renal glucosuria:* In this blood sugar level is normal, but renal threshold is lowered. No treatment is required. Patient is reassured.
2. *Alimentary glucosuria:* Glucose is excreted in urine after a rich carbohydrate diet. Due to increased absorption of glucose from intestine, hyperglycemia occurs for shorter period which becomes normal within 1-1½ hours.

Pathological Conditions

1. Diabetes mellitus.
2. Hyperthyroidism.
3. Hyperadrenalisin.

Ketone Bodies

These are acetone, acetoacetate, beta hydroxy butyric acid. They are formed from acetyl coA.

Ketonuria occurs in uncontrolled DM, high fat and low carbohydrate diet and starvation.

Bile Salts

Sodium and potassium salts of glycocholic acid and taurocholic acid formed from cholesterol. These are present in obstructive jaundice and sometimes in hepatocellular jaundice.

Bile Pigments

These are bilirubin and biliverdin. Bilirubin is formed from Hb in RES. In liver, it is conjugated with glucuronic acid and excreted in bile. Conjugated bilirubin appears in urine in obstructive and hepatocellular jaundice. Unconjugated bilirubin cannot pass through kidney as it is bound to albumin.

Physical Properties

Appearance:
Color:
Odor:
Specific gravity:
pH:

Chemical Properties

Heat and acetic acid test	On adding acetic acid, denatured protein gets precipitated, but gets dissolved on excess acidification	Presence of protein
Benedict's test	Colored ppt green/ yellow/orange/red color	Presence of reducing sugars
Rothera's test 3 mL soln + saturate with $(NH_4)_2 SO_4$ + 3 drops sodium nitroprusside + liq ammonia	Appearance of purple ring at the junction	Presence of ketone bodies
Hay's test 1st test tube—2 mL water + sulfur powder (on top) 2nd T T -2 mL soln + S powder	Sulfur powder present in the urine solution sinks to the bottom	Presence of bile salts
Modified Fouchet test 5 mL of urine + 1 mL $MgSO_4$ Δ—+ 10% $BaCl_2$ till max ppt obtained—filter-dry the filter paper—2 drops fouchets reagent	Blue/green color developed	Presence of bile pigments

- **What is functional and pathological proteinuria?**
  Functional proteinuria: It includes those conditions that are not related to any diseases. The protein excreted in urine is usually small and the condition is temporary. For example, Proteinuria following violent exercise, in pregnancy and after prolonged standing (orthostatic or postural proteinuria).
  Pathological proteinuria:
  Prerenal: Cardiac disease, ascites, tumor of abdomen, collagen vascular disease, severe hypertension, fever, convulsions, anemia, liver disease.
  Renal: Nephrotic syndrome: TB, kidney, glomerulonephritis.
  Postrenal: Inflammatory, degenerative, traumatic lesions of pelvis of kidney, ureter, urinary bladder, prostate, urethra.
- **What are Bence Jones protein?**
  They are light chains of immunoglobulins excreted in urines in cases of multiple myeloma. They are precipitated on heating urine from 40–60°C. On further heating turbidity disappears. Reappears on cooling.
- **What is the principle of Rothera's test?**
  The purple ring formed due to reaction of sodium nitroprusside with ketone bodies to form a complex ferropentacyanide.
- **Name the ketone body, which does not answer the Rothera's test.**
  Acetone and acetoacetate will answer the test. But β-hydroxyl butyrate does not give the answer.
- **What is the principle of Hay's test?**
  Bile salts will reduce the surface tension. Hence the test tube containing urine (bile salts) helps to sink down the sulfur powder.
- **What is Fouchet's reagent?**
  Fouchet's reagent is ferric chloride in trichloroacetic acid.
- **What is the principle of modified Fouchet's test?**
  The white precipitate obtained is $BaSO_4$. To this when reagent is added, $FeCl_3$ oxidizes bilirubin to biliverdin (green) and bilicyanin (blue).

QUANTITATIVE EXPERIMENTS

Changes in normal values in blood or changes in urinary values if measured quantitatively can be used for diagnostic as well as for prognostic purposes.

Normal value: Defined as amount of a particular constituent present in body fluids of a healthy normal individual.

Factors affecting normal value: Sex, type of individual-race, genetic variations diseases, etc.

Collection of blood samples: Blood samples are either capillary or venous. For the investigation of blood pH, blood gas analysis, hemoglobin concentration whole blood is taken. Serological investigation is done by separating the serum. This is done by taking the blood in a clean dry container and allowing it to clot under room temperature. After some time clot retracts and serum separates as supernatant layer this layer is removed. During separation CO_2 is lost and K+ and PO_4 move from cell to serum. Hence for electrolytes estimation plasma is required.

For preparing plasma, blood is collected in a container containing anticoagulant and centrifuged. Cells settle down and plasma separates. Serum does not contain fibrinogen, clotting factors, whereas plasma contains fibrinogen.

Some of the anticoagulants used in laboratory are heparin, EDTA, citrates, oxalates. For samples used for the estimation of glucose, specific agents which prevent glycolysis are required, i.e. NaF along with oxalates. Estimation with hemolyzed samples gives wrong results. If analysis is not carried out immediately, serum can be stored for a week at 4°C. In bilirubin estimation serum is protected from light since it is destroyed on exposure to light.

Collection of urine samples: For qualitative estimation single specimen is needed. But for quantitative estimation, 24 hour urine samples are required. For that it has to be collected in a container having HCl, thymol, chloroform, etc.

COLORIMETRY

Measurement of concentration of colored substances in solution is the basis of colorimetry. Colored solutions can absorb light rays of a particular wavelength. This is called as absorbance. This can be measured by photoelectric equipment.

Colorimetry is based on Beer-Lambert's Law which states that:

Beer's Law

It states that the amount of light absorbed is directly proportional to concentration of absorbing material.

Lambert's Law

It states that the amount of light absorbed depends on thickness of the medium.

It is expressed as $A = € \times b \times c$

A—absorbance/optical density

b—length of light passed

c—concentration of absorbing material

€—molar absorptivity constant.

Most of the clinical chemistry estimations are done by calorimetric/photometric method. A colored derivative of the compound to be measured is prepared, and its absorbance is measured using a photoelectric colorimeter. This value is compared to that of a standard of known concentration. The concentration can be calculated as:

$$\frac{\text{Optical density of test soln}}{\text{Optical density of standard soln}} = \frac{\text{Concentration of test soln}}{\text{Concentration of std soln}}$$

Concentration of test soln =

$$\frac{\text{OD of test soln}}{\text{OD of standard soln}} \times \text{concentration of standard solution}$$

ESTIMATION OF BLOOD SUGAR

Glucose Oxidase Method

It is an enzymatic method for estimation of blood glucose. It is highly specific and gives true glucose values.

Principle

$$\text{Glucose} \xrightarrow{\text{GO}} \text{Gluconic acid} + H_2O_2$$

$$H_2O_2 \xrightarrow{\text{Peroxidase}} H_2O + (O)$$

$$\text{Colorless chromogenic substrate} \xrightarrow{\text{O}} \text{colored dye}$$

Reagents

Working reagent, sample solution, standard solution, distilled water.

Procedure

- Take three test tubes and mark them as T, S, B for test, standard, and blank respectively.
- Add 1.5 mL of working reagent to all the three test tubes.
- Add 0.02 mL of test solution to 'T' and 0.02 mL of standard solution into 'S', mix well.

Calculation

	Blank	Test	Standard
Working reagent	1.5 mL	1.5 mL	1.5 mL
Test	–	0.02	–
Standard solution	–	–	0.02
Keep for incubation for 5 min at 37°C			
Distilled water	1.5 mL	1.5 mL	1.5 mL
Optical density at 505 nm	–	–	–

Optical density of test solution = T
Optical density of standard solution = S
Concentration of test solution = T/S × concentration of standard

Result

Concentration of glucose in the given sample = mg/dL

- **What is the normal blood glucose level?**
  Normal fasting blood glucose level is 70–110 mg/dL.
- **What is the clinical significance?**
  Hyperglycemia—Diabetes mellitus, hyperthyroidism, hyperpituitarism, emotional stress.
  Hypoglycemia—Insulin overdosage, insulin secreting tumors, hypothyroidism, hypopituitarism.
- **What are other methods to estimate blood glucose level?**
  Chemical method—Folin-Wu method. Nelson Somogyi method, Asatoor and King method, ortho toluidine method.
  Enzymatic methods—Glucose oxidase method and hexokinase method.
- **What are the other reducing substances in blood?**
  Glutathione, glucuronic acid, ascorbic acid, uric acid, homogentisic acid.
- **What is the wavelength used in this experiment?**
  505 nm.

ESTIMATION OF BLOOD UREA

Diacetyl Monoxime Method

Principle

When urea is heated with substances containing two adjacent carbonyl groups such as diacetyl, colored complexes, are formed. On heating in acidic medium; diacetyl monoxime decomposes to give hydroxylamine and diacetyl which condenses with urea.

Thiosemicarbazide and ferric ions are used as catalysts for the reaction.

Reagents

- *Mixed acid reagent:* Contains ortho phosphoric acid, con. H_2SO_4, $FeCl_3$.
- *Color reagent:* Contains diacetyl monoxime (DAM), thiosemicarbazide.
- *Stock urea standard:* 100 mg/100 mL.
- *Working reagent:* 1 mL/100 mL.

Procedure

- Take three test tubes and mark them as T, S, B for test, standard, and blank respectively.
- To S, add 1 mL of working urea standard soln; to T add 1 mL test solution, and to B, add 1 mL of distilled water.
- To all test tubes, add 2 mL of mixed color reagent and mix.
- To all test tubes, add 2 mL of mixed acid reagent and mix thoroughly.

Calculation

	B	*S*	*T*
Distilled water	1 mL	–	–
Diluted standard	–	1 mL	–
Test solution	–	–	1 mL
Mixed acid reagent	2 mL	2 mL	2 mL
Mixed color reagent	2 mL	2 mL	2 mL
Place all test tubes in boiling water bath for 20 minutes			
OD at 520 nm	0	?	?

Concentration of urea = T/S × concentration of standard.

Result

Concentration of urea in the given sample = ----- mg/dL.

Viva Questions

- **What is the normal blood urea level?**
  Normal serum urea level: 20–40 mg/dL.
- **What are various methods to estimate blood urea?**
  - *Enzymatic method using urease:* Nessler's method, Berthelot method, glutamate dehydrogenase method
  - *Nonenzymatic method:* Diacetyl monoxime method.
- **What is the disadvantage of this diacetyl monoxime method?**
  The color formed is not stable and less specific.
- **What is the wavelength used to measure OD in this experiments?**
  520 nm.
- **What are the conditions in which blood urea level is increased?**
  Prerenal causes—Dehydration, diabetic coma, shock, severe burns, fever.
  Renal causes—Acute glomerulonephritis, nephritic syndrome, chronic mercury poisoning.
  Postrenal causes—Enlargement of prostate, urinary calculi, malignant tumors of bladder/ureter.

- **Name the condition in which blood urea level is decreased.**
  In severe liver disease.
- **What is urea clearance? What is its significance?**
  Volume of plasma/blood which is completely cleared of urea by the kidney per minute
  Urea clearance = U × V/P
  U—concentration of urea in urine.
  V—volume of urine excreted per minute
  P—concentration of urea in plasma
  Normal value - 75 mL/min.

ESTIMATION OF SERUM CREATININE

Jaffe's Method

Principle

Jaffe's reaction—red colored tautomer of creatinine picrate is formed on adding alkaline picrate solution.

Reagents

- Creatinine standard solution
- Protein-free filtrate (prepared by - 1 mL serum + 1.5 mL DW + 0.5 mL 10% sodium tungstate soln + 1 mL H_2SO_4—keep for 10 min and filter)
- Picric acid
- NaOH, distilled water.

Procedure

- Take 3 test tubes; mark T, B and S.
- Add 3 mL of protein-free filtrate to T
- Add 3 mL DW to B
- Add 3 mL standard solution to S
- Then add 1 mL of picric acid and NaOH to all the 3 test tubes.

Calculation

	B	*S*	*T*
Protein-free filtrate	–	–	3 mL
Standard solution	–	3 mL	–
Distilled water	3 mL	–	–
NaOH	1 mL	1 mL	1 mL
Picric acid reagent	1 mL	1 mL	1 mL
Mix well, wait for 5 minutes			
OD at 520 nm	0	?	?

Concentration of test solution = T/S × concentration of standard

Result

Concentration of creatinine in a given sample = ----- mg/dL.

Viva questions

- **What other methods are used to estimate serum creatinine?**
  Chemical methods: Based on the reaction with alkaline picrate; e.g. Jaffe's method.
  Enzymatic method: Using enzymes such as creatininase, and creatine deaminase (these methods are expensive).
- **What is normal serum creatinine level?**

Age	*Serum creatinine*
<12 years	0.25–0.85
Adult male	0.7–1.5
Adult female	0.4–1.2

- **What is the wavelength used to measure OD in this experiment?**
  520 nm.
- **What is the significance of serum creatinine estimation?**
  - Sensitive indicator of GFR
  - Helps in early detection of functional impairment of kidney
  - Helpful in long-term monitoring of renal diseases.
- **What is creatinine clearance?**
  Volume of plasma which contains that amount of creatinine that is excreted in 1 minute by the kidneys
  Creatinine clearance $= \frac{U \times V}{P}$
  U—concentration of creatinine in urine (mg/dL)
  P—concentration of creatinine in plasma (mg/dL)
  V—volume of urine excreted per minute (mL/min)
- **What is creatinine co-efficient?**
  Urinary creatinine expressed in mg/kg body wt in 24 hours. Normal value is 20–28 mg/kg/day in males and 15–21 mg/kg/day in females.

ESTIMATION OF SERUM PROTEINS

Biuret Method

Principle

All proteins contain a large number of peptide bonds. When a solution of protein is treated with cupric ion in moderately alkaline medium, colored chelated complexes are formed between cupric ions and carboxvl and amino groups of the peptide bonds. An analogous reaction takes place between the cupric ions and the organic compound biuret (NH_2 CO NH CO NH_2). This reaction is, therefore, referred to as biuret reaction.

Reagents

1. *Biuret reagent:* Dissolve 9 gm of sodium potassium tartarate + 3 gm of $CuSO_4$ in 250 mL of 0.2N NaOH + 5 gm of KI—and make upto 1 L with 0.2N NaOH.

2. *Standard solution:* Concentration of standard—6 gm/ 100 mL.
3. Test serum.

Procedure

- Take 3 test tubes and label them as S, T and B
- Pipette out 0.1 mL serum in T
- Pipette out 0.1 mL of standard solution to S
- Add 0.1 mL DW into B
- Add 5 mL of biuret reagent to all the 3 test tubes.

Calculation

	B	*S*	*T*
Distilled water	0.1 mL	–	–
Standard solution	–	0.1 mL	–
Serum	–	–	0.1 mL
Biuret reagent	5 mL	5 mL	5 mL
Mix and keep for 10 minutes			
OD at 540 nm	0	?	?

OD of test solution: T
OD of standard solution: S
Concentration of test solution = T/S × con. of standard solution.

Result

The concentration of total protein in the given sample of serum is = ----- g/dL.

Viva Questions

- **What is the normal level of proteins?**
  Total proteins: 6–8 g/100 mL
  Albumin: 3.5–5.5 g/100 mL
  Globulin: 1.5–3 g/100 mL
  A/G ratio: 1.2–1.5.
- **What is the clinical significance of serum protein?**
  Serum proteins are increased in dehydration due to decreased water intake from excessive water loss occurring in vomiting, diarrhea, Addison's disease, or diabetic insipidus (DI).
  Multiple myeloma, total protein is increased to over 10 gm/dL; Rheumatoid arthritis infections, advanced tuberculosis and malignancies.
- **Name some conditions in which protein levels are decreased?**
  Nephrotic syndrome, severe burns, chronic liver disease, intestinal malabsorption, excessive bleeding, protein energy malnutrition, pregnancy.

ESTIMATION OF SERUM ALBUMIN

The ability of albumin to bind certain dyes like BCG provides a method for its quantitation.

Principle

Albumin present in serum binds specifically with bromocresol green at pH 4.1 to form a green-colored complex, with maximum absorbance at 620 nm. The intensity of which can be measured colorimetrically.

Reagents

BCG reagent
Albumin standard (4.5 g%).

Procedure

- Take 3 test tubes and label as T, S and B
- Pipette out 0.1 mL serum into T
- Pipette out 0.1 mL standard solution into S
- Add 0.1 mL DW into B
- Add 4 mL of BCG reagent to all the 3 test tubes.

Calculation

	B	*S*	*T*
Distilled water	0.1 mL	–	–
Standard solution	–	0.1 mL	–
Serum	–	–	0.1 mL
BCG reagent	4 mL	4 mL	4 mL
Mix well and keep it for 10 min			
OD at 620 nm	0	?	?

OD of test solution: T
OD of standard solution: S
Con. of serum albumin—OD of test/OD of standard × 4.5 g/dL

Result

Con. of albumin present in the given sample of serum = ... g/dL.

Viva Questions

- **Name two functions of albumin.**
  It acts as a binding and carrier protein. It is an osmotic regulator.

- **What is the normal serum albumin level?**
  3.5–5.5 g/dL.
- **What are the conditions in which albumin level is varied?**
  Increased: Dehydration
  Decreased:
  Excessive loss of albumin can occur in—Nephrotic syndrome, severe burns.
  Defective anabolism due to liver disease, malnutrition, muscular dystrophy.
  Increased catabolism of proteins as in fever and after injury, severe hemorrhage, early stage of shock.
- **What is Albumin/globulin ratio?**
  Albumin/globulin ratio is the ratio between the quantities of albumin by that of globulin present in the plasma/serum.
- **Name the conditions causing Albumin/globulin reversal?**
  Albumin/globulin ratio reversed in liver cirrhosis, multiple myeloma and in nephritic syndrome.

pH Meter

It is an electronic instrument used to measure the pH of a liquid. A typical pH meter consists of a special measuring probe (a glass electrode) connected to an electronic meter that measures and displays the pH reading.

SPOTTERS

REAGENTS

- Molisch reagent—α naphthol in alcohol
- Benedict's reagent—$CuSO_4$, Na_2CO_3, sodium citrate
- Barfoed's reagent—copper acetate in acetic acid
- Foulger's reagent—40% H_2SO_4 with stannous chloride in urea.
- Seliwanoff's reagent—resorcinol in HCl
- Ehrlich's reagent—paradimethyl amino benzaldehyde in HCl
- Fouchet's reagent—$FeCl_3$ in trichloroacetic acid
- Mixed acid reagent—orthophosphoric acid, concentrated H_2SO_4, $FeCl_3$
- Mixed color reagent—diacetyl monoxime, thiosemicarbazide.

TESTS

- *Molisch test:* Purple ring with green color below
- *Aldehyde test:* Purple ring with coagulum on top
  - For proteins containing amino acids with indole ring
- *Rothera's test:* Purple ring with white crystals of ammonium sulfate at the bottom.
  - Test for ketone bodies in urine
  (First 3 tests are ring test)
- *Benedict's test:* Green/yellow/orange/red precipitate
  - Test for reducing sugars
- *Biuret test:* Violet color for proteins
- *Specific urease test:* Slow development of pink color shows presence of urea.
- *Hay's test:* Yellow solution with sulfur particles at bottom
  - Test for bile salts
- *Modified Fouchet's test:* Filter paper with blue/green spot
  - Test for bile pigments
- *Schiff's test:* Filter paper with black spot
  - Test for uric acid
- *Xanthoproteic test:* Light yellow and desolutions
  - Test for aromatic amino acids
- *Millon's test:* Test for amino acids with phenol group
- Van den Bergh test
  - For detection of bilirubin
  - Reag A-sulfanilic acid in HCl
  - Reag B-sodium nitrite in water
- Clearance test
  $C = U \times V/P$
  U—Concentration of substance in urine
  V—rate of urine flow
  P—Concentration of substance in plasma.

SAMPLES

- *Define limiting amino acids. Name the limiting amino acids in the given food stuff.*
  Certain proteins are deficient in one or more essential amino acids. These amino acids which are deficient in the particular protein are called limiting amino acids.
  - Rice—Lys, Thr
  - Wheat—Lys, Thr
  - Bengal gram—Cys, Met
  - Tapioca—Phe, Tyr
  - Maize—Trp

NUTRITION

- *Define biological value of proteins.*
  It is the ratio between the amount of nitrogen retained and nitrogen absorbed during a specific interval.

$$BV = \frac{\text{Retained nitrogen}}{\text{Absorbed nitrogen}} \times 100$$

  - Egg—90
  - Milk—84
  - Wheat—58
  - Bengal gram—58
  - Rice—64

INDICATORS

(Range?, Color change?, What is it used for?)

- *Phenol red:* 6.4 (yellow)-8.4 (red)
  - Specific urease test.
- *Chlorophenol red:* 4.8-6.8
  - Heat coagulation test
- *Thymol blue:* 1.2 (red)-2.8 (yellow)
  - Specific sucrose test
- *Phenolphthalein:* 8.2 (colorless)-10 (pink)
  - Test for ammonia in urine, gastric acidity.
- *Bromocresol green:* 3.8 (yellow)-5.4 (blue)
  - Isoelectric precipitation for casein.

MICROSCOPY

- *Hemin crystals:* It is chemically hematin chloride and used to identify blood stains.
- *Osazone crystals (Figs 1A to C):*

Glucose, fructose and mannose: Give yellow colored needle shaped/'sheaves of corn' shaped osazone crystals

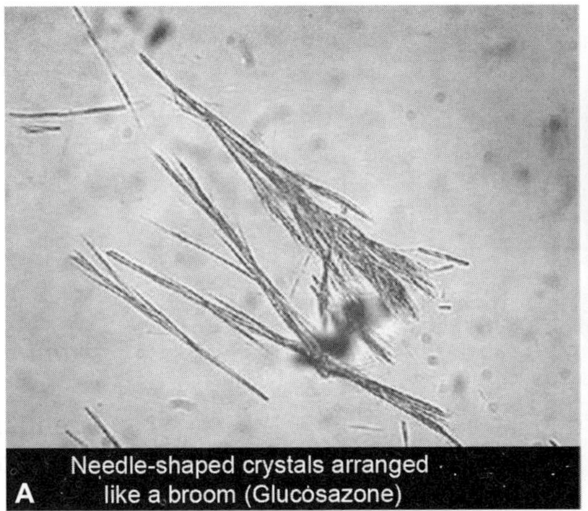

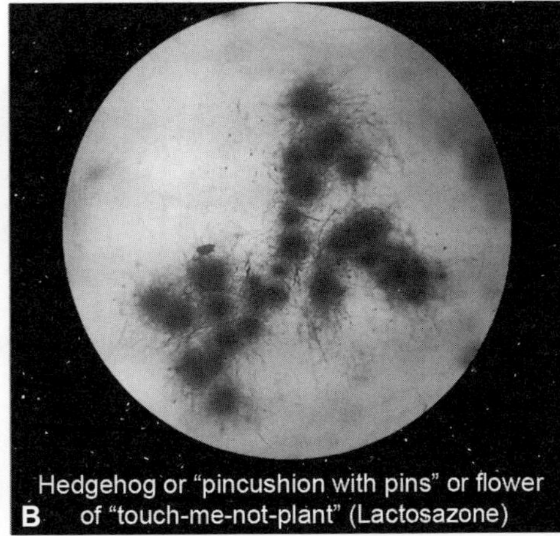

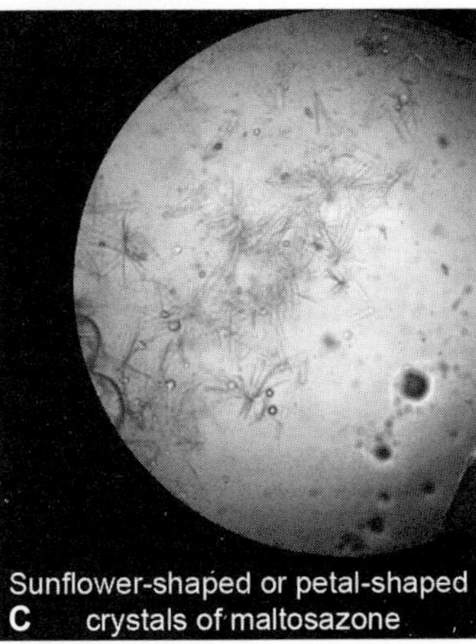

Figs 1A to C Osazone crystals (*For color version, see Plate 28*)

Lactosazone: Puff-shaped/cotton ball-shaped osazone crystals.
Maltosazone: Petal-shaped/sunflower-like crystals.

INSTRUMENTS

- *Folin-Wu tube*
  - It is used for the estimation of glucose
  - Proteins are precipitated by tungstic acid. The protein-free filtrate containing glucose reduces blue cupric ions of copper reagent to red cuprous oxide. The cuprous oxide reduces phosphomolybdic acid to phosphomolybdous acid
  - Folin-Wu tube has 3 parts: (i) bulbous part (capacity 4 mL); (ii) constricted neck—prevents auto-oxidation of reagents by atmospheric air; (iii) body—graduation at 12.5 mL–25 mL
- *Urinometer*
  - Used for measuring the specific gravity of urine
  - Normal specific gravity 1.015–1.025
  - It is a measure of osmolarity and indicates concentrating ability of kidneys
  - First morning sample is taken to measure specific gravity
  - *Decreased:* In excessive water intake, nephritis, pyelonephritis, diabetes insipidus, etc.
  - *Increased:* In diabetes mellitus, hepatitis, nephrosis, adrenal insufficiency
- *Ryles tube*
  - For aspiration of gastric juice during gastric function test.
  - Nasogastric feeding

    Significance of the markings: The end of the tube containing the 3 beads is inserted through the mouth of the person. The marking closest to that end is seen at the lip of the person.
    - *Marking:* When the tube reaches the cardiac end of stomach
    - *Marking:* Body of stomach
    - *Marking:* Pylorus of stomach
- *pH meter*
  - Used to measure pH using electrical potential difference created between 2 electrodes
  - It is based on the principle that when a glass membrane seperates 2 different solutions differing in pH, a potential difference is found to exist between 2 surface of the glass. The potential is measured against a standard calomel electrode.
- *Colorimeter*
  - Device used to measure optical density of a colored solution
  - It works on the principle of Beer-Lambert's law

    Types—analog and digital colorimeter
- *Electrophoretic apparatus*
  - Horizontal electrophoretic tank.
  - Used for SDS-slide/agarose gel electrophoresis
  - Electrophoresis is the analytical method frequently used in molecular biology and medicine for the separation and characterization of serum proteins, Igs, isoenzymes, nucleic acids, viruses
  - Electrophoretic apparatus consists of an electrophoretic tank to hold the buffer

    A: A separate M band (or myeloma band or monoclonal band) with a sharp narrow spike is seen. It indicates increased level of Ig molecules.

    C: Normal serum will be separated into 5 bands

    Albumin has maximum and gamma globulin have the minimum mobility in the electrical field. Movement is as follows—albumin, α1-globulin, α2-globulin, β-globulin, γ-globulin (Figs 2A to D)
- *Esbach's albuminometer*

  Use—rough estimation of total proteins in urine in 24 hours

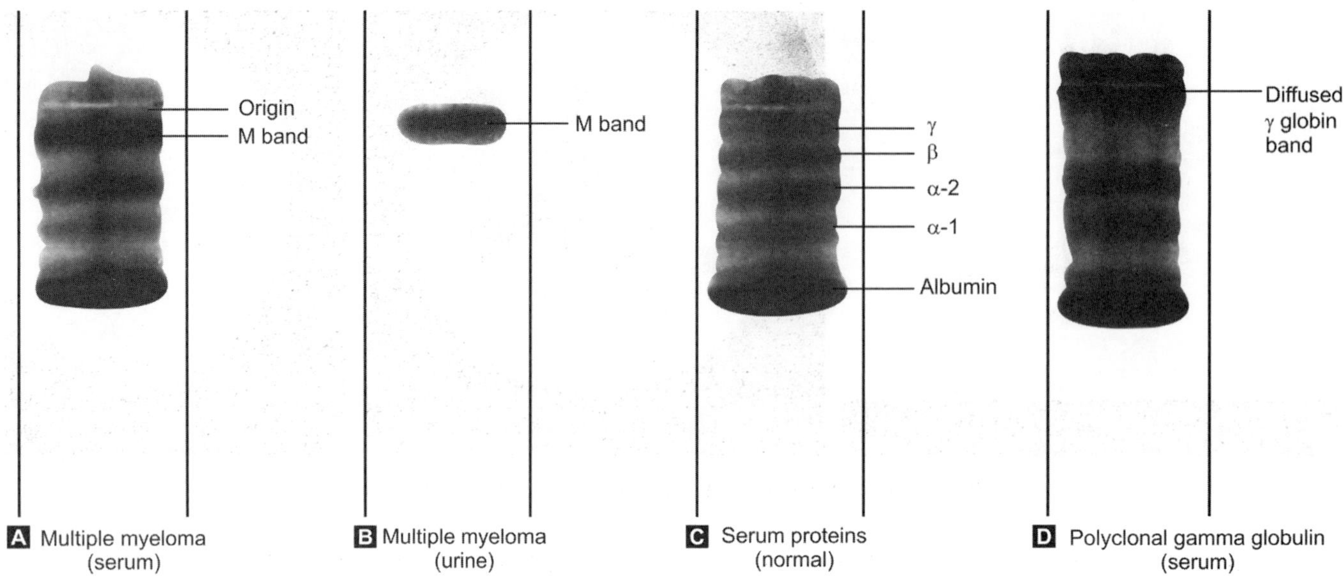

Figs 2A to D Electrophoretic apparatus

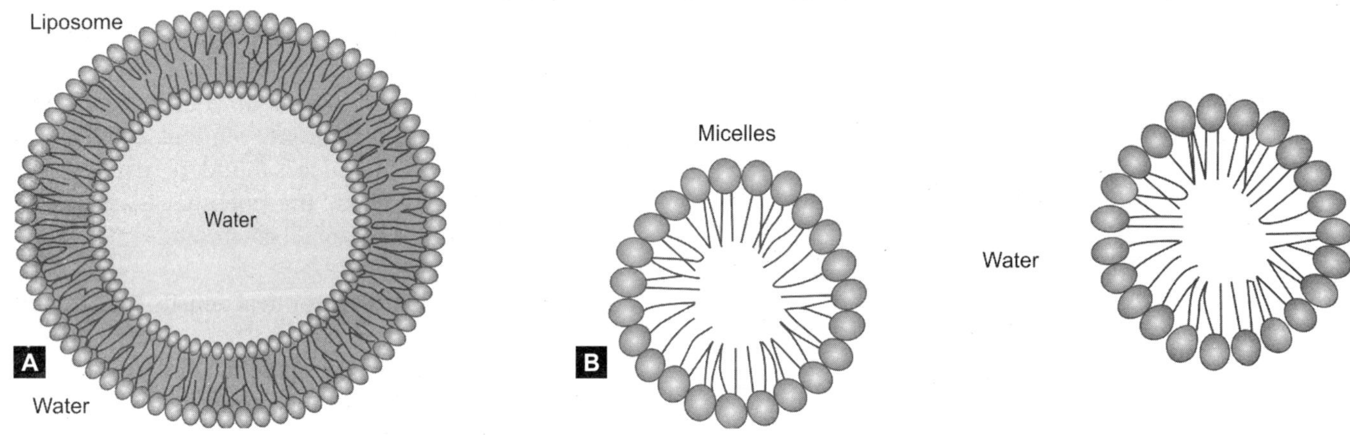

Figs 3A and B Therapy of liposomes

Markings and significance—urine up to marking 'U' and reagent up to 'R'.

- *Paper chromatography*
  2 phases—stationary phase—water held in filter paper (cellulose).
  Mobile phase—water + nonpolar solvent + acid/base.

DIAGRAMS

- *Liposomes:* These are carrier of proteins, protein, enzymes to target sites
  They are used in cancer chemotherapy, antimicrobial therapy, gene therapy (Figs 3A and B)
- *Micelle:*
  - These are molecular aggregations of phospholipids with hydrophobic part inside and hydrophilic part outside
  - These are involved in solubilization of lipids in aqueous media and help in digestion and absorption of lipids.
- *t-RNA:* It has 4 arms (Fig. 4):
  - Acceptor arm—capped with a sequence 'CCA' (5′–3′). The amino acid attached to the acceptor arm.
  - Anticodon arm—this arm, with the three specific nucleotide bases (anticodon), is responsible for the recognition of triplet codon of mRNA.
  - D arm—named due to the presence of dihydrouridine
  - TΨC arm—it contains a sequence of T, pseudouridine (represented by psi) and C
  - Variable arm—it is the most variable in t-RNA
- *Insulin (Fig. 5)*
  - It is a polypeptide hormone produced by the β-cells of islets of Langerhans of pancreas.
  - It is a hypoglycemic hormone
  - Biological importance
    - Increases glucose uptake
    - Increases glycolysis
    - Increases glycogenesis

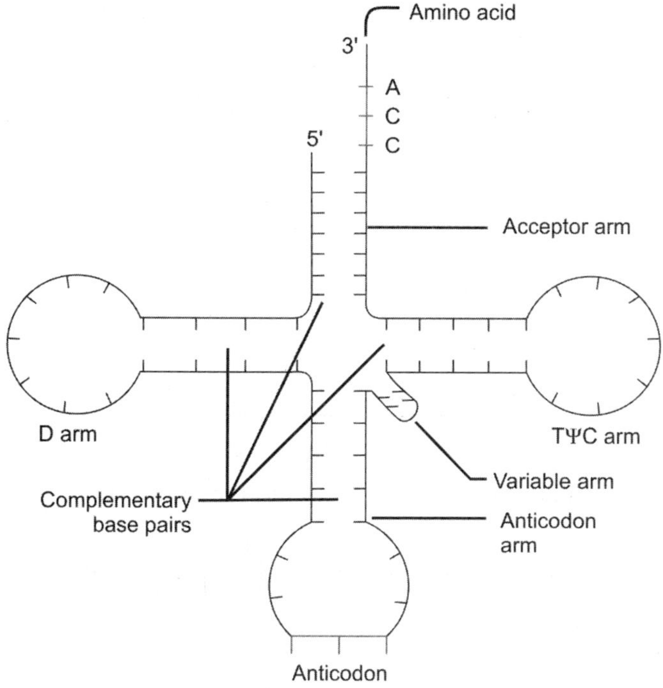

Fig. 4 t-RNA

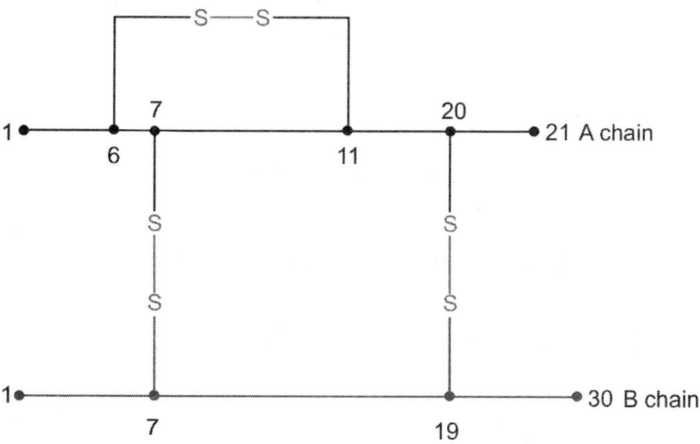

Fig. 5 Insulin

- Increases HMP shunt
- Decreases gluconeogenesis
- Decreases glycogenolysis

- *Immunoglobulin (Fig. 6)*
  All immunoglobulins have two heavy chains and two light chains held together by disulphide linkages and noncovalent interactions:
  IgG–secondary immune response
  IgA–secretory in function
  IgM–primary immune response
  IgE–anaphylaxis
  IgD–attached to B lymphocyte

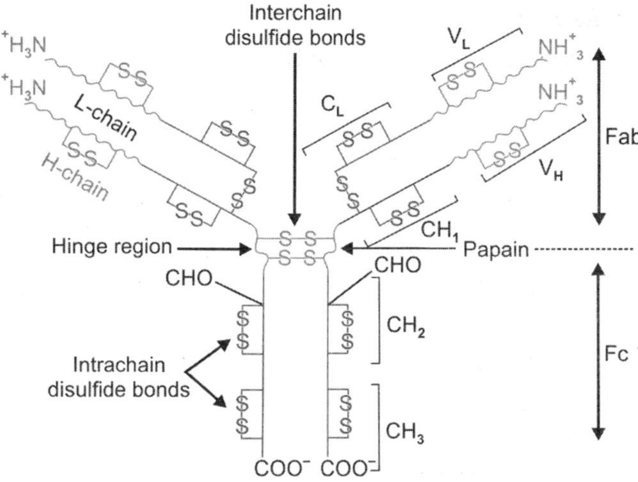

Fig. 6 Immunoglobulin

SPECTROSCOPY

- *Oxyhemoglobin:* Dark red (Fig. 7)
  - α-578 nm, β-540 nm

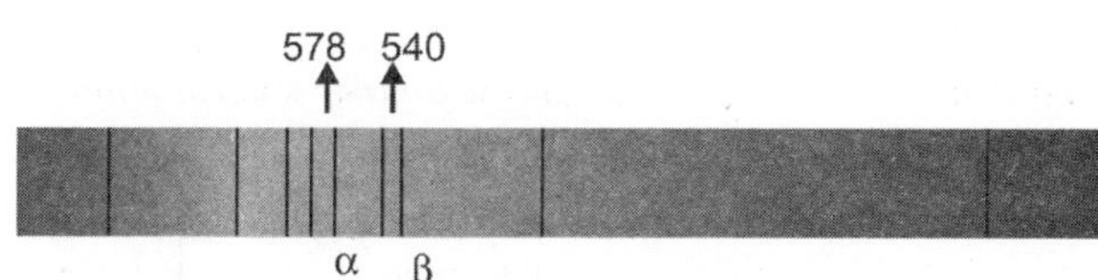

Fig. 7 Oxyhemoglobin (*For color version, see Plate 28*)

- *Deoxyhemoglobin:* Purple; plugged (Fig. 8)
  Single band at 565 nm

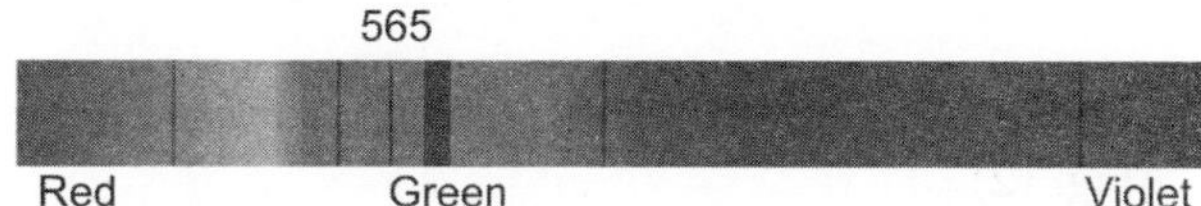

Fig. 8 Deoxyhemoglobin (*For color version, see Plate 28*)

- *Methemoglobin:* Cherry red (Fig. 9)

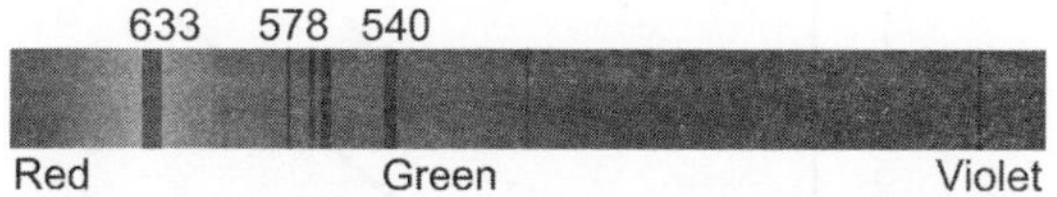

Fig. 9 Methemoglobin (*For color version, see Plate 28*)

  - A band in red with its center at 633 nm while white bands for oxyhemoglobin persist
- *Globin hemochromogen:* Dark red, plugged
  - Bands at 558 nm, 526 nm
- *Carboxyhemoglobin:* Pink (Fig. 10)
  - Bands at 572 nm, 535 nm

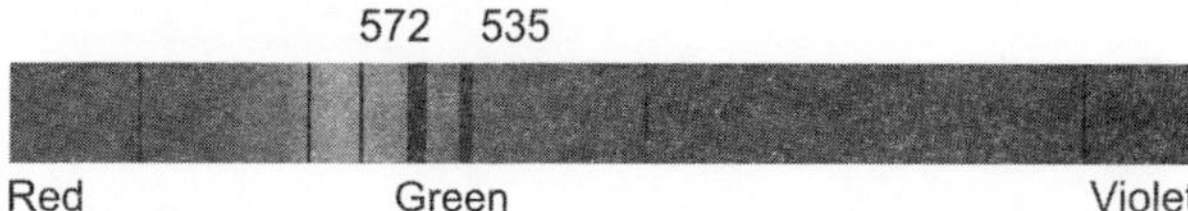

Fig. 10 Carboxyhemoglobin (*For color version, see Plate 28*)

GRAPHS

- Oral glucose tolerance test (Fig. 11)

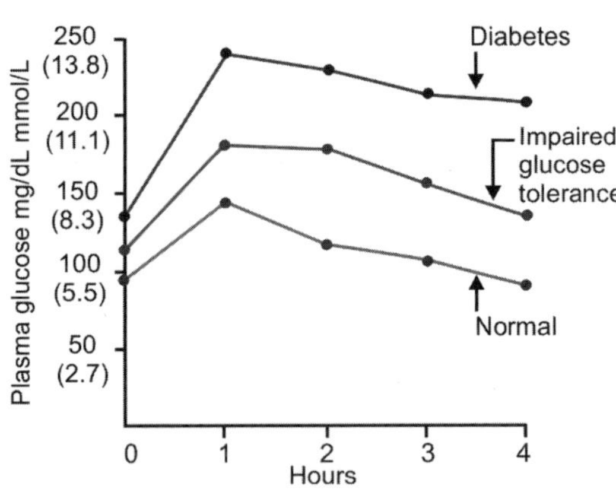

Fig. 11 Oral glucose tolerance test

Diagnostic criteria for oral glucose tolerance test

Condition	*Plasma glucose concentration as mmol/L (mg/dL)*		
	Normal	Impaired glucose tolerance	Diabetes
Fasting	< 110	< 126	>126
2 hours after glucose	< 140	< 200	>200

- Effect of enzyme concentration on enzyme velocity (Fig. 12)

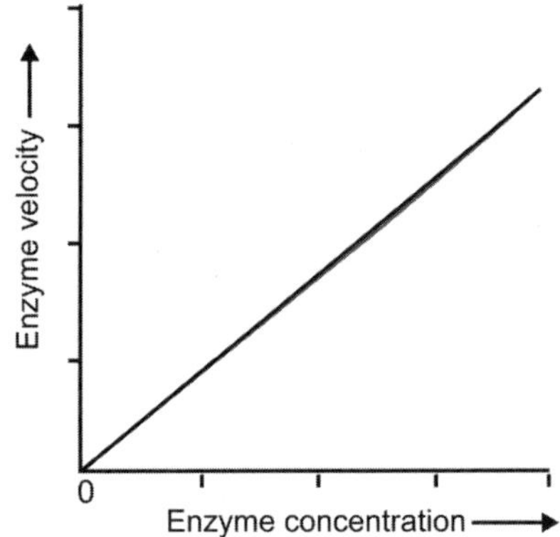

Fig. 12 Concentration and velocity of enzyme

- Effect of substrate concentration on enzyme velocity (Fig. 13)

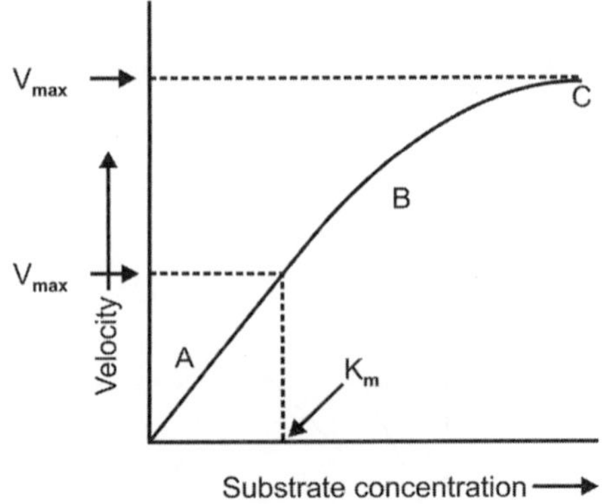

Fig. 13 Substrate concentration of enzyme velocity

- Line weaver curve/double reciprocal curve (Fig. 14)

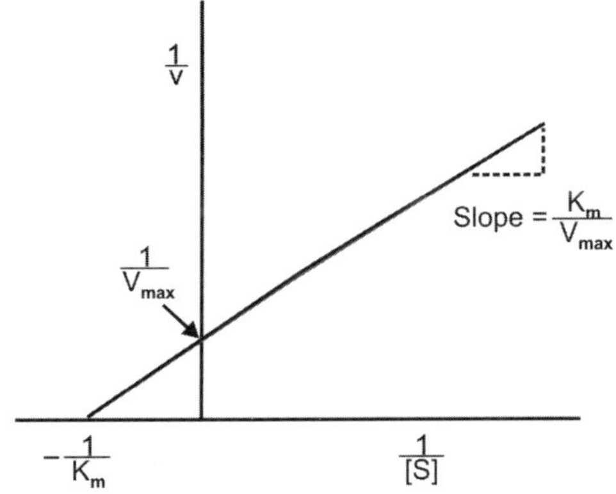

Fig. 14 Double reciprocal curve of enzyme

- Effect of pH of enzyme activity (Fig. 15)

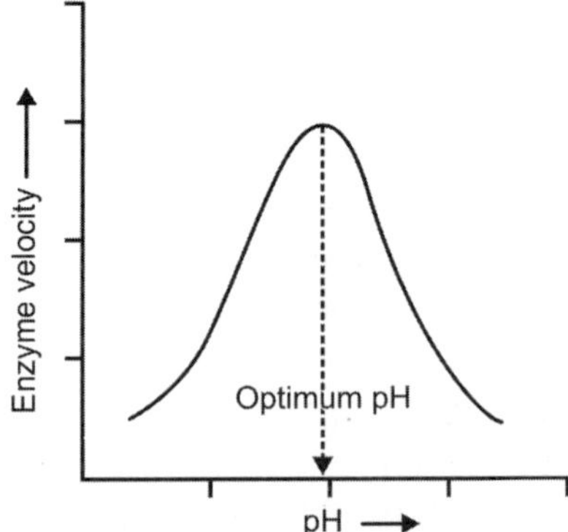

Fig. 15 pH of enzyme activity

- Effect of temperature on enzyme velocity (Fig. 16)

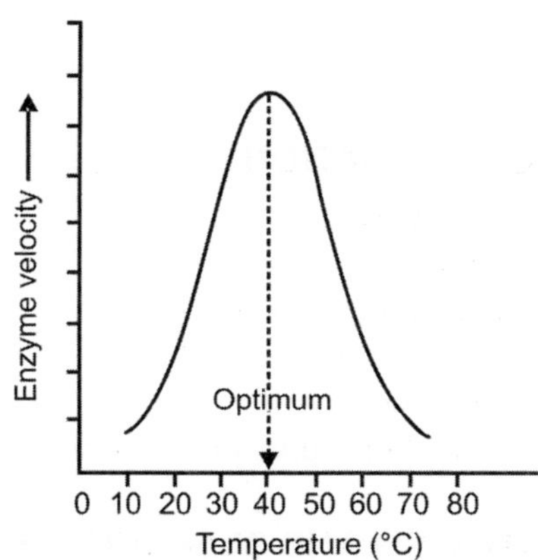

Fig. 16 Temperature effect on enzyme velocity

- Effect of enzyme on activation energy of a reaction (A, the substrate and B, is product, enzyme decreases activation energy (Fig. 17).

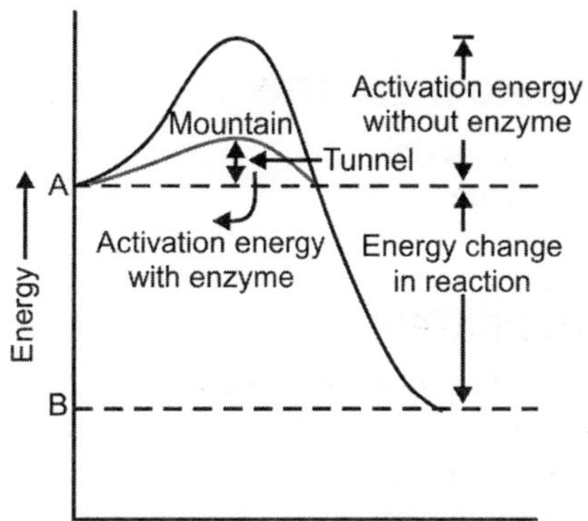

Fig. 17 Activation energy of enzyme

THEORY—VIVA VOCE

GENERAL BIOCHEMISTRY

- Fluid mosaic model
- Marker enzyme
- Ionophores.

CARBOHYDRATES

- Isomerism of monosaccharides
- Invert sugar
- Mucopolysaccharides
- Glucose transporters
- G6P DH deficiency
- Cory's bicycle
- Essential pentosuria
- Fructose metabolism
- Linkages in sucrose, maltose, lactose, starch, glycogen
- Cycles—steps and enzymes.

LIPIDS

- Classification of lipids
- Phospholipid
- Lecithin
- Chylomicron
- Liposome
- Fatty liver
- Ketosis
- Cholesterol
- Steps in β oxidation.

PROTEINS

- Structure of proteins
- Transamination
- Classification of proteins
- Steps in urea cycle
- Disorders of urea cycle
- Homocystinuria
- Maple syrup urine disease
- Polyamines
- Phenylketonuria
- Alkaptonuria
- Functions of cysteine
- Methionine metabolism.

ENZYMES

- Classification of enzymes
- Michaelis tendon theory
- Enzyme inhibitors
- Allosteric enzymes.

BIOLOGICAL OXIDATION

- Energetic of TCA cycle
- TCA cycle inhibitors
- Binding change mechanism
- High-energy compounds
- Chemiosmotic theory
- Inhibitors of oxidative phosphorylation.

HEME SYNTHESIS AND BREAKDOWN AND HEMOGLOBIN

- Heme synthesis
- Heme catabolism
- Porphyrias
- Jaundice
- Van den Bergh test
- O_2, CO_2 cycle
- ODC
- Thalassemia
- Sickle cell anemia.

CLINICAL ENZYMOLOGY AND BIOMARKERS

Enzyme markers for:

- Cardiac disease
- Hepatic diseases
- Bone disease
- Prostatic cancer
- Enzymes for therapeutic agents.

REGULATION OF BLOOD GLUCOSE, INSULIN AND DIABETES MELLITUS

- Regulation of glucose level
- Diabetes mellitus
- OGTT
- Reducing substances in urine
- Metabolic syndrome
- Diabetic ketoacidosis
- Glycated hemoglobin
- Metabolic derangement in diabetes.

VITAMINS

Fat-soluble vitamins:

- Wald's visual cycle
- Biochemical role of vitamin D, E, and K
- Night blindness.

WATER-SOLUBLE VITAMINS

- Beriberi
- Pellagra
- Biotin antagonists
- Functional role of vitamin B_{12}
- Folate trap.

MINERAL METABOLISM

- Ca—functions, regulation
- Fe-absorption
- Wilson disease
- Ceruloplasmin
- Fluorosis.

ENERGY METABOLISM AND NUTRITION

- Respiratory quotient
- Protein-energy malnutrition.

ACID-BASE BALANCE

- Maintenance of normal pH
- Henderson–Hasselbalch equation
- Anion gap
- Metabolic acidosis, alkalosis
- Respiratory acidosis, alkalosis.

FREE RADICALS AND ANTIOXIDANTS

- Free radical scavenging enzyme
- Antioxidants.

NUCLEOTIDES

- Gout
- Purine synthesis inhibitors
- Lesch-Nyhan syndrome
- Orotic aciduria
- Difference between CPS I and CPS II.

DNA-STRUCTURE AND REPLICATION

- Base pairing rule
- Wobble hypothesis
- Nucleosomes
- Telomere and telomerase.

TRANSCRIPTION AND TRANSLATION

- Types of RNA
- Steps of transcription and translation
- RNA polymerase
- Post-transcriptional and post-translational changes
- Spliceosomes
- Ribozymes
- Genetic code
- Polysomes
- Chaperons
- Inhibitors of translational changes
- Mitochondrial DNA.

MOLECULAR GENETICS AND CONTROL OF GENE EXPRESSION

- Mutations
- Apoptosis
- Prions
- Lac operon.

RECOMBINANT DNA TECHNOLOGY AND GENE THERAPY

- Recombinant DNA technology
- Vectors
- Gene therapy
- Retrovirus.

CANCER AND AIDS

- Oncogenic virus
- Proto-oncogene.

IMMUNOCHEMISTRY

- Structure and function of immunoglobulins
- Multiple myeloma
- Bence-Jones proteins
- Acute phase proteins.

CLINICAL BIOCHEMISTRY

- Liver, gastric and renal function tests
- Rf value
- Creatinine clearance
- Urea clearance
- Southern blot
- RFLP
- PCR
- Monoclonal antibodies
- Electrophoresis.

CHARTS FOR DISCUSSION

1. Urine of a newborn baby gives a positive Benedict's test.
   a. What are the test to be done to identify the sugar?
   b. What is the most likely reducing sugar to be present?
   c. Explain the biochemical basis of glycosuria?

   Diabetes Mellitus
2. A 60-year-old man was admitted with fever and severe diarrhea. He appeared severely dehydrated.

   Investigations

   pH–7.2; $PaCO_2$–40 mm Hg; bicarbonate ion–14 mm/L; pO_2–92 mm Hg
   a. What is the primary acid-base disorder in this patient?
   b. What is anion gap?

   Metabolic acidosis
3. A 30-year-old woman during her second pregnancy had a glucose tolerance test and results are: fasting glucose level–125 mg/dL, 1 hour glucose level–210 mg/dL, 2 hours value–170 mg/dL:
   - Comment on the GTT result.
   - What will be the result of Benedict's test with the urine sample collected along with each blood sample?
   - What is the importance of assessing the glucose tolerance in a pregnant lady?
   - How do you rule out lactosuria in this case?

   Gestational diabetes mellitus
4. A 6-month-old child was brought to the pediatric surgery department with recurrent vomiting and upper abdominal mass since 2 weeks.

   Investigations

   pH–7.55; bicarbonate ion–35 mmol/L; $PaCO_2$–40 mm Hg
   - What is the most likely acid-base disorder?
   - What is the mechanism to maintain body pH?

   Metabolic alkalosis
5. A 30-year-old female was seen in the emergency room with breathlessness.

   Investigations

   pH–7.55; Bicarbonate ion–25 mmol/L; PCO_2–25 mm Hg
   - What is the most likely acid-base disorder?
   - What are buffers?
   - Name the plasma buffers.

   Metabolic alkalosis
6. A comatose patient with tremors admitted in the hospital. His blood glucose level was 300 mg/dL. His urine was positive for both Rothera's test and Benedict's test
   - What is the diagnosis?
   - What are the lines of treatment?

   Diabetic ketoacidosis
7. A 50-year-old male complains of polyuria, polydipsia, polyphagia.
   - What is the most likely diagnosis?
   - How will you investigate?

   Diabetes
8. An apparently healthy man, on a routine check-up was found to have fast blood sugar of 80 mg/dL, and urine showed no abnormal constituents. After a heavy breakfast of one and half hours, his blood sugar was 140 mg/dL and urine sample at that time was positive for Benedict's test.
   - What is the diagnosis?
   - What are the other investigations?
   - What is the line of treatment?

   Renal glycosuria
9. A 40-year-old obese business executive, sought medical advice. He was a nonsmoker and nonalcoholic. He was fond of cheese, eggs and nonvegetarian food. The biochemical profile of the patient is as follows:
   - Serum triglyceride–144 mg/dL
   - Serum cholesterol–330 mg/dL
   - Fasting blood glucose–70 mg/dL
     - Comment on the biochemical profile.

       Hypercholesterolemia
     - What dietary modifications you would like to give to this patient?

       Decrease the intake of cholesterol
10. A 45-year-old man brought to the MES hospital complaining of chest pain. The ECG revealed ischemic changes.
    - What are the biochemical tests to be done immediately to establish the diagnosis?
    - How is the patient to be monitored during the next two weeks?
    - What is the advice regarding diet to be given to the patient?

    Acute myocardial infarction

11. Values of GTT test for a 55-year-old male as follows:

Time in hours	*Glucose (mg/dL)*	*Urine-Benedict's test*
0	85	Negative
0.5	130	Negative
1	150	Negative
1.5	125	Negative
2	87	Negative

- Comment on the result.
- Describe the procedure for long GTT.

12. A 65-year-old man weighing 85 kg goes for routine morning jogging. After 15 minutes, he complained of discomfort in the chest radiating to the arm, with profuse sweating and breathlessness and soon collapsed on the road. He was taken to casualty.
    - What is the probable diagnosis?
    - What are the biochemical investigations you will do to diagnose the condition?

    Myocardial infarction

13. One evening, a smart 40-year-old male business executive entertained a party in which much food and alcohol had been consumed. In the next morning, he woke-up with excruciating pain in ankle. He was admitted to the hospital. On examination he had fever. The ankle joint was swollen, and red, felt hot to touch, and was very tendor and stiff. No other joints were involved. Lymph glands were normal, not tendor. Routine peripheral smear revealed mild granulocytosis. The laboratory data were,
    Blood glucose-130 mg/dL; blood urea-38 mg/dL; serum creatinine-1 mg/dL; serum uric acid-10 mg/dL:
    - What is the most probable diagnosis?
    - Which part of this case history and laboratory data helped you to reach this diagnosis?
    - What is the origin and fate of uric acid?
    - What are the causes for primary and secondary hyperuricemia?
    - What is the short-term and long-term treatment for gout?

    Acute Gout

14. The laboratory results of a 50-year-old school teacher are given below:
    Random blood glucose-95 mg/dL; blood cholesterol-285 mg/dL.
    - Plasma T4-4 μg/dL (normal range—5-12)
    - Plasma T3-70 (normal range—120-190 ug/dL)
    - Plasma TSH-6 mlU/mL (normal range—0.5-4.5 mL/UmL)

    A. How will you interpret the result to arrive at a diagnosis?
    B. Why TSH has increased while T4 is lowered?
    C. What are the other physiological changes observed in this patient?
    D. Which of the laboratory results is crucial in making the diagnosis?

    Hypothyroidism

15. Investigations showed elevated levels of amylase and lipase.
    - What is the probable diagnosis?
    - Mention the hormones produced by the hormone.

    Acute pancreatitis

16. A patient was operated for intestinal obstruction. He had continuous gastric aspiration for the past 3 days. The arterial blood gas results of this postoperative patient are given below:
    Investigations
    pH-7.54; pCO_2-45 mm Hg; plasma bicarbonate-36 mmol/L; serum sodium-130 mmol/L; serum potassium-2.8 mmol/L; serum chloride-90 mmol/L
    - What are the abnormalities noted?
    - What is the significance of serum potassium in relation to acid-base status?
    - What is the significance of measuring urine chloride level in this patient?

    Metabolic alkalosis with hypokalemia

17. The following are the blood gas results of a patient who has been on a respirator for the past week.
    Investigations
    pH-7.5; pCO_2-24 mm Hg; pO_2-88 mm Hg; plasma bicarbonate-18 mmol/L
    - What is the acid-base status of the patient?
    - Explain the nature of the disturbance and the alteration in each parameter.
    - What is the nature of the compensatory change?

    Respiratory alkalosis

18. The following results were obtained by blood gas analysis on the arterial blood of a patient admitted in an unconscious state with suspected barbiturate poisoning.
    Investigations
    pH-7.24; pCO_2-60 mm Hg; HCO_3-27 mmol/L
    - What is the nature of acid-base disturbance? Explain.
    - Why barbiturates cause acid-base disturbance?

    Respiratory acidosis

19. The laboratory results of a 6-year-old boy are as follows:
pH–7.31; pO_2–94 mm Hg; pCO_2–35 mm Hg; plasma bicarbonate–20 mmol/L; sodium–138 mmol/L; potassium–3 mmol/L; chloride–112 mmol/L
- What is the nature of acid-base balance?
- Explain the abnormalities in electrolyte levels.

Acidosis

20. A 40-year-old woman was brought with history of right hypochondrial pain and generalized itching. On examination, she is jaundiced. Stools are clay colored and cannot flushed of easily, blood examination shows the following biochemical values. What is the probable diagnosis?
Investigation
BR total–6 mg%; BR direct–5.4 mg%; ALT–32 IU/L; AST–30 IU/L; ALP–500 IU/L
- Which jaundice?
- Give the urinary findings.
- Reason for itching.
  - **Obstructive jaundice** (presence of bile salts in blood is the reason for itching).

21. A 50-year-old female patient was admitted with generalized weakness, easy fatigability, itching, and jaundice since one month. On examination, the patient was emaciated and scratch marks were seen all over the body. She was jaundiced and a mass was palpable in the upper abdomen.
Investigations
Hb–12 gm%, reticulocyte count—1%.
Liver function tests
Blood: Serum bilirubin–18 mg; conjugated bilirubin–15 mg%; alanine amino transferase–13 IU/L; aspartate amino transferase–12 IU/L; alkaline phosphatase–64 KAU
Urine: Bile salts: ++; bile pigments: ++; urobilinogen-absent;
Stool: Clay colored.
a. What is the type of jaundice?

Obstructive jaundice

22. Analyze the data—BR total–5 mg%; BR direct–0.2 mg%; ALT–20 IU/L; AST–20 IU/L; ALP–80 IU/L.
- What is the probable diagnosis?
- Give the urinary findings in this case.

Hemolytic jaundice

23. A 40-year-old woman was admitted in the hospital with recurrent pain of abdomen. After 2 days, she developed jaundice. History revealed that pain aggravated after ingestion of fatty food. She also complained of itching
Urine: Bile pigments-++; bile salts-++; urobilinogen-absent
- What is the most likely cause?
- Explain the findings in urine.
- What is the type of jaundice?
- Which are the blood tests to be done to confirm diagnosis?
- If the patient has to undergo surgery, what liver function has to be done prior to surgery?

Obstructive jaundice

24. The following biochemical tests were ordered: TSH–20 mIU/L; T4–4 pmol/L; cholesterol–320 mgm/dL.
- What is your diagnosis?
- What is the cause of hypercholesterolemia?
- What is the treatment for the above condition?

Hyperthyroidism

25. Fructose-1-phosphate $\xrightarrow{//}$ glyceraldehydes + **DHAP** (refer fructose intolerance)
- Which enzyme crystallizes this reaction?
- Name the condition caused by the deficiency of this enzyme.
- Mention the signs and symptoms of this disease.

26. Tyrosine $\longrightarrow$ Homogentisic acid $\xrightarrow{//}$ Maleyl-acetoacetate
Tyrosine kinase (refer phenyl ketonuria)
- Name the enzyme deficient.
- Name the metabolite excreted in urine.
- What are the diagnostic tests?
- What is the reason for blackening of urine?

27. Galactose-1-phosphate + UDP galactose $\xrightarrow{//}$ UDP galactose + G1P
- Which enzyme is deficient in this condition?
- How will you diagnose the condition?
- What are the clinical features?
- What is the biochemical basis of management?

28. Hypoxanthine +PRPP $\xrightarrow{//}$ IMP + PPi
Refer Gout
- Name the enzyme deficient.
- Name the clinical condition.
- What is the mode of inheritance?
- What is the cause of renal failure in later stages of disease?

29. A mentally retarted 3-year-old child was brought to the pediatric casualty with convulsions and coma. The mother complained that the child has poor weight gain. The child was jaundiced. Liver and spleen were enlarged. Ophthalmologic examination showed cataract.
    Urine: Benedict's test was +ve; glucose oxidase test was negative.
    Galactosemia
    - Give the probable diagnosis.
    - Which is the enzyme deficient in this case?

30. A mother sought medical help for her child, with the complaint that diapers used for the child stained dark. Urine on exposure became dark.
    Investigations
    Benedict's test—positive; ferric chloride test—positive; glucose oxidase test—negative
    Phenylketonuria
    - What is your diagnosis?
    - What is the biochemical defect?

31. Homocysteine + serine —//→ cystathionine
    Refer homocystinuria
    - Name the enzyme catalyzing the reaction.
    - What is the clinical condition resulting from the deficiency of this enzyme?
    - Name the test to diagnose the condition.
    - What is the treatment?

NORMAL VALUES

Analyte	*Normal value*	*Increased in*	*Decreased in*
Alanine amino transferase (ALT)	10–35 IU/L	Liver disorders	
Aspartate amino trasnferase (AST)	8–20 IU/L	Myocardial infarction	
Alkaline phosphatase (ALP)	40–125 IU/L	Liver and bone diseases	
Total protein	6–8 g/dL	Multiple myeloma	Malnutrition
Albumin	3.5–5 g/dL		Cirrhosis, nephritic malnutrition
Globulin	2.5–3.5 g/dL	Multiple myeloma, liver disease	
Fibrinogen	200–400 mg/dL		
Bilirubin-total	0.2–8 mg/dL	Jaundice	
Bilirubin-conjugated	0–0.2 mg/dL	Obstructive jaundice	
Bilirubin-unconjugated	0.2–0.6 mg/dL	Hemolytic jaundice	
Bicarbonate	22–26 mEq/L	Alkalosis	Acidosis
Calcium	9–11 mg/dL	Hyperparathyroidism	
Chloride	96–106 mEq/L		
Sodium	136–145 mEq/L		
Potassium	3.5–5 mEq/L		
Creatinine	0.7–1.4 mg/dL	Renal failure	
Cholesterol-total	150–200 mg/dL	Diabetes, atherosclerosis, obstructive jaundice	

HDL	Male	30–60 mg/dL		
	Female	35–75 mg/dL		
LDL 30–39 years		80–175 mg/dL		
Triglycerides	Male	50–200 mg/dL		
	Female	40–150 mg/dL		
pH		7.4	Alkalosis	Acidosis
pH of urine		4.5–9.8		
pO_2		90–100 mm Hg		
pCO_2		35–45 mm Hg		
Glucose (fasting blood sugar)		70–110 mg/dL	Diabetes mellitus	
Random blood sugar (RBS)		140–200 mg/dL		
Hemoglobin	Male	14–16 mg/dL	Polycythemia	Anemia
	Female	13–15 mg/dL		
Urea		20–40 mg/dL	Kidney disease	
Uric acid		3.5–7 mg/dL	Gout	

Disease	*Deficient enzyme*
Acute intermittent porphyria	Uroporphyrinogen-I-synthetase
Albinism	Tyrosinase
Alkaptonuria	Homogentisic acid oxidase
Citrullinemia	Arginosuccinate synthetase
Crigler-Najjar syndrome	Defective conjugation of bilirubin
Cystathionuria	Cystathionase
Cystic fibrosis	Defective chloride channels
Fructose intolerance	Fructose-1-phosphate aldolase
Galactosemia	Galactose-1-phosphate uridyltransferase
Gilbert's disease	Defective uptake of bilirubin
Gaucher's disease	Beta glucosidase
Hartnup disease	Defective absorption of aromatic amino acids
Hereditary fructose intolerance	Aldolase B
Homocystinuria	Cystathionine synthase
Hyperammonemia	CPS 1 deficiency
Lesch-Nyhan syndrome	HGPRTase
Maple syrup urine disease	Branched chain keto acid decarboxylase
McArdle's disease	Muscle phosphorylase
Methylmalonic aciduria	Methylmalonyl CoA mutase
Niemann-Pick disease	Sphingomyelinase
Orotic aiduria	Orotidine 5 P decarboxylase
Pentosuria	Xylulose dehydrogenase
Phenylketonuria	Phenyl alanine hydroxylase
Tay-Sachs disease	Hexosaminidase
von Gierke's disease	Glucose 6 phosphatase
Wilson's disease	Copper transport protein

IMPORTANT PATHWAYS

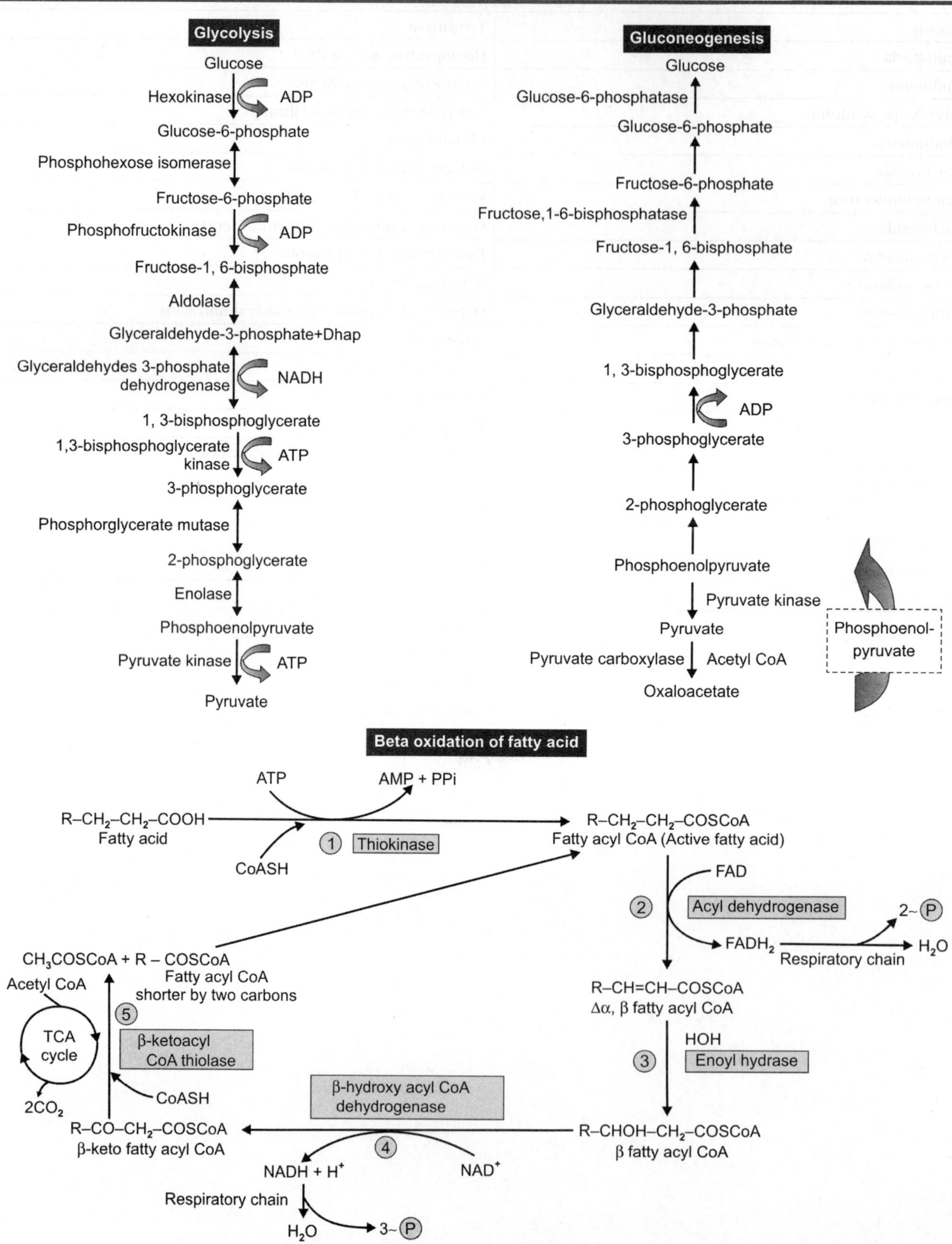

HMP Shunt Pathway

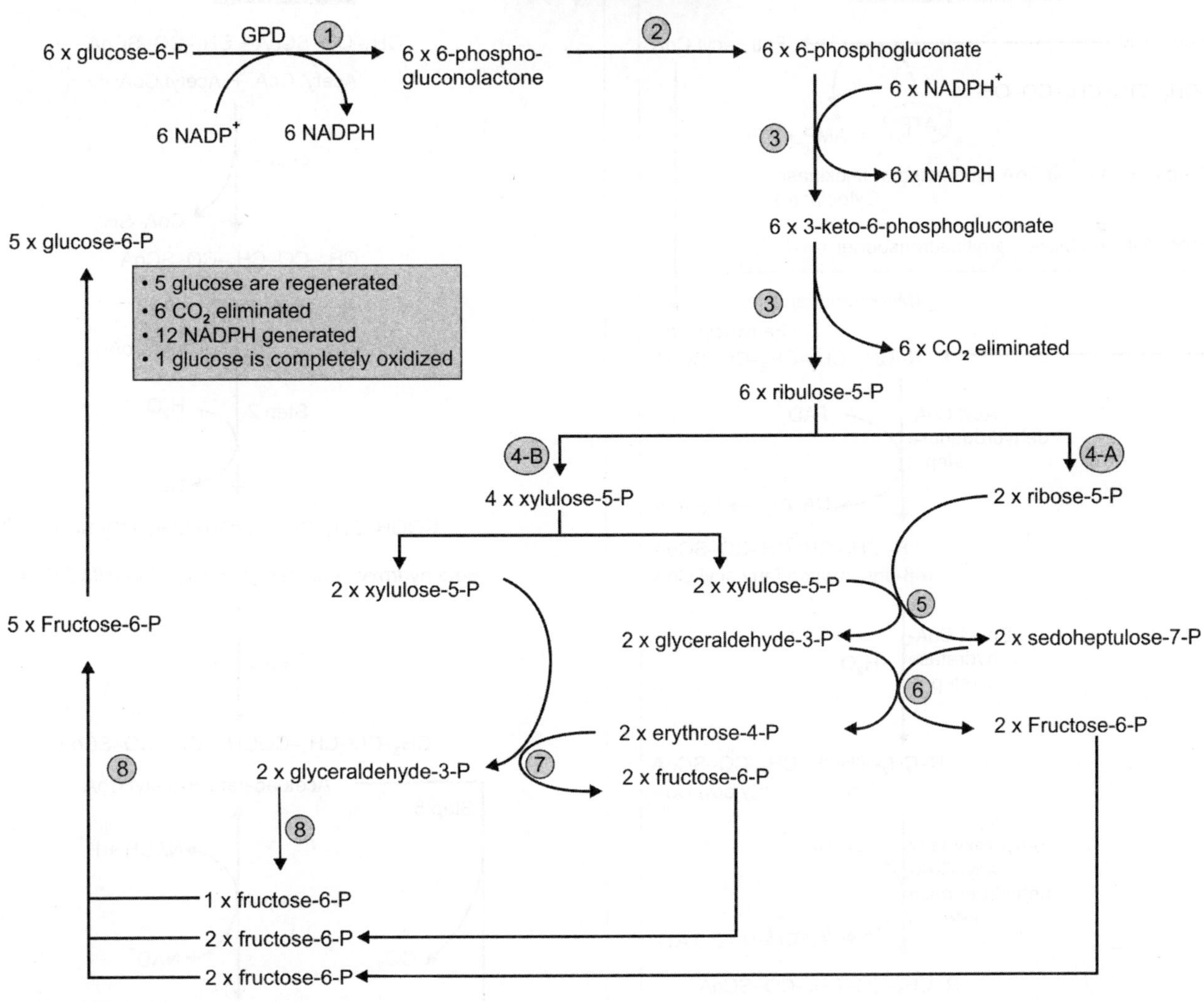

Enzymes:
1 = Glucose-6-phosphate dehydrogenase (GPO)
2 = Gluconolactone hydrolase
3 = 6-phosphogluconate dehydrogenase
4A = Isomerase
4B = Epimerase

5 = Transketolase
6 = Transaldolase
7 = Second transketolase
8 = Reversal or glycolysis

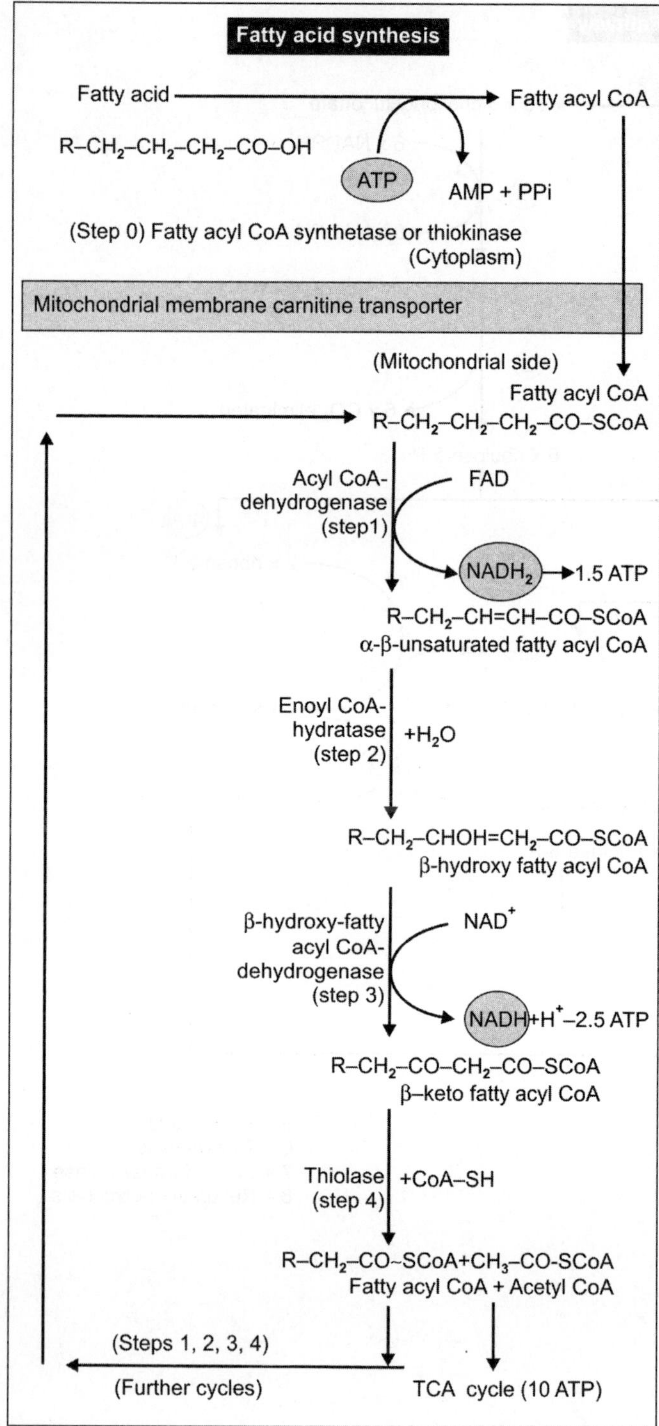
Fatty acid synthesis
Fatty acid
Fatty acyl CoA
R–CH2–CH2–CH2–CO–OH
ATP
AMP + PPi
(Step 0) Fatty acyl CoA synthetase or thiokinase
(Cytoplasm)
Mitochondrial membrane carnitine transporter
(Mitochondrial side)
Fatty acyl CoA
R–CH2–CH2–CH2–CO–SCoA
Acyl CoA-dehydrogenase (step1)
FAD
NADH2
1.5 ATP
R–CH2–CH=CH–CO–SCoA
α-β-unsaturated fatty acyl CoA
Enoyl CoA-hydratase (step 2)
+H2O
R–CH2–CHOH=CH2–CO–SCoA
β-hydroxy fatty acyl CoA
β-hydroxy-fatty acyl CoA-dehydrogenase (step 3)
NAD+
NADH+H+–2.5 ATP
R–CH2–CO–CH2–CO–SCoA
β–keto fatty acyl CoA
Thiolase (step 4)
+CoA–SH
R–CH2–CO~SCoA+CH3–CO-SCoA
Fatty acyl CoA + Acetyl CoA
(Steps 1, 2, 3, 4)
(Further cycles)
TCA cycle (10 ATP)

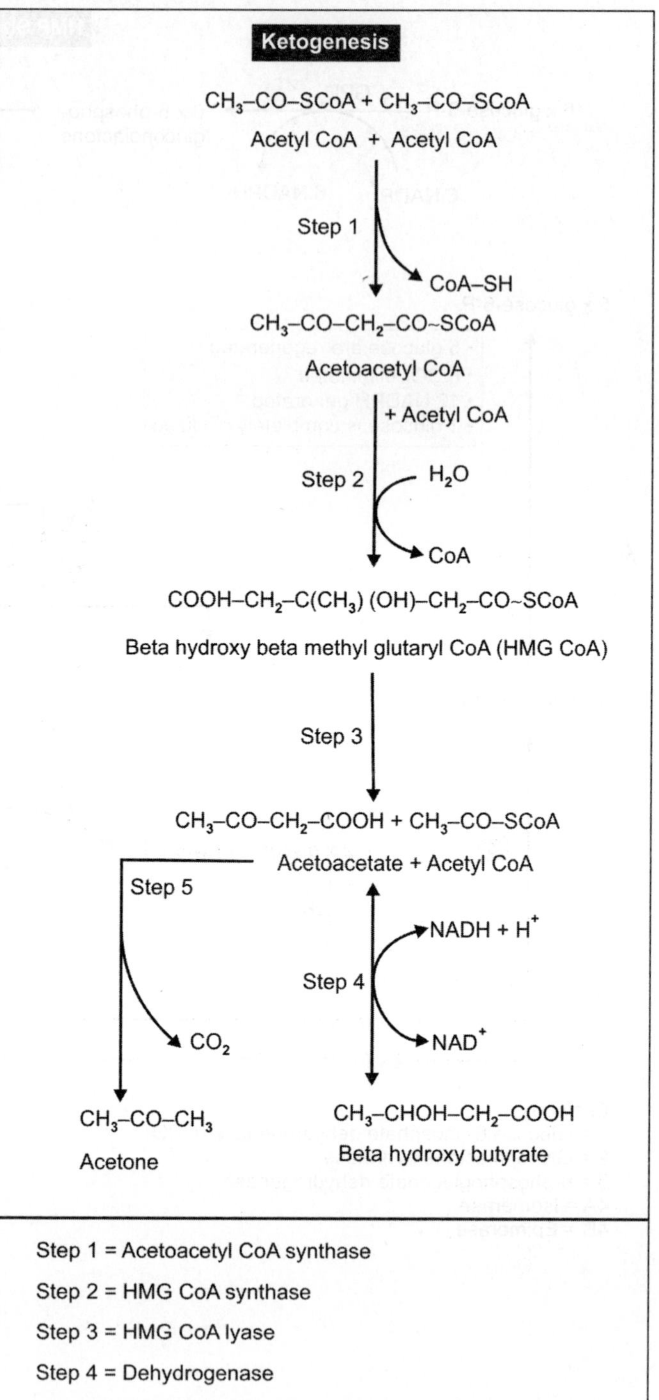
Ketogenesis
CH3–CO–SCoA + CH3–CO–SCoA
Acetyl CoA + Acetyl CoA
Step 1
CoA–SH
CH3–CO–CH2–CO~SCoA
Acetoacetyl CoA
+ Acetyl CoA
Step 2
H2O
CoA
COOH–CH2–C(CH3) (OH)–CH2–CO~SCoA
Beta hydroxy beta methyl glutaryl CoA (HMG CoA)
Step 3
CH3–CO–CH2–COOH + CH3–CO–SCoA
Acetoacetate + Acetyl CoA
Step 5
Step 4
NADH + H+
NAD+
CO2
CH3–CO–CH3
Acetone
CH3–CHOH–CH2–COOH
Beta hydroxy butyrate
Step 1 = Acetoacetyl CoA synthase
Step 2 = HMG CoA synthase
Step 3 = HMG CoA lyase
Step 4 = Dehydrogenase
Step 5 = Nonenzymatic and spontaneous

Cholesterol biosynthesis

Acetyl CoA + acetyl CoA

↓ Acetoacetyl CoA synthase

Acetoacetyl CoA

↓ HMG CoA synthase

HMG CoA

↓ HMG CoA reductase (2 $NADP^+$)

Mevalonate (6c)

↓

5-phosphomevalonate (6c)

↓

5-pyrophosphomevalonate (6c)

↓

3-phospho-5-pyrophosphomevalonate (6c)

↓

Isopentanyl pyrophosphate (5c)

↓

Dimethyl allyl pyrophosphate (5c)

↓

Geranyl pyrophosphate (10c)

↓

Farnesyl pyrophosphate (15c)

↓

Squalene (30c)

↓

Squalene epoxide (30c)

↓

Lanosterol (30c)

↓

Zymosterol (27c)

↓

Desmosterol (27c)

↓

Cholesterol (27c)

One-carbon metabolism

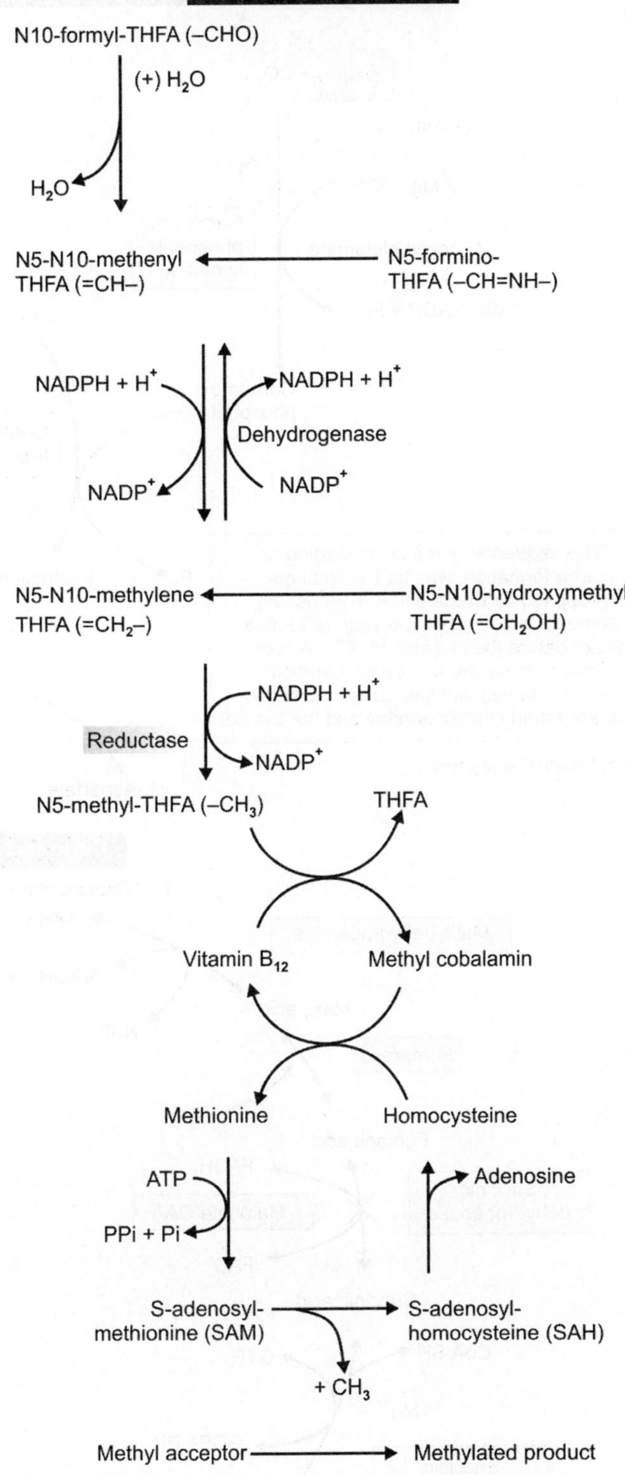

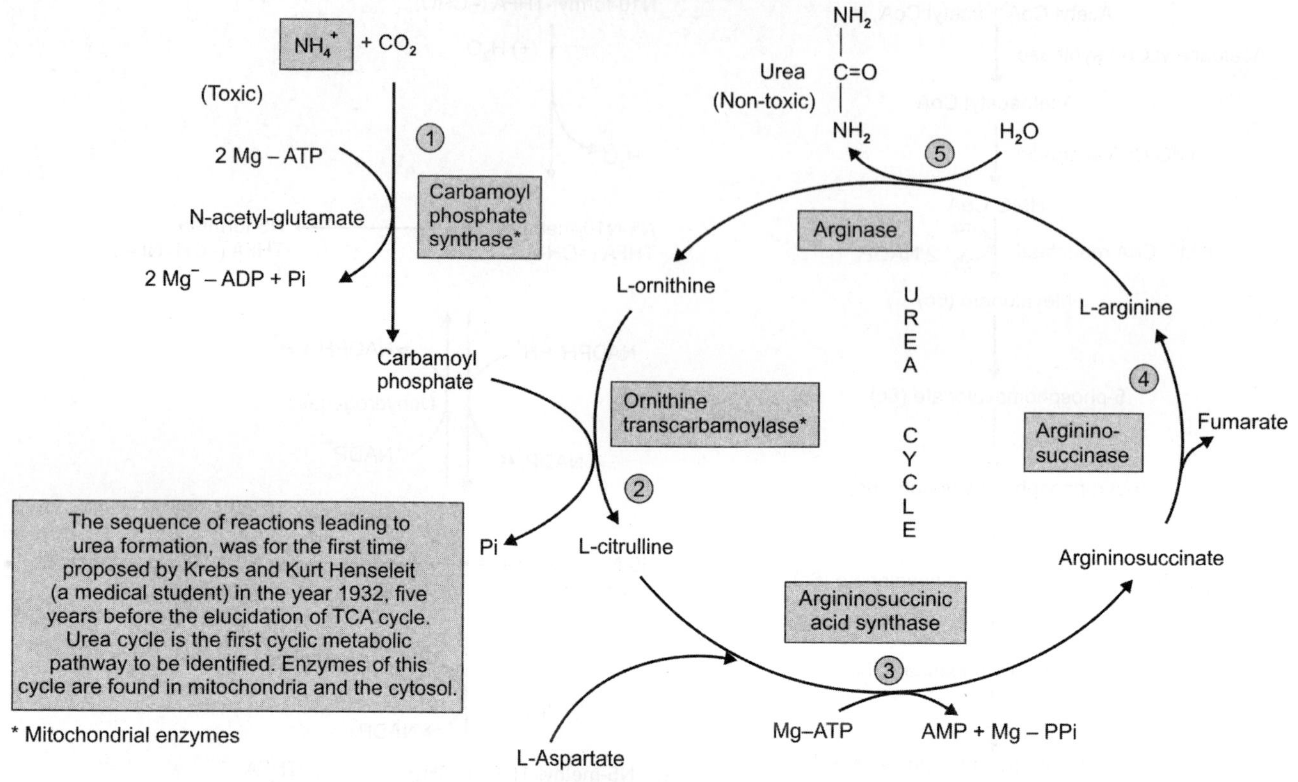
Urea cycle/Krebs-Henseleit cycle
NH4+ + CO2
(Toxic)
2 Mg – ATP
N-acetyl-glutamate
2 Mg– – ADP + Pi
1
Carbamoyl phosphate synthase*
Carbamoyl phosphate
NH2
C=O
NH2
Urea (Non-toxic)
H2O
5
Arginase
L-ornithine
L-arginine
UREA CYCLE
Ornithine transcarbamoylase*
2
Pi
L-citrulline
4
Arginino-succinase
Fumarate
Argininosuccinate
Argininosuccinic acid synthase
3
Mg–ATP
AMP + Mg – PPi
L-Aspartate
The sequence of reactions leading to urea formation, was for the first time proposed by Krebs and Kurt Henseleit (a medical student) in the year 1932, five years before the elucidation of TCA cycle. Urea cycle is the first cyclic metabolic pathway to be identified. Enzymes of this cycle are found in mitochondria and the cytosol.
* Mitochondrial enzymes

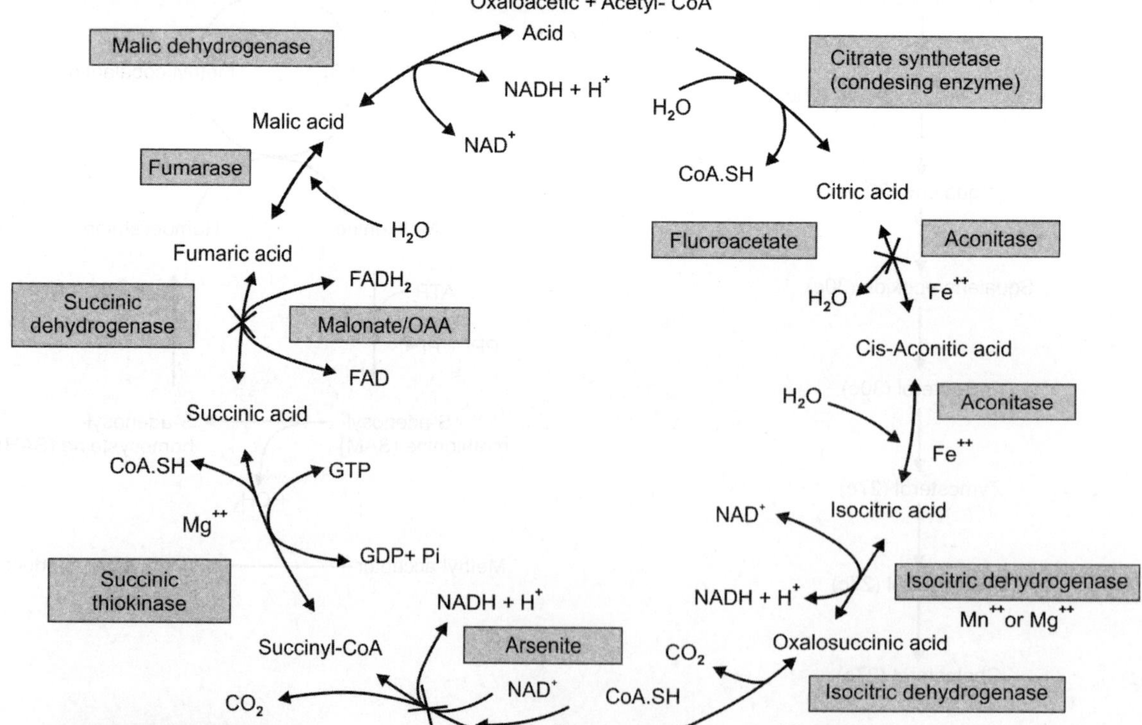
Citric acid cycle
Oxaloacetic + Acetyl- CoA
Acid
Malic dehydrogenase
NADH + H+
NAD+
Malic acid
Citrate synthetase (condesing enzyme)
H2O
CoA.SH
Citric acid
Fumarase
H2O
Fumaric acid
Fluoroacetate
Aconitase
H2O
Fe++
FADH2
Succinic dehydrogenase
Malonate/OAA
FAD
Succinic acid
Cis-Aconitic acid
H2O
Aconitase
Fe++
CoA.SH
GTP
Mg++
GDP+ Pi
Succinic thiokinase
NAD+
Isocitric acid
NADH + H+
Isocitric dehydrogenase
Mn++ or Mg++
NADH + H+
Succinyl-CoA
Arsenite
CO2
Oxalosuccinic acid
NAD+
CoA.SH
Isocitric dehydrogenase
CO2
TPP, FAD, Lipoic acid, Mg++
α-ketoglutaric acid
Mn++ Or Mg++
α-ketoglutaric dehydrogenase complex

Phenylalanine and tyrosine metabolism

Phenylalanine
↓ Phenylalanine hydroxylase
Tyrosine
↓ Tyrosine transaminase
Parahydroxy phenyl pyruvic acid
↓ Parahydroxyl phenylpyruvate hydroxylase
Dihydroxy phenyl acetic acid (Homogentisic acid)
↓ Homogentisic acid oxidase
Maleyl acetoacetic acid
↓ Maleyl acetoacetate isomerase
Fumaryl acetoacetic acid
→ Acetoacetic acid (Ketogenic P/W)
→ Fumaric acid (Glucogenic P/W)

Tryptophan metabolism

Tryptophan
↓ Tryptophan pyrrolase
N-Formyl kynurenine
↓
Kynurenine
↓
3-OH-Kynurenine
↓ Kynureninase → Alanine → Glucogenic
3-Hydroxy anthranillic acid
↓
Amino carboxy muconaldehyde
↓
Amino muconate aldehyde
↓
Keto adipic acid
↓
Acetoacetyl CoA
↓
Ketogenic

Heme synthesis

Succinyl CoA + Glycine
↓ ALA synthase
Delta amino levulinic acid (ALA)
↓ ALA dehydratase
Porphobilinogen (PBG)
↓ PBG deaminase, UPG III cosynthase
Uroporphyrinogen III (UPG III)
↓ Uroporphyrinogen Decarboxylase
Coproporphyrinogen III (CPG III)
↓ Coproporphyrinogen Oxidase
Protoporphyrinogen (PPG III)
↓ Protoporphyrinogen Oxidase
Protoporphyrin III
↓ Heme synthase
Heme

Enzyme deficiencies in porphyria

Glycine + Succinyl CoA
↓ (Enzyme 1) ALA-synthase
Delta amino levullinic acid (ALA)
↓ (Enzyme 2) ALA-dehydratase
Porphobilinogen (PBG)
↓ (3) PBG-deaminase → Acute intermittent porphyria
↓ (Enzyme 3b) UPG-III-co-synthase → Congenital erythropoietic porphyria
Uroporphyrinogen (UPG)
↓ (4) UPG-decarboxylase → Porphyria cutanea tarda
Coproporphyrinogen (CPG)
↓ (5) CPG-oxidase → Hereditary coproporphyria
Protoporphyrinogen (PPG)
↓ (6) PPG-oxidase → Porphyria variegata
Protoporphyrin
↓ (7) Heme synthase → Hereditary protoporphyria
Heme

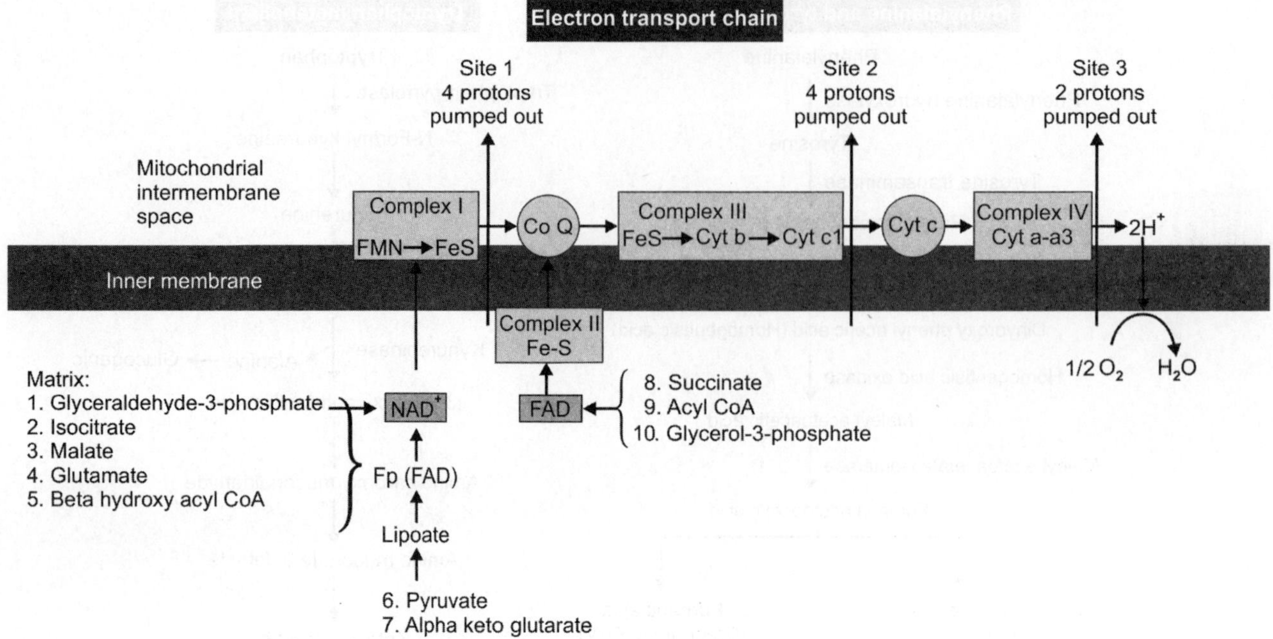
Electron transport chain
Site 1
4 protons
pumped out
Site 2
4 protons
pumped out
Site 3
2 protons
pumped out
Mitochondrial
intermembrane
space
Complex I
FMN→FeS
Co Q
Complex III
FeS→Cyt b→Cyt c1
Cyt c
Complex IV
Cyt a-a3
2H+
Inner membrane
Complex II
Fe-S
1/2 O2
H2O
Matrix:
1. Glyceraldehyde-3-phosphate
2. Isocitrate
3. Malate
4. Glutamate
5. Beta hydroxy acyl CoA
NAD+
Fp (FAD)
Lipoate
6. Pyruvate
7. Alpha keto glutarate
FAD
8. Succinate
9. Acyl CoA
10. Glycerol-3-phosphate

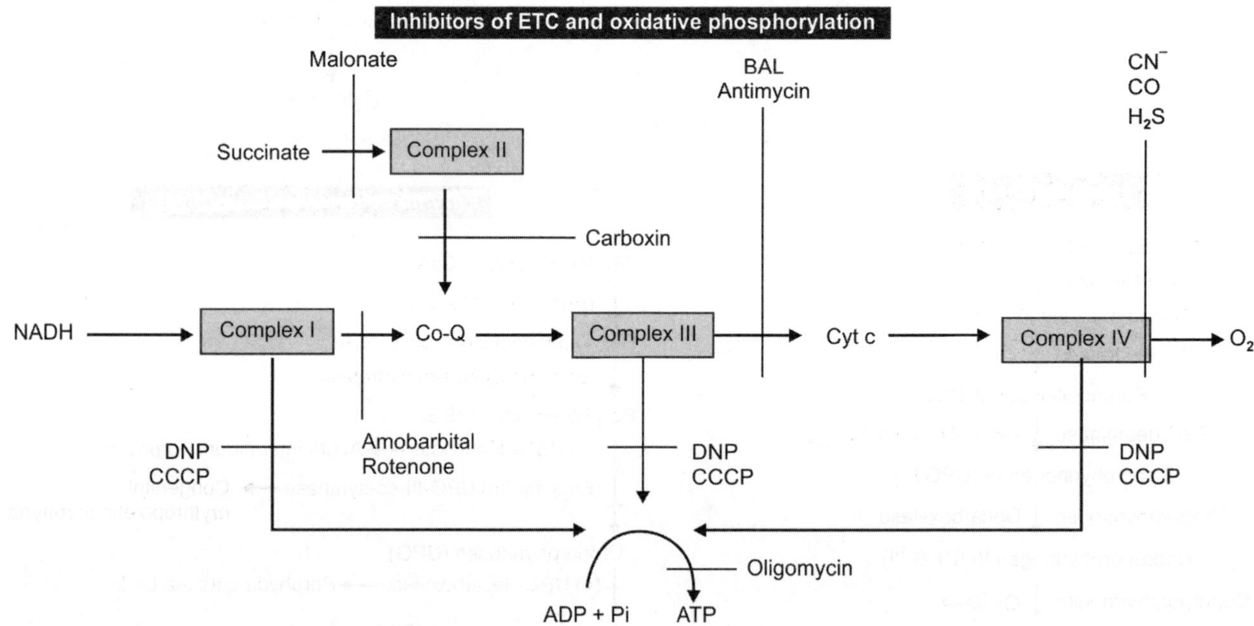
Inhibitors of ETC and oxidative phosphorylation
Malonate
Succinate
Complex II
Carboxin
BAL
Antimycin
CN-
CO
H2S
NADH
Complex I
Co-Q
Complex III
Cyt c
Complex IV
O2
DNP
CCCP
Amobarbital
Rotenone
DNP
CCCP
DNP
CCCP
Oligomycin
ADP + Pi
ATP

De Novo synthesis of purines

Step 0 Ribose-5-phosphate → (ADP) Phoshoribosyl pyrophosphate (PRPP)

Step 1 Glutamine + PRPP → 5-Phosphoribosyl-1-amine

Step 2 → (ADP) GAR

Step 3 → (THFA) FGAR

Step 4 → (ADP, Glutamine) FGAM

Step 5 → (ADP) AIR

Step 6 → ACAIR

Step 7 Aspartic acid (+) → (ADP) SAICAR

Step 8 → (Fumaric acid) AICAR

Step 9 → (THFA) FAICAR

Step 10 → IMP

Step 11 → (Fumaric acid)

Adenosine monophosphate (AMP)

Degradation of purine metabolites

Adenosine monophoshate → (H_2O; AMP-deaminase; NH_4^+) Inosine monophosphate

Inosine monophosphate → (H_2O; Phosphomonoesterase; Pi) Inosine

Adenosine → (H_2O; Adenosine-deaminase; NH_4^+) Inosine

Inosine → (Pi; PNP; R-1-P) Hypoxanthine

Guanosine → (Guanase; NH_4^+) Xanthosine

Guanosine → (Pi; PNP; R-1-P) Guanine

Hypoxanthine → ($H_2O + O_2$; Xanthine oxidase; H_2O_2) Xanthine

Xanthosine → (Pi; PNP; R-1-P) Xanthine

Guanine → (Guanase; NH_4^+) Xanthine

Xanthine → ($H_2O + O_2$; Xanthine oxidase; H_2O_2) Uric acid

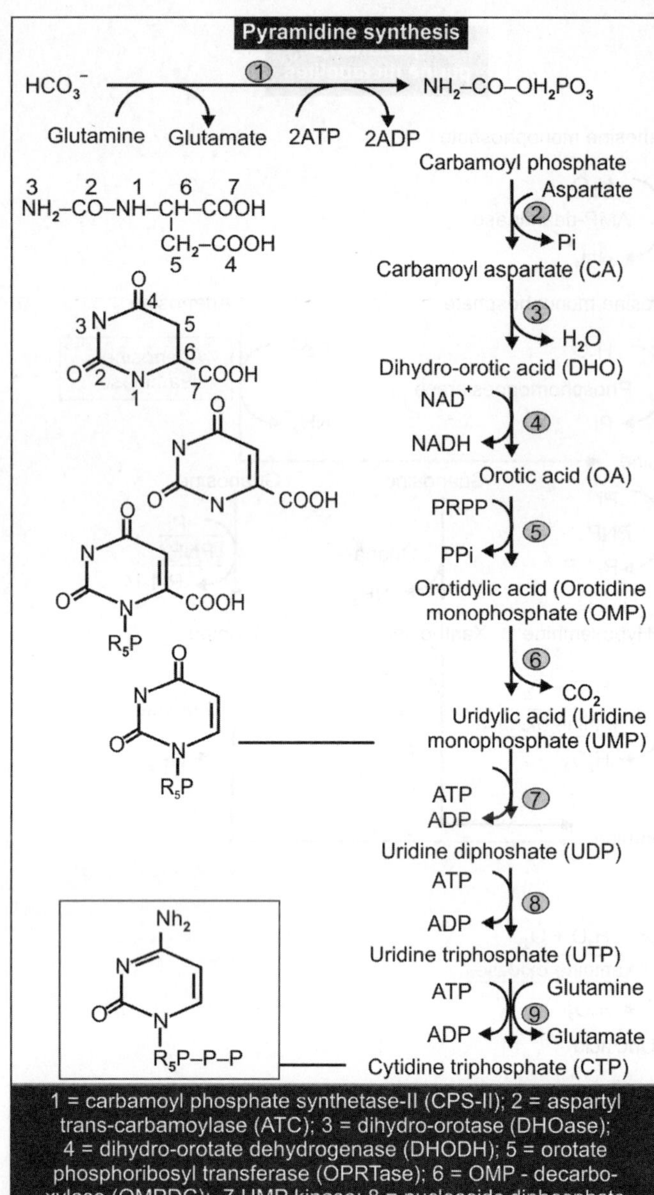
Pyramidine synthesis
HCO3⁻
NH2–CO–OH2PO3
Glutamine Glutamate 2ATP 2ADP
Carbamoyl phosphate
Aspartate
Pi
Carbamoyl aspartate (CA)
H2O
Dihydro-orotic acid (DHO)
NAD+
NADH
Orotic acid (OA)
PRPP
PPi
Orotidylic acid (Orotidine monophosphate (OMP)
CO2
Uridylic acid (Uridine monophosphate (UMP)
ATP
ADP
Uridine diphoshate (UDP)
ATP
ADP
Uridine triphosphate (UTP)
ATP Glutamine
ADP Glutamate
Cytidine triphosphate (CTP)
NH2–CO–NH–CH–COOH
CH2–COOH
COOH
R5P
Nh2
R5P–P–P
1 = carbamoyl phosphate synthetase-II (CPS-II); 2 = aspartyl trans-carbamoylase (ATC); 3 = dihydro-orotase (DHOase); 4 = dihydro-orotate dehydrogenase (DHODH); 5 = orotate phosphoribosyl transferase (OPRTase); 6 = OMP - decarboxylase (OMPDC); 7 UMP kinase; 8 = nucleoside diphosphate kinase; 9 = CTP synthetase

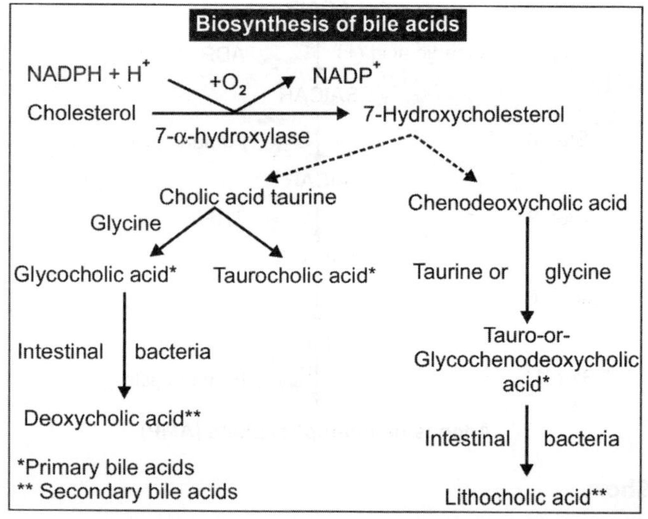
Biosynthesis of bile acids
NADPH + H+
+O2
NADP+
Cholesterol
7-Hydroxycholesterol
7-α-hydroxylase
Cholic acid taurine
Glycine
Chenodeoxycholic acid
Glycocholic acid*
Taurocholic acid*
Taurine or glycine
Intestinal bacteria
Tauro-or-Glycochenodeoxycholic acid*
Deoxycholic acid**
Intestinal bacteria
*Primary bile acids
** Secondary bile acids
Lithocholic acid**

MODEL QUESTION PAPER

FIRST MBBS DEGREE MODEL EXAMINATION—2013

Time: 3 hours **Max Marks: 50**

- Answer All questions
- Draw diagrams wherever necessary

PAPER I
ANATOMY

Long Essay **(10)**

1. A 52-year-old man presented with shortness of breath and coughing up small volumes of blood. Clinical examination revealed multiple dilated veins around the neck. A chest X-ray demonstrated a tumor mass involving the upper part of right lung and elevated right dome of diaphragm. Based on your anatomical knowledge, answer the following questions.
   - Compression of which structure in the chest by the tumor is responsible for dilated veins around the neck?
   - Mention the extent and relation in the mediastinum
   - Briefly describe the other structures related to the mediastinal surface of the right lung.
   - Injury to which structure is responsible for elevated diaphragm on the right side?
   - Briefly describe the broncho-pulmonary segments of lungs and their applied importance.

(1+2+3+1+3=10)

Short Essays **(3×5=15)**

2. Hip joint—articular surfaces, capsule and ligaments, muscles involved in appropriate movements of the joint.
3. Intermuscular spaces of scapular region—boundaries and contents and applied anatomy.
4. Intraembryonic mesoderm—formation, parts and derivatives.

Short Notes **(5×3=15)**

5. Fertilization.
6. Hamstring's muscles.
7. Left coronary artery.
8. Axillary lymph nodes.
9. Interosseous muscles of hand.

Short Answers **(3×2=6)**

10. Greater sciatic forarmen.
11. Klienfelter's syndrome.
12. Microscopic structure of hyaline cartilage.

Draw Diagrams **(2×2=4)**

13. Brachial plexus.
14. Longitudinal arches of foot.

PAPER II
ANATOMY

Long Essay **(10)**

1. A 35-year-old woman with four living children and history of all vaginal deliveries attended gynecological out-patient department with complaints of pelvic heaviness, a dragging sensation in the vagina, protrusion of a mass coming down from the vagina and backache. On examination, the condition was diagnosed as prolapse of uterus. With your knowledge of anatomy answer the following questions.
   - Anatomical position of non-gravid uterus
   - Peritoneal relations of uterus
   - Supports of uterus
   - Arterial supply of uterus
   - Lymphatic drainage of uterus (1+4+2+1+2=10)

Short Essays **(3×5=15)**

2. Corpus striatum.
3. Interior of larynx.
4. Lesser sac.

Short Notes **(5×3=15)**

5. Developmental descent of testis.
6. Pre-central gyrus of cerebrum.

7. Microscopic structure of pancreas.
8. Middle meatus of nose.
9. Spermatic cord.

Short Answers **(3×2=6)**

10. Motor and sensory innervation of tongue.
11. Bile duct.
12. Derivatives of mid gut.

Draw Diagrams **(2×2=4)**

13. Transverse section at the level of inferior colliculus of mid brain.
14. Anterior relations of right kidney.

PAPER I
PHYSIOLOGY

Long Essay **(10)**

1. A road traffic accident victim was found to be unconscious and breathing in an irregular rhythm. From your knowledge of physiology.
   - Name two types of periodic breathing.
   - Explain the neural regulation of respiration.
   - What is the mechanism of function of medullary chemoreceptors? (1+5+4=10)

Short Essays **(2×5 =10)**

2. Name the components of the enteric nervous system and outline its functions.
3. Describe the intrinsic pathway of coagulation. Mention one test for assessing it.

Answer Briefly **(5×3=15)**

4. Law of intestines.
5. Sickle cell anemia.
6. Non-renal functions of kidney.
7. Pathophysiology of peptic ulcer.
8. Cystometrogram.

Draw and Label **(2×2½=5)**

9. Splay.
10. Cardiac muscle action potential.

Explain the physiological basis of the following (5×2=10)

11. Korotkoff's sounds.
12. Alveoli are dry.
13. Skin is cold in hypovolemic shock.
14. Q wave in an ECG.
15. Steatorrhea in diseases that destroy exocrine pancreas.

PAPER II
PHYSIOLOGY

Long Essay **(10)**

1. A 50-year-old patient of hypertension suddenly developed weakness of right upper and lower extremities and difficulty in speaking following a brief episode of loss of consciousness. On examination motor tone of his right extremities was found to be increased. Answer the following questions based on your knowledge in physiology:
   - What would an examination of power and deep tendon reflexes of the patient reveal?
   - What would examination of the plantar reflex of the patient most likely reveal?
   - Explain the physiological basis of the findings of deep tendon reflexes in this patient?
   - What is the most likely clinical diagnosis of his condition? (2+2+5+1=10)

Short Essays **(2×5=10)**

2. Metabolic effects of insulin.
3. Denervation hypersensitivity.

Answer Briefly **(5×3=15)**

4. Accommodation reflex.
5. Pituitary dwarfism.
6. Parkinsonism.
7. Features of cerebellar lesions.
8. Ovarian cycle.

Draw and Label **(2×2½=5)**

9. Length-tension relationship in skeletal muscle.
10. Wald's visual cycle—flow chart.

Explain the physiological basis of the following (5×2=10)

11. Patients with sensory ataxia lose balance on closing their eyes.
12. Intra-uterine contraceptive devices prevent pregnancy.
13. Diaphragmatic pain is felt at the tip of the shoulder.
14. Patients of acromegaly may develop diabetes.
15. Cardiac muscle cannot be tetanised.

PAPER I
BIOCHEMISTRY

Essay **(10)**

1. Discuss the metabolism of phenylalanine.

Short Essays **(2×5=10)**

2. Digestion and absorption of lipids.
3. Describe glycogen metabolism.

Short Notes **(5×3=15)**

4. Mutarotation.
5. Essential fatty acids.
6. Isoenzymes.
7. Co-enzyme Q.
8. Fate of pyruvate.

Answer Briefly **(5×2=10)**

9. Regulation of cholesterol synthesis.
10. LDL receptor.
11. GABA.
12. Albinism.
13. Ketogenic amino acids.

Give Precise Answers **(5×1=5)**

14. What are epimers?
15. What is lecithin and mention its use?
16. Define iso-electric pH.
17. Name two transport proteins.
18. Mention two examples of biologically important peptides.

PAPER II
BIOCHEMISTRY

Essay **(10)**

1. Discuss in detail the mechanism by which kidney maintains the blood pH. What is meant by metabolic acidosis and how is it compensated. (1+6+3=10)

Short Essays **(2×5=10)**

2. Explain the degradation of heme.
3. Discuss the process of transcription in prokaryotes.

Short Notes **(5×3=15)**

4. Cytochrome p450.
5. List the different functions of plasma proteins.
6. Describe the Wald's visual cycle.
7. Antioxidants.
8. Discuss the base repair mechanism of DNA.

Answer Briefly **(5×2=10)**

9. Pellagra.
10. Factors affecting iron absorption.
11. DNA fingerprinting.
12. Define gout and name three drugs used to treat gout.
13. Orotic aciduria.

Give Precise Answers **(5×1=5)**

14. Mention two features of mitochondrial DNA.
15. List the functions of restriction endonucleases.
16. Define tumor markers and mention one example.
17. The normal albumin-globulin ratio and mention a condition in which it is reversed.
18. Mention the examples of partially acceptable missense mutation and unacceptable missense mutation.

Index

Page numbers followed by *f* refer to figure

I

J

K

L

M

N

O

P

R

S

T

U

V